Medical Management of Pulmonary Diseases

Clinical Guides to Medical Management

Consulting Editor

BURTON E. SOBEL, M.D.
Medical Center Hospital of Vermont
University of Vermont
Burlington, Vermont

Medical Management of Heart Disease, edited by Burton E. Sobel

Medical Management of Rheumatic Musculoskeletal and Connective Tissue Diseases, edited by Jan Dequeker, Gabriel Panayi, Theodore Pincus and Rodney Grahame

Medical Management of Atherosclerosis, edited by John LaRosa

Medical Management of Liver Disease, edited by Edward L. Krawitt

Medical Management of Pulmonary Diseases, edited by Gerald S. Davis; Associate Editors: Theodore W. Marcy and Elizabeth A. Seward

ADDITIONAL TITLES IN PREPARATION

Medical Management of Kidney and Electrolyte Disorders, edited by F. John Gennari

Medical Management of Pulmonary Diseases

edited by

Gerald S. Davis

University of Vermont College of Medicine
Burlington, Vermont

Associate Editors

Theodore W. Marcy
Elizabeth A. Seward

University of Vermont College of Medicine
Burlington, Vermont

MARCEL DEKKER, INC.   NEW YORK · BASEL

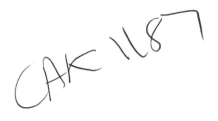

ISBN: 0-8247-6002-6

This book is printed on acid-free paper.

Headquarters
Marcel Dekker, Inc.
270 Madison Avenue, New York, NY 10016
tel: 212-696-9000; fax: 212-685-4540

Eastern Hemisphere Distribution
Marcel Dekker AG
Hutgasse 4, Postfach 812, CH-4001 Basel, Switzerland
tel: 41-61-261-8482; fax: 41-61-261-8896

World Wide Web
http://www.dekker.com

The publisher offers discounts on this book when ordered in bulk quantities. For more information, write to Special Sales/Professional Marketing at the headquarters address above.

Current printing (last digit):
10 9 8 7 6 5 4 3 2 1

PRINTED IN THE UNITED STATES OF AMERICA

We dedicate this book with our thanks to:

- Our spouses Karin, Kim, and John, who cheered and forgave us;

- Pam Carter, whose administrative support and hard work made this book possible;

- Our colleagues, who generously encouraged us and lightened our loads;

- Graham Garratt, in memorium, whose vision as a publisher made this series possible;

- Our authors, whose excellence and authority provided the substance of the book;

- Our patients with pulmonary diseases, who show us how much more we need to know.

Preface

The medical management of pulmonary disease has advanced dramatically in the last 30 years, progressing from a discipline that focused largely on tuberculosis to one that now includes a wide spectrum of acute and chronic illnesses. Three decades of concerted research into the pathophysiology of respiratory diseases are now offering new directions in the diagnosis and treatment of cystic fibrosis, asthma, lung cancer, and diffuse interstitial lung diseases. New technology offers practical, portable, cost-effective modalities for oxygen therapy, sleep apnea, and chronic mechanical ventilation. The care of patients with pulmonary disease is very gratifying, but it is also complex, challenging, and changing rapidly. We hope that this book will help practitioners offer better care and better outcomes to their patients.

This text has been designed to be useful in the clinical care of patients with pulmonary diseases, to be concise and readable, to be authoritative and current, and to focus on difficult but common problems in medical management. The emphasis is on accurate diagnosis and effective therapy, rather than epidemiology or pathophysiology of disease. This volume deals extensively with problems in the ambulatory care setting, with briefer attention to hospitalization. It serves as a useful guide for the practitioner to follow when confronted with a symptom, a sign, or a known disease of the respiratory system.

This book is directed to both the specialist and the generalist. Pulmonary disease specialists, fellows in training, and residents or students focusing on respiratory diseases will find the advice and opinions of experts useful in amplifying their own personal experiences. The general internist and the family practitioner will also find this book an important resource; Elizabeth A. Seward, an Associate Editor of this book and a practicing internist provided perspective and reviewed this text from this vantage point. Nurse practitioners, physician assistants, and respiratory therapists will also find it useful in approaching their patients.

The contributors to this volume are experts in their fields who are also practicing physicians. Their theoretical and scientific knowledge has been tested by the reality of clinical experience. They have been chosen for their abilities as teachers, their contributions as investigators, and their clarity as authors. They share with the reader their expertise in approaching difficult problems in the practice of pulmonary disease.

The style of this book is direct, readable, and declarative. The authors' opinions and advice are presented in a straightforward manner. Each concept is not referenced extensively in the text; rather, a list of suggested readings at the end of each chapter provides a source of more detailed information. Illustrations of radiologic, pathologic, and physiologic abnormalities highlight the text and tables summarize important topics concisely.

The symptoms, signs, diagnostic tests, and treatment modalities related to respiratory diseases overlap and intertwine among many different specific conditions. For this reason, the text is extensively indexed and cross-referenced. A chapter has been provided for each important topic, and these chapters are referred to, when relevant, in the discussion of various diseases. The book can be read in a linear fashion, beginning with Chapter 1 and ending with Chapter 45, but it is not necessary to do so. Readers may begin at whatever point their interests dictate or is relevant to the patient at hand. A symptom, a test result, or a known diagnosis will lead from that chapter to relevant information on further studies or appropriate treatments.

The book is divided into seven parts, each with several chapters. Part I provides a concise summary of the anatomy and physiology of the respiratory tract, including examples of abnormalities drawn from common diseases. It provides a background for the effects of disease. Part II discusses the symptoms and signs of pulmonary diseases, with a review of the medical history and the physical examination. It develops an approach to the diagnosis of specific diseases that will be presented in other chapters. Part III reviews common diagnostic tools that are used for patients with a variety of pulmonary problems. The principles and procedures for these studies are presented in detail, with illustrations drawn from specific conditions, as well as patterns of abnormalities that suggest particular diseases. The emphasis for some studies, such as lung biopsy, is placed primarily on indications, risks, likelihood of definitive findings, and effect on the patient, rather than the details of how the procedure is performed.

Common diagnostic and treatment dilemmas are presented in Part IV. These entities are not unique to a particular disease, but do lend themselves to a staged logical approach that results in a specific diagnosis. Algorithms for diagnosis and therapy are presented with each of them. Common therapies in pulmonary disease are presented in Part V. These modalities, such as oxygen therapy or management of respiratory failure, cut across the lines of specific diseases and are useful for a variety of patients. Discussions of particular disease states elsewhere in the book refer to this section, and then augment the information to make it specific.

Part VI presents important specific pulmonary diseases. In these chapters the experts present their opinions and advice on the detailed management of patients with asthma, COPD, sleep-disordered breathing, tuberculosis, and other conditions. Lung cancer is approached from the perspective of initial diagnosis, staging, and the issues that determine the best available therapy for an individual, with a focused summary of surgical, radiation, and chemotherapeutic treatment options. Respiratory disease in special settings is presented in Part VII, with emphasis on factors such as occupation or air travel that may cause or modify existing lung disease, and on conditions such as pregnancy or incidental surgery that may be greatly affected by pulmonary diseases. This section may be particularly valuable for specialists in disciplines other than internal medicine.

In an effort to be concise and focused, several areas of pulmonary disease have not been covered in this book. Critical care and respiratory diseases of children, as well as other topics such as nosocomial pneumonia, pulmonary manifestations of HIV/AIDS, or rare congenital conditions have been judged too specialized to be of broad interest.

This volume offers a concise but authoritative overview of respiratory illnesses and their management. We know it will be valuable to our colleagues in clinical practice and beneficial to their patients with pulmonary diseases.

Gerald S. Davis
Theodore W. Marcy
Elizabeth A. Seward

Contents

VII. Respiratory Disease in Special Settings

Contributors

Veena B. Antony, M.D.   Professor of Medicine and Pediatrics, Pulmonary Disease and Critical Care Medicine, Department of Medicine, Indiana University School of Medicine, Indianapolis, Indiana

T. Glen Bouder, M.D.   Assistant Professor of Medicine, Director, Medical Intensive Care Unit, Pulmonary Disease and Critical Care Medicine Unit, Department of Medicine, University of Vermont College of Medicine, Fletcher Allen Health Care, Burlington, Vermont

Sidney S. Braman, M.D.   Professor of Medicine, Department of Medicine, Brown University School of Medicine, Providence, Rhode Island

William J. Calhoun, M.D., F.C.C.P.   Associate Professor of Medicine, Director, Asthma, Allergy, and Airway Research Center, Pulmonary, Allergy, and Critical Care Medicine, Department of Medicine, University of Pittsburgh, Pittsburgh, Pennsylvania

Thomas V. Colby, M.D.   Professor of Pathology, Department of Pathology, Mayo Graduate School of Medicine, Mayo Clinic Hospital, Scottsdale, Arizona

James H. Dauber, M.D., F.C.C.P.   Professor of Medicine, Medical Director of Lung Transplantation, Pulmonary, Allergy, and Critical Care Medicine, Department of Medicine, University of Pittsburg, Pittsburgh Veterans Administration Medical Center, Pittsburgh, Pennsylvania

Scott F. Davies, M.D.   Professor of Medicine, Director, Division of Pulmonary and Critical Care Medicine, University of Minnesota Medical School, Hennepin County Medical Center, Minneapolis, Minnesota

Gerald S. Davis, M.D., F.A.C.P., F.C.C.P.   Professor of Medicine, Director, Pulmonary Disease and Critical Care Medicine Unit, Department of Medicine, University of Vermont College of Medicine, Fletcher Allen Health Care, Burlington, Vermont

Peter A. Dietrich, M.D.   Professor of Diagnostic Radiology, Department of Radiology, University of Vermont College of Medicine, Fletcher Allen Health Care, Burlington, Vermont

Patrick A. Dowling, M.D.   Clinical Assistant Professor, Pulmonary and Critical Care Medicine, Department of Medicine, University of Wisconsin, Madison, Wisconsin

Jeffrey D. Edelman, M.D.   Assistant Professor of Medicine, Pulmonary, Allergy, and Critical Care Division, University of Pennsylvania, Philadelphia, Pennsylvania

Stanley B. Fiel, M.D.   Professor of Medicine, Chief, Pulmonary and Critical Care Medicine, Medical College of Pennsylvania and Hahnemann University School of Medicine, Philadelphia, Pennsylvania

David E. Gannon, M.D., F.A.C.P., F.C.C.P.   Assistant Professor of Medicine, Director, Sleep Disordered Breathing Program, VT Regional Sleep Disorders Center, Pulmonary Disease and Critical Care Medicine Unit, Department of Medicine, University of Vermont College of Medicine, Fletcher Allen Health Care, Burlington, Vermont

William G.B. Graham, M.D.   Professor Emeritus of Medicine, Pulmonary Disease and Critical Care Medicine Unit, Department of Medicine, University of Vermont College of Medicine, Fletcher Allen Health Care, Burlington, Vermont

Gunnar Gudmundsson, M.D.   Department of Medicine, National University Hospital, Reykjavik Iceland

Richard A. Helmers, M.D.   Assistant Professor of Internal Medicine, Section Chair, Thoracic Diseases and Critical Care Medicine, Mayo Graduate School of Medicine, Mayo Clinic Hospital, Scottsdale, Arizona

William E. Hopkins, M.D., F.A.C.C.   Associate Professor of Medicine, Associate Chair for Clinical Affairs, Department of Medicine, Cardiology Unit, University of Vermont College of Medicine, Fletcher Allen Health Care, Burlington, Vermont

Gary W. Hunninghake, M.D.   Professor of Medicine, Director of Pulmonary, Critical Care, and Occupational Medicine, University of Iowa, Iowa City, Iowa

David H. Ingbar, M.D.   Professor of Medicine and Pediatrics, Director, Medical Intensive Care Unit and Respiratory Care, Pulmonary, Allergy, and Critical Care Division, University of Minnesota School of Medicine, Fairview University Medical Center, Minneapolis, Minnesota

Richard S. Irwin, M.D., F.A.C.P., F.C.C.P.   Professor of Medicine, Director, Division of Pulmonary, Allergy, and Critical Care Medicine, Department of Medicine, University of Massachusetts Medical School, UMass Memorial Health Care, Worcester, Massachusetts

Michael D. Iseman, M.D., F.A.C.P., F.C.C.P.   Professor of Medicine, Chief, Clinical Mycobacteriology Services; Girard and Madeline Beno Chair in Mycobacterial Diseases, Division of Infectious Diseases, University of Colorado School of Medicine, National Jewish Medical and Research Center, Denver, Colorado

David A. Kaminsky, M.D.   Assistant Professor of Medicine, Director, Pulmonary Function Laboratory, Pulmonary Disease and Critical Care Medicine Unit, Department of Medicine, University of Vermont College of Medicine, Fletcher Allen Health Care, Burlington, Vermont

Jason Kelley, M.D.   Professor of Medicine, Chief, Pulmonary and Critical Care Medicine, Texas A&M Health Sciences Center, Olin E. Teague VA Medical Center; Scott and White Clinics, Temple, Texas

Talmadge E. King, Jr., M.D., F.A.C.P., F.C.C.P.   Constance B. Wofsy Distinguished Professor, Chief, Medical Services; Vice-Chair, Department of Medicine, University of California, San Francisco General Hospital, San Francisco, California

Jeffrey S. Klein, M.D.   Associate Professor of Radiology, Chief of Thoracic Radiology, Department of Radiology, University of Vermont College of Medicine, Fletcher Allen Health Care, Burlington, Vermont

Joel N. Kline, M.D., F.A.C.C.P.   Assistant Professor, Division of Pulmonary, Critical Care, and Occupational Medicine, University of Iowa, Iowa City, Iowa

John W. Kreit, M.D.   Assistant Professor of Medicine, Division of Pulmonary, Allergy, and Critical Care Medicine, Department of Medicine, University of Pittsburgh, Pittsburgh, Pennsylvania

Louis A. Lanza, M.D.   Assistant Professor of Surgery, Department of Surgery, Mayo Graduate School of Medicine, Mayo Clinic Hospital, Scottsdale, Arizona

James C. Leiter, M.D.   Associate Professor of Physiology and Medicine, Chief, Section of Pulmonary and Critical Care Medicine, Dartmouth Medical School, Dartmouth-Hitchcock Medical Center, Lebanon, New Hampshire

Kevin O. Leslie, M.D., F.A.C.P.   Associate Professor of Pathology, Department of Pathology, Mayo Graduate School of Medicine, Mayo Clinic Hospital, Scottsdale, Arizona

Jing W. Liu, M.D., F.A.C.P., F.C.C.P.   Assistant Professor of Medicine, Associate Chief, Pulmonary Section, University of Virginia School of Medicine, Salem Veterans Administration Medical Center, Salem, Virginia

Robert G. Loudon, M.B., Ch.B., F.R.C.P.E.   Professor Emeritus of Internal Medicine, Pulmonary Disease, University of Cincinnati College of Medicine, Cincinnati, Ohio

J. Mark Madison, M.D.   Associate Professor of Medicine and Physiology, Associate Director, Pulmonary, Allergy, and Critical Care Medicine; Director, Pulmonary Diagnostic Laboratories, University of Massachusetts Medical School, UMass Memorial Health Care, Worcester, Massachusetts

Donald A. Mahler, M.D., F.A.C.P., F.C.C.P., F.A.C.S.   Professor of Medicine, Director of Fellowship Training Program, Pulmonary and Critical Care Medicine, Dartmouth Medical School, Dartmouth-Hitchcock Medical Center, Lebanon, New Hampshire

Theodore W. Marcy, M.D., F.C.C.P. Associate Professor of Medicine, Pulmonary Disease and Critical Care Medicine Unit, Department of Medicine, University of Vermont College of Medicine, Fletcher Allen Health Care, Burlington, Vermont

John J. Marini, M.D. Professor of Medicine and Chair of Academic Medicine, Chief, Pulmonary Disease and Critical Care Medicine, University of Minnesota, Regions Hospital, St. Paul, Minnesota

Kevin K. Matsuba, M.D. Clinical Instructor, Department of Radiology, University of Vermont College of Medicine, Fletcher Allen Health Care, Burlington, Vermont

Roberto Mejia, M.D. National Institute of Respiratory Diseases, Mexico City, Mexico

Raymond L.H. Murphy, Jr., M.D., Sc.D. Professor of Medicine, Chief, Pulmonary Service, Faulkner Hospital and Lemuel Shattuck Hospital, Tufts University School of Medicine, Boston, Massachusetts

Walter J. O'Donohue, Jr., M.D. Professor of Medicine and Associate Dean for Graduate Medical Education, Chief, Division of Pulmonary and Critical Care, Creighton University School of Medicine, Omaha, Nebraska

Todd R. Peebles, M.D. Clinical Instructor, Chief Resident, Diagnostic Radiology, Department of Radiology, University of Vermont College of Medicine, Fletcher Allen Health Care, Burlington, Vermont

Carrie A. Redlich, M.D., M.P.H., F.A.C.O.E.M., F.A.C.C.P. Associate Professor of Medicine, Occupational, Environmental Medicine Program and Pulmonary and Critical Care Section, Yale University School of Medicine, Yale–New Haven Hospital, New Haven, Connecticut

Herbert Y. Reynolds, M.D., F.A.C.P., F.C.C.P. J. Lloyd Huck Professor of Medicine, Chair, Department of Medicine, Pennsylvania State University, Milton S. Hershey Medical Center, Hershey, Pennsylvania

M. Patricia Rivera, M.D., F.C.C.P. Assistant Professor of Medicine, Co-Director, Pulmonary and Critical Care Medicine Program, University of North Carolina, Chapel Hill, North Carolina

Dudley F. Rochester, M.D. Professor Emeritus, Division of Pulmonary and Critical Care Medicine, Department of Medicine, University of Virginia School of Medicine, Charlottesville, Virginia

Robert M. Rogers, M.D. Professor of Medicine and Anesthesiology, Director, Comprehensive Lung Center, Division of Pulmonary, Allergy, and Critical Care Medicine, Department of Medicine, University of Pittsburgh, Pittsburgh, Pennsylvania

Milton D. Rossman, M.D. Professor of Medicine, Pulmonary, Allergy, and Critical

Care Division, Department of Medicine, University of Pennsylvania, Philadelphia, Pennsylvania

Jay H. Ryu, M.D., F.A.C.C.P. Associate Professor of Medicine, Department of Pulmonary and Critical Care Medicine, Mayo Medical School, Mayo Clinic, Rochester, Minnesota

Joseph L. Saraceno, D.O. Assistant Professor of Medicine, Pulmonary and Critical Care Division, Albany Medical Center, Albany, New York

David A. Schwartz, M.D., M.P.H. Professor, Director, Center for Environmental Lung Diseases; Associate Chair of Medicine, Division of Pulmonary, Critical Care, and Occupational Medicine, Department of Internal Medicine, University of Iowa, Iowa City, Iowa

Marvin I. Schwartz, M.D. James C. Campbell Professor of Pulmonary Medicine, Head, Division of Pulmonary Sciences and Critical Care Medicine, University of Colorado, Denver, Colorado

Roger H. Secker-Walker, M.B., F.R.C.P., F.A.C.P., F.C.C.P. Professor Emeritus of Medicine, Pulmonary and Critical Care Medicine Unit, Department of Medicine, University of Vermont College of Medicine, Burlington, Vermont

William P. Sexauer, M.D. Assistant Professor of Medicine, Pulmonary and Critical Care Medicine, Medical College of Pennsylvania and Hahnemann School of Medicine, Philadelphia, Pennsylvania

Shawn J. Skerrett, M.D. Associate Professor of Medicine, Division of Pulmonary and Critical Care Medicine, University of Washington, Seattle, Washington

Akshay Sood, M.B.B.S., M.P.H. Occupational, Environmental Medicine Program, and Pulmonary and Critical Care Section, Yale University School of Medicine, Yale–New Haven Hospital, New Haven, Connecticut

Simon D. Spivack, M.D., M.P.H., F.A.C.C.P. Associate Professor of Medicine, Pulmonary and Critical Care Division, Department or Medicine, Albany Medical College; SUNY School of Public Health, Albany Medical Center; Wadsworth Center, NY State Department of Health, Albany, New York

Diane E. Stover, M.D., F.C.C.P. Professor of Clinical Medicine, Chief, Pulmonary Service; Head, Division of General Medicine, Cornell University, Memorial Sloan-Kettering Cancer Center, New York, New York

Michael Unger, M.D., F.A.C.P., F.C.C.P. Clinical Professor of Medicine, Director, Pulmonary Cancer Detection and Prevention Program, Thomas Jefferson University, Jefferson Medical College, Fox Chase Cancer Center, Philadelphia, Pennsylvania

1

Anatomy of the Respiratory System

Theodore W. Marcy and Gerald S. Davis
University of Vermont College of Medicine
Fletcher Allen Health Care
Burlington, Vermont

OVERVIEW

To understand respiratory system disorders, one first must have an appreciation of the normal respiratory system, its functions, and how its anatomy serves those functions. To those who specialize in pulmonary medicine, one of its attractions is how these principles illuminate what we observe daily in patients. This chapter is an introduction to the function and anatomy of the respiratory system. Space constraints dictate that this chapter be a very brief overview. However, concepts mentioned here are further expanded in the chapters that immediately follow on respiratory muscles and control of ventilation, airflow, gas exchange, and host defense. They are then echoed in the chapters on diagnostic evaluation, specific disorders, and common therapies. Excellent chapters or monographs on anatomy and physiology are listed at the end of the chapter.

FUNCTION OF THE RESPIRATORY SYSTEM

Gas Exchange

The principal function of the respiratory system is to accomplish exchange of oxygen (O_2) and carbon dioxide (CO_2) between the atmosphere and the blood. The mitochodria that generate adenosine triphosphate by oxidative phosphorylation for metabolism consume a total of 250 mL/min of oxygen at rest in the normal adult. With exertion, oxygen consumption can rise to as high as 4000 mL/min in trained athletes. Unlike the digestive system, which consumes large quantities of calories intermittently and converts the excess to stores for times of fasting, the respiratory system cannot store significant amounts of oxygen in tissues. Instead, the respiratory system must tirelessly replenish the venous blood with oxygen. At the same time, the lung must excrete from the blood into the atmosphere carbon dioxide (CO_2) as a metabolic waste product. Carbon dioxide is also a major determinant of the extracellular fluid compartment's acid:base status. At rest, the normal individual's carbon dioxide production is about 200 mL/min. Carbon dioxide production will increase linearly as an individual moves from rest to moderate levels of exertion. However, the rate of carbon dioxide production will accelerate once the individual reaches a level of exercise that exceeds oxygen availability, at which point anaerobic metabolism causes the accumulation of lactate—a level of exercise termed the *anaerobic threshold*. In normal subjects, carbon dioxide production can approach 4000 mL/min with heavy exertion, an amount that would result in severe tissue acidosis if it were not excreted. Fortunately, the rate of excretion of carbon dioxide is directly proportional to minute ventilation, and the individual can increase carbon dioxide elimination by breathing faster and deeper. (The response to exercise is covered in greater detail in Chap. 9.)

The reserve of the respiratory system is such that normal subjects do not even approach their maximum minute ventilation at exhausting exercise; they are limited instead by cardiac output and by symptoms that protect the individual from exercising to the point of irreversible neuromuscular injury. On the other hand, even at rest, carbon dioxide in the blood builds up quickly and the oxygen saturation falls if we stop breathing for any appreciable length of time. Most of us become acutely uncomfortable if we hold our breath for just 60 s. There is no rest for the respiratory system: carbon dioxide and oxygen must be exchanged continuously.

Metabolic, Endocrine, and Biochemical Modification Functions

The pulmonary vascular bed is ideally situated to remove or transform circulating substances produced in the body or absorbed from the alimentary tract. The lung is interposed between the venous and arterial circulation and receives almost the entire venous drainage with the exception of the bronchial and Thebesian veins. Because of this anatomic relationship, the lung can serve as a mechanical filter for particulate matter such as thromboemboli, microorganisms, and injected talc. In addition, the huge surface area of the pulmonary endothelium (115 m^2) is arrayed with luminal enzymes and transport proteins that permit both intracellular and extracellular transformations of circulating proteins, peptides, and other active chemicals. An example is the conversion within the pulmonary endothelium of angiotensin I, a relatively inactive peptide, into the potent systemic vasoconstrictor angiotensin II. Other systemically active substances (e.g., serotonin, bradykinin, and prostaglandin E$_1$) are removed by the pulmonary endothelium.

A variety of pulmonary parenchymal cells are the source of substances that have both local and systemic effects. For example, macrophages and other parenchymal cells can release a variety of inflammatory cytokines that may contribute to the failure of other organs in patients with the acute respiratory distress syndrome (ARDS). Specialized cells within the pulmonary epithelium—the pulmonary neuroendocrine cells—secrete a variety of peptides and amines into the systemic circulation (e.g., substance P, calcitonin, somatostatin) that have, as yet, uncertain clinical significance. However, pulmonary neoplasms presumed to originate from these neuroendocrine cells are associated with a variety of important paraneoplastic syndromes including Cushing's syndrome, hypertrophic pulmonary osteoarthropathy, and the syndrome of inappropriate antidiuretic hormone (SIADH), illustrating the profound effects these substances can exert. (See Chaps. 7 and 32.)

Host Defense

The lung is in direct contact with a total of 10,000 L of inhaled air daily, and all of the microorganisms, hazardous gases, and particulates suspended in this air. The conducting airways and alveoli are endowed with overlapping mechanical, cellular, and immunological methods of clearing or neutralizing these foreign materials. Most of the time, the lung maintains its sterility and prevents entry of threatening substances to the circulation without invoking an inflammatory response that would injure the lung's delicate architecture. The details of these defense mechanisms, and the problems that occur when they fail are covered in subsequent chapters. (See Chaps. 5 and 18.)

Air Movement for Sound Generation and Other Behaviors

We sometimes forget the importance of the respiratory system in other human behaviors. The movement of air across the vocal cords allows speech—the unique human ability that facilitates rich interactions with others in our families and society. [One is reminded of how this is taken for granted when we struggle to understand an awake but intubated patient in the intensive care unit (ICU)]. The movement of air past the lips is essential for some forms of music (wind instruments), occupations (glass blowing), and, at least in the past, the study of chemistry and biology (mouth pipetting!). These activities illustrate the remarkable versatility of the respiratory system. While performing continuous and life-sustaining gas exchange, this movement of air simultaneously permits these voluntary behaviors. No wonder that respiratory disease can be so incapacitating.

STRUCTURE–FUNCTION RELATIONSHIPS

One method of understanding all of the anatomic structures comprised by the respiratory system is to organize them into one of two components of the respiratory system: the *gas-exchange organ* (the lungs and associated vasculature) and the *ventilatory pump* that moves air into (and at times out of) that gas-exchange organ. While obviously not a perfect system of classification, this division may aid in the formation of an appropriate differential diagnosis when one is confronted by a patient with impending respiratory failure. The variety of problems leading to respiratory failure from impairment of the gas-exchange organ and/or the ventilatory pump are covered in Chapter 19.

The Gas-Exchange Organ

Together, the right and left lungs weigh approximately 1000 g; they are about 24 cm in height in the normal adult at end expiration. The volume of gas remaining in the lungs at end expiration is called the functional residual capacity (FRC), and is approximately 2.5 L in the average individual. FRC, total lung capacity (TLC), and other lung volumes vary with the age, height, gender, and race of the individual. TLC in a normal-sized individual will approach 6 L. The blood volume at FRC is 400–500 mL, but this will also increase with deep inspiration. The combined alveolar-capillary membrane of the estimated 300 million alveoli in the lungs provide a large surface area (130 m²) for gas exchange. Within the lung parenchyma are the airways and blood vessels that transport air and blood to the alveoli, as well as the lymphatics, nerves, and supporting interstitium for these structures. The lungs are stabilized within the thorax by the right and left hila, where the pulmonary arteries and veins and the bronchi attach to the mediastinal structures of the heart and trachea. The hila also contain lymph nodes, which drain lymphatics arising from within the lung.

The lungs are wrapped in the pleural membranes much as a hand pushed into a balloon is surrounded by the balloon's surface contiguous with the hand (which is analogous to the visceral pleura), by the space inside the balloon (the pleural space), and by the other side of the balloon (the parietal pleura). The reflection of the mediastinal and visceral pleura forms the pulmonary ligament, which extends down from the hilum. The distance between the parietal and visceral pleura is only micrometers in dimension with a very small, difficult to measure volume of fluid that reduces frictional resistance of the two pleural surfaces during breathing. The pleural space in health remains largely free of significant fluid or air and acts to couple the lung's inward elastic recoil with the outward recoil of the chest wall. This dynamic equilibrium causes the pressure within the pleural space to be about 5 cm lower than atmosphere. This coupling allows the muscles that expand the thorax to also expand the lung. When this coupling is lost, as in a traumatic pneumothorax, the lung deflates and the thorax springs outward.

Moving outward from the hilum, the major bronchi and pulmonary arteries divide to form three lobes on the right and two lobes on the left, each surrounded by a visceral pleura that forms the major and minor fissures. Further out from the hilum, the bronchi and pulmonary arteries divide into segments of each of these lobes (Fig. 1). Continued division of the arteries and airways ends when they form a terminal respiratory unit, defined as the alveoli and alveolar ducts arising from a single respiratory bronchiole and surrounded by a connective tissue envelope within which the pulmonary veins drain the capillary blood (Fig. 2). Interwoven connective tissue fibers spiral back along the bronchi and attach to the hilum, conferring an elastic property to the lung that causes it to deflate passively after inspiration while at the same time tethering open the airways. This *axial*, or central-to-peripheral, orientation of lung structure is reflected in clinical and radiographic patterns of certain respiratory diseases. Pneumonias often obey segmental or lobar boundaries; obstruction of segmental or lobar bronchi causes segmental or lobar atelectasis; occlusion of segmental pulmonary vessels by thromboemboli will cause segmental atelectasis or tissue infarction.

The major components of the lung parenchyma are briefly described below.

Airways

The airway divides from the main carini to create, on average, 23 successive generations of airways out to the periphery of the lung (Fig. 3). The first 15 generations have cartilaginous plates and are called *bronchi*. The membranous *bronchioles* have no surrounding cartilage and are, instead, tethered open by the connective tissue of the lung, expanding and contracting with the respiratory cycle. Gas exchange begins just beyond the *terminal bronchioles* in the *respiratory bronchioles*, which have alveolar epithelium. The diameter of each new generation of airways is smaller than that of the prior generation, beginning with the trachea (2 cm), mainstem bronchi (1 cm), and segmental bronchi (0.5 cm—about the diameter of an aspirated peanut), until reaching the terminal bronchioles, beyond which airway diameter in further generations remains at 0.5 mm. Even though the airways be-

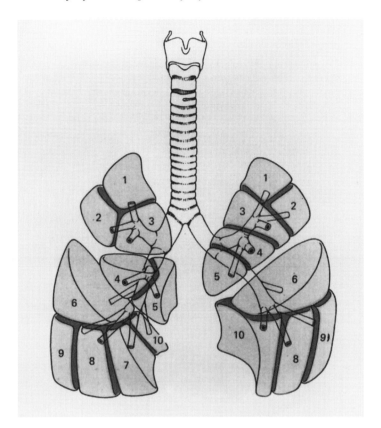

Figure 1   An exploded schematic diagram of the segmental anatomy of the right and left lungs with the lungs slightly turned inward to allow visualization of the posterior segments. Left and right upper lobes: (1) apical, (2) posterior, (3) anterior, (4) superior lingula (left), and (5) inferior lingula (left) segments. Right middle lobe: (4) lateral and (5) medial segments. Lower lobes: (6) superior (apical), (7) medial basilar (right only), (8) anterior basilar, (9) lateral basilar, and (10) posterior basilar segments. (From Weibel ER, Tayler CR. Functional design of the human lung for gas exchange. In: Fishman AP, ed. Pulmonary Disease and Disorders, 3d ed. New York: McGraw Hill, 1998.)

come smaller, the *total* cross-sectional area of the airway lumen is much greater in the periphery of the lung than it is at the trachea because the number of bronchi multiplies at each generation. This means that the linear velocity of air diminishes as it travels out into the distal airway, until gas movement in the terminal and respiratory bronchioles occurs primarily by diffusion and by the mixing generated by the heart's contractions. Most of the frictional resistance to airflow occurs in the cartilaginous bronchi. (See Chap. 3.)

Gas is inspired and expired through the same airways, leading to an inevitable amount of anatomic dead space, i.e., the volume within the airways from the mouth to the terminal bronchioles in which no gas exchange occurs and ventilated air is wasted. The anatomic dead space volume in an adult is estimated to be 150 mL.

The airways down to the terminal bronchioles are lined on their luminal surface by columnar epithelium. Half of these cells are covered on their surface by cilia—projections

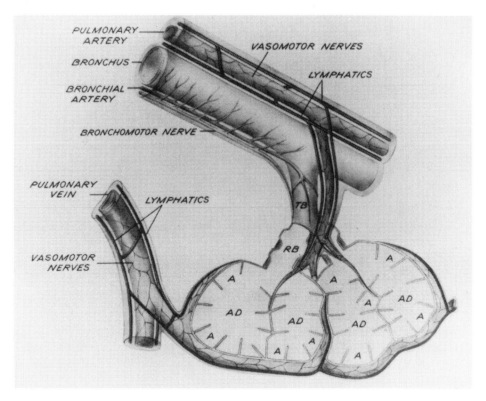

Figure 2 A simplified schematic of a terminal respiratory unit illustrating the relationship of the pulmonary arteries with the airways and the bronchial arteries. The alveoli (A) and the alveolar ducts (AD) branch from a respiratory bronchiole (RB), which arises from a terminal bronchiole. The pulmonary veins that drain the capillary plexus are within the loose connective tissue covering the terminal respiratory unit. Lymphatics and nerves travel both within the bronchoarterial sheath and along the pulmonary veins. (From Staub NC. Hum Pathol 1970; 1:419.)

that are 6 μm long, each with a microtubular array that confers coordinated movement. Cilia beat rhythmically within a gel-like mucous layer that traps inhaled particulates and other debris, acting to propel this mucus toward the mouth. This mechanism, called the *mucociliary escalator*, is an important component of host defense. Mucins, water, and solutes are secreted into the airway by interspersed secretory serous and goblet cells. The cartilaginous airways have larger secretory glands that extend down into the submucosa. The epithelial cells rest on a basement membrane, beneath which is a layer of spiraling connective tissue that extends out to the terminal respiratory unit. The connective tissue is covered, in turn, by bands of smooth muscle that encircle the airways out to the respiratory bronchioles. Autonomic nervous system innervation and mediators from resident mast and neuroendocrine cells as well as inflammatory cells alter the tone of these muscles, allowing for changes in airway circumference and regional ventilation.

Diseases that narrow or obstruct the airway lumen increase the frictional resistance of gas flow and lead to maldistribution of inspired air. These diseases are an important cause of respiratory symptoms and impairment. Emphysema is associated with destruction

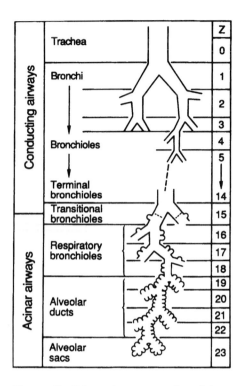

Figure 3 Schematic representation of the organization of the airways in human lungs, showing assignment to generations (z) of dichotomous branching beginning at the trachea (0) and ending at the alveolar sacs. (From Weibel ER. Design of airways and blood vessels considered as branching trees. In: Crystal RG, West JB, Barnes PJ, Weibel ER, eds. The Lung, Scientific Foundations, 2d ed. Philadelphia: Lippincott-Raven, 1977.)

of the connective tissue that tethers open the membranous bronchioles. Patients with chronic bronchitis have a thickened epithelium from hypertrophy of mucous glands. They also have excessive mucous secretion, further clogging the airway lumen. Asthma is characterized by inflammation of the airway epithelium with edema, excess mucous secretions, and diffuse contraction of the encircling smooth muscle (bronchospasm). These problems are discussed in greater detail in Chapters 26 and 27.

Blood Vessels

The pulmonary arteries accompany the bronchi, branching with them in their parallel course out into the parenchyma of the lung with roughly the same diameter as their paired airways (see above). These blood vessels transport venous blood from the right heart in high-capacitance vessels that have much less total resistance than the systemic circulation because their walls contain fewer elastic and smooth muscle fibers. Even though the blood flow through the pulmonary circulation equals left ventricular cardiac output, the pulmonary arterial system has a much lower mean pressure: 15 mmHg versus the systemic arterial mean pressure of 95 mmHg. The high-capacitance properties of the pulmonary circulation allow it to accommodate a high return of venous blood during exercise (up to

40 L/min in athletes) without significant increases in pulmonary pressures. Regional blood flow is dependent on hydrostatic forces (less blood flow to the apices than the bases), on lung inflation through the same tethering effect on the vessels as with the bronchioles, and on autonomic control of the encircling smooth muscle. The lumina of the blood vessels lined with endothelial cells containing numerous organelles that transform bioactive substances as described above.

The bronchioles, alveoli, and interstitium of the lung parenchyma receive substrates from the venous blood and sufficient oxygen from the inspired air to sustain their own metabolism. Only the larger bronchi and the visceral pleura require a separate arterial blood supply from the bronchial arteries arising from the thoracic aorta and/or the intercostals. The bronchial arterial system is, therefore, at systemic pressures. Most serious lower airway bleeding originates from the bronchial arteries that hypertrophy in areas of chronic inflammation or tumors. Embolism of the bronchial arteries under radiographic guidance is a therapeutic approach to life-threatening hemoptysis. (See Chap. 21.) Except for the bronchial arteries supplying the hilar structures, most of the bronchial arterial blood flow is drained by a peribronchial venous plexus that empties into the pulmonary veins, contributing to the small amount of normal, or physiologic, venous admixture into the left atrium (right-to-left shunt).

Alveoli

Efficient gas exchange is accomplished within the lung at the alveolar capillary membrane by combining a large airway surface area (130 m^2) with an extraordinarily thin (2-μm) barrier between the air and blood. The alveolus is not spherical but rather a complex geometric shape with flat sides and angulations at junctions. It is intimately connected with adjacent alveoli, with which it shares capillary endothelium (Fig. 4). In health, they remain open even at low lung volumes, but with airway obstruction or impaired regional lung inflation, they collapse (become atelectatic) and are difficult to reexpand.

Each alveolus consists of a thin septum that contains vascular endothelium (endothelial cells), epithelial lining cells on the air side (type I alveolar cells), and their respective basement membranes (Fig. 4). Therefore, the barrier for oxygen and carbon dioxide diffusion is four cell membranes (two for each cell) and two fused basement membranes. Type I alveolar cells have a very large surface area with markedly attenuated cytoplasm, very tight junctions between cells, and few mitochondria or intracellular organelles. The alveoli also contain cuboidal type II alveolar cells that, in contrast to type I cells, contain large numbers of mitochondria and intracellular organelles. These cells transport fluid and electrolytes into and out of the alveoli. They also synthesize, store, and secrete surfactant, a combination of phospholipids and proteins that spreads into a thin epithelial lining fluid on the epithelial surface of the alveolus. The epithelial lining fluid (ELF) markedly reduces the surface tension along the alveolar wall, a force acting to collapse these tiny spheres. In addition, the ELF contains substances that enhance local defense against foreign substances within the alveolar space. The type II cells also transform and divide to replace damaged type I cells.

The endothelial cells of the alveolar capillary membrane do not have as large a surface area and the junctions between cells are less tight, allowing inflammatory cytokines, neutrophils, and other inflammatory cells of local host defense into and out of the interstitium. There is also solute and fluid flux across the capillary into the interstitium and, eventually into the alveolar space, that is cleared by active solute transport by alveolar type II cells. Pulmonary edema occurs if there is elevated hydrostatic pressure within the

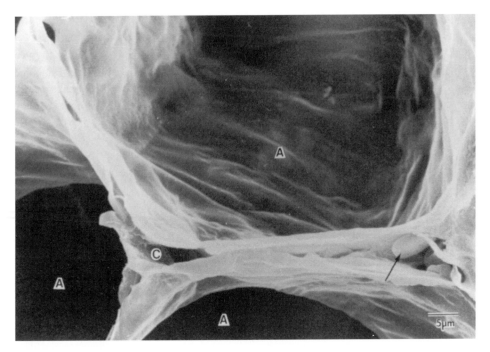

Figure 4   An electron micrograph of a perfusion-fixed normal rat lung illustrating the microscopic detail of the alveolar septum with a capillary (C) split longitudinally across three alveoli (A). Remaining red blood cells within the capillary give a sense of the scale (arrow). (From Staub NC, Albertine KH. Anatomy of the lung. In: Murray JF, Nadel JA, eds. Textbook of Respiratory Medicine, 2d ed. Philadelphia: Saunders, 1994.)

capillaries that increases fluid flux into the interstitium and alveolar space or if the alveolar capillary membrane is more permeable because of injury. Lymphatics originating at the junction between respiratory and terminal bronchioles drain extravasated fluid back to the systemic venous system via progressively larger lymphatic vessels and the lymph nodes of the lung, hilum, and mediastinum. The larger lymphatic vessels contain smooth muscle that pumps the lymph through one-way valves to the hilum against elevated central venous pressures. Disorders of lymphatic drainage (for example, lymphoma and lymphangioleiomyomatosis) cause accumulation of lymph fluid in the pleural space—a so-called chylous effusion. (See Chaps. 17 and 29.)

   Other cells reside in or near the alveolar space. Alveolar and interstitial macrophages (histiocytes) and lymphocytes provide local host defense and help clear particulates that reach the alveolar level. Mast cells release histamine and other mediators that are important in regulating vascular permeability and the inflammatory response. Fibroblasts and other interstitial cells synthesize collagen and elastin fibers that provide the structural integrity to this system of airways and blood vessels. Inflammatory and infectious diseases that involve the lung parenchyma disrupt the fragile alveoli, impairing normal gas exchange. The lung usually repairs itself, but in some chronic disease processes (for example, idiopathic pulmonary fibrosis) restructuring fails and the normal alveolar architecture is replaced by fibrosis and scarring, with permanent diminution of the gas-exchange surface.

Nerves

The autonomic nervous system innervates the lung with parasympathetic fibers from the
vagus nerve and sympathetic fibers from the upper thoracic and cervical ganglia (see Table
1). Afferent nerves are part of the cough reflex and provide input about lung stretch and
inflation to the respiratory control centers. (See Chaps. 2 and 5.) Efferent nerves influence
the smooth muscle tone of the airways and blood vessels, altering regional ventilation and

Table 1   Innervation of the Lung and Thorax

Autonomic innervation

	Nerve		Functions
Parasympathetic	Vagus nerve (cranial nerve X)	Afferents	Irritant (cough) receptors, stretch (inflation) receptors, C fibers (parenchymal tissue distortion)
		Efferents	Airway constriction, increased glandular secretion, dilatation of pulmonary vasculature
Sympathetic	Preganglionic from spinal cord of T1 to T6 to sympathetic trunks	Efferents	Airway relaxation, inhibition of glandular secretion, constriction of pulmonary vasculature
	Postganglionic fibers from upper four to five paravertebral ganglia to pulmonary plexus		

Skeletal muscle innervation

Muscle	Nerve	Nerve roots	Function
Diaphragm	Phrenic nerve	C 3–5	Inspiration
Sternocleidomastoids	Cervical and cranial nerves	Cranial nerve XI C 1–2	Inspiration
Scalenes	Cervical nerves	C 4–6	Inspiration
Intercostals	Thoracic spinal nerves	T1–12	Inspiration and expiration
Pectoralis	Thoracic spinal nerves	C 6–8	Expiration
Transversus thoracis	Thoracic spinal nerves	T 2–6	Expiration
Rectus abdominis	Thoracoabdominal branches	T 6–12	Expiration
External and internal abdominal obliques	Thoracoabdominal branches of thoracic spinal nerves	T 6–12	Expiration
Transversus abdominis	Thoracoabdominal branches	T 6–12	Expiration

perfusion. This activity can contribute to bronchospasm. Efferent autonomic activity can also modify the secretion of mucus and solute from secretory glands.

The Ventilatory Pump

As marvelous as the lung is, it is entirely useless as an organ for gas exchange unless it is replenished with fresh gas on a continuous basis. The task of the ventilatory pump is to move air from the atmosphere into the lung against the forces of frictional resistance from the airways and lung tissue, and the elastic recoil of the lung parenchyma and chest wall. Elastic recoil is a property of the lung conferred by its network of collagen and elastic fibers, which allow the lung to deflate passively without active muscle contraction while simultaneously tethering open the airways. However, during coughing or with the increased ventilatory requirements of exertion, the ventilatory pump generates a positive pressure relative to atmosphere to achieve active exhalation. It is not possible to point to any one organ or region to identify the ventilatory pump. Instead, it functions by the coordinated efforts of several different systems and structures that range in location from the abdominal musculature to the central nervous system.

Thoracic Cage

Air enters the lung because the space encompassed by the bony structures of the thorax is expanded by the force of the inspiratory muscles. Because of the coupling effects of the pleural space described above, this also expands the lung, creating the pressure gradient across the lung (transpulmonary pressure) that drives inspiratory airflow. The thorax consists of 12 pairs of ribs that articulate with the thoracic vertebral bodies posteriorly, and, except for the eleventh and twelfth pair, are attached to the sternum anteriorly. Contraction of the diaphragm compresses the abdominal contents, increasing the craniocaudal dimension of the thorax. Even when the individual is at rest, the intercostal muscles running between the ribs are active, preventing the upper thorax from moving inward with the force of the descending diaphragm. Some of the inspiratory muscle force of the diaphragm acts to move the lower articulated ribs outward in a motion, much like that of a bucket handle, that expands the thoracic cage. The upper ribs are moved upward and outward by the accessory muscles of respiration—the scalenes, the sternocleidomastoids, and the muscles of the shoulder girdle and neck. These accessory muscles become active when there is an increased ventilatory load from either a high minute ventilation requirement or because of increased resistive or elastic forces. For example, patients with emphysema often utilize accessory muscles of respiration at rest.

The compliance of the thorax, defined as the change in the dimension of the chest for a given amount of inspiratory muscle force, is diminished with the thoracic cage deformities of kyphosis or scoliosis, both of which are risk factors for acute or chronic hypercapnic respiratory failure. A traumatic fracture of the ribs in two locations causes this rib segment to move inward with inspiration, a condition called a *flail chest*, which decreases the efficiency of inspiratory efforts and can contribute to respiratory failure, especially if the patient has other pulmonary injuries or disease.

Respiratory Muscles

The inspiratory muscles of respiration mentioned above are all skeletal, striated muscles— the only skeletal muscles essential for life. They share with all striated muscles the property that their degree of force generation is related to the length of the muscle at rest and to the nerve firing frequency. In normal subjects, the diaphragm has a resting tone that places it at an optimal length for maximal force generation at the end of expiration. A problem that contributes to the breathlessness and limited ventilatory reserve of patients with emphysema is that their chests are markedly hyperinflated from air trapping. At the end of expiration, the diaphragm is shortened and not at an optimal length for force generation. In addition, the thoracic cage is less compliant at these lung volumes. One of the proposed benefits of surgery to reduce lung volume is that the removal of emphysematous lung returns the diaphragm and the thoracic cage to more optimal dimensions.

The muscles that generate an active expiratory effort include the intercostals, the clavicular head of the pectoralis, and the transversus thoracis, the latter being muscles that run down the inner aspect of the anterior thorax from the second through sixth ribs to the sternum. Collectively, these muscles pull the ribs downward and inward. In addition, the muscles of the abdominal wall push the abdominal contents forcibly upward, raising the diaphragm. Together, these muscles can generate intrathoracic pressures of 100 to 200 mmHg and a 500-mph outward linear velocity of air. Loss of expiratory muscle function from cervical or thoracic spinal cord injury or neuromuscular disease can lead to poor secretion clearance, atelectasis, and pneumonia. Interestingly, the expiratory muscles can be recruited to perform, in effect, inspiratory work during times of high ventilatory loads. Active expiratory efforts compress thoracic volume below its resting volume; relaxation of these muscles at the end of exhalation allows the chest cage to expand passively outward, contributing to inspiration.

Muscle Innervation

As striated muscles, the muscles of respiration are innervated with peripheral nerves that initiate depolarization and muscular contraction (Table 1). The diaphragm is innervated by the right and left phrenic nerves, which arise from the fourth cervical nerve with contributions from the third and usually the fifth cervical segments. The phrenic nerves descend anterior to the medial border of the scalene muscles into the mediastinum, traveling anterior to both hilum and between the pericardium and mediastinal pleura before attaching to the diaphragm. Unilateral diaphragmatic paralysis can occur by injury to these nerves from trauma, malignancies in the hilar region, or neuromuscular disease. Unilateral and occasionally bilateral phrenic nerve paralysis has occurred as a complication of the cold cardioplegia used for open heart surgery.

The sternocleidomastoid muscles are innervated by the eleventh cranial nerve and the first and second cervical nerves. Therefore, these accessory muscles of inspiration can, with training, partially compensate for bilateral phrenic nerve paralysis due to high cervical cord injury. The other respiratory muscles are innervated from spinal nerves, as outlined in Table 1. All of the peripheral nerves are vulnerable to neurotoxins (botulism), demyelinating conditions (Guillain-Barré syndrome), chronic or degenerative neurological diseases that affect the nerve itself (e.g., polio or amyotrophic lateral sclerosis), and neuromuscular transmission (e.g., myasthenia gravis).

Central Respiratory Controller

The coordinated firing of these peripheral nerves is controlled by respiratory centers in the pons and medulla of the central nervous system. These centers, in turn, are influenced by multiple inputs, including vagal afferents from peripheral chemoreceptors and lung stretch receptors, central chemoreceptors on the ventral surfaces of the medulla, and input from the cerebral cortex. Afferents from joint proprioceptors may allow the respiratory centers to increase minute ventilation during exertion in advance of changes in arterial carbon dioxide and oxygen. The redundancy of input into the respiratory centers helps protect the organism from the effects of damage to any one of the inputs. Patients with bilateral lung transplants, and therefore no vagal afferents, have remarkably normal respiratory patterns and responses. The complexity of respiratory control is examined in greater depth in Chapter 2.

SUMMARY

The respiratory system serves a life-sustaining metabolic function with a remarkable ability to be adaptable and tolerant to different environments. It applies its capacity to move air to less critical but still useful activities such as speech. Its structure is necessarily complex and, therefore, vulnerable despite built-in reserves and redundancies. Respiratory symptoms are associated with practically every major systemic disorder. Respiratory pathophysiology encompasses practically the full range of scientific inquiry: from the physics of gas flow to the molecular biology of cell membrane transport. The chapters that follow further explore the respiratory system in both health and disease.

SUGGESTED READING

1. Murray JF. The Normal Lung, 2d ed. Philadelphia: Saunders, 1986.
2. Netter FH. Respiratory system. In: The Ciba Collection of Medical Illustrations, Vol. 7. West Caldwell, NJ: Ciba-Geigy Corp., 1980.
3. Staub NC, Albertine KH. Anatomy of the lung. In: Murray JF, Nadel JA, eds. Textbook of Respiratory Medicine, 2d ed. Philadelphia: Saunders, 1994.
4. Weibel ER, Tayler CR. Functional design of the human lung for gas exchange. In: Fishman AP, ed. Pulmonary Diseases and Disorders, 3d ed. New York: McGraw-Hill, 1998.
5. West JB. Respiratory Physiology—The Essentials, 5th ed. Baltimore: Williams & Wilkins, 1995.

2

Muscles, Nerves, and Central Control of Respiration

James C. Leiter

Dartmouth Medical School
Dartmouth–Hitchcock Medical Center
Lebanon, New Hampshire

RESPIRATORY MUSCLES AND NERVES

Muscles of the Ventilatory Pump

The diaphragm is the primary muscle of inspiration. The diaphragm functions well only when active in harmony with other respiratory muscles and when the mechanical characteristics of the respiratory system are well matched to the capacity of the diaphragm (and other muscles of respiration) to perform work. The parasternal, scalene, and external intercostal muscles aid the diaphragm during inspiration at rest. During exercise, the pattern of intercostal muscle activation changes to enhance inspiratory forces; additional accessory muscles of the upper chest and neck, such as the sternocleidomastoids, may become active during inspiration. The diaphragm is innervated by the phrenic nerves, which originate from cervical nerves C3–C5, travel over the anterior scalene muscles, and dive into the thoracic cavity adjacent to the subclavian arteries and veins. Within the thoracic cavity, the nerves run along the lateral aspects of the pericardium until they ramify over the surface of the diaphragm. The intercostal muscles are innervated segmentally by intercostal nerves. The accessory muscles are innervated by a variety of nerves originating from the eleventh cranial nerve or cervical or intercostal nerves.

The diaphragm consists of a central tendon in the shape of a dome (Fig. 1). Costal fibers of the diaphragm run along the outer rim of the central tendon and insert along the rib cage. Crural fibers of the diaphragm originate along the posterior and medial aspects of the central tendon and insert posteriorly along the spine. The costal diaphragmatic muscles are oriented axially and apposed to the chest wall. The action of the costal diaphragm pulls the central tendon down and the rib cage up toward the head as the lower rib cage expands. Furthermore, the area of costal apposition is subjected to abdominal pressures, which are positive during inspiration; therefore, the rib cage tends to move outward along the insertion of the costal fibers during inspiration. Crural diaphragmatic fibers have no significant effect on the rib cage in normal situations but pull the central tendon down during inspiration. Therefore, the inspiratory actions of crural and diaphragmatic contraction are independent but parallel. The contraction of the crural and costal

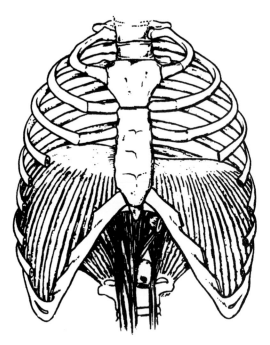

Figure 1 The location of the diaphragm within the thoracic cavity at the end of expiration. The insertion of the crural parts of the diaphragm is shown along the spine, and the costal parts of the diaphragm insert along the lower border of the rib cage. (From Rochester DF, Arora NS, Braun NMT. Maximum contractile force of human diaphragm, determined in vitro. Trans Am Clin Climatol Assoc 1981; 83:200–208.)

parts of the diaphragm probably originates in different cervical segments from different populations of phrenic motor neurons, and stimulation of these parts of the diaphragm may be controlled independently. Parallel but independent activation increases the strength of the diaphragm and permits a wider repertoire of respiratory activities. For example, the esophagus passes through the crural diaphragm, and we can swallow, burp, or vomit—while the crural diaphragm is relaxed—without compromising costal diaphragmatic function.

The parasternal muscles lift the "bucket handles" of the upper ribs laterally and outward, and the scalenes, which insert on the first two ribs, lift the entire rib cage outward and rostrally, a so-called "pump-handle" movement. The intercostal muscles have variable effects on the rib cage depending on the orientation of the muscle fibers, lung volume, and the rostral-to-caudal pattern of activation. Hence, it is not possible to state unequivocally that external intercostal muscles are inspiratory and internal intercostal muscles are expiratory. For example, activation of external intercostal muscles has an inspiratory effect at low lung volumes but an expiratory effect at high lung volumes. Furthermore, the extent of external intercostal muscle activation expands in a rostral-to-caudal direction as respiratory drive and minute ventilation increase. The actual movement of the chest wall during resting breathing is modest, with little discernible inspiratory action, but the activation of the parasternal, scalene, and intercostal muscles also stiffens the rib cage and prevents paradoxical inward movement of the rib cage during inspiration. Stiffening of the rib cage is not a minor issue; quadriplegic patients lack intercostal muscle activation and demonstrate paradoxical, inward rib cage movement with each inspiration. These patients are susceptible to respiratory failure after only modest insults despite normal diaphragmatic function. The accessory muscles fix or lift the shoulder girdle during inspiration and augment inspiration. Fixation of the shoulder girdle also improves the mechanical function of the intercostal muscles and diaphragm. As respiratory drive increases, the inspiratory actions of the parasternal, scalene, and intercostal muscles increase. When the diaphragm is weak or at a mechanical disadvantage, the inspiratory activation of accessory muscles may be apparent even at rest.

Expiration is passive during resting breathing and driven solely by the elastic recoil of the respiratory system. This does not mean, however, that all respiratory muscles are inactive. The duration of expiration is usually longer than one would predict based on the mechanical characteristics of the respiratory system alone. Expiration is retarded and slowed by two mechanisms. First, the inspiratory activation of the diaphragm persists during the early phase of expiration. Therefore, the elastic recoil of the respiratory system must stretch the incompletely relaxed diaphragm, which slows expiration, in addition to propelling gas out of the lungs. Second, relaxation of the major laryngeal abductor, the posterior cricoarytenoid, and activation of laryngeal adductors, such as the thyroarytenoid, narrow the laryngeal orifice and increase expiratory resistance, which also prolongs expiratory time.

Activation of expiratory muscles also shortens expiratory time, and, more importantly, increases the force of expiration and the expiratory flow rate. Active expiration is powered by the abdominal muscles, the rectus abdominis, the transversus abdominis, the external and internal oblique muscles, and the internal and external intercostal muscles, depending on lung volume and the pattern of intercostal muscle activation. Expiration becomes active when respiratory drive increases—for example, during exercise. During exercise, expiratory muscle force may drive lung volume below the relaxation volume of the respiratory system and thereby augment the subsequent inspiratory force by the passive, inspiratory recoil of the respiratory system toward the relaxation volume. Expiratory muscles are also active during expulsive maneuvers such as coughing, sneezing, and vomiting and during the Valsalva maneuver (forced expiration against a closed glottis) accompanying a bowel movement.

Muscle Fatigue

Muscle fatigue is a diminution in muscle capacity, either the generation of force or the velocity of contraction, that can be restored by rest. Muscle activities that result in fatigue can be described by a rectangular hyperbole (Fig. 2) in which the duty cycle of the contraction is plotted as a function of the force of contraction. The duty cycle is the fraction of each respiratory cycle during which contraction occurs or the ratio of inspiratory time to total respiratory cycle time (T_I/T_{TOT}), and the force of contraction is the average transdiaphragmatic pressure during each effort (Pdi) expressed as a fraction of the maximum Pdi (Pdi max). The curve describes a diaphragmatic tension-time index in which all combinations of duty cycle and relative transdiaphragmatic pressure to the right and above the curve are fatiguing. The further above and to the right of the curve any combination of Pdi/Pdi max and T_I/T_{TOT} are, the more rapidly the muscle fatigues. There is an inverse relationship between Pdi and T_I/T_{TOT}: a prolonged duty cycle at a relatively low Pdi can be as fatiguing as more forceful contractions of relatively short duration. The curve in

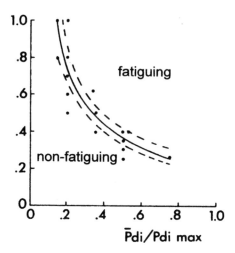

Figure 2   The duty cycle (T_I/T_{TOT}) has been plotted as a function of the average diaphragmatic force during a contraction expressed as a fraction of the maximal force (Pdi/Pdi max). All combinations of T_I/T_{TOT} and Pdi/Pdi max to the right and above the curve are fatiguing, and any combination of T_I/T_{TOT} and Pdi/Pdi max to the left of the curve can be performed indefinitely without fatigue. The dashed lines indicate the 95% confidence interval about the curve. (From Bellemare F, Grassino A. Evaluation of human diaphragm fatigue. J Appl Physiol 1982; 53:1196–1206.)

Figure 2 was generated over a small, fixed range of flow rates, but the metabolic need of the muscle also depends on the inspiratory flow rate; high flow rates are inversely related to the transdiaphragmatic pressure that can be sustained without fatigue. Respiratory muscle fatigue may occur when inspiratory flow, the duty cycle, and/or the Pdi are excessive. Furthermore, if the diaphragm is weak to begin with (low Pdi max), then any given level of Pdi will be a greater fraction of Pdi max. Therefore, the risk of fatigue may be reduced by correcting factors, such as hypophosphatemia and acidemia, that reduce the force of diaphragmatic contraction and by fostering diaphragm strength by ensuring good nutrition. The tidal volume, inspiratory flow rate, and Pdi determine the rate of energy consumption, but this is only half of the equation. Factors that reduce the rate of energy supply may also contribute to fatigue of respiratory muscles. Reduced diaphragmatic oxygen delivery by virtue of hypoxemia or reduced diaphragmatic blood flow may promote muscle fatigue at levels of Pdi, inspiratory flow, and duty cycle that would not otherwise be fatiguing.

In the presence of muscle fatigue, the central respiratory controller may try to optimize muscle function. Decreasing the size of the tidal volume can reduce Pdi and the energy consumption of each breath. Hence, rapid shallow breathing is often seen in the presence of respiratory muscle fatigue. However, respiratory frequency must increase to maintain alveolar ventilation when the tidal volume falls, and the energy consumption per unit time may actually increase. The central controller appears to reduce the fatiguing potential of each particular muscle contraction, but at the cost of an increased number of muscle contractions and increased energy consumption over time. This strategy cannot be sustained and hypoventilation and ventilatory failure may develop despite reduced energy consumption of each breath.

A more effective strategy in the face of respiratory muscle fatigue is to alternate the pattern of inspiratory muscle activation so that either the diaphragm or intercostal and accessory muscles provide the major inspiratory force. In this way, the diaphragm may rest when the intercostal and accessory muscles are active and vice versa. The mechanism whereby the central controller optimizes the force of each contraction and alternates the pattern of respiratory muscle activation is unknown, but the result is prolonged respiratory muscle endurance.

"Other" Respiratory Muscles

Traditionally, analysis of respiratory muscle function has been restricted to the diaphragm, intercostal muscles, and accessory muscles of the neck and shoulder girdle. However, the muscles of the soft palate, tongue, ventral surface of the neck (the sternohyoid, for example), and the larynx are also activated in synchrony with the respiratory cycle. The upper airway of humans is unique among mammals because of humans' capacity for speech. The acoustic requirements of speech necessitate a large supraglottic space to modulate the relatively simple tones produced by the vocal cords.

The epiglottis and the larynx, which are closely adjacent to the nasal choanae at the back of the nose in most mammals, have descended in humans, and the pharynx is elongated. The pharynx is not supported by any rigid structures in humans, and inspiratory activation of the muscles of the tongue and those attached to the hyoid bone stiffens and dilates the pharynx, preventing upper airway collapse during inspiration, when the transmural pressure in the extrathoracic airway is negative. The pharynx possesses some intrinsic rigidity, and the inspiratory activation of upper airway muscles that dilate and stiffen the airway may be absent at rest. However, if the airway is narrowed as a result of obesity and fat deposition around the pharynx, if nasal resistance is elevated, or if inspiratory flow rates are high, then the more distal pharyngeal transmural pressure will be decreased and the dilating action of upper airway muscles may be essential to maintain upper airway patency. Furthermore, the airway may be more susceptible to collapse during sleep, when activation of upper airway muscles diminishes, as discussed below.

CENTRAL CONTROL OF RESPIRATION

For the purposes of this discussion, the reader need only know that the central respiratory controller is in the medulla and pons. Two types of sensory information are used by the central respiratory controller to regulate ventilation: (1) mechanical feedback from the lungs, chest wall, and muscles of respiration and (2) chemosensors monitoring the P_{O_2} and P_{CO_2}.

Mechanical Receptors

Receptors within the lung fall into three categories: slowly adapting receptors, rapidly adapting receptors, and C fibers. Both slowly adapting and rapidly adapting stretch receptors are myelinated, whereas C fibers are unmyelinated and possess no specialized nerve endings. All of these fibers travel to the central nervous system in the vagus nerve.

Slowly adapting receptors resemble the arterial baroreceptors in that they respond to stretch. The firing rate of slowly adapting receptors increases as lung volume increases and, as the name suggests, there is little adaptation (little reduction in the firing rate as the stimulus is maintained). The slowly adapting receptors are close to smooth muscle in the extra- and intrathoracic lower airways. The slowly adapting receptors provide volume-related afferent feedback that is essential in the Hering-Breuer reflex. The Hering-Breuer reflex has two manifestations. First, if the airway is obstructed at the onset of inspiration, the duration of the inspiratory effort is prolonged and the amplitude of phrenic nerve activity is increased. The lack of activation of the stretch receptors seems to indicate that the respiratory controller should continue inspiratory efforts if lung volume is not increasing. Second, if the airway is obstructed at the end of inspiration, preventing expiration, or if the lung is artificially inflated above the end-inspiratory volume, the duration of expiration is prolonged. In this setting, increased slowly adapting receptor activity seems to indicate that the respiratory controller should not start a new inspiration before the gas associated with the previous inspiration has been exhaled. The Hering-Breuer reflex has been examined in innumerable studies of anesthetized animals, but there is little evidence that it actively controls inspiratory and expiratory time during wakeful, resting breathing in humans.

There are other aspects of the Hering-Breuer reflex that may still be important. The Hering-Breuer reflex is usually thought of in terms of effects on respiratory timing, but the activation pattern of the respiratory muscles is also modulated by lung stretch. During a normal inspiration, the rate of rise of phrenic nerve activity diminishes; the growing volume of stretch-related information indicates to the respiratory controller that inspiration is proceeding normally and phrenic activity may increase at a more leisurely pace (in reality, stretch-related activity may actively inhibit phrenic nerve activity). During airway obstruction, the absence of growing stretch receptor information indicates a need for vigorous effort and the rate of rise of phrenic nerve activity is steeper. More striking than the rate of rise of phrenic nerve activity is the rate of rise of upper airway muscle activity, which tends to dilate the airway and, under usual circumstances, alleviate any airway obstruction (Fig. 3). Hence, the Hering-Breuer reflex can be seen as an integrated response to airway obstruction—leading to longer and more vigorous inspiration and dilation of the upper airway. The action of the Hering-Breuer reflex to relieve airway obstruction has probably been far more important evolutionarily than simply controlling inspiratory and expiratory duration.

Rapidly adapting receptors, also called *irritant receptors*, are associated with the airway epithelium. These receptors respond to mechanical deformation, but the firing rate adapts and diminishes quickly even as the stimulus is maintained. Rapidly adapting stretch receptors also respond to chemicals, smoke, and dust—hence the designation irritant receptors. Histamine is among the chemicals that activate rapidly adapting receptors, but whether histamine modifies receptor output directly or modifies the mechanical properties of the environment of the receptor and thereby changes the receptor output is not clear. Stimulation of rapidly adapting receptors in the large bronchi and trachea may produce coughing, mucous secretions, and bronchoconstriction. This may be a protective response; irritants may be expelled in the mucus by coughing, and bronchoconstriction narrows the airway and increases the shear stress of air flowing over the epithelial surface, thereby helping propel the mucus toward the mouth.

C fibers, also called J receptors, are divided into pulmonary and bronchial C fibers based on the latency of the excitation of the fibers after injection of chemicals such as capsaicin (the substance responsible for the hot sensation in hot peppers) into the circulation. Fibers with a short latency after injection into the right heart are pulmonary C fibers, and fibers activated with a short latency after injection into the left heart are bronchial

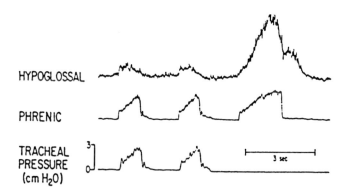

Figure 3 The integrated activity of the phrenic nerve and the hyoglossal nerve, which innervates the tongue—a muscle that often demonstrates inspiratory activity to stiffen and dilate the upper airway—and the tracheal pressure from a decerebrate cat are shown as functions of time. Inflation was withheld on the third breath; therefore, tracheal pressure remains zero. Note that the duration of inspiratory phrenic nerve activity is increased on the third breath, but note also the very large increase in hypoglossal compared to phrenic nerve activity. The prolongation of inspiratory activity and the marked increase in upper airway muscle activation relative to the increase in diaphragm activation are all part of the Hering-Breuer reflex. (From Bartlett D Jr, St John W. Influence of lung volume on phrenic, hypoglossal and mylohyoid nerve activities. Respir Physiol 1988; 73:97–110, with kind permission of Elsevier Science-NL, Sara Burgerhartstraat 25, 1055 KV Amsterdam, The Netherlands.)

C fibers. When stimulated, C fibers produce rapid shallow breathing, bradycardia, and hypotension. Endogenous chemicals capable of stimulating C fibers include histamine, bradykinin, serotonin, and prostaglandins; these are chemicals that may be released in asthma, by interstitial edema, or by pulmonary embolism.

There are also a variety of receptors in the joints, tendons, and muscles of the chest wall that provide afferent feedback related to the volume of the chest, the rate of change of volume (flow), and the load on respiratory muscles. Furthermore, the phrenic nerve contains efferent fibers that provide information about the load on the diaphragm.

Once again, it is important not to neglect the upper airway, in which there are mechanical receptors, irritant receptors, and flow receptors (which probably sense temperature and are cooled by increased inspiratory airflow). All of these receptors contribute to respiratory control and participate in sneezing, coughing, and other protective reflexes. For example, negative pressure in the upper airway, as occurs during upper airway obstruction, increases activation of upper airway muscles that tend to dilate the upper airway and alleviate any obstruction. There are also sensors that reduce respiratory output. The main elements of the dive reflex, apnea and bradycardia, are elicited by cold, wet stimulation in the region of the trigeminal nerve distribution on the face. In what may be a less vigorous manifestation of the dive reflex, cool air directed toward the face may reduce respiratory drive. This may be the mechanism whereby some patients are made more comfortable by breathing cooler air or having cool air blown on their faces.

The receptors in the upper airway, lung, and chest wall and the muscles of respiration provide multiply redundant information to the respiratory controller so that the load on the respiratory system, the state of muscle contraction, the volume of the respiratory sys-

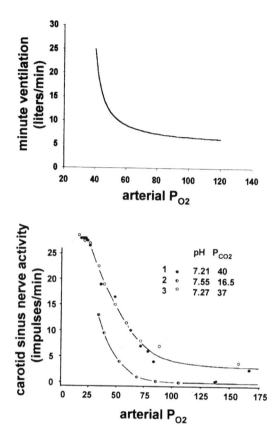

Figure 4 Ventilation (upper panel) and carotid sinus nerve activity (lower panel) have been plotted as a function of the Pa_{O_2}. Note the similar response profiles of ventilation and carotid sinus nerve activity. In the lower panel, the interactive effect of Pa_{CO_2} and Pa_{O_2} on integrated carotid sinus nerve activity is shown. The numbers at the end of each line are the Pa_{O_2} for that particular response curve. At any level of Pa_{O_2}, carotid sinus nerve activity increases as the Pa_{CO_2} increases. This interaction between hypercapnia and hypoxia originates in the carotid body. (Lower panel from Hornbein TF, Roos A, Griffo A. Quantitation of chemoreceptor activity: interaction of hypoxia and hypercapnia. J Neurophysiol 1961; 24:561–568.)

tem, the rate of airflow, and the presence of foreign substances in the airways can be incorporated into an appropriate ventilatory output.

Peripheral Chemoreceptors

The ventilatory response to hypoxia originates primarily from the carotid bodies in humans. The shape of the ventilatory response to hypoxia is shown in Fig. 4. The ventilatory response (panel A) closely follows the pattern of discharge of the carotid sinus nerve (panel B). The ventilatory response to Pa_{O_2} in humans is flat above 100 torr but rises rapidly at a Pa_{O_2} of about 60 torr. This is approximately the P_{O_2} at which the oxygen content of blood starts to fall steeply on the oxyhemoglobin dissociation curve. This coincidence probably reflects evolutionary selection to respond to hypoxia at a time when the content of oxygen is falling rapidly rather than a mechanistic connection: the carotid body senses the partial pressure of oxygen, not oxygen content. Blood flow in the carotid body is among the highest in any organ in the body on a per-gram basis. As a result, the arteriovenous P_{O_2} difference is small, and the carotid body tissue P_{O_2}, which chemoreceptors sense, closely approximates the Pa_{O_2}. Within the carotid body, the hypoxic response is probably generated by hypoxia-sensitive potassium channels in type I carotid body cells. Under well-oxygenated conditions, the type I cells are hyperpolarized. In a dose-dependent manner, the type I cells depolarize as the partial pressure of oxygen drops within the carotid body. Cytoplasmic vesicles in type I cells contain catecholamines, and when type I cells depolarize, vesicles are released and probably stimulate the carotid sinus nerve endings. The exact mechanism whereby potassium channels sense P_{O_2} remains unresolved.

The carotid body is also sensitive to acid stimuli. Carbon dioxide is the most common and potent acid stimulus. The effects of P_{CO_2} and other acid stimuli are probably mediated through changes in intracellular pH of type I cells. Furthermore, there is an interaction between P_{CO_2} and P_{O_2} at the level of the carotid body. For any given Pa_{O_2}, the carotid sinus discharge and ventilation are higher if the Pa_{CO_2} is also elevated (Fig. 4, panel B).

The carotid body contributes only modestly to respiratory drive under resting conditions, and what drive the carotid body does not seem to be essential. Ventilation is well maintained when breathing 100% oxygen, which reduces carotid sinus nerve activity to nil. Moreover, the carotid bodies have been removed as part of a misguided therapy for individuals with asthma. Following this procedure, individuals lack a response to hypoxia (admittedly a handicap), the hypercapnic ventilatory response is slightly reduced, the breath-holding time is prolonged, and the initial ventilatory response to exercise is slightly altered. However, resting ventilatory function is remarkably normal: there is no hypoventilation; the steady-state response to exercise is normal; and no other long-term adverse ventilatory consequences are apparent.

Central Chemoreceptors

The hypercapnic ventilatory response is linearly related to the end-tidal or arterial P_{CO_2} (Fig. 5) and originates from stimulation of chemoreceptors in the brainstem. There have been three main controversies in studies of central chemoreceptors, which persist to this day. What is the stimulus: arterial pH, the pH of cerebrospinal fluid, interstitial pH of brain tissue or intracellular pH (pHi)? Do carbon dioxide and fixed acids, such as hydrochloric or lactic acid, have independent effects on chemoreceptors? Last, where are the chemoreceptors within the brainstem? There is still debate, but the intracellular pH within the chemoreceptors is probably the main stimulus to central chemoreceptors. The importance of pHi as the stimulus to central chemoreceptors was first emphasized at the beginning of the twentieth century, but the pHi hypothesis fell out of favor and extracellular pH (pHe) was thought to be the stimulus. In the last 30 years, the putative chemoreceptor stimulus has migrated from pHe of bulk cerebrospinal fluid to pHe of the interstitium of the brain tissue, to the pHe-pHi gradient across chemoreceptor cell membranes, and finally back to the pHi of chemoreceptor cells. Carbon dioxide is often a more potent stimulus than a fixed acid even when acidity of the arterial pH is equivalent. However, carbon dioxide diffuses more readily through cell membranes and may alter pHi more effectively for similar changes in extracellular or arterial pH. Hence, if the site of the central chemoreceptor stimulus is intracellular, there is no consistent evidence that fixed acids and carbon

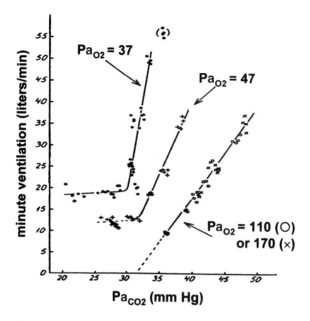

Figure 5 Ventilation has been plotted as a function of Pa_{CO_2}. The ventilatory response to hypercapnia was studied at different Pa_{O_2} levels to demonstrate the interaction between hypoxia and hypercapnia. Note the linear change in ventilation as Pa_{CO_2} increased; the increase in ventilation at any Pa_{CO_2} as the Pa_{O_2} was reduced; and the increased slope of the hypercapnic ventilatory response as Pa_{O_2} was reduced. The interaction between hypercapnia and hypoxia demonstrated here incorporates the interaction between hypercapnia and hypoxia in the carotid body but includes a more powerful interaction originating in the central nervous system. (From Nielson M, Smith H. Studies on the regulation of respiration in acute hypoxia, with an appendix on respiratory control during prolonged hypoxia. Acta Physiol Scand 1952; 24:293–313.)

dioxide have independent actions. Knowing the exact stimulus within neurons and the location of the stimulus has been difficult, since chemoreceptor cells with a clear respiratory function have yet to be identified unequivocally. Hypotheses about the location of chemoreceptor cells within the central nervous system have also been changing recently. In 1943, Julius Comroe found evidence of chemoreceptor sensitivity distributed throughout much of the medulla. Subsequent investigations focused attention on areas at or very near the surface of the ventrolateral medulla. But here also, recent investigators have found evidence of more widely distributed chemoreceptor sites within the medulla and even into the pons. Hence, the ventrolateral surface of the medulla may contain chemosensitive areas, but other sites within the brainstem also seem to be sensitive to carbon dioxide.

Just as there is an interaction between the P_{O_2} and P_{CO_2} in the carotid body, there is an interaction between hypercapnia and hypoxia, but this interaction reflects the central integration of carotid body afferent information and central chemoreceptor activity in the brainstem. For any level of hypoxia, the resting ventilation is elevated and the response to hypercapnia is accentuated (in Fig. 5, note that the slope of the hypercapnic response is steeper as the oxygen level falls). Unlike the peripheral chemoreceptors, the central chemoreceptors are quite important in moment-to-moment control of ventilation. The chemoreceptors seem to provide a tonic excitatory influence that sustains ventilation. This is most apparent in sedated or anesthetized subjects, in whom it is possible to suppress or suspend measurable respiratory activity by hyperventilating the subject, thereby reducing the P_{CO_2} and the stimulus to breathe.

INTEGRATED CONTROL

Respiratory Sensations

We are usually unaware of the interplay among chemical control of ventilation; afferent feedback from the lungs, upper airway, and chest wall; central respiratory processes in the brainstem; and cortical influences—all of which determine our respiratory output at a particular time. However, if asked, normal subjects appear to have access at a cortical level to much of the information driving ventilation, even though we rarely attend to it. Normal subjects are remarkably good at estimating the size of tidal volumes, respiratory force developed, and effort expended. Subjects can detect accurately that a 0.6-L breath is larger than a 0.3-L breath in the same proportion that a 1.2-L breath is larger than a 0.6-L breath. Subjects are also good at estimating the size of added respiratory loads. The afferent information available to subjects is redundant. Patients who have had bilateral lung transplants (and therefore bilateral pulmonary vagotomies) are as good as normal subjects at estimating the size of respiratory loads. Similarly, quadriplegics who lack afferent information from the chest wall and patients who have had laryngectomies and lack afferent information from the upper airway can estimate the size of added respiratory loads well. Hence, no single source of afferent information is essential, and any set of afferents from the chest wall or vagus is sufficient.

It is particularly interesting that subjects can, if asked, estimate the sense of effort—how hard they are trying—independent of the sense of inspiratory force generated. The sense of effort differs from the actual force developed or work done and is the perception of the extent of voluntary activation of skeletal muscles. The sense of effort probably originates from activation of the sensory cortex concurrently with activation of the muscles of contraction. This copy of the pattern of muscle activation sent to the sensory cortex has been called an "efference" copy, since the sense of effort is proportional to the efferent activation of the muscles. The sense of effort provides an internal measuring stick against which the actual force developed can be compared. For example, as fatigue develops in a muscle, the sense of effort and the size of the central command to the muscle increase, but the actual force developed diminishes. The utility of an efferent sense of effort against which the actual force developed can be checked should be obvious. If the match between the sense of effort and the force developed is unexpectedly poor (too much effort for too little gain), alternate strategies can be adopted to accomplish the task, or one may decide that the effort is not worth it and give up as a form of protection against injury. In many circumstances but not all, breathing is uncomfortable when the subject must exert disproportionate effort for a particular respiratory output.

Dyspnea, "an uncomfortable sensation of breathing," is among the most common respiratory complaints. The sensation of dyspnea probably derives from a comparison between the outgoing motor command and afferent feedback from receptors described above. For example, patients with muscle weakness may be dyspneic because the sense of effort is large but tidal volume produced and the afferent feedback disproportionately small. Asthmatics may have a mismatch between the sense of effort and the actual tidal volume produced, but they complain of other sensations as well, such as chest tightness, which may derive from stimulation of irritant receptors. Hence, the character of dyspnea in different illnesses may reflect the particular set of receptors stimulated.

Automatic and Behavioral Respiratory Control

Hypoxia acting through the carotid bodies, hypercapnia acting through central chemoreceptors, and mechanical afferent information from the lungs and chest wall provide the fundamental inputs driving ventilation. But the factors controlling ventilation are richer and more varied than these inputs alone. Respiration is unusual among automatic functions in that there is the possibility of volitional control in a way not possible for other automatic activities. At a simple level, one cannot hold one's heartbeat (with rare exceptions) or suspend digestion, but most of us can hold our breath without great difficulty if not for a particularly long time. On a more elegant and complex level, we can modify respiration to talk and sing or use respiratory muscles to stabilize the chest wall and muscles of posture as we lift heavy objects. The transition between these volitional and automatic respiratory functions is seamless and, with minor exceptions, volitional control of respiratory function acts through the machinery of automatic control; for example, those neurons within the brainstem that automatically shape the pattern and frequency of each breath are probably actively inhibited during a breath-hold.

The presence of two interacting control mechanisms becomes apparent when one system is impaired or the interaction between the control mechanisms is interrupted. These "experiments of nature" are extremely rare but instructive. The "locked in" syndrome is caused by a bilateral brainstem infarct in the ventral pons that destroys the corticospinal tracts through which higher volitional centers in the cortex communicate with the automatic respiratory controller in the medulla and caudal pons. These patients have no volitional control over respiration, and their respiration is monotonously regular. Hence, much of the moment-to-moment variation in respiration, which is absent in these patients, derives from the bombardment of the automatic respiratory controller by a host of stimuli originating above the pons, whether the stimuli are visual, auditory, or generated within the central nervous system volitionally. These suprapontine stimuli provide a variable, but persistent excitatory stimulus to respiration during breathing. Hence, hyperventilation and hyperoxia—which remove excitatory inputs from the carotid body and central chemoreceptors and reduce stimulation of the automatic respiratory mechanism—do not normally terminate respiratory activity; the background of suprapontine influences sustains respiration when chemical stimuli are reduced. In the locked-in syndrome, there is no mechanism through which suprapontine stimuli can be transmitted to the respiratory controller, and apnea develops after modest hyperventilation in patients with brainstem abnormalities impairing communication between higher centers and the respiratory controller such as the locked-in syndrome (Fig. 6).

"Ondine's curse," central alveolar hypoventilation, is the mirror image of the locked-in syndrome. Ondine, a mythological character, placed a curse upon her mortal husband after he jilted her. Her curse was that he must consciously direct every bodily function, including those that had previously been automatic. In patients with Ondine's curse, suprapontine stimuli communicate effectively with the respiratory controller, but mechanisms sustaining automatic ventilation are impaired. The common denominator of brainstem lesions producing Ondine's curse is a loss or marked reduction of sensitivity to carbon dioxide. Hypoxic sensitivity may or may not be lost. Respiration is usually

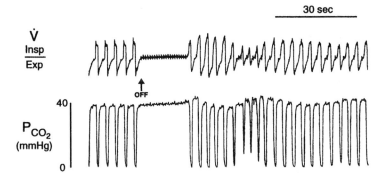

Figure 6 Inspiratory and expiratory airflow and the end-tidal P_{CO_2} from a patient with the locked-in syndrome are shown above. To the left of the "off" arrow, the patient was passively ventilated sufficiently to reduce his P_{CO_2} by 2 torr. When the ventilator was turned off, he did not immediately resume breathing as a normal, waking subject would. Hence, very mild hypocapnia reduced the patient's respiratory drive, and without suprapontine influences to sustain respiration, the patient had a prolonged apnea. (From Heywood P, Murphy K, Corfield DR, Morrell MJ, Howard RS, Guz A. Control of breathing in man; insights from the "locked-in" syndrome. Respir Physiol 1996; 106:13–20, with kind permission of Elsevier Science-NL, Sara Burgerhartstraat 25, 1055 KV Amsterdam, The Netherlands.)

adequately sustained during wakefulness; there may be hypoventilation and carbon dioxide retention, but the pattern of respiration is not monotonously automatic nor are there prolonged apneas. The variability of respiratory output, typical of normal people during wakefulness, may persist in patients with Ondine's curse as well. However, at the onset of sleep, respiration becomes irregular, with long apneic periods, and profound hypercapnia and cyclic episodes of hypoxia develop (Fig. 7). Once the excitatory suprapontine influences accompanying wakefulness are lost, the instability of the respiratory control system

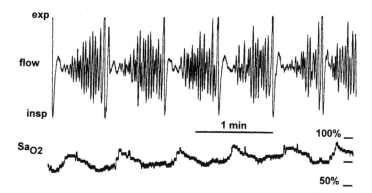

Figure 7 A polysomnographic record during stage 2 sleep from a patient with a brainstem tumor in which airflow and oxyhemoglobin saturation are shown over 3 min. Note the repetitive pattern of apneas and hyperventilation associated with recurrent hypoxemia. This patient's respiratory pattern was regular and nonapneic during wakefulness.

is unmasked during sleep. The tonic excitatory influences from central chemoreceptors that normally support regular activity of the respiratory controller are lost in patients with Ondine's curse. The hypoxic drive is alinear (drops off quickly as the Pa_{O_2} rises above 60 torr), and hypoxia alone cannot sustain regular respiration during sleep.

Although Ondine's curse and the locked-in syndrome are rare, the abnormalities apparent in patients with these syndromes reveal a control system with multiple inputs. The multiplicity of inputs promotes a stable respiratory output in all conditions. If the automatic or volitional input to the respiratory controller is lost, the system is less robust: regular respiratory output is not maintained under all conditions and prolonged apneas may occur in certain circumstances (Figs. 6 and 7 above).

Respiration During Sleep

As discussed above, resting ventilation during wakefulness is driven by input from central chemoreceptors, the carotid body, afferents from the lung and chest walls, and nonrespiratory sensory information from the outside world, which contributes to our level of arousal and activation of the reticular activating system. Endogenous cortical activity may also increase our level of arousal. The sum of these excitatory stimuli has been called the *waking stimulus*. During non–rapid eye movement (NREM) sleep, the waking stimulus and volitional inputs to respiratory control are lost. The ventilatory stimulus depends solely on chemical and neuromechanical factors integrated within the brainstem, and there is an overall reduction in central respiratory drive associated with a drop in metabolic rate. Throughout the body, the tone of most skeletal muscles decreases during NREM sleep, but activation of the diaphragm is immune to the inhibitory effects of sleep. The diaphragm and accessory muscles of respiration may actually show greater activation during NREM sleep. This phenomenon emphasizes again the importance of interactions between the muscles of the upper airway and the muscle of the ventilatory pump. During NREM sleep, activation of upper airway muscles decreases and upper airway resistance increases. Increased upper airway resistance places a load on the respiratory system, and accessory muscles are activated to respond to the increased upper airway resistance. Automatic control of ventilation results in a regular, invariant respiratory pattern when NREM sleep is well established. The end-tidal P_{CO_2} (PET_{CO_2}) increases during NREM sleep. The increase in PET_{CO_2} is derived in part from reduced central drive. However, the added load on the respiratory system secondary to increased upper airway resistance contributes to the increased PET_{CO_2} as well. The ventilatory response to carbon dioxide is reduced in NREM sleep. The ventilatory response to hypoxia is reduced in men, but a reduction in hypoxic responsiveness in women has not been found consistently.

During rapid eye movement (REM) sleep, when dreaming occurs, it has been said that suprapontine stimuli dominate the respiratory drive, as they do during wakefulness, but automatic, metabolic control of ventilation is absent during REM sleep. This is probably an overstatement. The hypoxic and hypercapnic ventilatory responses are reduced below NREM levels, but chemical control of breathing is not ablated completely during REM sleep. Rather, suprapontine influences and metabolic factors both contribute to respiratory drive during REM sleep. The respiratory pattern is more variable than NREM sleep, more like wakefulness, but still influenced by the level of P_{CO_2} and P_{O_2}.

REM sleep is associated with skeletal muscle atonia, but the diaphragm is spared and remains active. The reduction in skeletal muscle activity varies inversely with the nonrespiratory function of the muscle. Muscles with predominantly respiratory function

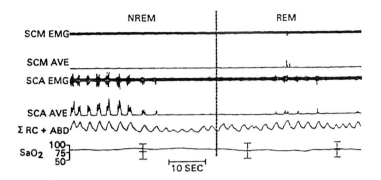

Figure 8   The unprocessed and average activity of the sternocleidomastoid muscle (SCM EMG and SCM AVE, respectively), the unprocessed and average activity of the scalene muscle (SCA EMG and SCA AVE, respectively), the sum of the ribcage and abdominal displacement (Σ RC + ABD), and the oxyhemoglobin saturation (Sa_{O_2}) are shown in a patient with COPD during NREM and REM sleep. Note the drop in muscle activity during REM sleep and the associated drop in Sa_{O_2}. (From Johnson MW, Remmers JE. Accessory muscle activity during sleep in chronic obstructive pulmonary disease. J Appl Physiol 1984; 57:1011–1017.)

(e.g., the diaphragm) are less inhibited during sleep, whereas muscles with respiratory input but a significant nonrespiratory function lose the respiratory input entirely. Hence, accessory muscles of the neck and shoulder girdle and intercostal muscles, which have a postural function, lose the respiratory drive during REM sleep. Furthermore, REM sleep is associated with direct inhibition of spinal motor neuron activity of postural muscles. Therefore, the electromyographic (EMG) activity of accessory muscles of respiration and intercostal muscles is reduced during REM sleep (loss of both respiratory and posture-related excitation) out of proportion to activation of the diaphragm. If ventilation is dependent on activation of the accessory or intercostal muscles, as it may be in some patients with chronic obstructive pulmonary disease (COPD) in whom diaphragm function is compromised, significant hypoventilation may result during REM sleep. This can be seen in Fig. 8. (See also Chap. 31.)

    In summary, the central respiratory controller integrates a variety of inputs to generate a pattern of ventilatory output appropriate for the varied demands placed upon the respiratory system. Volitional control of ventilation is possible, but we need not consistently think about breathing. An automatic mechanism—responsive to chemical information (carbon dioxide and oxygen), afferent information from the chest wall, pulmonary and upper airway receptors, and suprapontine influences reflecting behavior and the state of wakefulness or sleep—sustains ventilation when we are inattentive to this vital function. The respiratory output is variable among states but robust, and the pattern of activation of respiratory muscles is carefully titrated to the particular load on the respiratory system.

SUGGESTED READING

1. Berger AJ, Mitchell RA, Severinghaus, JW. Regulation of respiration. N Engl J Med 1977; 297:92–97, 138–143, 194–201.
2. Cherniack NS. Respiratory dysrhythmias during sleep. N Engl J Med 1981; 305:325–330.

3. Manning HL, Schwartzstein RM. Pathophysiology of dyspnea. N Engl J Med 1995; 333:1547–1553.
4. Nattie EE. Central chemoreception. In: Dempsey JA, Pack AI, eds. Regulation of Breathing. New York: Marcel Dekker, 1994:473–510.
5. Roussos C, Moxham J, Bellemare F. Respiratory muscle fatigue. In: Roussos C, ed. The Thorax. New York: Marcel Dekker, 1995:1405–1461.
6. Xie A, Bradley TD. Respiratory muscle activity during sleep. In: Roussos C, ed. The Thorax. New York: Marcel Dekker, 1995:1373–1404.

3
Principles of Air Movement Into and Out of the Lung

David A. Kaminsky
University of Vermont College of Medicine
Fletcher Allen Health Care
Burlington, Vermont

INTRODUCTION

All cells require oxygen (O_2) for production of energy, and likewise must rid themselves of carbon dioxide (CO_2) produced by cellular respiration. Since both O_2 and CO_2 are gases, they move around simply by following relative pressure gradients between areas. The respiratory system continually replenishes fresh air and the circulation continually carries gases by bulk transport to optimize these pressure gradients for gas exchange between the environmental air (relatively high in O_2 and low in CO_2) and the tissue capillary blood (relatively high in CO_2 and low in O_2).

The respiratory system does its part in this process by continually moving fresh gas containing oxygen into the lung where gas exchange takes place and removing waste gas from the lung back to the environment. The respiratory system is composed of the chest wall and respiratory muscles, which together serve as the pump, and the lungs themselves, which serve as the conduits for air movement and provide the interface for gas exchange between blood and air. The capacity of the respiratory system to move air is enormous. Under basal conditions, cycling at 15 breaths per minute and moving 500 mL with each breath, the respiratory system moves 7.5 L/min of air, or 10,800 L/day—a daily volume equivalent to that of a home swimming pool! Under conditions of metabolic stress or exercise, the respiratory system can easily increase this capacity by tenfold or more.

This chapter reviews the basic static and dynamic properties of the chest wall and lung, including the airways, and the relationship of these properties to how air is moved into and out of the lung. General physical principles rather than specific mathematical relationships are emphasized, although some specific formulas are found in a brief appendix for interested readers. Throughout the chapter, the principles of air movement are related to common clinical conditions associated with pulmonary disease.

FORCES INVOLVED IN AIR MOVEMENT

Boyle's Law

Air, being a mixture of gases, moves about simply: it passively follows gradients of pressure established around it. To move air from the environment into the lung, the respiratory system must generate a reduced pressure in the lung relative to atmosphere, and to move the air out, the opposite pressure gradient must be created. These pressure gradients are generated by changing the volume of the respiratory system, as pressure (P) and volume (V) must change in opposite directions according to Boyle's law: PV = constant (Fig. 1). Thus, during inspiration, the chest wall and muscles expend energy to increase the volume of the respiratory system, which abruptly drops alveolar pressure relative to atmospheric pressure and causes air to flow into the lung. During expiration, the respiratory muscles relax, allowing the elastic recoil of the lung to increase alveolar pressure and therefore expel air back to the environment, which returns the chest wall and lung to their resting position (functional residual capacity, or FRC).

Static Properties

The force that the respiratory muscles must generate to increase lung volume is determined by the static and dynamic properties of the chest wall and lung. The static properties, or properties under conditions of no airflow, are simply the elastic properties of the chest wall and lung (Fig. 2). The elastic properties of the chest wall are related to the inherent elasticity of the skin, muscles, bones, and connective tissue of the chest wall. The chest

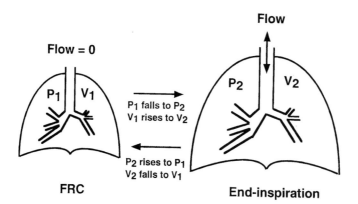

Boyle's Law: $P_1V_1 = P_2V_2$

Figure 1 Boyle's law: how we breathe. Boyle's law is a special condition of the universal gas law, which states that PV = nRT, where P = pressure, V = volume, n = number of moles, T = temperature and R = constant. Under conditions of constant temperature, PV is constant for a given quantity of gas. Starting with an initial P = P_1 and V = V_1, any changes in P and V must be balanced by a new set of conditions, P_2, V_2, such that $P_1V_1 = P_2V_2$. Applied to the lungs at FRC, as V_1 rises to V_2, P_1 must fall to P_2, causing air to flow in; hence, lung volume increases during inspiration. Likewise, at the beginning of exhalation, as V_2 relaxes to V_1, P_2 must rise to P_1, causing air to flow out; hence, lung volume falls during expiration.

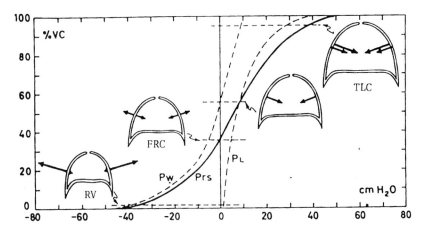

Figure 2 Static pressure-volume curves of the lung (P_l), chest wall (P_w), and their sum, the total respiratory system (P_{rs}). The drawing of respiratory system depicts the lung (inner line) encased by the chest wall (outer line), with directions and magnitudes of force at various lung volumes depicted for each. Moving from left to right, at residual volume (RV), the lung exerts minimal inward recoil force and the chest wall exerts a strong outward force, yielding a P_{rs} of about -40 cmH$_2$O; at FRC, approximately 40% of vital capacity (VC), lung and chest wall forces are equal and opposite and P_{rs} = zero H$_2$O; at approximately 60% VC, chest wall forces equal zero and the lung's elastic recoil is unopposed, yielding a P_{rs} of about 10 cmH$_2$O; at TLC, both lung and chest wall want to recoil, giving a P_{rs} of near 60 cmH$_2$O. (Adapted from Agostoni E, Hyatt RE. Static behavior of the respiratory system. In: Handbook of Physiology, Sec. 3. *The Respiratory System*. Vol. III. *The Mechanics of Breathing*, Part I. Bethesda, MD: American Physiological Society, 1986, Fig. 3.)

wall's elastic properties at FRC act to try to expand the chest wall outward to a final position occupying a volume equivalent to approximately 60% of total lung capacity (TLC). In conditions such as severe kyphoscoliosis or morbid obesity, these elastic forces are increased and hence the natural equilibrium point for the chest wall is reduced to some volume below this level. Accordingly, the respiratory muscles must generate greater force to increase thoracic volume above this point, which may increase the work of even quiet, normal breathing.

The elastic properties of the lung are more complex, because the lung not only contains elements of muscle and connective tissue but also has surface tension at the air–alveolar cell interface that serves as an additional impediment to increase in volume. The elasticity is often described directly but is also commonly described by the reciprocal of elasticity, or compliance. Thus, a very elastic lung has a low compliance, and a poorly elastic lung has a high compliance. The lung's elastic properties act to reduce the lung to a minimum volume. Thus, FRC represents the equilibrium point between the chest wall's tendency to expand outward and the lung's tendency to recoil inward when the respiratory muscles are relaxed.

The major component of the lung's static recoil is surface tension. If each alveolus is considered a sphere, then the surface tension of that alveolus is governed by the law of LaPlace, which states that the pressure necessary to distend the sphere is proportional to the surface tension and inversely related to the radius (Fig. 3). Thus, the smaller the sphere, the greater the pressure necessary to keep the sphere from collapsing under conditions of constant surface tension. This would be a critical problem in the lung, because

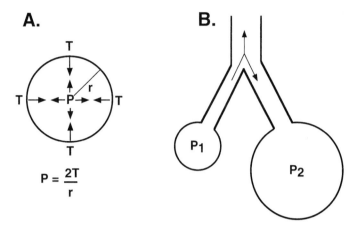

Figure 3 The law of LaPlace. A. The generalized law of LaPlace for a sphere describes the interaction of surface tension (T), transmural distending pressure (P), and sphere radius (r), as $P = 2T/r$. B. As a consequence of this relationship, smaller alveoli have higher transmural pressures (P_1) than larger alveoli (P_2) for a given level of surface tension, and so small alveoli would collapse and empty, at least in part, into the larger alveoli. This situation is minimized by the presence of surfactant (see text).

with each cycling of breath, small alveoli would develop higher internal pressures than larger alveoli and would therefore empty into these larger alveoli. Widespread alveolar collapse would ensue, with resulting severe consequences for gas exchange. This problem is ameliorated because the alveolar lining fluid contains surfactant, a complex combination of phospholipid and protein, which has the unique property of lowering surface tension at reduced alveolar volumes. This phenomenon results in a relatively constant internal pressure among alveoli of different sizes and thus stabilizes the lung.

The presence of surfactant also allows the lung to remain inflated at relatively lower distending pressures than would otherwise be allowed by native surface tension forces at the air–liquid interface. These significant surface tension forces are the major determinant of the hysteresis of the lung, which is the difference in the pressure–volume relationship during inspiration versus expiration (Fig. 4). Lung hysteresis means that higher pressures are required to achieve a given lung volume during inspiration than are required during expiration. Thus, compared with an air-filled lung without surfactant, the air-filled lung lined with surfactant can be inflated at significantly lower transmural pressures. When surfactant function is deficient, as in the infant respiratory distress syndrome, alveolar collapse is common, with detrimental effects not only on gas exchange but also on the requirement for large pressures to inflate the lungs.

Dynamic Properties

The lung also has dynamic forces that must be overcome to change lung volume. These forces are primarily due to the flow-resistive properties of the airways, although there is some contribution from tissue-resistive properties (known as *tissue viscosity*) as well. At low flow rates, stream lines of airflow are parallel and flow is said to be laminar. Laminar flow is mainly found in the periphery of the lung, where flow rates are low and proportional

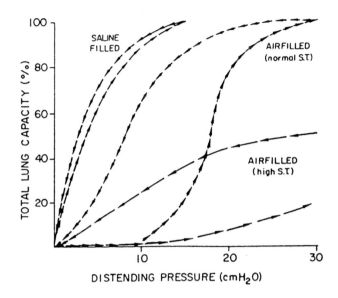

Figure 4 Pressure-volume curves for a saline-filled lung, an air-filled lung lined with surfactant with normal surface tension (ST), and an air-filled lacking surfactant with high ST. Hysteresis is seen as the area between the inflation and deflation curves, as depicted by the arrows. Notice the greater hysteresis of the air-filled lungs compared to the saline-filled lung lacking significant surface tension forces, and also the effect of surfactant of lowering the distending pressure for any given volume of the air-filled lung due to reduction of surface tension forces. (From Light RW. Mechanics of respiration. In: George RB, Light RW, Matthay MA, Matthay RA, eds. Chest Medicine. Baltimore: Williams & Wilkins, 1990, Fig. 3.7.)

to driving pressure. At higher flow rates, stream lines become disorganized and chaotic, a situation known as *turbulent flow*. Even during quiet, normal breathing, turbulent flow occurs in the trachea and larger airways and also at the junction between branching airways. It requires more energy to maintain turbulent than laminar flow, and turbulent flow rates fail to increase in direct proportion to driving pressure because of the inherent loss of energy in maintaining turbulence. Whether flow will be laminar or turbulent can be predicted by the Reynold's number (see Appendix).

For laminar flow, airway resistance varies inversely with the fourth power of the radius according to Poiseuille's law (see Appendix). Hence, if airway radius is halved, resistance increases 16-fold. Since flow varies directly with the pressure gradient and inversely with the resistance, a higher pressure must be generated to maintain a given flow rate in the presence of higher resistance. This situation is commonly found in asthma and accounts, in part, for why asthmatics must work harder to breathe.

Most total airway resistance below the vocal cords is found in the first eight generations of larger airways (i.e., of >2 mm in diameter); accordingly, 80% of airway resistance is in these airways (Fig. 5). Since flow in these larger airways is additionally turbulent and turbulent flow requires more energy than laminar flow, disorders of the large airways, such as tumors or foreign bodies, may quickly lead to respiratory muscle fatigue and respiratory failure.

While the airways smaller than 2 mm each individually offer increased resistance compared with individual larger airways (because of their smaller radii), the total airway

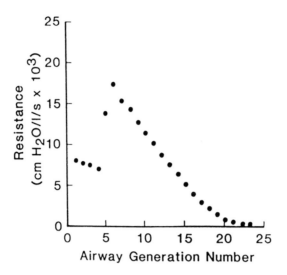

Figure 5   Relationship of airway resistance and airway generation number. Total airway resistance is much higher in the more central than the peripheral airways, with the highest resistance in generations 5–8. (From Taylor, AE, Rehder K, Parker JC. Clinical Respiratory Physiology. Philadelphia: Saunders, 1989, Fig. 7-5.)

resistance (R_{total}) derived from these parallel, small airways is calculated as the sum of their *inverse* resistances (i.e., $1/R_{total} = 1/R_a + 1/R_b + 1/R_c +, \ldots$, for airways a, b, c, etc.). With resistance summed in this way and with there being so many small airways, very little contribution to *total* airway resistance is found in the lung periphery. This is part of the reason why standard tests of pulmonary function may be inadequate for detecting subtle or early changes in small airway physiology: i.e., by the time the FEV_1 has dropped, substantial abnormality may exist in the small airway region of the lung.

AIR MOVEMENT INTO THE LUNG

Changes in Volume, Pressure, and Flow

Now that general principles have been discussed, the actual events involved in moving air into the lung will be described. At FRC, the lung and chest wall are in equilibrium, each exerting approximately 5 cmH$_2$O pressure in opposite directions against each other (Fig. 6). Assuming patent airways, pressure in the alveoli at this time is equal to atmospheric pressure, defined as zero cmH$_2$O. Following contraction of the diaphragm, and to a lesser extent the other muscles of inspiration including the intercostals and sternocleidomastoids, the chest cavity increases in volume, causing pleural pressure to become more subatmospheric. The *trans*pulmonary pressure, or pressure difference across the alveoli as seen from the inside (alveolar pressure minus pleural pressure), is now positive, causing the alveoli to expand. The increase in alveolar volume causes alveolar pressure to become subatmospheric, and air flows into the lung. At the point at which the inspiratory muscles cease contracting but have not yet begun to relax, a positive transpulmonary pressure is maintained, holding the alveoli inflated at their new end-inspiratory volume. Since alveolar

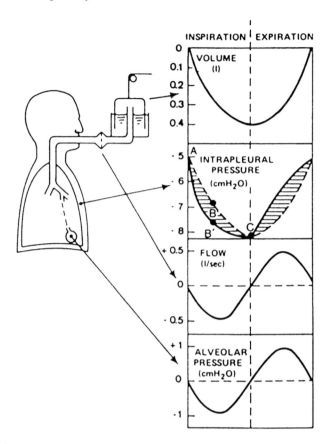

Figure 6   Changes in volume, pressure, and flow during a breathing cycle. Beginning at FRC, alveolar pressure = atmospheric pressure (= 0) and hence flow = 0. Intrapleural pressure falls as inspiration begins, causing alveolar pressure to fall and inspiratory flow to begin, gradually increasing lung volume. As alveolar pressure approaches atmosphere again, flow decreases and eventually stops at end-inspiration, with end-tidal volume now achieved. These events are reversed during expiration as the respiratory muscles relax, less negative pleural pressure is generated, and expiratory flow with reduction in volume is achieved. The shaded area on the intrapleural pressure tracing (line AB'C) depicts the extra force needed to overcome airway and tissue resistance in addition to lung elastic recoil. (From West JB, Respiratory Physiology—The Essentials, 4th ed. Baltimore: Williams & Wilkins, 1990, Fig. 7.13.)

volume is no longer increasing, the pressure difference between atmosphere and alveoli rapidly diminishes to zero, at which point airflow ceases. Inspiration has now ended.

Role of Respiratory Muscles in Determining TLC

The limit of lung volume increase with inspiration is determined by the strength of the respiratory muscles relative to the forces they have to overcome (Fig. 7). The maximal volume of the lung, TLC, occurs when the ability of the inspiratory muscles to generate force can no longer overcome the inward recoil force exerted by the chest wall and lung. With muscle weakness, as in myasthenia gravis or multiple sclerosis, the maximum force

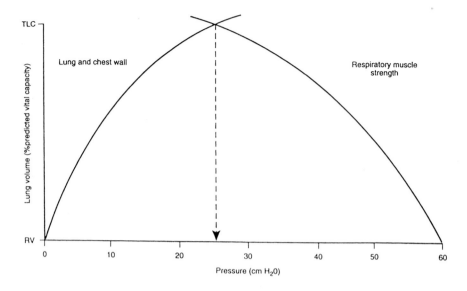

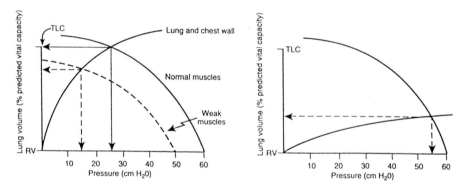

Figure 7 Relationship between lung volume and pressure generated by the lung and chest wall system and the respiratory muscles. Top: As lung volume increases from RV, the lung and chest wall gradually build up recoil pressure, while the force-generating capacity of the inspiratory muscles decreases. When the respiratory muscles have generated the same force as the lung and chest wall system exert, TLC has been reached. Bottom left: In respiratory muscle weakness, the pressure curve for the respiratory muscles is shifted down and to the left, yielding a new intersection with the lung and chest wall curve at a lower TLC and lower pressure at TLC (seen by dashed lines). Bottom right: In lung diseases of reduced compliance, the lung and chest wall curve is shifted down and to the right, yielding a new intersection with the respiratory muscle curve at a lower TLC and a higher pressure at TLC (shown by dashed lines). (From Leff AR, Schumacker PT. Respiratory Physiology: Basics and Applications. Philadelphia: Saunders, 1993, Fig. 1-7.)

generated by the muscles is reduced and, therefore, the TLC is decreased, even though the intrinsic elastic properties of the lung and chest wall may be normal. With decreased lung compliance, as in interstitial fibrosis, maximal lung inflation (TLC) is decreased because of increased inward recoil of the lung, not because of any inherent weakness of the respiratory muscle.

Distribution of Inspired Air Due to Gravity

Now it is important to consider how the air that has been drawn into the lung is distributed throughout the airways and alveoli. Just like the entire body, the lung is under the influence of gravity, especially when in the upright position. This causes the intrapleural pressure to be less subatmospheric at the base of the lung than at the apex. Accordingly, alveoli at the base of the lung are relatively smaller at FRC than are those at the apex but are situated on a steeper part of the pressure-volume curve for the whole lung compared to those at the apex (Fig. 8). Therefore, basilar alveoli expand more on inspiration than apical alveoli, causing more air to flow to the base than the apex. This situation helps optimize gas exchange, since more blood flow goes to the base than to the apex, allowing better matching of ventilation and perfusion (see Chap. 4).

At lung volumes below FRC, approaching residual volume (RV), the situation may be entirely different (Fig. 8). At low lung volumes, the intrinsic elastic recoil of the lung is less, resulting in less negative pleural pressures at the lung base; in fact, even positive pressures may occur. This results in actual closure of some alveoli and airways in the most gravity-dependent regions of the lung at very low lung volume. Now when inspiration begins, the initial quantity of air will ventilate the apex of the lung more than the base. This is of little consequence in normal, healthy individuals, because normal, quiet breathing does not take place at such low lung volumes. However, effectively the same situation arises if lung elastic recoil is reduced by disease (e.g., emphysema) or by aging, leading to more widespread basilar airway closure. In these situations, ventilation may

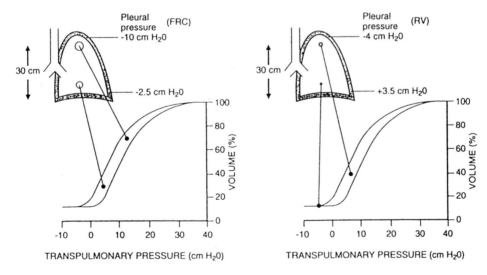

Figure 8   Effect of pleural pressure gradient on distribution of ventilation at FRC (left) and RV (right). At FRC, pleural pressures are more subatmospheric at the lung apex compared with the base, putting the apex on a higher and less steep portion of the pressure-volume curve for the lung. Small increases in transpulmonary pressure thus lead to larger changes in volume for the basilar regions than for the apical regions. At RV, basilar regions are under superatmospheric pressure and may even be closed, such that small increases in transpulmonary pressure result in increased ventilation to the apical rather than the basilar regions. (From Leff AR, Schumacker PT. *Respiratory Physiology: Basics and Applications.* Philadelphia: Saunders, 1993, Fig. 1-22.)

actually be greater to the apical regions of the lung than to the bases, causing more mismatching of ventilation and perfusion and impairment of gas exchange.

Distribution of Inspired Air Due to Time Constant Inequalities

Another important reason for uneven ventilation is the inhomogeneity of local resistance and compliance in the lung, especially in disease states (Fig. 9). For example, two areas of lung may have different compliances but substantially similar resistances. In this situation, the more compliant region will receive more air in a given period of time (e.g., the respiratory cycle) than the less compliant region. Similarly, if two regions have equivalent compliance but different airway resistances, then the region with lower resistance will receive more air in a given period of time. The components of resistance (R) and compliance (C) together (the product RC) determine the "time constant" for the region of lung specified, a measure of how quickly that region will fill and empty. When time constants are long, either due to increased compliance or increased resistance, the region of lung will take more time to fill and likewise more time to empty. The opposite holds true for

A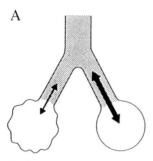

Regional changes in elasticity

B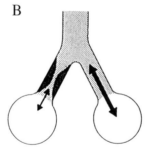

Regional obstruction

C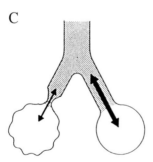

Regional dynamic compression

Figure 9 Causes of uneven ventilation due to time constant inequalities. In panel A, reduced elasticity in the alveolar unit on the left results in less driving force and less ventilation than in the unit on the right. In panels B and C, airway narrowing in the unit on the left has the same effect because of increased time constants. (From Forster RE, DuBois AB, Briscoe WA, Fisher AB. The Lung: Physiologic Basis of Pulmonary Function Tests, 3d ed. Chicago: Year Book, 1986, Chap. 3, Fig. 21.)

regions of short time constants. Thus, ventilation will be distributed unevenly in the lung due to time constant inequalities, with shorter time constant regions filling and emptying more quickly and the overall lung filling and emptying occurring in a sequential rather than a synchronous manner. This situation may arise in any type of airways disease or heterogeneous parenchymal disease. In chronic obstructive pulmonary disease (COPD), for example, regions of lung with high resistance (bronchitis) or high compliance (emphysema) will be less well ventilated than other, relatively more normal regions. Such inequalities also give rise to falls in overall compliance with increasing respiratory frequency (so-called *frequency-dependence of compliance*). As breathing frequency increases, areas of lung with long time constants are unable to fill or empty completely, resulting in less volume change for a given change in pressure—a decrease in dynamic compliance. The loss of compliance with higher respiratory rates causes an increase in the work of breathing and hence can quickly lead to respiratory muscle fatigue.

Finally, additional factors also determine the distribution of ventilation. At the acinar level, gas movement no longer occurs by bulk flow and instead is governed by simple diffusion. Usually, diffusion is very rapid and complete in healthy, small airways. However, diffusion may be less complete if distances are increased or obstruction is present, as in emphysema or chronic bronchitis. Additionally, the distribution of gas is affected by the way in which the mechanical movements of alveoli affect each other (so-called *interdependence*). Gas movement also takes place via collateral channels and is affected by the beating of the heart. All of these factors may be affected by various disease states, with consequences for the distribution of ventilation.

Dead Space Ventilation

Now that air has entered and distributed itself into the lung according to the factors described above, gas exchange takes place between the gas present in the alveolar regions (at and beyond the level of the respiratory bronchioles) and the surrounding capillary blood. However, this gas represents only approximately 70–80% of the total air inspired. The air that does not participate in gas exchange is called *dead space ventilation*, since it resides within the volume of lung occupied only by conducting airways (Fig. 10A). This volume, often referred to as the *anatomic* dead space, is commonly estimated at 150 mL, or, when expressed in mL, as equivalent to the person's ideal weight in pounds. It can be measured directly by performing a nitrogen washout analysis, a test sometimes referred to as Fowler's method (see Appendix). Since the volume of the conducting airways is essentially unchanged over the course of a breath, the proportion of each breath occupied by dead space ventilation varies inversely with the tidal volume. In other words, for the same total ventilation per minute (minute ventilation), larger tidal volumes at slower respiratory frequencies result in less relative dead space ventilation as compared with smaller tidal volumes at more rapid frequencies and are therefore more efficient at effecting gas exchange.

However, not all air that enters the respiratory bronchioles and alveoli participates in effective gas exchange. For example, in emphysema, many regions may be relatively well ventilated but poorly perfused due to capillary destruction (Fig. 10B and C). Such regions are also a dead space functionally, and, together with the anatomic dead space, determine the total area of lung serving as a true dead space not participating in gas exchange. This total area is termed the *physiological* dead space. In healthy lungs, the anatomic and physiological dead spaces are similar in volume, but in disease states, the

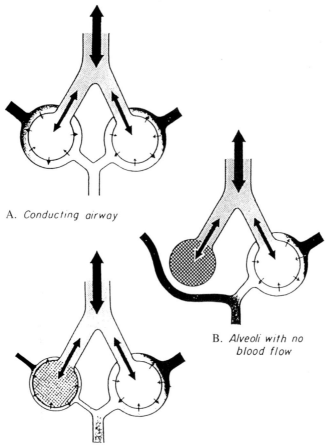

A. *Conducting airway*

B. *Alveoli with no blood flow*

C. *Ventilation in excess of blood flow*

Figure 10 Types of respiratory dead space. In panel A, anatomic dead space is depicted by the shaded conducting airway regions that do not participate in gas exchange. In panels B and C, physiological dead space is seen as the sum of the anatomic dead space and regions of poorly matched ventilation and perfusion, resulting in wasted ventilation. (From Forster RE, DuBois AB, Briscoe WA, Fisher AB. The Lung: Physiologic Basis of Pulmonary Function Tests, 3d ed. Chicago: Year Book, 1986, Chap. 3, Fig. 12.)

physiological dead space usually exceeds the anatomic dead space. The physiological dead space in healthy individuals usually accounts for 25–35% of the minute ventilation and is measured by directly sampling both arterial and expired gas for CO_2, a technique known as *Bohr's method* (see Appendix).

The gas that reaches the respiratory bronchioles and alveoli is collectively referred to as the *alveolar ventilation* ($\dot{V}A$). This is the gas that participates in gas exchange and thus is involved in determining the ultimate blood gas composition of CO_2 and O_2. The Pa_{CO_2} is determined by the ratio of CO_2 production to the amount of alveolar ventilation ($Pa_{CO_2} \propto \dot{V}_{CO_2}/\dot{V}A$). Thus, any process that increases CO_2 production (e.g., increased metabolic states) or reduces alveolar ventilation (e.g., increased physiological dead space or overall hypoventilation) can lead to hypercarbia. The Pa_{O_2} is determined by the more complex interaction of factors described by the alveolar air equation and is the subject of the next chapter (Chap. 4).

AIR MOVEMENT OUT OF THE LUNG

Changes in Pressure, Volume, and Flow

Amazingly, all of the above described events take place within the inspiratory portion of one, single breath, which takes about 1–2 s! Following these events, the respiratory muscles relax, releasing their influence on changes in pleural pressure (Fig. 6). Transpulmonary pressure abruptly becomes less positive (i.e., less pressure keeping the alveoli distended) as the elastic recoil of the lung raises alveolar pressure above atmospheric pressure and air flows out of the lung. As the air traverses from the distal airways to the more proximal ones, the total cross-sectional area of the airways decreases dramatically and velocity of airflow increases. This increase accounts for the eventual transition of laminar flow back to turbulent flow in the larger airways. In addition, as the velocity increases, intra-airway pressure falls, according to the Bernoulli effect (Fig. 11). This fall in pressure becomes important when one is considering forced exhalations (see below).

Factors Affecting Expiratory Airflow

Expiratory airflow may be affected by both intrinsic airway resistance as well as lung elastic recoil. Recall that flow varies as driving pressure divided by resistance. Therefore, in states of increased elastic recoil, such as pulmonary fibrosis, airflow may be increased due to increased driving pressure; in states of decreased elastic recoil, such as emphysema, airflow may be diminished due to decreased driving pressure. Likewise, increased airway resistance, such as found in asthma, will also diminish airflow. These effects become more

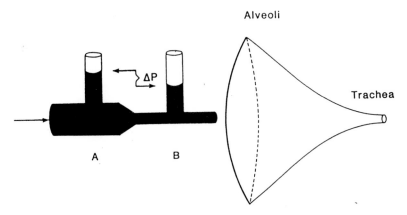

Figure 11 The Bernoulli effect during airflow. On the right is shown a schematic of the relative areas of the alveoli and small airways compared to the trachea and larger airways. Since net area decreases as air flows from the periphery of the lung outward, the velocity of air must increase. As shown by the tube analogy on the left, such acceleration from A to B leads to a drop in internal pressure (ΔP), known as the Bernoulli effect. (From Taylor AE, Rehder K, Parker JC. Clinical Respiratory Physiology. Philadelphia: Saunders, 1989, Fig. 7-1.)

pronounced and clinically important during states of high minute ventilation (such as exercise) or with forced exhalations. During high flow states, intra-airway pressure falls, as described above. At the same time, the respiratory muscles may become active during exhalation and exert an additional positive pressure on the airways. Together, these factors combine to cause collapse of noncartilaginous airways and thus limitation of airflow (Fig. 12). Flow limitation occurs during forced maneuvers at volumes below approximately 70% of TLC. At higher lung volumes, parenchymal tethering of the airways is thought to prevent significant airway collapse. The theoretical limit to airflow can be predicted from wave speed theory, which describes the relationship between flow in a nonrigid tube and the cross-sectional area and transmural pressure of the tube.

Consequences of Airflow Limitation

There are two important consequences of severe airflow limitation, such as may occur in severe asthma or COPD. First, airflow may be so markedly reduced that patients' normal tidal breathing becomes subject to flow limitation (Fig. 13). In this situation, patients have no physiological reserve for increasing their minute ventilation and therefore may be severely limited in their capacity for exercise or any increase in activity. Second, be-

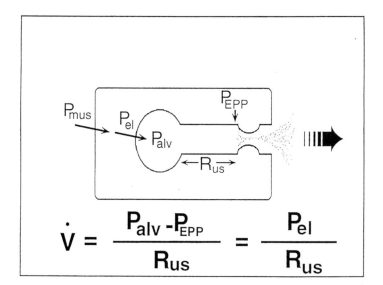

Figure 12 Airflow limitation due to airway collapse on forced expiration. Airflow occurs because of a pressure gradient developed between the alveolar space (Palv) and the atmosphere. Palv is the sum of lung elastic recoil pressure (Pel) and respiratory muscle pressure (Pmus). Pmus is exerted all along the path of the airway, so at some point, the pressure external to the airway (Pmus) will equal the pressure internal to the airway, a point known as the equal pressure point (EPP). At the EPP, the distensible airway will begin to collapse. Since factors below the EPP will not contribute to modifying airflow, flow ($\dot{V}$) is governed by driving pressure (Palv − P_{EPP} = Pel + Pmus − Pmus = Pel) and resistance in the airways upstream from the EPP (Rus), or $\dot{V}$ = Pel/Rus. Hence, any disease process that either increases Rus or decreases Pel will result in reduced airflow. (From Kaminsky DA, Irvin CG. Lung function in asthma. In: Barnes PJ, Grunstein MM, Leff AR, Woolcock AJ, eds. *Asthma*. Philadelphia: Lippincott-Raven, 1997, Fig. 8A.)

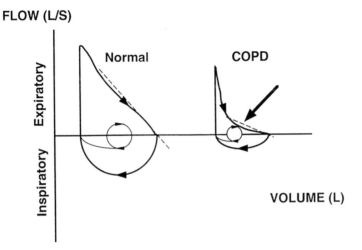

Figure 13 The effects of airflow limitation on tidal breathing in severe COPD. On the left is the normal tidal volume loop (thin line) and forced flow-volume loop (thick line). Notice that there is additional room between tidal expiration and forced (airflow-limited) expiration. The limits of airflow are depicted by the diagonal dashed line. On the right is what happens during severe airflow limitation. In this situation, tidal breathing abuts the limits of airflow on the forced expiratory maneuver (large arrow), leaving no ability to increase airflow further.

cause of severe time constant inequalities (excessive resistance or compliance) or overt airway collapse on expiration, there may be incomplete emptying of lung units, with consequent air trapping and lung hyperinflation. This problem may lead to increased work of breathing, hemodynamic compromise, and risk of barotrauma.

WORK OF BREATHING

What is the work required to move air into and out of the lung? *Work* is usually defined as a force acting through a distance. In the respiratory system, it is commonly defined as the product of pressure and volume. The work of breathing may be illustrated by depicting the area under the curve of a volume-pressure diagram (Fig. 14). Such a diagram summarizes the total work necessary to overcome both static (elastic) and dynamic (viscous) forces in the respiratory system as a whole. For example, total work is increased in asthma due to increased work of overcoming increased flow resistance, while total work is increased in interstitial fibrosis because of the increased work of overcoming increased elastic forces (Fig. 14).

When estimates are made of the work of breathing based on oxygen consumption, total work of breathing consumes less than 5% of total resting oxygen consumption. This value may increase to 30% or more in patients with significant respiratory system disease. The work of breathing also increases disproportionately in disease states as the level of minute ventilation is increased, thereby dramatically limiting activity level (Fig. 15).

The work of breathing may also alter the pattern of breathing. For any given level of alveolar ventilation, there is an optimal respiratory rate and tidal volume that minimizes

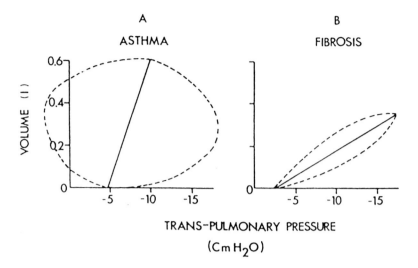

Figure 14 The work of breathing in asthma (A) and interstitial fibrosis (B), as depicted by the area of a pressure-volume (PV) diagram (in this case, transpulmonary pressure is recorded as a negative number representing pleural pressure minus alveolar pressure). In asthma, there is a normal amount of elastic work of breathing (area bounded by the volume axis and the solid PV line); however, severe airway narrowing results in an increase in the flow-resistive work of both inspiration (area bounded by the dashed line to the right of the solid line) and expiration (area bounded by the dashed line to the left of the solid line). Notice that the expiratory flow work loop falls outside the limits of elastic work (dashed line portion to the left of the volume axis), indicating that active expiratory muscle force must be used to generate expiratory flow. In fibrosis, elastic work is greatly increased as shown by a shift of the solid PV line down and to the right, with an increase in the elastic work area (area bounded by the volume axis and the solid line); however, flow-resistive work (area within the dashed lines) is normal. (From Cherniack RM. Pulmonary Function Testing. Philadelphia: Saunders, 1977, Fig. 2-19.)

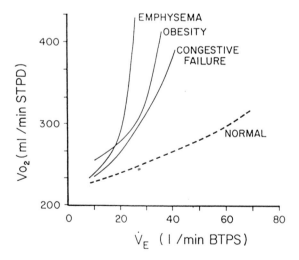

Figure 15 Increased energy expenditures in normal and diseased respiratory states. The plot shows the level of oxygen consumption in relation to the minute ventilation. Notice the markedly increased energy requirement of increased minute ventilation in emphysema, obesity, and congestive heart failure compared with the normal condition. (From Cherniack RM. Pulmonary Function Testing. Philadelphia: Saunders, 1977, Fig. 2-21.)

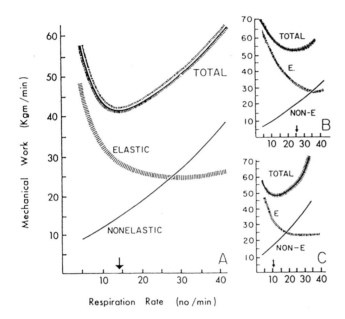

Respiration Rate (no /min)

Figure 16 Relationship between work of breathing and respiratory rate for normal (A) and diseased conditions (B, increased elastic work; C, increased nonelastic or flow-resistive work). In the normal condition, total work is minimized at a respiratory rate of approximately 12–14 breaths per minute (small arrow). In increased elastic work, such as interstitial fibrosis, total work is minimized with higher respiratory rates (and hence smaller tidal volumes for a given level of minute ventilation). In increased flow-resistive work, slower rates and higher tidal volumes are more efficient. (From Cherniack RM. Pulmonary Function Testing. Philadelphia: Saunders, 1977, Fig. 2-20.)

the total work. As seen in Fig. 16A, when respiratory rate is too high, the energy required to overcome nonelastic (flow-resistive) forces increases (and the total amount of ventilation must increase as more ventilation is wasted with each breath). If respiratory rate is too low, flow-resistive work is reduced but larger tidal volumes are necessary to achieve adequate minute ventilation, and this increases the amount of work necessary to overcome elastic forces of the respiratory system. Disease states that alter the static or dynamic properties of the respiratory system will also affect the optimal pattern of breathing. Rapid, shallow breathing minimizes the work of breathing in restrictive disorders (Fig. 16B), while slower, deeper breathing is more efficient in obstructive disorders (Fig. 16C).

SUMMARY

The principles of air movement into and out of the lung are the principles of physics. Air passively follows gradients of pressure established by the respiratory system. The chest wall serves as the supporting structure and pump of the respiratory system and the lung as the conduit for air movement and the interface for gas exchange. Both gravity and regional differences in resistance and compliance influence the distribution of air within the lung during inspiration. Some of the inspired air is necessarily wasted in the physiological dead space. During expiration, several factors influence expiratory airflow, with airflow limitation leading to significant problems associated with air trapping and hyperinflation. All of these factors combine to influence gas exchange and determine the ultimate work of breathing—endpoints that may be altered in various disease states. From these principles, symptoms and signs of pulmonary disease based on the alteration of movement of air into and out of the lung are better understood.

ACKNOWLEDGMENT

The author would like to thank John Evans, Ph.D., for his thoughtful review of the manuscript.

APPENDIX

Reynolds Number

The Reynolds number (Re) is a dimensionless number that predicts whether flow will be laminar or turbulent:

$$Re = \frac{2rvd}{\eta}$$

where r = radius, v = average velocity, d = gas density and η = viscosity. Therefore, as gas is more dense, travels more rapidly, travels in a more narrow tube, or is less viscous, Re will be greater. When Re >2000, turbulent flow is expected. Re exceeds 2000 in the trachea, even during quiet breathing; hence flow is turbulent. As flow proceeds to the periphery, cross-sectional area increases greatly, allowing velocity to decrease, which overall lowers Re to <2000; hence flow is laminar.

Poiseuille's Law

Poiseuille's law describes the relationship between flow and pressure under laminar flow conditions in a tube:

$$V = \frac{\Delta P \pi r^4}{8 \eta L}$$

where ΔP = pressure drop along the tube, V = flow rate, r = tube radius, η = fluid viscosity, L = length of tube. Since resistance (R) = $\Delta P/V$,

$$R = \frac{8 \eta L}{\pi r^4}$$

Thus, R varies with viscosity and the length of the tube, and inversely with the fourth power of the radius.

Anatomic Dead Space Calculation (Fowler's Method)

The dead space is found by analyzing the concentration of nitrogen in the expired air following a full, deep inhalation of pure oxygen. The nitrogen concentration rises as the dead space is washed out, and eventually reaches a slightly rising plateau, representative of the alveolar space. The dead space is determined conventionally by the volume at which half the dead space nitrogen gas has been expired.

Physiological Dead Space Calculation (Bohr's Method)

Taking advantage of the fact that all of the expired CO_2 comes from the alveolar gas and not from the dead space, the amount of CO_2 in the expired gas can be measured and related to the total amount of expired gas to determine the difference, that being the dead space. In mathematical terms:

$$\frac{\dot{V}d}{Vt} = \frac{P_{A_{CO_2}} - P_{E_{CO_2}}}{P_{A_{CO_2}}}$$

where Vd is the dead space, Vt the tidal volume, $P_{A_{CO_2}}$ is the partial pressure of CO_2 in the alveolar gas (estimated by $P_{a_{CO_2}}$, the partial pressure of arterial CO_2), and $P_{E_{CO_2}}$ is the partial pressure of CO_2 in the expired air (measured with a rapid gas analyzer).

SUGGESTED READING

1. Bates DV. Respiratory Function in Disease, 3rd ed. Philadelphia: Saunders, 1989.
2. Cherniack RM. Pulmonary Function Testing. Philadelphia: Saunders, 1977.
3. Forster RE, DuBois AB, Briscoe WA, Fisher AB. The Lung: Physiologic Basis of Pulmonary Function Tests, 3d ed. Chicago: Year Book, 1986.
4. Leff AR, Schumacker PT. Respiratory Physiology: Basics and Applications. Philadelphia: Saunders, 1993.
5. Taylor AE, Rehder K, Hyatt RE, Parker JC. Clinical Respiratory Physiology. Philadelphia: Saunders, 1989.
6. West JB. Respiratory Physiology—The Essentials, 4th ed. Baltimore: Williams & Wilkins, 1990.

4

Principles of Blood Flow, Gas Exchange, and Oxygen Delivery

Jason Kelley
Texas A&M Health Sciences Center
Olin E. Teague VA Medical Center
Scott and White Clinics
Temple, Texas

INTRODUCTION

The complementary functions of pulmonary blood flow, gas exchange, and the delivery of oxygen to peripheral tissues are considered and reviewed in this chapter. Individual disease states are alluded to in this chapter, but only by way of illustrating key physiological principles. The reader is referred to the other relevant chapters for more detailed discussions of the individual disease states.

BLOOD FLOW

The Pulmonary Circulation

Efficient gas exchange, the uptake of oxygen and elimination of carbon dioxide, is the primary function of the lungs and depends on the normal functioning of the pulmonary circulation. Anatomically, the pulmonary circuit consists of the pulmonary arteries and arterioles, the capillary network where gas exchange occurs, and the pulmonary veins, which direct oxygenated blood to the left heart. The pulmonary circulation guides the entire cardiac output into a thin film located in the alveolar walls, where gas exchange rapidly takes place. Each capillary is approximately 10 μm in diameter, slightly wider than a red blood cell. In the aggregate, the alveolar–capillary interface has been estimated to be as broad as 100 M^2.

In addition to the pulmonary circulation, portions of the lung receive blood flow via the bronchial circulation. The bronchial arteries provide nutrient blood to most of the central structures of the lung, including the bronchi, bronchioles, pulmonary nerves, lymphatics, and pulmonary arteries. The bronchial arteries receive blood from the aorta and therefore are systemic vessels functioning at systemic pressures. The bronchial circulation is probably critically important in fetal development and plays a critical role in certain chronic lung disorders, including cystic fibrosis and neoplasms. On the other hand, it is clear that the normal adult lung can function normally without a bronchial circulation.

Table 1 Vascular Pressures in the Pulmonary
and Systemic Circulation

Vessel/chamber	Pressures (mmHg)
Right atrium	3
Right ventricle	22/4
Pulmonary artery	20/10
Left atrium (mean)	5
Aorta	120/75
Resistances (mmHg/L/min)	
Pulmonary vascular resistance	1.4
Systemic vascular resistance	13–14

Hemodynamics of the Pulmonary Circulation

The pulmonary circulation is a low-pressure circulation. In this respect it differs importantly from the high-pressure systemic circulation; this distinction is a key to understanding many aspects of altered circulatory physiology. Despite its low pressures compared with the systemic circulation (Table 1), the pulmonary vasculature allows passage of the entire cardiac output through the lungs. The mean pulmonary artery pressure is 14–15 mmHg.* The pressure difference across the pulmonary vascular bed is usually less than 5 mmHg when cardiac output is at its basal level, and rises only modestly as cardiac output increases. This small pressure gradient moves 5–6 L of blood through the circuit every minute.

Resistance in the pulmonary circulation is proportional to the arteriovenous pressure difference across the lungs and inversely proportional to flow through the lung vasculature. This relationship is expressed in Eq. (1):

$$R_{PV} = \frac{P_{PA} - P_{LA}}{\dot{Q}_T} \tag{1}$$

where measurement units = mmHg/L/min.

In this equation, R_{PV} is the pulmonary vascular resistance, P_{PA} is the pulmonary artery pressure on the right side of the pulmonary circulation, P_{LA} is the left atrial pressure, and $\dot{Q}_T$ is the cardiac output. Total pulmonary blood flow is nearly identical to the cardiac output except when an intracardiac shunt is present.

Pulmonary vascular resistance has the capacity to fall below the normal value when either pulmonary arterial or venous pressures rise. This occurs because, under conditions of normal cardiac output, many pulmonary vessels, particularly those in the upper zones of the lungs, are not conducting blood flow. As flow rises, these vessels are recruited to conduct flow. Moreover, all of the pulmonary vessels are relatively distensible and can dilate passively to accommodate greater blood flow when pressure rises.

Because the alveoli and the pulmonary vessels are mechanically interdependent, vascular resistance is partially controlled by lung volume and therefore varies during the respiratory cycle. For small, distensible vessels in close proximity to airways, resistance

---

* By convention, units of blood pressures are given in mmHg; all units of gas pressures and partial
  pressures are given in cmH_2O.

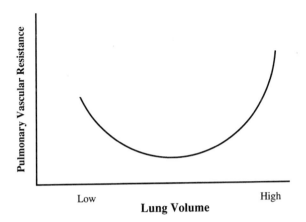

Figure 1 Relationship between lung volume and pulmonary vascular resistance. At low lung volumes, the extra-alveolar vessels have less traction forces to distend them and resistance rises. At high lung volumes, resistance in pulmonary capillaries (alveolar vessels) is compromised by high alveolar pressures. Lowest pulmonary vascular resistance occurs at intermediate lung volumes. The figure assumes constant blood flow independent of lung volume.

is lowest at mid-lung volumes; at lower lung volumes these vessels become narrowed; at high lung volumes, the distensible capillaries are collapsed by the high intraalveolar pressures (Fig. 1).

However, not all pulmonary vessels are so obviously influenced by the swings in alveolar pressure. In this regard, physiologists distinguish between *alveolar* and *extra-alveolar* vessels. Alveolar vessels are those that are close enough to alveolar tissue to be directly influenced by the intra-alveolar pressures. Capillaries are clearly alveolar vessels in that they are thin-walled and directly exposed to alveolar pressures, but it is not clear where the transition between alveolar and extra-alveolar vessels occurs. Extra-alveolar vessels can be separated either by anatomic considerations and functional issues. Arteries, arterioles, venules, and veins are all surrounded by a connective tissue sheath which buffers them from alveolar pressure; this sheath is in communication with the pleural pressures.

GAS EXCHANGE

Physics and Chemistry of Gases

The amounts of individual components of gas mixture (or dissolved in blood or tissue) can be expressed in several ways. These include the fractional concentration, the partial pressure, and the content. The fractional concentration (F) is the fraction that a particular gas constitutes in a mixture. By convention, fractional concentration is expressed as a decimal fraction or as a percent. F is used to describe gas mixtures but not gases in solution; F_I is the fractional concentration of a particular gas in inspired gas, e.g. $F_{I_{O_2}}$ is the fractional concentration of oxygen in an inspired gas mixture. Nitrogen is the most abundant component of (dry) atmospheric air, making up 79.0% of the total. The fractional concentration of oxygen in atmospheric air is 20.9%. Carbon dioxide makes up only 0.04% of atmospheric air.

The partial pressure of a gas (P) is the amount of pressure that the gas exerts in a gas mixture or in a liquid. The atmospheric gas pressure at sea level is 760 mmHg, the average barometric pressure. It falls to 632 mmHg at 1500 m (e.g., in Denver, Colorado) and 525 mmHg at 3050 m. The partial pressure of an inhaled gas is the product of the fractional concentration (F_I) and the local barometric pressure (P_B). Thus, the partial pressure of oxygen in dry gas at sea level is:

$$P_{O_2} = 0.21 \cdot 760 \text{ mmHg} = 159 \text{ mmHg} \tag{2}$$

In biological systems, moisture is always present and therefore water vapor pressure must be further taken into account. Gas inhaled into the upper airways rapidly becomes completely humidified. At the normal body temperature of 37° C, the partial pressure of water vapor is 47 mmHg. The water vapor pressure is independent of barometric pressure but depends markedly on the temperature. The partial pressure of an inspired gas after it becomes fully humidified in the airway is given as:

$$P_I = F_I \cdot (P_B - P_{H_2O}) \tag{3}$$

where measurement units = mmHg. For example, at sea level the partial pressure of oxygen in humidified inspired gas is:

$$P_{I_{O_2}} = 0.21 \cdot (760 - 47) = 149 \text{ mmHg} \tag{4}$$

The content of a gas is expressed as the volume of gas per unit volume of fluid or tissue. The relative contents of several gases within a fluid such as plasma are not necessarily proportional to their partial pressures. For example, O_2 and CO_2 have quite different solubilities in plasma. If a degassed sample of plasma is exposed to a gas mixture of O_2 and CO_2 that are initially at the same partial pressure, considerably more CO_2 will dissolve in the plasma than O_2.

The Alveolar Gas Equation

The normal P_{O_2} in arterial blood is slightly less than 100 mmHg when a healthy young adult calmly breathes ambient air at sea level. Note that the P_{O_2} measured in arterial blood is significantly lower than the P_{O_2} in inspired gas [Eq. (3)]. The difference between these two values, referred to as the *alveolar-arterial oxygen difference*, is largely a consequence of the partial pressure of the carbon dioxide (Pa_{CO_2}) that continuously flushes into the alveoli from the venous blood.

The importance of the alveolar-arterial difference for oxygen to the clinician is that it represents the best index of gas exchange efficiency of the lungs. Following the alveolar-arterial difference over time indicates to the clinician the progress of a disease course. The relationship between P_{O_2} and P_{CO_2} in the alveoli is mathematically complex. Moreover, although samples of arterial blood can be obtained conveniently, samples of alveolar gas cannot be conveniently or safely obtained for determination of the PA_{O_2}. However, the alveolar oxygen level can be estimated using the alveolar gas equation:

$$PA_{O_2} = F_{I_{O_2}} \cdot (P_B - P_{H_2O}) - PA_{CO_2} \cdot \left[F_{I_{O_2}} + \frac{(1 - F_{I_{O_2}})}{R} \right]$$

where measurement units = mmHg, $F_{I_{O_2}}$ is the fraction of O_2 in inspired air, and PA_{CO_2} is the mean alveolar P_{CO_2}. R is the respiratory exchange ratio; it corrects for the fact that slightly more oxygen is removed from alveolar gas than the carbon dioxide that is added, a reflection of normal body metabolism. The value of R is $\dot{V}_{CO_2}/\dot{V}_{O_2}$ and is usually close to 0.8 for subjects eating a diet with a normal fat and carbohydrate content. The alveolar gas equation can be simplified for use at the bedside as follows:

$$PA_{O_2} = PI_{O_2} - \frac{PA_{CO_2}}{0.8}$$

Furthermore, because the arterial P_{CO_2} is nearly identical to the alveolar P_{CO_2}, the value obtained from a blood gas sample can be substituted in the equation. The key variables required to solve this equation can be determined from an arterial blood sample obtained at a known FI_{O_2}. The normal alveolar–arterial difference for oxygen is no more than 8 mmHg in young adults breathing air at sea level. It normally increases to twice this value in healthy elderly people as a consequence of worsening ventilation/perfusion ($\dot{V}/\dot{Q}$) imbalance. Recumbency, advancing age, and other factors widen the alveolar–arterial difference in seemingly normal subjects.

About half of the normally small alveolar–arterial difference occurs as a result of normal shunting of blood through minor intrapulmonary circulations; the remaining difference is a consequence of $\dot{V}/\dot{Q}$ mismatch. Note that this value obtains only for subjects breathing room air; the alveolar–arterial difference is higher when the subject is breathing oxygen. This determination is most useful at the bedside, because an abnormal alveolar–arterial difference points to intrinsic lung disease but is not diagnostically revealing.

Hypoxemia and Hypercapnia

From the physiologist's perspective, hypoxemia can be classified as being a consequence of either hypoventilation, a widened alveolar–arterial difference, or both. The characteristics of hypoventilation are an inappropriately elevated Pa_{CO_2} and reduced alveolar ventilation. Hypoventilation represents a problem in control of ventilation and not a problem with the gas exchange capacity of the lungs. Under these circumstances the alveolar–arterial difference for O_2 is normal. Hypoventilation is usually a consequence of extrapulmonary abnormalities such as central nervous system structural disorders, narcotic use, or respiratory muscle dysfunction.

The physiological causes of a widened alveolar–arterial difference are threefold: $\dot{V}/\dot{Q}$ perfusion inequality, shunt, and altered diffusion capacity. From the clinician's perspective, most patients with hypoxemia and a widened alveolar–arterial difference have a $\dot{V}/\dot{Q}$ abnormality. Patients demonstrating pure intrapulmonary shunts as a cause of their hypoxemia are not often encountered outside of the intensive care unit. Patients whose hypoxemia can be traced to an isolated diffusion abnormality are even rarer. Although identification of the physiological cause of hypoxemia can be most helpful in its management, it rarely points to a specific diagnosis by itself. Indeed, most disease processes resulting in hypoxemia involve more than one physiologic cause.

Patients with both intrinsic lung disease and hypoventilation of nonpulmonary causes can present with blood gases reflecting both disorders. An example might be a patient with unrecognized chronic obstructive pulmonary disease who is given excessive doses of respiratory depressant narcotics postoperatively.

Ventilation-Perfusion Mismatch

Blood flow through the lungs is anatomically inhomogeneous. The effects of gravity on the low-pressure pulmonary circulation are to create a vertical gradient of blood flow such that most flow is to the lowest—i.e., most dependent—lung regions. The relationship between total ventilation and total perfusion through the lungs as a whole can be described in the $\dot{V}/\dot{Q}$ ratio:

$$\frac{V}{\dot{Q}_T} = \frac{5 \text{ L/min}}{6 \text{ L/min}} = 0.83 \tag{7}$$

where there are no specific measurement units. The blood flow per unit of lung tissue in the upright position is about six- to tenfold greater in the lung bases than in the uppermost portions of lung tissue. A parallel vertical gradient for ventilation also occurs but is less pronounced. In consequence of these two gradients, there is both more perfusion and more ventilation to the lung bases than to the apices.

Both ventilation and perfusion are increased in the lowermost lung zones. However, because there is a larger gradient for blood than for alveolar air, the upper zones have relatively more ventilation than perfusion; conversely, in the lower zones perfusion is relatively greater than ventilation. These gradients notwithstanding, it would be incorrect to assume that ventilation per unit lung volume is greater in the apices than in the bases. (Fig. 2).

Uptake of oxygen and elimination of carbon dioxide within the lung would be optimal if there were perfect mixing of incoming venous blood in all the capillaries coursing through the alveolar walls with the gas in the adjacent alveoli. However, the effects of gravity on a low-pressure pulmonary circulation and the different densities of alveolar

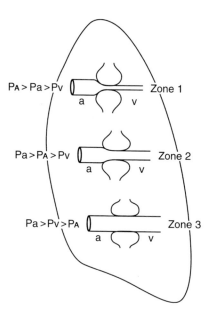

Figure 2   The pull of gravity in the upright lung results in uneven relationships between ventilation and perfusion. West and colleagues have provided a schematic way of demonstrating the perfusion and ventilation of the lungs and the resulting $\dot{V}/\dot{Q}$ relationships by describing three zones in which the $\dot{V}/\dot{Q}$ relationships differ. Up in zone 1, the highest local pressure lies within the alveoli, resulting in no effective perfusion of capillaries. Down in zone 3, the arterial pressure is the highest pressure, assuring flow that is independent of airway pressure.

gases, blood, and tissue place limits on the gas exchange process. Additionally, small amounts of shunted blood pass through the lungs without becoming oxygenated. As a result, a small degree of deoxygenation occurs in even the healthiest lungs. This small amount of normal shunt accounts for part of the alveolar–arterial difference for oxygen.

The relationships between pressures within various compartments of the lungs determine the hemodynamic pressure and flow relationships. The key pressures involved are the pulmonary arterial and venous pressures and the effective airway pressure. The latter is of importance because compliant alveolar walls can compress pulmonary capillaries and impair normal blood flow. Based on the relationships between these three pressures, it is convenient to think of the upright lungs as having three hemodynamic zones. In the uppermost zone (zone 1), alveolar pressure exceeds the extremely low pulmonary arterial pressure and pulmonary venous pressures; therefore, there is no blood perfusion to this zone. Because there is no blood flow in zone 1, this uppermost portion of the lung does not normally contribute to gas exchange. Because of its high $\dot{V}/\dot{Q}$ ratio, zone 1 is an alkaline environment with a high P_{O_2} and a very low P_{CO_2}.

Zone 2, the central portion of the lungs, is a transitional area in which the pulmonary arterial pressure exceeds alveolar pressure but the latter still exceeds venous pressure. As one moves down this transitional zone from the border of zones 1 to 3, blood flow progressively increases. In zone 3, the lowermost zone, both arterial and venous pressures exceed alveolar pressure, so flow is purely a function of the arterial–venous pressure difference. Most of the gas exchange function of the lung takes place in zone 3.

Regulatory mechanisms within the normal lungs act to optimize the mixing of blood and air. Like the airways, large and medium-sized pulmonary vessels are endowed with smooth muscle capable of regulating luminal caliber. The normally low pulmonary vascular resistance can be actively modulated by contraction of these muscular pulmonary vessels. Resistance can also change passively as a consequence of changes in the pressures and flows in the right and left sides of the heart as well as by intrapulmonary blood volume. Local oxygen levels are the strongest determinants of vasoconstriction; other factors include acidosis, high CO_2, serotonin, histamine, and catecholamines. The molecular mechanisms by which hypoxia mediates pulmonary vasoconstriction remain unclear.

Under normal conditions, transient vasoconstriction in vessels feeding small areas of atelectatic lung where oxygen content is low serves to divert blood away toward more normally oxygenated areas. Such redistribution does not normally result in pulmonary hypertension because of the vast capacitance of the pulmonary circulation. However, when a diffuse disease state involves much or all of the lung, hypoxic vasoconstriction can no longer suffice to maintain the normal alveolar–arterial difference, pulmonary hypertension ensues, and the right heart fails.

Intrapulmonary Shunts

A shunt is a vascular channel that allows desaturated venous blood to enter the arterial side of the circulation without passing through the gas exchange portions of the lungs. Normal but tiny shunts occur and account for a portion of the normally small alveolar–arterial difference. These include (1) the bronchial circulation, which returns some deoxygenated blood via the pulmonary veins to the left atrium, and (2) the thebesian veins, which direct some of the coronary venous blood directly into the left ventricle.

True shunts are infrequently encountered outside the critical care unit. Examples include congenital cardiac defects, isolated pulmonary arteriovenous malformations

(AVM), or multiple AVMs in the hereditary hemorrhagic telangiectasia (HHT; Osler-Weber-Rendu) syndrome. They can be distinguished from $\dot{V}/\dot{Q}$ disorders by having hypoxic subjects breathe pure oxygen briefly. When a shunt is present, no amount of oxygen will correct the high arterial–alveolar difference for oxygen; this feature distinguishes true shunts from hypoxemia caused by $\dot{V}/\dot{Q}$ disorders and diffusion disorders; in these latter conditions, a high inspired oxygen will correct the low Pa_{O_2}.

An intrapulmonary or intracardiac shunt can also be demonstrated by radionuclide imaging. Macroaggregated albumin labeled with technetium (the same isotopic preparation used in pulmonary perfusion scans) is injected into the venous circulation. A gamma counter scans over the cerebrum, kidneys, or other highly vascularized organs. If significant radionuclide is present, it has clearly not been appropriately filtered during its passage through pulmonary circulation. Echocardiography after the injection of blood mixed with CO_2 bubbles can also be used to identify intracardiac right-to-left shunts.

Breathing 100% oxygen corrects arterial oxygen desaturation caused by $\dot{V}/\dot{Q}$ disorders, but not those caused by intrapulmonary shunts. This physiological concept, while important, is often difficult to apply at the bedside for a number of reasons. Tight-fitting masks reliably delivering 100% oxygen are hard to manage, and the process of breathing high levels of oxygen can rapidly promote atelectasis, further worsening underlying pulmonary disorders. Sometimes there is additional concern that high levels of oxygen, even when briefly applied, can promote oxygen toxicity or hypoventilation and hypercapnia.

The flow of blood through a shunt can be estimated using the so-called shunt equation (Fig. 3):

$$\frac{\dot{Q}s}{\dot{Q}T} = \frac{Cc'_{O_2} - Ca_{O_2}}{Cc'_{O_2} - C\bar{v}_{O_2}} \tag{8}$$

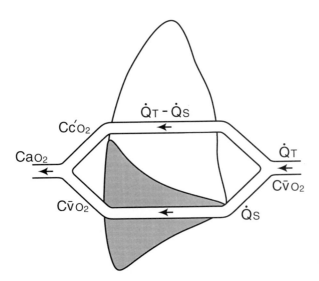

Figure 3 Effect of intrapulmonary shunt on oxygen delivery. Blood flowing through diseased region of lung (shaded area) does not become enriched with oxygen: its oxygen content remains at the venous level ($C\bar{v}_{O_2}$). The oxygen content in the blood passing through normal portion of lung ($\dot{Q}T - \dot{Q}s$) rises normally from $C\bar{v}_{O_2}$ to Cc'_{O_2}. The oxygen content of the mixed blood when it reaches systemic arteries (Ca_{O_2}) will be intermediate between $C\bar{v}_{O_2}$ and Cc'_{O_2}.

where there are no specific measurement units. In this equation, $\dot{Q}s$ is the flow through the shunt; the shunt fraction ($\dot{Q}s/\dot{Q}T$) is the fraction of the total cardiac output ($\dot{Q}T$) that flows through a nonoxygenating shunt. Of the three oxygen content values needed to solve this equation, Cc'_{O_2} (oxygen content of end-capillary blood) must be assumed. Ca_{O_2} and $C\bar{V}_{O_2}$ can be calculated from P_{O_2} determinations of an arterial blood specimen and a simultaneously obtained sample of mixed venous blood, respectively. The latter requires the presence of a right heart catheter.

Diffusion Disorders

Several laws describe the diffusion of respiratory and other gases through tissues or membranes. The transfer of a gas through a tissue barrier is proportional to its area and to the partial pressure difference across the barrier and inversely proportional to the barrier thickness. In addition, a diffusion constant describes the physicochemical properties of the barrier for any gas crossing the barrier. The diffusion constant is proportional to the solubility of the gas in the barrier tissue and inversely proportional to the square root of the molecular weight of the gas. The area of transfer in the case of the lung is as much as 100 M^2; the thickness of the alveolar-capillary barrier is no more than 0.3–0.5 μm. The diffusion of CO_2 is about 20 times greater than that for oxygen, even though the two molecules are of similar molecular weight.

The diffusing capacity of the lung for oxygen is the quantity ($\dot{V}_{O_2}$) that diffuses across the alveolar-capillary membrane per unit time as a function of the differential pressure gradient for oxygen on the two sides of the membrane ($PA_{O_2} - Pc_{O_2}$):

$$\dot{D}L_{O_2} = \frac{\dot{V}_{O_2}}{PA_{O_2} - Pc_{O_2}} \tag{9}$$

where measurement units = mL/min · mmHg. Gases that have low solubility in blood are said to be "perfusion-limited." Examples include nitrous oxide and the inert gases such as helium. Conversely, gases such as O_2 and carbon monoxide (CO) are avidly bound by blood components and the kinetics of their transfer from alveolus to blood are described as "diffusion-limited."

The flow of blood through the pulmonary capillaries under conditions of a normal cardiac output takes about 0.75 s. Oxygen takes only about 0.25 s to equilibrate with capillary blood, about one-third of the transit time of red cells. During exercise, the dwell time of red cells in gas exchange capillaries is reduced to 0.25 s, just barely an adequate time for complete equilibration of O_2. However, in the diseased lung, the transfer of gas may be slowed resulting in arterial desaturation.

The diffusion capacity ($\dot{D}L$) is measured in the clinical laboratory using a tracer gas with diffusion properties similar to oxygen (see Chap. 9). As mentioned previously, isolated diffusion abnormalities are rarely a cause of hypoxemia. Even with exercise, a maneuver that shortens the dwell time of erythrocytes in pulmonary capillaries, diffusion limitations only become a cause of hypoxemia at altitude with reduced oxygen partial pressure (see Chap. 42).

Case Examples

The following cases illustrate several of the points made in the preceding discussion.

Case 1

You are called about a 22-year-old woman who has just been brought to a local emergency department (ED). She is described to you only as being comatose. An arterial blood gas sample obtained upon her arrival indicates a pH of 7.28, a Pa_{O_2} of 64, and a Pa_{CO_2} of 64 as she breathes air. The physician's assistant who contacts you is impressed with the level of hypoxemia and suggests that such a low Pa_{O_2} could only be encountered in patients with severe lung disease. You are asked to determine how to proceed with the evaluation.

Comment   Using the alveolar gas equation, you determine that her Pa_{O_2} must be 69 mmHg (assume that R is 0.8 and assume that she is indeed breathing air). This value is less than 5 mmHg above the determined Pa_{O_2} and therefore you surmise that she currently has no pulmonary disorder. The cause of the coma and the further management should be based on a search for nonpulmonary causes of hypoventilation.

Case 2

You visit a patient in the intensive care unit who has no history of pulmonary disease but who has just been admitted for an acute myocardial infarction. Although the chest x-ray is normal, an arterial blood gas sample obtained while the patient breathes 35% oxygen has a pH of 7.45, Pa_{O_2} of 78, and Pa_{CO_2} of 32. The surgeon is pleased that the patient appears to have no pulmonary problems.

Comment   You note that when these values are put into the alveolar gas equation, there is a great difference between the alveolar P_{O_2} and the arterial P_{O_2}. The alveolar–arterial difference normally increases as the inspired oxygen concentration rises; nevertheless, this is an inordinately high difference and points to intrinsic lung disease. You advise the patient's surgeon and point out that the radiographic appearance of the lungs may underestimate the physiological derangements. Indeed, after this patient undergoes a period of diuresis, the alveolar–arterial difference narrows and the patient is able to sustain a physiologically acceptable Pa_{O_2} while breathing progressively lower levels of oxygen.

OXYGEN TRANSPORT AND DELIVERY

Oxygen Transport

Oxygen is transported in arterial blood mostly in conjunction with hemoglobin (oxyhemoglobin). Even when alveolar gas and end-capillary blood are in equilibrium with regard to partial pressures of a particular gas, the amount ("content") of gas in a given volume of alveolar gas or blood is markedly different. The oxygen content (CO_2) of blood [generally expressed as milliliters of O_2 per 100 mL of blood or as volume percent (vol %)], is the amount of oxygen contained in a given volume of blood. A small amount of the oxygen in blood is dissolved in plasma; a much greater proportion is bound to the hemoglobin within red cells.

The maximum amount of oxygen that can be carried by hemoglobin, the oxygen-carrying capacity (Cap) is a function of the concentration of hemoglobin and the oxygen-binding properties of the hemoglobin. Each gram of normal hemoglobin can carry about 1.4 mL of oxygen. Thus a hemoglobin concentration of 15 g/dL provides an oxygen-carrying capacity (O_2Cap) of 1.4 mL/g · 15 g/dL = 21 mL/dL (vol%).

The oxygen saturation (S) of blood is a dimensionless unit of relative concentration usually expressed as a percentage. It is the ratio of actual saturation to the maximal saturation:

$$S\ (\%) = \frac{O_2\ \text{content}}{O_2\ \text{Cap}} \cdot 100 = \frac{C_{O_2}}{O_2\ \text{Cap}} \cdot 100 \qquad (10)$$

where there are no specific measurement units. At a partial pressure of 100 mmHg, arterial blood is normally 97% saturated.

The Oxyhemoglobin Dissociation Curve

Oxygen in the alveolar space diffuses rapidly across the alveolar capillary membrane and into the plasma within the capillaries. From there it crosses the red blood cell membrane and binds to hemoglobin. Plasma itself carries very little oxygen; almost all the oxygen carried in blood is bound to hemoglobin. The relationship between the P_{O_2} and the amount of oxygen carried in blood is described in the oxyhemoglobin desaturation curve (Fig. 4).

Oxygen saturation can be estimated accurately at the bedside using a pulse oximeter. However, when the saturation falls below 90%, the accuracy of these devices suffers. The nonlinear nature of this curve assures that peripheral tissues can take up considerable oxygen without reducing the saturation significantly. In consequence, the driving pressure for unloading oxygen—the difference in partial pressures—remains high. For example, delivery of blood oxygenated to P_{O_2} values greater than about 80 mmHg fails to increase the oxygen saturation of blood substantially. Hence mixtures of equal amounts of blood at 60 and 100% oxygen saturation would yield a stream of blood that would contain oxyhemoglobin at 80% saturation. This would yield an arterial P_{O_2} of only 45 mmHg. In this example, it would be incorrect to average the two P_{O_2} values. This is a direct consequence of the nonlinear relationship between partial pressure and saturation.

The oxyhemoglobin saturation curve can be modulated by disease states and other factors. When hemoglobin becomes more avid for oxygen, the central portion of the curve

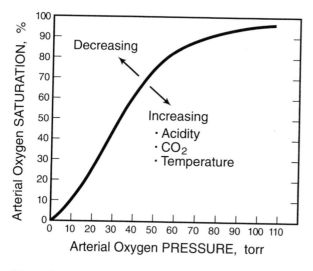

Figure 4 The normal oxyhemoglobin dissociation curve relates the saturation of hemoglobin with oxygen (or the O_2 content of hemoglobin) to the P_{O_2}. The curve is for standard conditions (pH 7.40, temperature 37°C). The point at which normal hemoglobin is 50% saturated with O_2, the P_{50}, is a convenient way to describe the curve. The P_{50} is normally 26.6 mmHg but varies considerably as the curve shifts to the right or left.

shifts to the left; conversely, when hemoglobin binds oxygen less avidly, the curve moves to the right but retains its sigmoid shape. Agents and circumstances which move the curve to the right include acidosis, fever, hyperthyroidism, and hypercapnia. These moderating influences generally act by increasing the concentration of 2,3-diphosphoglycerate within red blood cells. The oxyhemoglobin curve applies to venous as well as to arterial blood. Note that venous blood, being slightly more acidic than arterial blood gives up its oxygen more freely. Chronic hypoxia also raises the intracellular 2,3-diphosphoglycerate and enhances unloading of oxygen in tissues.

The oxygen-carrying capacity of abnormal forms of hemoglobin is reduced. This statement applies to altered forms of normal hemoglobin such as methemoglobin and carboxyhemoglobin as well as to genetically distinct forms of hemoglobin.

The amount of oxygen dissolved in plasma is only a tiny portion of the total oxygen in blood. For each 100 mmHg of P_{O_2} there is 0.3 mL oxygen per deciliter dissolved in blood (0.3 vol%). Hence less than 2% (0.3 ÷ 21.3) of the oxygen in arterial blood is dissolved in plasma.

Oxygen Delivery and Consumption

Oxygen delivery ($\dot{D}_{O_2}$) is given as the product of the cardiac output and the O_2 content of arterial blood (Table 2):

$$\dot{D}_{O_2} = \dot{Q}_T \cdot Ca_{O_2} \tag{11}$$

$$\dot{D}_{O_2} = 5 \text{ L/min} \cdot (21 \text{ mL/dL}) = 1050 \text{ mL/min} \tag{12}$$

where measurement units = mL/min.

Oxygen consumption by the body ($\dot{V}_{O_2}$) is the difference between the amount of O_2 delivered to peripheral tissues and the amount returning to the right heart (arteriovenous oxygen content difference ($Ca_{O_2} - C\bar{v}_{O_2}$). It is approximately 250 mL/min or 3.6 mL/kg/min. It is the product of the cardiac output and the arteriovenous oxygen content difference:

$$\dot{V}_{O_2} = \dot{Q}_T \cdot (Ca_{O_2} - C\bar{v}_{O_2}) \tag{13}$$

where measurement units = mL/min.

The $C\bar{v}_{O_2}$ can be determined using a right heart catheter. Mixed venous blood has an oxygen content ($C\bar{v}_{O_2}$) that is normally about three-quarters of the arterial oxygen content value. Hence the extraction of oxygen during the passage of blood through the systemic circulation is normally about 25% at rest. $\dot{V}_{O_2}$ can also be calculated in the pulmonary function laboratory by determining the loss of oxygen when a subject breathes from a closed circuit. Note that under normal circumstances, the amount of oxygen delivered to the peripheral tissues far exceeds the oxygen consumption.

Table 2 Oxygen Delivery and Consumption

Parameter [Symbol]	Formula
O_2 delivery to tissues [$\dot{D}_{O_2}$]	$\dot{Q}_T \cdot Ca_{O_2}$
O_2 leaving tissues and returning to lungs	$\dot{Q}_T \cdot C\bar{v}_{O_2}$
Arteriovenous O_2 content difference [$(a - \bar{v})O_2$]	$Ca_{O_2} - C\bar{v}_{O_2}$
O_2 consumption [$\dot{V}_{O_2}$]	$\dot{Q}_T \cdot (Ca_{O_2} - C\bar{v}_{O_2})$

When the lungs are functioning normally, the mixed venous blood oxygen content has no effect on the P_{O_2} of arterial blood. However, when lung disease is present, oxygen consumption may become a significant determinant of arterial oxygenation. Blood returning to the right heart from the systemic circulation is desaturated below a point from which the diseased lungs can fully reoxygenate it. It should be emphasized that when lungs are normal there is no such linkage between oxygen consumption and arterial oxygenation.

The Fick equation [rearranged from Eq. (13)] uses the oxygen consumption and arteriovenous O_2 content difference to calculate the cardiac output ($\dot{Q}_T$):

$$\dot{Q}_T = \frac{\dot{V}_{O_2}}{Ca_{O_2} - C\bar{v}_{O_2}} \tag{14}$$

where measurement units = L/min. The Fick equation is often used in the critical care unit to validate cardiac output measurements made by right heart catheter using the thermodilution method.

Case

A 58-year-old man is brought to the emergency room with pallor, anemia, and angina. You find out that he has lived a reclusive life on a very poor diet, possibly the explanation of his low hematocrit of 12% (hemoglobin concentration 4 g/dL). The ED physician expresses genuine surprise that despite the patient's anemia, his O_2 saturation as determined by a pulse oximeter was 96% even before he was given supplemental oxygen. This O_2 saturation has been confirmed by a blood gas analysis yielding a Pa_{O_2} of 92 mmHg.

Comment

The ED physician has confused the indices of O_2 saturation and Pa_{O_2} with the more physiologically relevant parameters of O_2 content and the O_2-carrying capacity of blood (Table 2). While the indices cited are normal, the Ca_{O_2} can be calculated as 1.4 mL/g · 4 g/dL · 0.96 = 5.6 mL/dL blood. Note that this is barely a quarter of the normal O_2 content of blood and likely puts the patient at risk of angina. Clearly the patient will benefit from restitution of the O_2-carrying capacity by transfusion of packed red blood cells. The already high O_2 saturation cannot be effectively improved upon with supplemental oxygen.

CARBON DIOXIDE CLEARANCE

The principles that govern the clearance of CO_2 from the blood differ in important details from those that apply to the uptake of oxygen. CO_2 is transported in blood in three forms: dissolved in plasma, as ionized bicarbonate, and bound to proteins (notably hemoglobin). If is far more soluble (20-fold more) than O_2 in plasma; hence plasma carries a significant portion of the total CO_2 transported in blood. The other two transport mechanisms take place within red blood cells. CO_2 is converted to bicarbonate ion after reacting with H_2O to form carbonic acid (H_2CO_3), a reaction that is catalyzed by the enzyme carbonic anhydrase present in red blood cells. Carbonic acid rapidly dissociates to H^+ and HCO_3^-. This is quantitatively the most important form of CO_2 transport in the blood. CO_2 forms carbamino compounds by combining with the amine groups of hemoglobin and other circulating proteins. The binding of CO_2 to hemoglobin is more closely linear than is the case for oxygen. Hence there is practically no upper limit, as there is for oxygen, to the amount of CO_2 that can be cleared from the bloodstream.

SUGGESTED READING

1. American Physiology Society. The Respiratory System. Vol. 4. Sec. 3. Bethesda, MD: APS, 1987:147–172.
2. Leach RM, Treacher DF. The pulmonary physician and critical care: 6. Oxygen transport: the relation between oxygen delivery and consumption. Thorax 1992; 47:971–978.
3. Leff AR, Schumacher PT. Respiratory Physiology: Basics and Applications. Philadelphia: Saunders, 1993.
4. Murray JF. The Normal Lung: The Basis for Diagnosis and Treatment of Pulmonary Disease, 2d ed. Philadelphia: Saunders, 1986.
5. Riley RL, Cournand A. ''Ideal'' alveolar air and the analysis of ventilation-perfusion relationships in the lungs. J Appl Physiol 1949; 1:825–847.
6. Samsel RW, Schumacher PT. Oxygen delivery to tissues. Eur Respir J 1991; 4:1258–1267.
7. West JB, Dollery CT, Naimark A. Distribution of blood flow in isolated lungs: relation to vascular and alveolar pressures. J Appl Physiol 1964; 19:713–724.
8. West JB. Respiratory Pathophysiology—The Essentials, 4th ed. Baltimore: Williams & Wilkins, 1992.
9. West JB. Respiratory Physiology—The Essentials, 5th ed. Baltimore: Williams & Wilkins, 1995.

5

Host Defense Mechanisms of the Lung

Herbert Y. Reynolds
Pennsylvania State University
Milton S. Hershey Medical Center
Hershey, Pennsylvania

INTRODUCTION

Humans can live in a great variety of habitats. Some may be natural but possess a polluted atmosphere, while others are transiently extreme, such as in the air, where airline passengers breathe pressurized air, under water, where scuba divers breathe compressed gases, or in an intensive care unit, where patients on assisted ventilation breathe oxygen-enriched air. Whatever the challenge, the respiratory system is amazingly adaptable and efficient in oxygenating blood, eliminating waste gases, and protecting itself at various environmental extremes. This task of eliminating or minimizing adverse effects from inhaled airborne particles or toxic gases is a breath-to-breath effort involving components spaced along the entire respiratory tract from the portals of air entry to the alveolar epithelial surface (Fig. 1). Pollutants are not always external but can be present in nasooropharyngeal secretions that may be aspirated into the airways or as microbial toxins carried in blood that perfuses the lung's vasculature. Nonetheless, injury to the lung from airborne toxins or from proliferation of bacteria on the mucosal surface of the airways is surprisingly infrequent for healthy people. Exposure to microbes, however, is incessant.

Aside from nuisance viral infections of the upper tract that humans experience often, serious infection with bacteria or opportunistic microbes is uncommon. Repeated infections are unusual and suggest that some component in the defense apparatus is not functioning in an optimal way. A clinician must recognize when a pattern of recurrence or propensity for certain infections develops in a patient, so that an impairment in host defense will be considered and steps taken to diagnose the condition and to initiate appropriate therapy. This chapter will primarily review the major components of respiratory host defenses. Table 1 outlines various syndromes and diseases where there is a deficiency or malfunction of an airway structure or cellular and/or immune component of host defense. At the end of the chapter, a case of a patient with repeated respiratory infections is presented to illustrate the evaluation of such patients. The "Suggested Reading" list

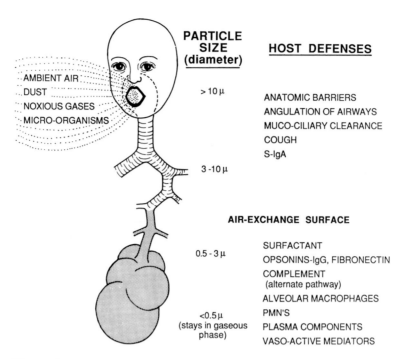

PARTICLE SIZE (diameter)

HOST DEFENSES

AMBIENT AIR
DUST
NOXIOUS GASES
MICRO-ORGANISMS

> 10 μ

ANATOMIC BARRIERS
ANGULATION OF AIRWAYS
MUCO-CILIARY CLEARANCE
COUGH
S-IgA

3 -10 μ

AIR-EXCHANGE SURFACE

0.5 - 3 μ

SURFACTANT
OPSONINS-IgG, FIBRONECTIN
COMPLEMENT
(alternate pathway)
ALVEOLAR MACROPHAGES

<0.5 μ
(stays in gaseous phase)

PMN'S
PLASMA COMPONENTS
VASO-ACTIVE MEDIATORS

Figure 1 A dynamic interplay exists between the influx of particles and potentially injurious substances in inhaled air or in aspirated nasopharyngeal and gastric secretions and the various defense components spaced along the respiratory tract designed to eliminate or neutralize the toxicity and harm of intruders. (Modified from Reynolds HY. Host-defense impairments that tend to respiratory infections. Clin Chest Med 1987; 8:339–358).

Table 1 Diseases of Host Defense Organized by the Component of Host Defense Presumed to Be Altered or Impaired

Level of host defense	Identified defects	Examples of syndromes or diseases
1. Anatomic barriers	Impaired swallowing and glottic closure	Central nervous system disorders: cerebrovascular disease; seizure disorders; degenerative diseases (e.g., Parkinson's disease)
		Neuromuscular diseases (e.g., amyotrophic lateral sclerosis, polymyositis)
	Congenital or acquired anatomic defects of the tracheobronchial tree	Congenital bronchial cartilage deficiency (Williams-Campbell syndrome)
		Tracheobronchomegaly (Mounier-Kuhn syndrome)
		Yellow-nail syndrome (lymphedema, bronchiectasis, yellow nails due to ? lymphatic obstruction)

Table 1 Continued

Level of host defense	Identified defects	Examples of syndromes or diseases
		Pulmonary sequestration (non-functioning pulmonary tissue supplied by an anomalous artery)
		Relapsing polychondritis
	Bypass of anatomic barriers	Tracheostomies and endotracheal tubes
2. Mucociliary clearance	Inherited ultrastructural defects of the cilia	Immotile cilia syndrome (ciliary dyskinesia syndrome). Includes Kartagener's syndrome (bronchiectasis, sinusitis, and situs inversus)
	Viscid mucous	Cystic fibrosis
	Miscellaneous disorders	Young's syndrome (infertility from obstructive azoospermia, sinopulmonary infections, and impaired mucociliary clearance with normal cilia, no cystic fibrosis)
3. Immunological mechanisms	Humoral	Congenital agammaglobulinemia (Bruton's)
		Selective deficiency in subclasses of IgG
		Common variable immunodeficiency
		IgA deficiency (either alone or combined with IgG subclass deficiencies)
		Complement deficiencies
	Cellular	DiGeorge syndrome (absent thymus)
	Congenital	
	Acquired	Purine nucleoside phosphorylase deficiency
		Ataxia-telangiectasia syndrome
		Severe combined immunodeficiency
		Wiskott Aldrich syndrome
		Human immunodeficiency virus infection
		Lymphomas
		Iatrogenic immunosuppression
4. Phagocytic cells	Neutropenia	Primary (rare), or secondary (common)
	Impaired generation of toxic oxygen radicals	Chronic granulomatous disease
	Impaired fusion of lysosomal granules	Chediak-Higashi syndrome
	Impaired chemotaxis (? impaired lymphocyte regulation)	Hyperimmunoglobulin E syndrome (Job's syndrome)

refers the interested reader to more in-depth discussions of these disorders. The reader is also referred to Chap. 34.

Awareness that a coordinated system of defense existed in the respiratory tract was heightened and made popular as a research area through systematic animal and human research. Subsequently, many investigators have contributed to the description of the components of the system. The author has reviewed this general topic previously and is indebted to many colleagues; their collective help is appreciated greatly.

OVERVIEW

As illustrated in Fig. 1, a human inspires ambient air that can be loaded with aerosolized microbes, dust particles, and noxious gases. Nasooropharyngeal secretions or regurgitated gastric contents can also enter the airways, especially by aspiration, which may occur in normal people during sleep. Aerosolized particles of small size, between 1 and 3 μm, can be carried to the alveolar surface in the inhaled airstream. Many microbes are of this critical size. Protecting against this influx is a complex network of anatomic barriers, mechanical clearing devices, and a cellular-humoral immunological system. Several different mechanisms are operant in each segment of the airways, such that redundancy is part of this fail-safe, interactive system. As an example, a microbe attempting to attach to a tuft of cilia on an airway epithelial cell might be coughed away, brushed away by beating cilia, detached by a secretory immunoglobulin antibody that interposes a proteinaceous barrier, or captured by a surface macrophage. A similar scenario can occur in the nasal passages. Sneezing can forcefully dislodge a foreign object that alights on the nasal mucosa, rhinorrhea can wash it away, or secretory IgA antibody can neutralize it or prevent adherence.

For brevity, nasal defenses are not reviewed, but they are important because sinusitis, middle ear infections, rhinitis, and nasal obstruction from polyps characterize many of the diseases to be discussed. Moreover, therapeutic control of the nasal part of the illness is almost always needed to gain similar control over the lower airway problem.

Anatomic barriers in the nose, pharynx, larynx, and conducting airways (trachea down to the respiratory bronchioles) combine to do several things that minimize the entry of foreign objects, particles, and nasopharyngeal secretions into the major airways. Reflex closure of the glottis largely prevents aspiration. Angulation and branching of air passages divert the airstream causing particulates to deflect and impact on the mucosal surface at bifurcations. Intermittent cough clears the airways but probably does not remove debris from the alveolar surface. Ciliary action continuously sweeps mucus and debris up along the airways, which is then swallowed or expectorated as needed.

Host protection mechanisms embedded within the airway lining and mucosa, depicted in Fig. 2, merge two roles of defense: (1) physical removal or neutralization of microbes or allergens or (2) initiation of an immunological response to an antigen(s), whereby antibodies are formed or cells activated so that immune readiness is established for future challenge. However, this immune response can become inappropriately excessive and stimulate allergic cells and mediators creating hypersensitivity reactions or asthma. Learning to modulate immune reactions that would promote host protection but not create airway disease is an area ripe for important research advances.

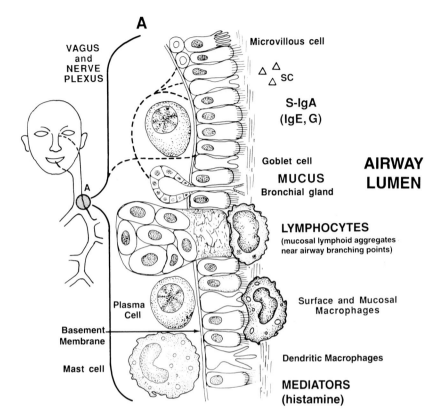

Figure 2 Enlargement A represents a portion of the mucosal and submucosal surface of the major conducting airways as found along the trachea and bronchi further down. The pseudostratified epithelium is depicted as a single layer of cells but is much more complex. Abbreviations: SC, secretory component; S-IgA, secretory immunoglobulin A; IGE, G, immunoglobulins E and G. (Modified from Reynolds HY. Pulmonary host defenses—state of the art. Chest 1989; 95:223–230S.)

Conducting Airways

This segment of the respiratory tract extends from the subglottic area where the trachea begins down to the respiratory bronchioles that connect with the alveolar structures. As mentioned, the multiple, dichotomous branching of the airways causes particles gliding in the laminar flow of air to deflect at corners and impact against the mucosa of ciliated epithelial mucosal cells and mucus-secreting cells. The mucociliary apparatus and cough largely remove them. However, the conducting airways also contain an elaborate immune system that is essential for secondary protection of the lungs, if the more mechanical components do not perform a complete job.

As illustrated in Fig. 2, which depicts a portion of the wall of a major airway, the lining surface that includes the submucosa and mucosa is very complex. The outer layers of the bronchial walls secrete substances onto the mucosal surface. These secretions have been recovered for analysis by selective airway washings or by bronchoalveolar lavage. In the deeper level of the submucosa beneath the lamina propria, bronchial glands and goblet cells interspersed in the epithelium produce mucus that acts as a lubricant of sorts for the cilia to move in, as well as creating a protective film to cover the airway surface. Excessive irritation from toxic fumes, microbes or their secretory products, allergic reactions, and inflammation stimulate secretion of mucus that can become excessive and viscous. This is designated as sputum when expectorated. Inappropriate fluid regulation from defects in cell channels, as found with cystic fibrosis, further alters mucosal secretions.

Beneath the mucosal surface reside lymphocytes and mast cells that make up important parts of the immunological system. Lymphocytes can be dispersed along the submucosal space or reside as collections within discrete structures identified as lymphoid tissue. Several distinctions should be made. Lymphocytes that differentiate into B cells and plasma cells are involved with production of immunoglobulin molecules, especially IgA, the predominant immunoglobulin in the conducting airway secretions. In contrast to serum IgA, which is primarily monomeric, most IgA in secretions is dimeric—two IgA molecules polymerized by J chain—and is associated with secretory component, a protein that binds with dimeric IgA during the process of active secretion of IgA by epithelial cells. The resulting complex is termed *secretory IgA* (sIgA). Other immunoglobulins can be identified in lesser amounts in the respiratory tract. IgG, including all four subclasses, is produced locally and can also transudate from circulating serum immunoglobulin. Small amounts of IgE are present in respiratory secretions even in normal subjects. IgE bound to high-affinity IgE receptors on resident mast cells located in the epithelium can, in turn, link to inhaled antigen. The antigen binding triggers the release of histamine and other mediators that are important in the immediate and late-phase responses to antigen challenge.

A variety of lymphoid structures are in contact with the respiratory tract—adenoidal-tonsillar tissue, lung hilar lymph nodes, intrapulmonary nodules, bronchial associated lymphoid tissue (BALT), lymphoid aggregates, and detachable lymphocytes on the alveolar surface. These last lymphocytes account for about 5% of the alveolar surface cells retrieved with lung lavage. Lymphocytes are also clustered in the mucosa of distal airways around branching points in loose aggregations of cells that do not have a very defined architectural structure, as is found in a lymph node. Along large bronchi, lymphocytes can be organized into discrete structures as BALT, though the presence of BALT is very species-dependent and is sparse in humans. Dendritic cells are numerous in the epithelium of distal airways, constituting about 1% of the cell types in the epithelium near the respiratory bronchioles and on the alveolar surface. These macrophage-like cells process antigens and seem similar to macrophages as antigen-presenting cells to lymphocytes, initiating an immune response.

The conducting airways terminate with the respiratory bronchioles that connect with the acinar ducts and then with the alveoli. This is a fascinating portion of the respiratory tract because the bronchioles create a choke point for airflow and contain important immunological structures. Lymphatic vessels originate here and provide drainage for alveolar epithelial lining fluid and egress for cells, such as alveolar macrophages and lymphocytes, that go to regional lymph nodes. The density of dendritic cells is high in the nearby epithelial layer and lymphoid aggregates are close by. Because the flow of air virtually ceases at this location in the airways, contact with antigen can be high and immune responses may be facilitated, occasionally to the detriment of the host. For example, bronchiolitis obliterans—a potentially life-threatening inflammatory disorder of the lung—is recognized to occur with infection and with forms of diffuse interstitial pneumonitis, connective tissue diseases, graft-versus-host reactions, and noxious fume exposure.

Defects in the host defense mechanisms of the conducting airways can lead to recurrent infections that can eventually result in irreversible scarring and deformation of the bronchi. Bronchiectasis is characterized by high-resolution computed tomography (HRCT) findings of bronchial wall thickening and luminal dilatation (see Chap. 11). The clinical manifestations are airflow limitation, chronic cough, and expectoration of mucopurulent and tenacious sputum. These may be the initial symptoms and findings that lead to the recognition of acquired or congenital defects in humoral immunity, ultrastructural defects in the cilia, or cystic fibrosis.

ALVEOLAR SPACE–AIR EXCHANGE SURFACE

The respiratory tract is designed to effectively oxygenate the blood and eliminate waste gases. Host defenses assist this process by cleansing ambient air so that it is largely devoid of noxious gases, particles, and microbes. The process is not perfect, but the lower airways of normals are reasonably sterile, and purified, humidified air reaches the alveolar surface. As depicted in Fig. 3, upper respiratory tract (URT) defenses and aerodynamic filtration eliminate all but a few microorganisms. Those that elude URT defenses must pass the gauntlet of many others in the alveolar spaces. However, there may be a few microbes indigenous to the alveoli that can be activated and cause infection. As an example, *Pneumocystis carini* may reside in alveolar type I cells, and immunosuppression, corticosteroid therapy, or malnutrition may permit proliferation and illness.

In general terms, there are three levels of alveolar defense: (1) resident cellular and soluble components of the alveoli; (2) immune activation of resident macrophages; and (3) recruitment of other inflammatory and immune effector cells. These levels of defense can be mounted selectively or together to form a full inflammatory reaction. Bacteria, as an example, can bump along alveolar walls with respiration and acquire coating with the epithelial lining fluid (ELF). ELF is a complex mixture of surfactant, serum proteins, immunoglobulins, cytokines, histamine, nitric oxide, and other materials. Fragments of fibronectin, surfactant, and IgG can serve as opsonins. With inflammation and the influx of plasma proteins, complement components can enter the alveoli and become opsonins. The value of opsonization is that this promotes receptor-mediated attachment to phagocytes, facilitating ingestion. Also, certain antibody opsonins can fix complement and initiate a lytic process that might destroy the microbe. These mechanisms are particularly important for clearing encapsulated bacteria, especially if type-specific antibody is present. The organisms may be lysed, or their phagocytosis by alveolar macrophages and polymorphonuclear neutrophils (PMN), may be expedited by opsonization.

Lymphocytes can be detached from the alveolar surface with lung lavage; when analyzed, the T lymphocytes are a mixture of T helper cells (CD4) and suppressor cells (CD8) in an approximately 1.5:1 ratio. Other important subsets of lymphocytes are natural killer (NK) cells (probably inactive in normals), and B cells and plasma cells that produce immunoglobulins. Some microbes can exist within macrophages as intracellular pathogens, either obligatory or facultative. A macrophage must be in a heightened or activated state in order to kill or contain these microbe(s) effectively. Activation can be created by stimulatory effects from cytokines produced by nearby lymphocytes. A subset of T lymphocytes (T helper cells) can activate macrophages with interleukin 1 and other cytokines. Thus, macrophage activation is an important response for the lung's containment of *Mycobacterium tuberculosis, Legionella pneumophilia, Pneumocystis carinii*, an array of important viruses (cytomegalovirus and the human immunodeficiency virus), and cer-

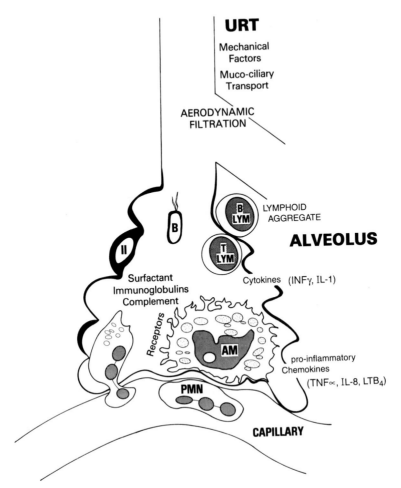

Figure 3 Clearance of bacteria (B) that escape the upper respiratory tract (URT) and reach the alveolus (represented by enlargement of one) is complex. A bacterium deposited in an alveolus may encounter three different but coordinated sets of immunological materials that can destroy it— opsonins or complement factors that hasten phagocytosis or create lysis, activated macrophages stimulated by cytokines from nearby lymphocytes, and other inflammatory phagocytic cells, usually polymorphonuclear neutrophils (PMN), attracted into the alveolar space by proinflammatory chemokines produced locally by macrophages primarily. (Modified from Reynolds HY. Respiratory infections may reflect deficiencies in host defense mechanisms. Disease-A-Month 1985; 31:1–98).

tain fungi. If the macrophages alone cannot contain a particular intracellular organism, an added option by the host is to mount a granulomatous response.

A large inoculum of microbes, or microbes of special virulence, requires additional phagocytes to control the alveolar infection. PMNs are recruited into the alveoli. One mechanism for attracting PMNs into the alveoli is by secretion of chemotactic substances that cause an influx of PMNs from a pool of marginated cells that are adherent to the vascular side of the endothelium of lung capillaries. Alveolar macrophages produce three major chemotactins: tumor necrosis factor, interleukin-8, and leukotriene B_4. Other cells in the airway mucosa can also secrete some of these cytokines. The exact signal(s) that initiate recruitment of PMNs by the alveolar macrophage or other cells is unclear. Macrophages can also reverse the process with a substance that inhibits PMN function. The lungs (and the host generally) seem especially susceptible to aerobic gram-negative bacilli and fungi when the host is leukopenic and immunocompromised. Thus, PMN may be required to suppress colonization and infection with *Pseudomonas aeruginosa* and *Aspergillus* sp., as examples.

RECOGNITION AND CHARACTERIZATION OF DEFECTS IN HOST DEFENSE

Selective malfunction of one or more of the host defenses of the respiratory tract, whether from a congenital or an acquired process, may predispose to recurrent sinopulmonary infections (Table 1). Some deficiencies, if correctly diagnosed, are amenable to replacement therapy or to preventive strategies that can reduce morbidity. Abnormalities in host defense should be suspected if a patient has recurrent sinopulmonary infections, severe pneumonia, evidence of significant sequelae from such episodes (e.g., bronchiectasis), or an opportunistic infection. The type of infection will provide clues as to the type of host defense abnormalities that may be present and will guide subsequent diagnostic evaluation as well as preventive strategies (Table 2). Because many host defense defects are genetic disorders, a family history of similar illness should be sought.

The evaluation should include a detailed history that provides information regarding the health status of siblings, the possibility of infertility, HIV risk factors, or a striking change in respiratory health that may signal the onset of an acquired abnormality. Preliminary screening tests might include microbial cultures of respiratory secretions, a sweat chloride test, and quantitative serum immunoglobulins, including subclasses of IgG. Subsequent testing, depending on initial findings, may include subtyping of blood lymphocytes, secretory IgA sampled in parotid fluid or nasal wash samples, assessment of ciliary clearance with an aerolized tracer, nasal mucosal biopsy for electron microscopic ultrastructural analysis of cilia or sperm motility in males, and documentation of bronchiectasis by HRCT. An evaluation by an otolaryngologist may be helpful to assist in the assessment and management of recurrent sinusitis, nasal polyps, and otitis media. A clinical case is presented to illustrate these concepts.

Table 2 Altered Host Defenses and Associated Pulmonary Infections

Type of host defense defect	Associated infections
Humoral (B lymphocyte) deficiency	Encapsulated bacteria: *Streptococcus pneumoniae, Haemophilus influenzae*
Cellular (T lymphocyte) deficiency	Bacteria: *Mycobacterium* species, *Nocardia asteroides, Legionella* species
	Viruses: Cytomegalovirus
	Fungi: *Cryptococcus neoformans, Histoplasma capsulatum, Coccidioides immitis*
	Protozoa: *Pneumocystis carinii*
Granulocytopenia or functional granulocyte impairment	Bacteria: *Pseudomonas aeruginosa, Klebsiella pneumoniae, Staphylococcus*
	Fungi: *Aspergillus* species

Case Presentation*

A 29-year-old single male was referred for complaints of coughing up small amounts of bright red blood every few days for the preceding several months. He reported similar episodes of recurrent hemoptysis over a 15-year interval. Radiographic evidence of bronchiectasis in his left upper lung and a bulla in his right lower lobe were present ever since an episode of pneumonia at age 14.

On review of his medical history, he had had respiratory infections since infancy—for which he often received antibiotics—including recurrent otitis media, bronchitis, and probably sinusitis. Infections were less frequent after he went to school and were not incapacitating until the severe pneumonia at age 14 years. As a child, he had mumps and chickenpox. He was a life-long nonsmoker. Nasal polyps were removed several years before this evaluation, and maxillary sinus drainage was done twice. He had no known allergies. He worked in an office and had no obviously hazardous environmental exposures. There were no significant family illnesses except that both of his parents had asthma. His sister and a younger brother had been healthy, although his brother had recently developed asthma.

At age 17 years, he was evaluated thoroughly for recurrent bronchitis and pneumonia. A sweat chloride test to evaluate for cystic fibrosis was normal. An open lung biopsy of the left midlung was initially interpreted as consistent with eosinophilic granuloma and he was treated with oral corticosteroids for several years. Later review of the slides judged the process to have been bronchiolitis obliterans with organizing pneumonia (BOOP) (see Chap. 29). During the preceding 10 years, his health had remained generally stable except for episodes of self-limited hemoptysis and bouts of upper or lower respiratory tract infections for which he had taken a variety of broad-spectrum oral antibiotics.

On examination, he was a thin, pale, energetic-appearing male. His weight was 64 kg and height 169 cm; vital signs were normal. Positive findings included nasal septal deviation and polyps observed in both nostrils, left minithoracotomy scar, clear lungs on auscultation, no cardiac abnormalities, no abdominal organomegaly, and prominent clubbing of his digits and toes but no cyanosis.

He brought medical records that included pertinent test results from 3 to 5 years previously. An antineutrophil cytoplasmic antibody (ANCA), rheumatoid factor, and antinuclear factor were all negative. The erythrocyte sedimentation rate was 18 mm/h; sputum cultures were negative for acid-fast bacilli; liver function tests were normal; and the complete blood count (CBC) showed a hematocrit of 32%, a hemoglobin of 11.4 g, a white cell count of 8000/UL, and an MCV of 89.

Before planning further evaluation, it was important to formulate a reasonable differential diagnosis based on the patient's detailed history and extensive medical records. In summary, this young adult had a lifelong history of recurrent respiratory infections involving the upper and lower respiratory tracts as well as bronchiectasis as the probable cause of his intermittent hemoptysis. However, there was no unifying diagnosis to explain his propensity for sinopulmonary infections. The frequency and chronicity of his infections suggested a fundamental defect in his immune defenses but not a life-threatening one.

---

* I gratefully acknowledge the patient's consent to include his case summary in the chapter, as well as his review of the presentation for accuracy.

Because of his youth and unmarried status, risk factors for HIV infection, recreational drug use, travel exposure, and medication allergies were rigorously excluded. Patients who have chronic hemoptysis usually accept and deal with its occurrence, so the frightening aspects of a first-time hemoptysis were not present. Therefore, management and further diagnostic evaluation could be orderly and not done under emergency conditions. An immediate bronchoscopy was not indicated. This patient said that every time he presented to a new pulmonologist with his history of hemoptysis, he was advised to have fiberoptic bronchoscopy. He thought he had received 10 such procedures.

Approach to Management and Diagnosis

The first consideration was to minimize the patient's cough and hemoptysis and to quiet down the inflammatory locus in his bronchiectatic airways responsible for the latest episode. Use of a mild cough suppressant (benzonatate USP); a 5-day course of trimethoprim/sulfamethoxazole; and some reduction of his strenuous work and exercise regimen were suggested. He was instructed about what to do if unusually severe hemoptysis should occur. Further diagnostic evaluation was based on a broad differential diagnosis including ciliary defects causing ciliary dyskinesia, cystic fibrosis, and deficiencies in humoral immunity, particularly deficiencies in IgA and/or subclasses of IgG.

Defects in mucociliary clearance are associated with otitis media, sinusitis, bronchitis, and bronchiectasis. Inherited disorders of ciliary function are referred to as the *immotile cilia syndrome*, though the term *ciliary dyskinesia syndrome* is more accurate, as the cilia in these disorders may have some movement. The ultrastructural defect of these immotile or dyskinetic cilia is usually the absence of dynein arms in the central core of the cilium, though other ultrastructural defects have also been reported. Kartagener's syndrome is a subset of the immotile cilia syndrome, defined by the triad of bronchiectasis, sinusitis, and *situs inversus* in association with absent dynein arms. This patient did not have situs inversus, but this does not exclude a ciliary disorder. Further diagnostic tests that were considered included examining a semen specimen for immotile spermatozoa or electron microscopy of nasal mucosal scrapings to look for ciliary ultrastructural abnormalities. A semen specimen would also evaluate for Young's syndrome—a combination of obstructive azoospermia and repeated sinopulmonary infections with no ultrastructural defects of the cilia and a normal sweat chloride test. These patients usually present in infertility clinics, as their respiratory problems are usually mild. The basis of impaired mucociliary clearance in patients with Young's syndrome is not known.

Cystic fibrosis (CF) seemed possible in this patient, although he had never had any digestive problems, had no family history, and had a reportedly normal sweat chloride analysis at age 17 years. *Pseudomonas* sp. had only recently been isolated from sputum cultures. Was this still a tenable diagnosis? Most patients with CF have, in addition to recurrent otitis media, sinusitis, lung infections, and nasal polyposis—a suggestive family history—although a firm diagnosis in distant relatives and siblings may not be established. Patients who are diagnosed with CF at an older age have usually had few gastrointestinal problems in infancy. Frequent respiratory infections usually direct attention to the diagnosis, especially if mucoid *Pseudomonas aeruginosa* is isolated from sputum cultures. A few CF patients can have normal sweat electrolytes. On the other hand, sweat chloride can be increased in a variety of other diseases and in older subjects. Although considerable progress has been made in elucidating the genetic defect responsible for the abnormal transport of electrolytes across epithelial cell membranes, genotyping for the cystic fibrosis transmembrane conductance regulator (CFTR) alone does not suffice to make the diagnosis conclusive because of the many mutations and the effect of counteracting gene mutations. Only the combination of two cystic fibrosis mutations combined with a compatible clinical manifestation or family history is sufficient for diagnosis. Retesting sweat electrolytes, and performing genotyping would be reasonable in the case presented. If these were inconclusive, sinus films to evaluate for pansinusitis, nasal potential-difference measurements, and semen testing with subsequent testicular biopsy to document obstructive azoospermia would be indicated (see article by Stern in Suggested Reading).

The patient had not had any formal evaluation of his humoral and cellular immunity. Skin tests that would assess delayed-type reactivity and measurement of serum immunoglobulins had apparently not been done. Two types of immunoglobulin deficiency could be considered: (1) an absence of IgA, specifically secretory IgA that is secreted onto the mucosal surfaces, or (2) IgG deficiencies, including deficiency of one or more of the IgG subclasses. It is probably not the deficiency in immunoglobulins per se that leads to repeated infections but rather the presence of impaired antibody responses to foreign proteins and polysaccharides. For example, isolated IgA deficiency is the most common of the primary immunodeficiency disorders (1 in 700 persons). The absence of IgA, however, may have little consequence and remain unrecognized, as it is not often associated with infections.

Recurrent upper and lower tract respiratory infections are found in some patients who have low serum IgA levels. In the absence of serum IgA, no detectable levels of secretory IgA are found. In contrast, even with a normal amount of serum IgA, secretory IgA can be absent because the secretory component is missing and the immunoglobulin cannot be transported onto the mucosal surface. The susceptibility of subclasses of IgA– IgA_1 and IgA_2 to enzymatic degradation in the mucosal secretions might be a factor promoting colonization of certain bacteria.

While IgA is the predominant immunoglobulin in the conducting airways, IgG is the major immunoglobulin in the alveolus and accounts for as much of 10% of the total protein recovered from alveolar lavage. Not surprisingly, then, repeated pneumonias can be the presenting problem of acquired and congenital disorders associated with low levels of IgG in the serum. Absence of one or more of the four subclasses of IgG has been associated with repeated pulmonary infections even if the total concentration of serum IgG is normal. Certain IgG subclass deficiencies can be linked with selective IgA deficiency, possibly explaining repeated infections in these patients. A deficiency of IgG_2 is important, as antibodies generated against capsular polysaccharide antigens from common bacteria such as *Haemophilus influenzae* type B, *Streptococcus pneumoniae*, and *Pseudomonas aeruginosa* are found in this subclass. Among 65 patients (4) with bronchiectasis of undetermined etiology, 31 patients (48%) had low serum values for one or more subclasses of IgG, with 19 being deficient in IgG_2; only three were for IgG_4. Normal values for concentrations of IgG subclasses can vary from laboratory to laboratory, and apparent ''deficiencies'' may be laboratory artifacts. As the purpose of immunoglobulin replacement therapy is to compensate for impaired antibody formation rather than just to correct a deficiency, this therapy should be reserved for those patients with demonstrated inability to form antibodies in response to antigen challenge. The physician must also remember that there is a risk of anaphylactic transfusion reactions to intravenous infusions of immunoglobulin in IgA deficient patients.

Other possible defects were considered for this patient. Several syndromes could reasonably be excluded based on the nature of the patient's infections and health status.

Although he had had respiratory infections from infancy, he developed and grew normally. The broad category of severe primary congenital immunodeficiency states is very unlikely, given his age and relatively localized sites of infection. For example, a defect in the complement pathway (classical) generating C_3b is associated with episodes of septicemia with encapsulated bacteria. Illness from pneumococcal sepsis (*Streptococcus pneumoniae*) or meningococcemia (*Neisseria meningitis*) often herald this deficiency. When a primary phagocytic disorder is present, the affected person may have recurrent pyogenic abscesses, especially involving the skin and hair areas. For the case described, such host defects did not fit the pattern of isolated sinopulmonary infections.

Dénouement

The outcome of this patient's case was resolved in an unexpected way. After an initial evaluation, an assessment of his humoral immunity seemed appropriate because this was the one area of host defense that had not been evaluated. A humoral immunodeficiency was a reasonable explanation for the recurrent sinus infections and bronchiectasis. A complete blood count, quantitative serum immunoglobulins, and IgG subclasses were obtained (Table 3).

About a week later, the patient began to have copious hemoptysis of bright red blood and felt light-headed upon standing. He was slightly orthostatic and his hematocrit was 17% (30% before). After stabilization and transfusion of two units of packed erythrocytes, a chest radiograph revealed a new consolidation in the left midlung area. A chest CT demonstrated bilateral tubular bronchiectasis in both lungs, but more extensive in the left upper lung; the prior 3-cm cavity in the right lower lobe was noted. However, in the posterior segment of the left upper lobe, a new cavity was found with a nodular tissue density within it. This lesion was consistent with a mycetoma, or "fungus ball." Fiberoptic bronchoscopy revealed blood coming from the left mainstem bronchus; coughing precluded a thorough inspection of other airways. In order to stop the bleeding and hemoptysis, selective bronchial artery embolization was considered. However, because of the extent of possible bronchiectatic-site bleeding and the apparent fungus ball in the left upper lobe, it was decided to perform a surgical excision of the left upper lobe.

The patient underwent a successful thoracotomy for removal of the left upper lobe and recovered without postoperative problems. The pathologist's findings included bronchiectatic airways, an inflammatory mass described as an aspergilloma within a distorted lobar bronchus, and several large vessels adjacent in the cavity. Erosion of one of these vessels or bleeding from granulation tissue in the bronchiectatic cavity's wall could have been the source of bleeding.

Table 3 Serum Immunoglobulin Values of the Patient in the Case Presentation

Interval	IgM	IgA	IgG	G_1	G_2	G_3	G_4
Initial visit	124 mg/dL (45–250)	164 mg/dL (85–385)	493 mg/dL (564–1765)				
			660 mg/dL (620–1475)	396 (350–1100)	168 (100–800)	46 (10–200)	10 (2–250)
6 weeks			691	354	156	38	10
Postsurgery							
1 year	—	—	723	427	237	42	14
2 years	—	—	723	454	207	49	12

The patient did well after surgery and had no further hemoptysis. Although his serum IgG values were low and the IgG$_4$ quite low, a decision was made not to begin intravenous IgG replacement therapy immediately. Rather, it was elected to see how he did following the lung resection and to observe the IgG levels. He has done well in the 3 years since surgery. He has not been troubled by lung infections and has had no hemoptysis. For his nasal polyposis, he was prescribed a regimen of intranasal corticosteroids and cromolyn plus a decongestant. Immunization with pneumococcal vaccine was done, and yearly influenza vaccines have been administered.

In conclusion, this patient's propensity for sinopulmonary infections was probably related to a relative deficiency of IgG. His serum levels of IgG subclasses have remained low although stable for several years. He has not had further difficulty with infections. The decision to follow him without any immunoglobulin replacement therapy has seemed appropriate.

SUGGESTED READING

1. Beck CS, Heiner DC. Selective immunoglobulin G$_4$ deficiency and recurrent infections of the respiratory tract. Am Rev Respir Dis 1981; 124:94–96.
2. Buckley RH, Schiff RI. The use of intravenous immune globulin in immunodeficiency diseases. N Engl J Med 1991; 325:110–117.
3. Davis PB, Drumm ML, Konstan MW. Cystic fibrosis—state of art. Am J Respir Crit Care Med 1996; 154:1229–1256.
4. DeGracia J, Rodrigo MJ, Morell F, Vendrell M, Miravitlles M, Cruz MJ, Codina R, Bofill JM. IgG subclass deficiencies associated with bronchiectasis. Am J Respir Crit Care Med 1996; 153:650–655.
5. Liles WC, Van Voorhis WC. Review: nomenclature and biologic significance of cytokines involved in inflammation and the host immune response. J Infect Dis 1995; 172:1573–1580.
6. Reynolds HY, DiSant'Agnese PA, Zierdt CH. Mucoid *Pseudomonas aeruginosa*—a sign of cystic fibrosis in young adults with chronic pulmonary disease. JAMA 1976; 236:2190–2192.
7. Reynolds HY. Host defense impairments that lead to respiratory infections. Clin Chest Med 1987; 8:339–358.
8. Reynolds HY. Integrated host defenses against infections. In: Crystal RC, West JB, Weibel ER, Barnes PJ, eds. The Lung: Scientific Foundations, 2d ed. Philadelphia: Lippincott-Raven, 1997:2352–2365.
9. Reynolds HY. Lung inflammation: normal host defense or a complication of some diseases? Annu Rev Med 1987; 38:295–323.
10. Reynolds HY. Respiratory infections may reflect deficiencies in host defense mechanisms. Disease-A-Month 1985; 31:1–98.
11. Rosen FS, Cooper MD, Wedgewood RJP. The primary immunodeficiencies. N Engl J Med 1995; 333:431–440.
12. Rossman CM, Forrest JB, Lee RMKW, Newhouse MT. The dyskinetic cilia syndrome—ciliary motility in immotile cilia syndrome. Chest 1980; 78:580–582.
13. Stern RC. The diagnosis of cystic fibrosis—current concepts. N Engl J Med 1997; 336:487–491.
14. Sturgess JM, Chao J, Turner JAP. Transposition of ciliary microtubules—another cause of impaired ciliary motility. N Engl J Med 1980; 303:318–322.
15. Sturgess JM, Chao J, Wong J, Aspin N, Turner JA. Cilia with defective radial spokes—a cause of human respiratory disease. N Engl J Med 1979; 300:53–56.
16. Walzer PD. *Pneumocystis carinii*—pneumonia in patients without human immunodeficiency virus infection—editorial. Clin Infect Dis 1997; 25:219–220.

6

The Respiratory System: History

Gerald S. Davis and Theodore W. Marcy
University of Vermont College of Medicine
Fletcher Allen Health Care
Burlington, Vermont

Information gathered from the patient provides essential clues to diagnosis and an invaluable guide to the progression of pulmonary diseases. Although time-consuming, a detailed and carefully recorded respiratory history is an essential part of the evaluation and medical management of a patient with respiratory disease. This chapter provides an overview of obtaining and interpreting historical information from patients and their families. It is closely linked with other chapters that deal with specific symptoms such as dyspnea (Chap. 14) or cough (Chap. 15). Each chapter about specific diseases also discusses the symptoms of that disorder. The information on obtaining an occupational and environmental exposure history supplements the chapters on occupational parenchymal lung diseases (39), hypersensitivity pneumonitis (40), and occupational and environmental airways disease (38).

The information provided by patients is, by its nature, "subjective," not "objective." It is colored by the perceptions, fears, and hopes of the patients, their friends, and their families. Because it is their view of the truth, it will be modified by their educational background, mood, and memory. Nonetheless, their perceptions of symptoms are of great importance, because these sensations are what bother them and bring them to medical attention. Regardless of whether the practitioner views a symptom as trivial or life-threatening, the patient views the complaint as worthy of relief.

SYMPTOMS OF RESPIRATORY DISEASE

Dyspnea

Difficulty breathing (shortness of breath, dyspnea) is the cardinal symptom of respiratory disease. Chapter 14 presents the physiological basis and evaluation of dyspnea in detail. The practitioner should inquire about dyspnea in an open-ended manner in order to gain an overview of the patient's symptoms (e.g., "Do you ever feel short of breath?"). A series of focused questions should then expand the information by defining the timing, duration, environmental surroundings, severity, and associated symptoms that characterize dyspnea for this patient, as listed in Table 1.

Table 1 Patient Information About Dyspnea

Time of onset
Stable or progressive since onset
Association with exertion
Degree of exertion needed to produce symptoms
Occurrence at rest
Occurrence at night
Continuous and predictable, or intermittent
Occurrence in particular environments
Associated symptoms
Actions that provide relief
Time required for recovery

The beginning of the symptoms of dyspnea can be dated with precision by some patients with acute illnesses or with rapidly changing diseases. For many patients with chronic respiratory diseases, such as emphysema or idiopathic pulmonary fibrosis, the onset of symptoms was insidious, and they cannot recall exactly when impairment began. An episode of unusually intense exercise or activity may unmask symptoms for many patients with gradually progressive disease. Swimming in the summertime, a mountain hike, deer hunting, household relocation, or a major housecleaning may uncover symptoms hidden by a more sedentary lifestyle. Patients often have difficulty estimating whether their dyspnea is stable or changing. Helping them to recall specific, recurrent activities and comparing performance may focus these symptoms.

Dyspnea is associated with exertion in almost all instances, since increased metabolic demands require increased respiration. Dyspnea associated with exertion may be caused by a high level of work of breathing imposed by flow resistance or low compliance, respiratory muscle weakness, inefficient (wasted) ventilation, and/or hypoxia as perfusion-ventilation matching worsens with increased pulmonary blood flow. Consequently, patients almost always report their symptoms of dyspnea in the context of effort or exertion. Dyspnea at rest is usually a symptom of severe respiratory impairment and marks the end stages of all chronic lung diseases. Acute episodes of asthma, laryngeal dysfunction syndrome, pulmonary edema, or exacerbations of chronic obstructive pulmonary disease (COPD) can produce episodes of dyspnea at rest.

It is useful to relate symptom severity to the intensity of exertion needed to produce it, and common activities can be used to calibrate symptoms. Stair climbing (e.g., ''Do you stop on the stairs, stop at the top, stop with packages?''), walking up hills, walking on the level (''Do you go more slowly than your friends, stop to rest, sit down to rest?''), and housework-or job-related tasks (''Do you make the beds, do laundry, carry packages, lift boxes?'') provide common, frequently repeated opportunities for exertion. Specific activities and the severity of symptoms (''Do you stop or keep going?'') should be recorded. A detailed discussion of symptoms will provide an understanding of how a patient has modified his or her lifestyle to accommodate dyspnea (''What have you stopped doing because of your breathing?''), and accordingly what impact lung disease has had on their lives (''What would you like to do if your breathing was better?'').

Dyspnea that occurs during sleep (nocturnal dyspnea) or immediately upon awakening implies particular causes and may provide important clues to diagnosis. The horizontal body position (orthopnea) may suggest cardiac pulmonary edema, severe emphysema with diaphragmatic compression from the abdomen, or gastroesophageal reflux. Sudden awakening with a gasp or snort may reflect obstructive sleep apnea. Asthma that is poorly controlled often causes nocturnal symptoms and may present as awakenings, awareness of wheezing during awakening for other reasons, or difficulty breathing upon arising in the morning. A spouse, roommate, or sleeping partner can provide valuable insight about nocturnal symptoms.

The symptoms of dyspnea associated with chronic destructive or fibrotic lung diseases are usually predictable for the patient and relatively constant from day to day. A particular task will elicit similar symptoms every day. Most patients experience "good days" and "bad days" related to weather, mood, or other factors, but the actual variation in performance ability is usually slight. Conversely, asthma or other intermittent respiratory diseases may change substantially in severity at different times.

Dyspnea that develops in some environments but not in others may provide important clues to the cause. Allergic asthma with recognized exposures to pets, pollens, or other specific allergens provides an obvious link between dyspnea and the environment. Occupational airways disease caused by very low concentrations of odorless chemicals or sensitizing organic materials may have an equally important but less obvious link to environmental exposure. Asthma dominated by a "late" reaction or hypersensitivity pneumonitis that peaks 4–8 h after exposure may be hard to link with the specific exposure that triggered the response. The association, or lack of association, between dyspnea and environmental exposures should be sought and recorded.

Patients with a wide variety of acute and chronic lung diseases will report difficulty breathing upon exposure to cold air, irritants such as chemical fumes or tobacco smoke, and strong odors such as perfume or spices. These symptoms are rarely due to true allergy but rather are a nonspecific irritant response that appears to be common to many respiratory diseases.

Dyspnea may be accompanied by other respiratory symptoms that worsen its impact or provide clues to diagnosis. Wheezing and dyspnea are usually linked in diseases with airflow obstruction. Chest wall or intercostal muscle pain may follow intense breathing efforts. Cough often precipitates dyspnea. Dizziness, light-headedness, faintness, or weakness may accompany dyspnea, particularly if hypoxia, hyperventilation with hypocarbia, or cardiac disease with inadequate cardiac output is the cause.

It is useful to obtain information about the strategies a patient has developed to relieve dyspnea. If the degree of difficulty breathing is purely associated with the intensity of exertion, most patients will respond by cutting back on the speed or intensity of their activities. It is surprising how many patients continue to rush to exhaustion at their former healthy pace and then stop to catch their breath. The advice to walk, climb, or work at a slower pace that does not produce dyspnea may be valuable to them. Relief of dyspnea with medications, such as beta-adrenergic bronchodilators, nitroglycerin, or oxygen, may be helpful in suggesting a possible cause for dyspnea. The lack of relief with medications may also be valuable information.

The time required for recovery from dyspnea may help guide diagnosis and therapy. Breathlessness caused by a high work of breathing or hypoxia associated with exertion usually resolves quickly after the effort ceases, and the patient returns to baseline within one or two minutes. Bronchospasm triggered by exertion (exercise-induced asthma) usually requires 5-10 minutes exertion to induce it, and persists for 10-30 minutes if untreated. Therapeutic oxygen may speed recovery time following exercise hypoxia, as well as relieve the hypoxia during the actual exertion.

Cough

The pathophysiology, features, and treatment of cough are dealt with in detail in Chap. 15. Collecting information about cough is a key element in the respiratory history, as summarized in Table 2. Although objective tests to measure cough have been developed for research studies, no means to measure its intensity or frequency are available for clinical use; thus the patient's description is the only information available. A spouse or friend may have observed cough frequency and can provide additional information. As with dyspnea, the timing of the onset of cough should be sought, and whether it began abruptly or insidiously. The time of day that coughing occurs should be explored, since it may be a clue to a nocturnal respiratory disorder (see above). Cough upon awakening in the morning is typical of chronic bronchitis or bronchiectasis, as the patient "clears out" from his or her chest the secretions that have accumulated overnight. Cough associated with chronic interstitial lung disease may occur throughout the day. It is sometimes important to distinguish whether cough is the only or dominant symptom of a respiratory disorder or whether it is just one of many problems in a symptom complex.

Cough is often triggered by specific activities, usually exertion, laughing, or prolonged speech. Telephone conversation is particularly difficult for some patients. Cough paroxysms that occur during meals or while drinking liquids should raise concern over swallowing difficulty and aspiration. Specific environments may trigger coughing, and most patients who cough will develop symptoms upon exposure to cold air or to intense irritants. Strong odors (perfume, after-shave lotion), chemical fumes (cleansers, solvents, petroleum products), dusts and smoke (sweepings, wood fires, tobacco), and a variety of other irritants often cause coughing. It is important for the practitioner to understand the activities and environmental exposures that cause cough in order to understand the impact of this symptom on the patient.

A patient may cough just once or twice, as though "clearing his throat," and this pattern of coughing often causes them little interruption of other activities. This pattern of coughing is often seen with chronic airways disease of any type or with postnasal drainage. Paroxysms of coughing that last up to several minutes can be physically and socially disabling and prevent other activities while the coughing spell lasts. Interstitial lung disease is often accompanied by paroxysms of cough, although this symptom is not specific for these diseases. Chronic cough may be more annoying or worrisome to family, friends, and coworkers than to the patient; some patients will be forced by their companions to seek medical attention for cough. The pattern and severity of coughing and its impact on other activities should be recorded.

Other symptoms often accompany cough. Breathlessness may follow a cough paroxysm, wheezing may precede or follow coughing, and sputum production is often the pur-

Table 2   Patient Information About Cough

Time when the cough began
Activities and environments that trigger cough
Prolonged paroxysms, or intermittent coughs
Severity of cough
Impact on other activities
Associated symptoms
Actions that provide relief

pose of the cough. Patients with frequent or intense coughing may develop headache, costochondral pain, intercostal muscle pain, or neck and back pain. Spontaneous rib fracture due to coughing is not uncommon in the elderly or those with osteoporosis due to steroid therapy. Cough syncope is rare, but a feeling of faintness or dim vision is common among patients with severe cough. Bladder stress incontinence is a particularly troublesome symptom associated with cough and is very common among older women.

Patients try a variety of strategies in their attempts to relieve coughing. Throat lozenges, hard candy, hot tea, and other food or beverages are often employed to help alleviate cough. Understanding the strategies that work or do not work for each patient may be useful in diagnosing and treating their cough.

Although the health care provider can obtain extensive information about cough symptoms, the features of coughing are almost entirely nonspecific and are generally not helpful in establishing a specific cause or diagnosis (see Chap. 15). Nonetheless, this information may help to elucidate the impact of respiratory disease on the patient and can be used as a guide to disease progression or improvement with therapy.

Wheezing

Wheezing is a musical, continuous sound associated with airflow during expiration and/ or inspiration. Patients are usually aware of wheezing and report a sensation of ''tightness in the chest,'' ''chest pressure,'' ''chest heaviness,'' and difficulty drawing air into or out of the chest. Many patients hear audible musical breathing sounds in their chests, and their companions may also report hearing them wheeze. Parents, spouses, roommates, or sleeping partners may describe the patient's wheezy breathing during sleep. The timing, severity, activities, exposures, associated symptoms, and relief strategies that accompany wheezing should be sought out, as described for dyspnea and cough.

The symptom (or sign) of wheezing implies turbulent or obstructed flow of air through the conducting airways. Although wheezing is the hallmark of asthma, a wellworn adage states that ''all that wheezes is not asthma.'' Within the lower respiratory tract, inflammation or fibrosis within and around bronchi (sarcoidosis, chronic bronchitis), secretions within the airway lumen (bronchiectasis), airway collapse during expiration (emphysema), foreign bodies, extrinsic airway compression, and intraluminal tumor masses can all cause wheezing. Diseases in the larynx or upper airway (tumors, edema, enlarged thyroid gland, laryngeal dysfunction syndrome) can also produce wheezing, sometimes with a harsher tone and an inspiratory emphasis referred to as *stridor*. The symptom of wheezing is often paralleled by distinctive physical examination findings and can be quantitated by direct measurements of airflow.

Sputum Production

Expectoration of mucoid or purulent secretions from the lower respiratory tract is a common symptom of respiratory disease. Normal bronchial mucus (with alveolar epithelial lining fluid) is clear or translucent, glassy, and minimal in quantity. Increased production of mucus occurs in most acute or chronic inflammatory lung diseases, particularly those involving primarily the airways. Normal mucoid sputum changes color to become white, then yellow, and finally green as neutrophils or eosinophils are recruited into the respiratory secretions, die, release peroxidase and other enzymes, and the debris is oxidized in air. It is believed that the intensity of sputum purulence (white $\rightarrow$ yellow $\rightarrow$ green) is

Table 3 Patient Information About Sputum Production

Time when sputum production began
Time of day when sputum is greatest
Color of sputum (clear, white, yellow, green, red)
Bloody sputum (hemoptysis)
Quantity of sputum per day (spoonfuls, cups)
Odor of sputum (foul, fecal)
Mucous plugs or bronchial casts

related to both the abundance of leukocytes and the residence time in the airway before expectoration. Thus, some patients describe daily sputum that is slightly colored upon awakening and then remains white for the rest of the day.

Acute lower respiratory infections are usually associated with cough and the production of sputum that may initially be white and then becomes yellow or green as the illness progresses. Sputum production may continue for weeks, finally tapering off long after the acute illness and its other signs have resolved. Both diffuse inflammatory airways diseases (bronchitis, asthma, cystic fibrosis) and localized conditions (bronchiectasis, pneumonia) can cause sputum production. Sputum is usually not a prominent feature of the diffuse interstitial lung diseases.

Symptoms of sputum production should be recorded in terms of the onset, the time of day it occurs, the quantity of sputum produced per day (teaspoons, tablespoons, quarter cup, full cup), and the color of the sputum at various times (clear, white, yellow, green). A particularly foul or fecal odor should be noted, as it may be associated with anaerobic infection or lung abscess. Mucoid plugs are common in asthma, and distinctive brown-black bronchial casts or "rubber band" mucous plugs are typical of allergic bronchopulmonary aspergillosis. Blood imparts its distinctive red color to sputum and is usually noticed by patients. Smaller quantities of blood may tinge sputum pink, darken its yellow color, or create a brown hue that is less obvious. The management of coughing up blood is discussed in Chap. 21.

Chest Pain

Pains in the chest may accompany other respiratory symptoms or occur alone. The timing, location, quality, and severity of pain should be carefully noted. Table 4 lists features of chest pain to be elicited in the history. A key issue will always be whether the pain could represent myocardial ischemia; thus features of angina pectoris should be sought specifically. After one determines that the pain is *not* substernal, compressive, radiating to the left arm or neck, brought on by exertion or stress, and associated with nausea or sweating, then additional features can be examined. Esophageal pain can also produce similar symptoms, whether from esophageal spasm or acid reflux. Chest pain associated with respiratory diseases usually arise from the bony thorax, the muscles that move the thoracic cage, the pleural surfaces, or the mediastinum. The lung itself rarely causes pain, although some patients describe deep pain or "heaviness" with lung cancer, pulmonary infarction, and other diseases. Pain arising from enlarged mediastinal lymph nodes with pressure on adjacent structures is sometimes described in sarcoidosis or lymphoma.

Chest wall pain typically occurs with movement, respiration, or coughing. The intensity may change with body position and is at its worst immediately after lying down or

Table 4 Features of Noncardiac Chest Pain

Location (central, lateral, posterior, bilateral)
Quality (dull, sharp, burning)
Constant or intermittent
Timing of pain
Associated with respiration
Associated with movement
Related to body position
Activities that bring on pain
Associated symptoms
Actions that provide relief from pain

sitting up, with gradual abatement over several minutes. The pain may be described as ''pleuritic'' in nature, meaning that it resembles pleurisy; it hurts with a deep breath in or out and is absent when the chest is motionless. Any conditions that injure or inflame the chest wall structures can cause pain of this sort. Rib fractures or intercostal muscle strain, common with severe coughing, can mimic irritation of the pleural membrane. Costochondral inflammation (costochondritis) is usually anterior, tender on palpation, and may be associated with a dull ache as well as sharp pain with movement.

True pleurisy is believed to be caused by inflamed pleural membrane surfaces rubbing against one another with respiration or movement. Pleural fluid may separate the inflamed membranes, and pain often decreases as fluid accumulates regardless of cause. The fluid may shift as the patient lies down or sits up, creating new areas of membrane contact and pain. Severe pleural pain can be excruciating and may require narcotic medications for relief. Nonsteroidal anti-inflammatory drugs are helpful and usually are sufficient for the treatment of pleural pain.

Pericardial pain associated with acute pericarditis may mimic pleurisy or accompany it. Pericardial pain is often reported as severe and persistent following a change in body position, then abating until position changes once more. Pain with respiration and sometimes with chest wall movement (twisting, bending) can occur with pericarditis as well, presumably caused by the friction of pleural surfaces against the inflamed pericardium. The pain of pericarditis may be quite difficult to distinguish from pleural pain, and diagnostic studies are usually required.

The features of chest pain may provide important clues to the cause but must be linked with other aspects of the history, with the physical examination, and with other tests. In many instances it is not possible to distinguish chest wall from pleural pain by history alone, and additional studies must be undertaken.

Upper Respiratory Symptoms

Symptoms related to the nasal passages, paranasal sinuses, throat, and larynx (the upper respiratory tract) may accompany disease in the lower respiratory system. Questions should be directed to the symptoms listed in Table 5. Complaints referable to the upper respiratory tract are particular common as the cause, or as the result, of chronic cough. The importance of this area is highlighted in Chaps. 15 and 16 dealing with cough and sinusitis.

Nasal congestion, obstructed airflow through the nose, and mucoid rhinorrhea may

Table 5 Symptoms of Upper Respiratory Tract Disease

Nasal congestion and obstructed air flow
Nasal discharge (mucoid, purulent, or bloody rhinorrhea)
Sinus pressure or pain
Postnasal drainage
Sore throat, tonsillar pain or swelling
Hoarse voice
Dysphagia

---

be associated with chronic allergic rhinitis and nasal polyposis—conditions that require specific treatments. Sinus congestion, pressure, or pain, and mucopurulent drainage may reflect acute or chronic sinusitis. Both rhinitis and sinusitis can be the cause of postnasal drainage, an important cause of chronic cough, sore throat, and hoarseness. Chronic sinusitis and/or allergic rhinitis are common partners of asthma and usually require simultaneous treatment for effective symptom control. Pathology in the larynx may cause coughing as well as hoarse voice and other local symptoms. Dysphagia may result in cough or hoarseness. Repeated gastroesophageal reflux, with acid reaching the level of the larynx, is believed to be an important cause of cough and to produce laryngeal erythema and other changes that suggest the diagnosis. In all instances, evaluation of the patient with cough requires careful questioning and examination regarding the upper respiratory tract.

Constitutional Symptoms

Respiratory diseases may produce systemic effects and constitutional symptoms. A thorough review of organ systems is essential, as discussed below. Although individual constitutional symptoms may accompany particular respiratory diseases, most are entirely nonspecific. Constitutional symptoms related to respiratory disease are summarized in Table 6. Generalized fatigue, poor energy, depression, and slowed cognition often are experienced with chronic hypoxia, and improve with oxygen therapy (see Chap. 22). These symptoms—along with anorexia, weight loss, and cachexia—are common features of lung cancer but may occur in the late stages of any severe lung disease. Patients with chronic pulmonary infection (tuberculosis, lung abscess, chronic cavitary histoplasmosis), severe emphysema, or advanced idiopathic pulmonary fibrosis often experience marked cachexia and report severe fatigue and weight loss.

Fever is common with acute infectious or inflammatory lung disease but is relatively rare with chronic diseases. Persistent daily fevers should prompt a search for chronic infection or neoplasm, as other causes are rare. Weight gain may reflect inactivity as a

Table 6 Constitutional Symptoms Associated with Respiratory Diseases

---

Fatigue, loss of energy
Anorexia, weight loss, cachexia
Fever
Night sweats
Weight gain
Excessive daytime somnolence

---

result of exertional dyspnea. Excessive daytime somnolence is an important symptom of sleep apnea. Thus questions regarding energy, fatigue, sleep, changes in appetite or body weight, and fever are an essential part of the respiratory evaluation.

Review of Systems

A survey of complaints referable to each of the major body organ systems is an important part of the complete respiratory disease evaluation. Constitutional symptoms are frequently associated with pulmonary diseases, as discussed above. Within each body system, specific symptoms may be part of a systemic disease involving the lungs or may be the consequence of a primary respiratory disease. Heart disease can cause dyspnea, cough, and other symptoms similar to those produced by lung disease; thus a careful cardiac history is essential. Gastrointestinal complaints of ''heartburn,'' ''acid indigestion,'' or ''water brash'' may reflect gastroesophageal reflux and be the cause of cough or asthma. Rheumatological symptoms are important because of the associations between many of the collagen-vascular diseases and diffuse parenchymal lung disease (see Chap. 29). Orthopedic impairments place an additional burden on respiratory work with walking or movement. Neurological diseases may be associated with respiratory muscle impairment, dysphagia with aspiration, or disordered control of breathing. Each organ system should be surveyed.

PAST MEDICAL HISTORY, FAMILY HISTORY, AND SMOKING

Past Medical History

Past medical events, or the absence of any previous ill health, affect both the diagnosis and therapy of current respiratory disease. A detailed past medical history is essential in order to understand current complaints. For example, recurrent episodes of lower respiratory infection, rather than a single episode of pneumonia, may imply a generalized impairment of pulmonary host defense mechanisms (see Chap. 5) or a localized anatomic problem such as bronchiectasis.

The past medical history for respiratory disease patients should include recording of (1) any past respiratory illnesses or chronic respiratory diseases, (2) serious medical illnesses in other organ systems, (3) previous hospitalizations, (4) major surgical operations, (5) past experiences with anesthesia, and (6) difficulties with pregnancy or childbirth. The detail with which this information is collected will be guided by the nature and severity of the current complaint, the age of the patient, and other factors.

Family History

A family history of respiratory disease is key information for interpreting a present illness. Open-ended questions regarding any family members with lung disease are useful for general screening proposes. Lung disease in family members may identify a common environmental exposure, such as tuberculosis or antigens responsible for hypersensitivity pneumonitis. Many lung diseases have well-recognized inheritance patterns, and unique molecular genetic alterations have been identified for several of them. Specific inquiries for a family history of cystic fibrosis, emphysema (alpha$_1$-protease inhibitor deficiency), idiopathic pulmonary fibrosis, hereditary hemorrhagic telangiectasia, lung cancer, or tuberculosis exposure are important if the patient presents with compatible disease.

Tobacco Smoking History

Smoking is the source of much of the respiratory disease seen throughout the world. Information about past or current tobacco smoking is essential for all patients with respiratory complaints. Even if the patient does not have a disease directly linked to tobacco as a cause—such as chronic bronchitis, emphysema, or lung cancer—smoking will adversely influence both the symptoms and the successful treatment of most other respiratory diseases.

The smoking history should identify the never smoker as well as the former smoker and current smoker. Cigarette, pipe, and cigar use should be noted; the ages of starting and stopping should be recorded. The total cumulative cigarette smoke exposure dose may be a useful estimate of the severity of chronic obstructive pulmonary disease, although there is great individual variation in the response. Total exposure is usually expressed in cigarette "pack-years," calculated as the number of packs of cigarettes smoked per day multiplied by the number of years the person has smoked. Thus, a person who began smoking at age 16, averaged $1\frac{1}{2}$ packs per day, and is still smoking at age 58 would have accumulated 63 pack-years of cigarette exposure.

Exposure to second-hand smoke should be noted for nonsmokers. Contact with tobacco smoke in the home or workplace may worsen asthma or other inflammatory airway diseases. Substantial exposure to second-hand or sidestream tobacco smoke has been identified by epidemiological studies as a risk factor for lung cancer among individuals who have never smoked.

OCCUPATIONAL AND ENVIRONMENTAL EXPOSURE HISTORY

A complete occupational and environmental history is essential in order to establish a correct diagnosis of lung disease due to inhalant exposure and also to exclude diseases due to inhaled materials. Complete documentation is required in order to obtain disability or compensation because of occupational lung disease (see Chap. 41). Workers may or may not know what exposures they have experienced. For example, railroad linemen may be unaware of asbestos in brake linings, automobile painters may not recognize isocyanate polymerizing agents, and agricultural workers may not identify specific organic materials as related to their symptoms. It is critical to understand exactly what tasks the worker has performed and what materials he or she has contacted and not merely to record the name of the job or industry. Detailed analyses of industries and exposures are presented in the chapters on occupational lung disease (Chaps. 38, 39, and 40).

The initial occupational history can be obtained in an open-ended manner ("What type of work have you done?"). A more detailed history is recorded by having the patient list each job and worksite with dates in sequence from the beginning of their working lifetimes. This approach often stimulates memories and elicits details that are not produced by the open question. The elements of an occupational and environmental exposure history are summarized in Table 7.

Specific exposures should be explored if other findings suggest particular types of

Table 7 Occupational and Environmental Exposure History

Current work title, industry, and employer
Nature of the work performed
Fumes, dusts, chemicals, or other inhalants in the workplace
Chronological listing of all jobs since childhood
Tobacco smoking history
Type of home residence
Heating and/or air conditioning systems in the residence
Hobbies with exposure to fumes, dusts, or inhalants
Exposure to barns, farms, livestock
Pets in the home

---

pulmonary disease. For example, a patient with diffuse pulmonary fibrosis and digital clubbing should be questioned carefully for any possible exposure to asbestos, while a patient with asthma might be questioned about current exposures to organic dusts or chemical polymerizing agents. The practitioner must have extensive knowledge about many different industries and the lung diseases that they cause in order to obtain a detailed history of this sort. Referral to a specialist in pulmonary disease or occupational medicine is often justified for this reason.

An association between respiratory symptoms and work should be examined. This link will be obvious in some instances, as symptoms develop promptly upon exposure. For example, an immediate (early) asthma reaction to western red cedar or toluene diisocyanate is likely to be recognized by the carpenter or the car painter. Workers who develop respiratory symptoms at home at the end of the workday may fail to associate them with the occupational exposure. Thus reactions that are delayed 4–8 h after the exposure—as may occur with a late asthma reaction or with hypersensitivity pneumonitis—may not be linked with their cause. Chronic diseases with a gradual onset may be related to continuous or daily exposure to sensitizing agents or may be the result of a mineral dust exposure that occurred decades previously.

Workers should be questioned in detail about the timing of their symptoms. As presented by Kline and Schwartz in Chap. 38, on occupational airway disease, dyspnea, wheezing, or cough may increase across the work shift or may be maximum on Mondays and gradually decrease as the week progresses. Evening symptoms on days with particular or unusual work exposures may help identify the cause. Freedom from symptoms while away from the workplace (weekends, vacations, alternate job assignments) is as notable as symptoms on the job. As with other groups of respiratory symptoms, information should be sought about fever, constitutional symptoms, the duration of symptoms once they develop, and what measures help to relieve symptoms.

The symptoms of occupational asthma, hypersensitivity pneumonitis, and industrial bronchitis are linked to current exposures. These conditions worsen if exposures increase, and the symptoms disappear when exposure stops. Years of exposure may go by before the worker becomes sensitized or symptoms develop, but current symptoms are almost always linked with ongoing current exposure. Thus, when one of these conditions is suspected, detailed information should be collected about the current job and the exposures to dusts or fumes that go with it.

The symptoms of mineral-induced diffuse interstitial lung disease are gradual in onset and usually slow in progression. For coal workers' pneumoconiosis, asbestosis, silicosis, and other diseases caused by inorganic particles and fibers, the symptoms do not develop until prolonged cumulative inhalation exposure has taken place, usually decades after the exposure began, and in some instances not until decades after the exposure ends. For these reasons, the historical information collected from pneumoconiosis patients should focus on the exact details of work exposures that occurred 20–40 years previously.

Environmental exposures that occur in the home or through hobbies should be examined as diligently as those in the workplace. Hypersensitivity pneumonitis can develop from moldy hay used to feed riding horses or from avian antigens spread by pet parakeets or homing pigeons. Home carpentry and furniture refinishing can cause asthma from exposure to cedar or varnish hardeners. Pottery making or stone sculpture carving can produce enough exposure to cause silicosis, although rarely. The family members of asbestos or beryllium workers may develop lung diseases from substances brought into the home on work clothes. Home insulation can cause substantial exposure to asbestos, with consequent pleural or parenchymal lung disease.

A detailed chronological work and exposure histories are not needed for every patient. Often the nature of their disease or their bland job exposure allow occupational lung diseases to be excluded.

MEDICATION USE HISTORY

Current Medications

The treatments and medications a patient is receiving currently for any and all medical problems are essential components of the respiratory history. Many drugs can cause severe lung disease, whether idiosyncratic adverse effects (pulmonary infiltrates with eosinophilia) or expected dose-related effects (bleomycin). For each medication, the brand name (or generic name), route, dose, and frequency prescribed should be listed. Topical and ophthalmic preparations must be included, since they can be absorbed systemically. For example, eyedrops causing beta-adrenergic blockade can worsen asthma. Current respiratory medications, whether scheduled or used intermittently, should be listed. Prescription and nonprescription medications for any other medical conditions should be recorded. The key points in a medication history are listed in Table 8.

Many patients use herbal, naturopathic, or traditional medicines to augment the allopathic prescription medications offered by their physicians. Their use of multivitamins, high-dose single vitamins, and herbal or organic products should be noted. This information is important because these preparations may create side effects or interact with pre-

Table 8 Medication History

Current respiratory medicines (dose, frequency)
Current medicines for all other conditions
Herbal or naturopathic medicines
Complaints or adverse effects of current medications
Medication use techniques
Compliance with medications
Previous experiences with respiratory medicines
Allergies or adverse reactions to medications

scribed therapy. It is also important because gathering this information recognizes the patients' beliefs and their participation in their treatment.

Undesirable side effects from medications should be sought and noted. Inhaled corticosteroids may cause sore throat, hoarse voice, or oral candidiasis. Theophylline may cause wakefulness, tremor, nausea, and other adverse effects. Oral corticosteroids and cytotoxic agents carry many unpleasant and sometimes dangerous side effects. The perception and severity of adverse effects from drugs may influence greatly the patient's willingness to comply with treatment as prescribed.

Medication Use and Compliance

Correct technique for the use of a metered-dose inhaler (MDI) is an essential skill for patients receiving inhaled medications. Spacer devices, breath-triggered MDI canisters, and updraft air-powered nebulizers may help to improve technique and effective delivery for patients who have difficulty with standard MDI units. It is of vital importance to instruct patients in the proper techniques for administering inhaled medications and then to observe their skills and document proper usage.

It is useful to inquire whether patients have had previous experience with treatments for their current complaint. A favorable response to medication in the past may predict future success. For example, an antibiotic that provided prompt relief with no adverse effects during a previous episode of acute bronchitis may be a wise choice for the future. It is also useful to know about medicines that a patient believes were not effective or previously caused unpleasant effects.

Compliance with medication usage is a problem for virtually all patients with chronic diseases. Gathering information about how a patient is actually taking medications is an essential part of the respiratory history. Very direct questions ("You are taking your medicine the way I prescribed it for you, aren't you?") will usually lead to affirmative, sometimes fabricated responses. A nonjudgmental open-ended question ("How do you take each of these medicines?") is preferable. One should also inquire whether a patient has stopped taking any medicines, either because of adverse effects, apparent lack of efficacy, inconvenience, or expense. It has been estimated that patients with chronic illnesses and multiple medications achieve appropriate drug dosing on fewer than 50% of days, and that only about 15% of patients achieve appropriate therapy on greater than 80% of days. It is helpful to have patients bring all of their current medicines with them to an office visit and then to have them indicate exactly how and when they take each one. The disparity between the prescribed or planned usage and the actual usage is often remarkable!

Drug Allergies and Previous Adverse Events

Allergic or anaphylactic reactions to any drugs should become a prominent part of the patient's medical record. Previous experiences with drugs that caused adverse events should also be recorded. It may be difficult for a patient to know with certainty whether an adverse reaction to a drug involved true allergy (e.g., hives and wheezing immediately upon taking penicillin), an idiosyncratic response (e.g., erythromycin hepatotoxicity), or a dose-related expected effect (e.g., bleeding while receiving warfarin). The health care provider should record the details of the adverse event ("Codeine made me nauseous!")

not just the patient's conclusion about the cause (''I'm allergic to codeine!''). Subsequent experiences with similar agents should also be noted.

CONCLUSIONS

A large amount of useful information can be gained by asking patients about their diseases, how they have treated them, and what impact they have on their daily lives. Armed with this information, the practitioner can help them to manage their pulmonary diseases more successfully. Obtaining a complete and useful respiratory system history is time-consuming and requires considerable knowledge in many fields as well as diligence in pursuing many questions. The effort is worthwhile.

SUGGESTED READING

1. Chung KF, Lalloo UG. Diagnosis and management of chronic persistent dry cough. Postgrad Med J 1996; 72:594–598.
2. Cochrane GM. Compliance and outcomes in patients with asthma. Drugs 1996; 52:12–19.
3. Corlett AJ. Aids to compliance with medication. BMJ 1996; 313:926–929.
4. Irwin RS, Curley FJ, French CL. Chronic cough: the spectrum and frequency of causes, key components of the diagnostic evaluation, and outcome of therapy. Am Rev Respir Dis 1990; 141:640–647.
5. Kohler CL, Davies SL, Bailey WC. Self-management and other behavioral aspects of asthma. Curr Opin Pulm Med 1996; 2:16–22.
6. Manning HL, Schwartzstein RM. Pathophysiology of dyspnea. N Engl J Med 1995; 333:1547–1553.
7. Patrick H, Patrick F. Chronic cough. Med Clin North Am. 1995; 79:361–372.
8. Piirila P, Sovijarvi AR. Objective assessment of cough. Eur Respir J 1995; 8:1949–1956.
9. Seamens CM, Wrenn K. Breathlessness: strategies aimed at identifying and treating the cause of dyspnea. Postgrad Med 1995; 98:215–216.
10. Widdicombe JG. Neurophysiology of the cough reflex. Eur Respir J 1995; 8:1193–1202.

7

Physical Examination of the Respiratory System and Thorax

Gerald S. Davis and Theodore W. Marcy
University of Vermont College of Medicine
Fletcher Allen Health Care
Burlington, Vermont

This chapter reviews the basic tools of physical examination of the thorax. Examples of specific diseases are used to illustrate patterns but do not provide a comprehensive summary of abnormalities. The physical findings related to specific respiratory diseases are presented in the individual chapters discussing these diseases. A more detailed approach to the physics of lung sounds and their application to diagnosis is offered in Chap. 8. There is no substitute for directly seeing, feeling, or hearing the physical findings of human pathology. This chapter may serve as an adjunct to or reminder of the real thing.

INSPECTION

Physical examination of the patient with respiratory disease begins at first contact. The apparent degree of difficulty breathing, ease of speech, rapidity of movement, speed walking, cough, audible wheezing, and general appearance of vigor or ill health are often evident as the patient enters the examination room. In some instances, a diagnosis of respiratory disease can be made about a stranger across a room or riding on a bus. These clues to the nature of a pulmonary disorder should not be ignored but rather focus and direct the traditional quartet of inspection, palpation, percussion, and auscultation.

The patient's appearance, apparent age, hygiene, and general state of health should be noted. Difficulty breathing, coughing, noisy respiration, pursed-lip breathing, or obvious distress should be recorded. Breathing is usually not apparent in healthy subjects who are dressed and sitting quietly; thus obvious respiration at rest is abnormal. Most people can comfortably speak 20–30 words in a phrase. A shortened length of phrase while speaking is an indication of dyspnea, weakness, or reduced vital capacity. These features of the respiratory examination can be assessed with the patient dressed—during initial contact or while obtaining the history.

For direct examination, the patient should be seated comfortably on an examining table or bed with feet hanging down. The patient should not sit with her legs extended, as this will require holding herself with the abdominal muscles or by other supports and will change normal respiratory patterns. In both office and hospital, it is desirable to have the patient turn to sit on the side of the examining table or the bed. This position allows the practitioner to stand directly behind the patient in order to examine and compare both sides of the chest simultaneously. The patient should sit in as relaxed a position as possible, with shoulders and hips placed symmetrically. If possible, the hands should rest in the lap, and not be supporting the patient. Bracing with the hands will fix the shoulders and limit assessment of the use of the accessory muscles. Ideally, the patient should be naked above the waist for thorough examination of the thorax, as any clothing will impair inspection and prevent accurate percussion and auscultation. A hospital-style gown that opens in the back can be provided for modesty or warmth and moved aside as needed.

Cyanosis—a bluish discoloration of the lips, face, fingers, or toes—reflects the presence in the skin of blood bearing blue-red desaturated hemoglobin rather than blood with the bright cherry-red color of hemoglobin that is well saturated with oxygen. Cyanosis should be noted if it is present but is not often a useful or reliable sign. Cyanosis is a more accurate index of peripheral venous stasis, poor cardiac output, or peripheral vasoconstriction than of arterial oxygen desaturation. Children who have played too long at the beach or swimming pool are routinely cyanotic but not hypoxic. Cyanosis may be particularly difficult to assess under fluorescent artificial light. Because of its wide availability, low cost, and accuracy, digital oximetery should be utilized routinely to directly measure oxygen saturation for all respiratory disease patients, regardless of whether or not cyanosis is suspected.

The Appearance of the Thorax

In normal subjects the thorax is symmetrical and the spine is straight in the midline of the posteroanterior plane. A slight dorsal anterior curve (kyphosis) of the spine complements the posterior curve (lordosis) of the lumbar spine. The trachea and sternum are centered in the midline. The thorax expands and deflates symmetrically with respiration in both the anterior and the lateral planes in normal subjects.

The visible trachea in the neck may shift from the midline as a result of either traction or pressure on the intrathoracic structures. Unilateral thyroid enlargement, unilateral mediastinal masses or lymph nodes, large pleural effusions, or pneumothorax with tension may push the trachea away from the side of disease. Lobar atelectasis, unilateral fibrosis, or surgical pneumonectomy may pull the trachea toward the side of the problem. Any deviation of the course of the trachea should be noted.

Many diseases can produce asymmetry and dysfunction of the thoracic skeleton. Congenital deformities creating protrusion of the sternum (pigeon breast, pectus carinatum) or depression of the sternum (funnel chest, pectus excavatum) may be cosmetically displeasing to the patient but rarely compromise respiration unless they are severe. Adolescent spinal scoliosis may cause few respiratory problems at a young age but become limiting in the elderly. Severe kyphoscoliosis and/or rotoscoliosis compromises breathing substantially and often causes progressive respiratory failure and cor pulmonale as patients reach their later middle years. Chest wall deformities resulting from trauma, surgery, or unilateral lung disease can also produce impairment of the chest bellows and disordered ventilation. Severe kyphosis associated with osteoporosis and aging can cause similar problems, particularly when linked with emphysema or other parenchymal lung diseases. Any asymmetry, deformity, or abnormal appearance of the chest wall structure or movement should be recorded.

Normal Quiet Breathing

Inspect the movement of the chest during quiet breathing, as this will reflect the patient's degree of difficulty. In healthy subjects, the mouth is closed or slightly opened for nasal breathing. Normal respiration is evident with careful observation of the naked subject, as gentle thoracic cage and abdominal movements can be seen. With normal quiet breathing, the primary muscles of inspiration (the diaphragm and the intercostal muscles) are used predominantly. The accessory muscles of respiration (strap muscles of the neck, shoulder girdle, rectus abdominis) are not utilized or only tense slightly to fix the position of the thoracic cage. The thorax is stationary or moves outward slightly with inspiration, while the abdomen expands as the diaphragm descends. The thoracic and abdominal movements are synchronous and coordinated. The shoulders and neck are quiet and do not appear to participate significantly in breathing. Expiration is passive and hardly apparent. Expiration requires a slightly longer time than inspiration, and there may be substantial pauses between breaths. Normal people breathe at rest 8–15 times each minute. The respiratory rate at rest without speaking should be recorded.

Increased Work of Breathing or Respiratory Distress

The primary muscles of respiration are used more vigorously and the accessory muscles are recruited as the work of breathing increases. The ribs expand outward more obviously with inspiration. The shoulders lift to expand the thorax; the neck, jaw, and lower face become tense; the mouth opens; the back straightens; and the excursions of the abdomen increase. In slim patients, particularly those with inspiratory airflow obstruction, retraction of the intercostal spaces and supraclavicular fossae appears with inspiration. Expiration may also be obvious, showing tensing of the abdominal musculature, forceful descent of the shoulders, and compression of the thorax by the intercostal muscles. Expiration may be rapid with diseases that increase lung elastic recoil, or greatly prolonged in diseases with air flow limitation. The use of accessory muscles of respiration should be assessed by inspection, possibly aided by palpation as described below.

Paradoxical breathing is an important sign of respiratory muscle weakness or respiratory failure (see Chap. 19). Respiratory paradox can often be assessed more easily with the patient supine or semirecumbent rather than seated. With paradoxical breathing, the thorax and abdomen move in opposite directions rather than in unison. This sign usually represents severe diaphragmatic fatigue in the patient with respiratory failure who does not have a primary neuromuscular disease. The chest wall and accessory muscles assume dominant responsibility for breathing, while the diaphragm relaxes or contracts dyssynchronously. With inspiration, the thorax expands and the shoulders rise, while, at the same time, the abdomen sinks. On occasion, some diaphragmatic contraction may occur and bulging of the abdomen may be seen after chest expansion is complete. This process leads to very inefficient breathing because the abdominal contents, rather than inspired air, move to fill the negative-pressure space created in the thorax. With expiration, a reverse pattern is seen and the abdomen may bulge as the chest is compressed.

Different patterns of paradoxical respiration may be seen in patients with primary neuromuscular diseases, depending on which muscle groups are involved. For example, patients with midcervical spine injuries may have preserved diaphragmatic function but a loss of intercostal and accessory muscle function. In these patients, inspiration is exclu-

Table 1   Features of Digital Clubbing

Thickening of the soft tissues of the distal phalanx
Downward curve to the nail plate
Loss of cuticle angle (Lovibond's angle)
Softening of the tissue proximal to the nail plate
Hyperemia and warmth of the fingertips

sively diaphragmatic, and the chest sinks passively as the abdomen expands. Expiration is largely or exclusively passive and depends on the elastic recoil of the lung.

The impression of respiratory distress should always be recorded. The use of accessory muscles, active expiration, or paradoxical breathing should be noted. Worsening of these signs may be an important feature of deteriorating respiratory failure, while improvement in these signs reflects improving strength and respiratory reserve.

DIGITAL CLUBBING

An alteration of the shape and characteristics of the tips of the fingers and toes known as "clubbing" is an important sign associated with several specific lung diseases. Digital clubbing is also seen with congenital heart diseases of the types that cause right-to-left shunting and chronic hypoxemia, sometimes seen with hepatic fibrosis, and may be associated with other conditions rarely. The features of digital clubbing are summarized in Table 1, and are illustrated in Fig. 1.

An early change of clubbing is softening of the tissues beneath and proximal to the nail plate, so that the nail seems to float and feel spongy when pressed. Another early change is a loss of the normal 160-degree angle between the nail plate and the soft tissue of the cuticle, or Lovibond's angle. As clubbing progresses, this angle straightens to 180 degrees or more and may become inverted to form part of a smooth curve from the skin

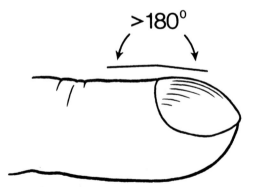

Figure 1 Digital clubbing. Nail clubbing is characterized by thickening of the tips of the digits, softening of the tissues beneath the nail plate, and a downward curved shape to the cuticle and nail. The root of the nail and the nail bed is normally at angle of 160 degrees, but with digital clubbing this angle is lost and may become reversed to greater than 180 degrees.

across the nail. The nail plate achieves a rounded, downward-curved shape that is often the most obvious sign of clubbing. The soft tissues of the tip of the finger or toe become thickened so that the distal phalanx is thicker than the middle phalanx. Additional changes can include redness and warmth of the fingertips, presumably reflecting increased blood flow. All fingers and toes are usually involved, although early changes may be more apparent in some digits than others.

Digital clubbing is part of the symptom complex known as hypertrophic osteo-arthropathy, characterized by distal extremity bone tenderness, arthralgias predominantly in the wrists and ankles, and clubbing. The tenderness along the distal shafts of the long bones of the extremities is explained by new growth of the periosteum at these sites. This can be detected by elevation of the periosteal membrane along the distal tibia, radius, or ulna seen on bone radiographs or by increased radiotracer uptake at these sites seen on bone scintigraphy. Clubbing is often seen alone, while the other features of the syndrome are less common.

Clubbing of the fingertips is virtually painless, although patients sometimes report stiffness and clumsiness. The other features of hypertrophic osteoarthropathy may be quite disabling, with severe aching and soreness of the affected joints and bony sites. The full-blown syndrome of hypertrophic osteoarthropathy is fairly common in patients with lung cancer and may require specific therapy. Primary treatment of the tumor often reduces the symptoms. Nonsteroidal anti-inflammatory drugs may help relieve the arthropathy. Local radiotherapy, pamidronate, or subcutaneous octreotride have been utilized in a few severe resistant cases.

Digital clubbing, sometimes with symptomatic hypertrophic osteoarthropathy, is common with all cell types of bronchogenic carcinoma (see Chap. 32). Clubbing is *not* seen as a feature of emphysema or chronic bronchitis alone; thus the finding of digital clubbing in a patient with chronic obstructive pulmonary disease (COPD) should always prompt a search for neoplasm. Tumors arising outside of the chest do not (as a rule) cause clubbing, but isolated pulmonary metastasis may produce the condition. Clubbing is virtually universal among patients with cystic fibrosis (see Chap. 34) and it usually progresses in parallel with the severity of suppurative lung disease. Bronchiectasis without cystic fibrosis can also produce clubbing, and the two features appear to parallel one another in severity. Clubbing can be found in patients with chronic bacterial lung abscess, but it is surprisingly rare among patients with cavitary tuberculosis. Clubbing is a common finding among patients with idiopathic pulmonary fibrosis and has been linked (loosely) with the rapidity of disease progression and/or the extent of smooth muscle proliferation evident on lung biopsy (see Chap. 29). Clubbing is also a common feature of asbestosis (see Chap. 39). The finding is very rare with all other chronic diffuse parenchymal lung diseases, although it is reported occasionally. Thus, sarcoidosis, bronchiolitis obliterans, eosinophilic granuloma, and interstitial pneumonitis with collagen-vascular diseases almost never manifest digital clubbing. It is entirely unclear why asbestos produces clubbing frequently, while silica, coal, talc, and other minerals do so very rarely. Recent reports describe occasional cases of digital clubbing attributed to human immunodeficiency virus (HIV) or acquired immunodeficiency syndrome (AIDS) infection.

Clubbing occurs with a variety of diseases that do not involve lung tissue, as listed in Table 2. Congenital heart disease with venous-arterial right-to-left shunts involving the heart or the great vessels cause digital clubbing in almost all cases. Chronic liver disease, particularly hepatitis or hepatic fibrosis, can cause clubbing. Occasional cases have been

Table 2 Diseases Associated with Digital
Clubbing and Hypertrophic Osteoarthropathy

Pulmonary diseases
    Bronchogenic carcinoma[a]
    Extrathoracic cancer metastatic to lung[a]
    Mesothelioma[a]
    Cystic fibrosis
    Bronchiectasis[a]
    Chronic lung abscess
    Idiopathic pulmonary fibrosis
    Asbestosis
    Arteriovenous malformations
Cardiovascular diseases
    Congenital heart disease (venous-arterial shunt)
    Aortic prosthetic grafts (infected)[a]
Miscellaneous
    Congenital/hereditary
    Liver disease with fibrosis[a]
    HIV infection
    Other diseases (rarely)

---

[a] Hypertrophic osteoarthropathy is common.

described in patients who had infected or noninfected prosthetic aortic vascular grafts and in patients with Takayasu's arteritis. Hereditary digital clubbing may develop in childhood and persist for life with no evidence of associated disease; a dominant pattern of inheritance within the family is usually found.

The pathophysiology of clubbing, and why it appears in certain conditions but not others, is not understood. It has been theorized that the responsible growth-promoting substance(s) could be produced locally in the lung at sites of tumor, inflammation, or infection. Alternatively, substances could be produced systemically that are normally deactivated by passage through the pulmonary circulation but allowed to reach the arterial circulation when major right-to-left shunts are present. Clubbing is reversible and sometimes regresses after successful treatment of a primary lung cancer or following lung transplantation for idiopathic pulmonary fibrosis.

The physical sign of digital clubbing should always be recorded, and it may be helpful to note the severity of clubbing for individual digits. Similarly, the absence of clubbing is an important finding, and should be recorded for patients with COPD, chronic diffuse parenchymal lung disease, occupational lung diseases, or chronic infections of the lung.

PALPATION

Palpation of the chest, neck, and extremities is used to assist inspection in assessing pulmonary diseases. Palpation will be used to explore sites of reported pain, tenderness, or a newly discovered mass and to examine the neck, supraclavicular fossae, and axillae for enlarged lymph nodes.

Hands placed lightly against the chest can sometimes feel the low-pitched vibrations of secretions in large airways (rhonchi, see below) more easily than these sounds can be heard. Palpation may detect the subtle "crunch" of subcutaneous emphysema (air in chest wall soft tissues) associated with spontaneous or iatrogenic pneumothorax or pneumo-mediastinum. Hands placed lightly around the base of the neck can sometimes perceive tensing of the sternocleidomastoid muscles with inspiration that exceeds normal and represents a subtle indication of the use of accessory muscles of respiration.

The symmetry of expansion of the chest can be gauged visually by standing behind the patient, placing the hands lightly just below the shoulder blades, and observing their excursions with inspiration and expiration. Slight inequality between the right and left sides can sometimes be appreciated more easily by the examiner watching and feeling his or her own hands than by visual inspection alone. Asymmetry in the resting position of the thorax or during inspiration can be seen with a pneumothorax, a large pleural effusion, or lobar atelectasis (see details below and in Table 3).

Tactile fremitus, the palpation of vibrations generated with speech, is used to assess the intensity of transmission of centrally generated sounds through the lung parenchyma. Either the flat palm of the hand or the ulnar edge of the hand and fifth digit are placed against the lower posterior lung fields or other sites of interest. Both sides of the chest are usually assessed simultaneously and symmetrically for comparison. The patient is instructed to speak repeatedly in a rather loud, deep voice that creates reproducible vibrations. Repeating the number "ninety-nine . . . ninety-nine" is easy and reliable. In a normal subject, the examiner will perceive a light vibration that is the same on both sides. The vibration disappears as the hands are moved below the diaphragm or over the shoulders. The intensity of vibration varies greatly with the loudness of speech, the pitch of the voice (women with high-pitched voices may generate minimal tactile fremitus), the thickness of the chest wall (obese subjects may generate little fremitus), and the location on the chest (greatest near the trachea).

Sound generated centrally, speech in the larynx, must travel through air, tissue, and several air/tissue interfaces before reaching the hands or ears of the examiner. Because air is a relatively poor conductor of sound vibrations and because air/solid interfaces absorb substantial sound wave energy, central sounds are transmitted poorly to periphery and the chest wall. Water or tissue is an efficient conductor of sound, and transmits vibrations more intensely than air. Consolidation of alveolar spaces with fluid or collapse of airless lung increase the transmission of sounds originating centrally, while overexpansion of lung tissue diminishes transmission. As a result of these phenomena, tactile fremitus is usually increased over a consolidated region of lung such as the site of a lobar pneumonia. Fremitus is decreased or absent over lungs with severe emphysema or local sites of large bullae.

Disease states that create additional air/water interfaces or that increase tissue mass outside of the lung parenchyma usually cause a decrease in tactile fremitus. A central obstructing tumor may create partial atelectasis but usually causes decreased tactile fremitus over the portion of the chest distal to the obstruction. Pleural effusion moves the lung away from the chest wall and causes decreased fremitus. Pneumothorax produces greatly reduced or absent fremitus.

Tactile fremitus need not be tested in every patient, but it is a useful tool for helping to sort out physical findings in conjunction with other maneuvers (see "Synthesis," below). It is particularly helpful in distinguishing consolidation from pleural effusion (see Table 4 and Figs. 2 and 3) and defining the border between a pneumonia and a parapneumonic effusion. Decreased fremitus may be useful in the global assessment of a patient with emphysema as a means of estimating the degree of destruction of lung tissue.

Table 3 Patterns of Physical Findings in Selected Diseases[a]

Disease	Inspection	Palpation	Percussion	Auscultation
Pneumonia	Respiratory distress, tachypnea	Local increased tactile fremitus	Local dullness (slight)	Bronchial breath sounds; localized crackles; whispered pectoriloquy
Pleural effusion	Normal; slight ipsilateral expansion	Local decreased tactile fremitus	Local dullness	Decreased breath sounds; pleural rub
Emphysema	Pursed lip breathing; hyperinflation; use of accessory muscles	Diffusely decreased tactile fremitus	Diffuse hyperresonance	Decreased breath sounds; prolonged expiration; wheezing
Asthma	Normal (variable distress, accessory muscles)	Normal	Normal (hyperresonance)	Wheezing, prolonged expiration
Pneumothorax	Respiratory distress; tracheal shift	Ipsilateral decreased tactile fremitus	Ipsilateral hyperresonance	Ipsilateral decreased/absent breath sounds
Idiopathic pulmonary fibrosis	Digital clubbing; tachypnea	Normal (increased fremitus)	Normal (high diaphragms)	Bibasilar crackles (high, end-inspiratory)
Atelectasis	Normal (ipsilateral inspiratory delay)	Decreased fremitus (shift of trachea to affected side)	Local dullness	Decreased breath sounds
Paralyzed diaphragm	Normal	Normal	High diaphragm; no respiratory shift in level of dullness	Absent breath sounds at lung base (high diaphragm) (crackles, egophony)

[a] Findings in parentheses are variable or uncommon.

Table 4 Conditions with Changes in Tactile Fremitus[a]

Increased tactile fremitus
  Thin chest wall, deep voice
  Pneumonia
  Atelectasis without central obstruction
Decreased tactile fremitus
  Thick chest wall, high voice
  Diffuse emphysema
  Localized bulla
  Pneumothorax
  Central bronchial obstruction
  Pleural effusion

---

[a] Abnormalities may be localized over sites of disease.

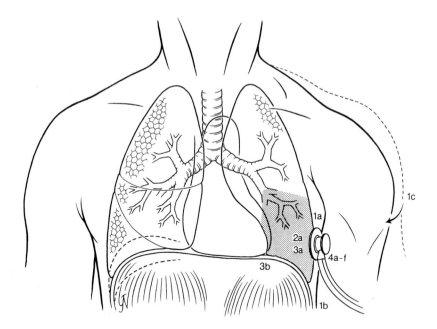

Figure 2 Pneumonia with consolidation. The physical findings of pneumonia are illustrated, although not all signs are always present: (1) **Inspection**—Decreased expansion of the affected side; decreased diaphragm movement; splinting of the affected side; (2) **Palpation**—increased tactile fremitus over the consolidated area; palpable rhonchi (occasionally); (3) **Percussion**—decreased resonance over affected area; decreased diaphragm movement; and (4) **Auscultation**—crackles (rales, crepitations); rhonchi; bronchial breath sounds; egophony; whispered pectoriloquy; pleural friction rub.

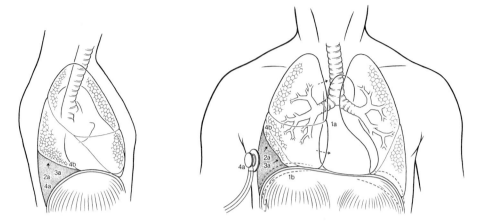

Figure 3 Pleural effusion. The physical findings associated with pleural effusion are shown: (1) **Inspection**—Mediastinal shift away from the disease process; diminished diaphragmatic movement on the affected side; (2) **Palpation**—Absent tactile fremitus over the effusion; (3) **Percussion**—Dullness over the effusion; (4) **Auscultation**—Absent breath sounds over the effusion; bronchovesicular breath sounds, egophony immediately above the effusion.

PERCUSSION

Percussion strikes the chest a sharp, tapping blow to create a drum-like sound. Percussion, or, more correctly, "mediate percussion," uses a finger, plate or "plectrum" laid against the chest as a surface to strike against, and then a finger of the opposite hand or a "percussion hammer" to strike the blow. Small, rubber-tipped hammers and thin metal, wood, or tortoiseshell plectrums were commonly used in former times. Currently, percussion is almost always performed with the hands alone, but these other tools may help examiners who find the technique difficult.

The art of percussion was first described by Leopold Auenbrugger (*On Percussion of the Human Chest* . . . , 1761) and popularized by Corvisart, physician to Napoleon I, in the early years of the nineteenth century. Auenbrugger, the son of an innkeeper in Graz, Austria, returned from his medical studies in Vienna and observed his father judging the level of wine in his cellar casks by tapping on them. The student applied this concept to the human chest filled with pleural fluid and later published his findings, "submitting to my brethren the fruits of seven years' observation and reflection."

The nondominant hand is placed lightly against the patient's chest at the site to be percussed, and the distal interphalangeal joint of the second finger is struck sharply with the tip of the second digit of the dominant hand. Each site of interest is usually struck two or three times in succession at a rate of about 60–100 beats per minute to create, reproduce, and characterize the tone. The key to successful percussion is a loose finger and wrist of the striking hand. The blow should be struck from the elbow, with the wrist and hand relaxed. A usefully loud drum-like sound is produced by the sharpness of the tap, not the force of the swing.

A percussion tap generates a local sound just beneath the strike, and the quality of the sound reflects the nature of the underlying tissues. In a normal subject, percussion over the lungs in the midback or over the upper chest creates a sound described as "resonant,'' over the liver as ''dull,'' and over the stomach with air as ''tympanic'' (like a tympani drum). The lung fields of a subject with a thin chest wall will sound more resonant, while those in a subject who is obese or very muscular will sound more dull.

Disease within the thorax alters percussive tone predictably. Emphysema creates destruction of lung tissue and hyperinflation, resulting in ''hyperresonance'' over the lung fields. Pneumothorax may create localized or ipsilateral hyperresonance. Pleural effusion, and occasionally dense consolidation, produce localized dullness. The border between the resonant air-filled lung and the denser abdominal contents below the diaphragm marks the position of the diaphragm. To assess diaphragmatic movement and thus to test for paralysis, the patient is instructed to take a full, deep breath and hold it. The border of dullness in the midscapular line is then defined by percussion and may be marked with a pen dot. The patient is then told to exhale entirely and hold it. The new border of dullness is defined and marked again. In normal subjects, the posterior border of dullness will move up at least 1 cm and often as much as 3 cm between full inspiration and full expiration. It may be difficult to define a precise border of dullness and/or to detect movement in subjects who are obese, in those with severe emphysema, or in patients with pneumonia or pleural effusion.

Percussion is particularly useful in several specific instances. It can be used routinely to assess hyperinflation (hyperresonance) in patients with COPD. Percussion is essential when used with other signs to define landmarks and assess the upper border of pleural fluid in patients undergoing thoracentesis. It is helpful in screening patients for unilateral diaphragmatic paralysis.

AUSCULTATION

The sounds created by air moving into and out of the lungs are evaluated by auscultation. Chap. 8 presents in detail the physics governing the creation and analysis of these sounds, their characteristics, and their implications in health and disease. This section emphasizes how to perform auscultation rather than the sounds that are heard with it.

The Stethoscope

When first developed in France by Réné Théophile Hyacinthe Laënnec (1781–1826), the stethoscope revolutionized and made practical the auscultation of lung sounds. Before Laënnec, ''immediate'' auscultation was performed by the examiner placing his ear directly against the chest of the patient. Aside from issues of modesty or hygiene, sound was transmitted poorly to the ear of the listener. Laënnec utilized a rolled sheaf of paper, and then a thick-walled tube of wood with a funnel shape at the distal end, to interpose an amplifying device between the chest and the ear. His *Treatise on Diseases of the Chest and on Mediate Auscultation*, published in 1818, reported great improvements in the fidelity and loudness of lung sounds and described many of the characteristic findings we recognize today. His bulky wooden tube evolved over a century into a smaller and more finely turned trumpet-like device crafted of wood, bone, or hard rubber and finally into the current device with a metal head and earpieces joined by plastic or rubber tubes.

The modern stethoscope is a precisely designed and manufactured acoustic device, and an instrument of high quality transmits lung and heart sounds distinctly and loudly to the examiner. Lung sounds are predominantly in the higher frequency range. The firm, thin stethoscope diaphragm held lightly against the chest is optimized for this range of lung and heart sounds. The bell of the stethoscope head utilizes the patient's skin as a loose diaphragm and is optimal for the transmission of cardiac sounds in the lower-frequency ranges. A high-quality stethoscope is essential for accurate and sensitive auscultation of lung sounds and is a worthwhile investment, since price generally follows quality. Inexpensive stethoscopes, particularly the ones sold in bulk for obtaining blood pressure, are nearly useless for auscultation of the lungs, as they miss most of the higher-frequency sounds. Electronic stethoscopes are available for practitioners with reduced hearing acuity.

Performing Auscultation

Auscultation is best performed standing behind the seated patient, positioned as described above for inspection of the chest. If necessary, auscultation can be performed with the patient sitting up and leaning forward in bed. Patients who cannot sit up may be examined semi-recumbent or supine by rolling from side to side in order to expose the back. A relaxed body position for the examiner as well as the patient will be helpful.

The stethoscope diaphragm is placed lightly against the skin of the chest with just enough pressure to create a firm seal. A series of locations should be surveyed over both the right and left lung. The "auscultatory triangle" is located just medial and caudal to the tip of the scapula—a relative gap formed by the borders of the latissimus dorsi, the trapezius, and the rhomboideus major muscles; breath sounds can be heard most clearly at this site. Additional sites for a survey examination include the lung base in the midscapular line and the midaxillary line, the posterior apex above the scapula, the axilla, beneath the breast anteriorly, and the upper chest above the breast and the bulk of the pectoral muscle. Most examiners prefer to compare the right and the left lungs at each site before moving on to the next site. Two or three complete breath cycles should be heard at each site.

The pattern of breathing is essential to understanding the findings of auscultation. The quality of breath sounds is always assessed with the patient breathing normally and quietly, not taking a full deep breath. The patient must open his mouth, relax the throat, and attempt not to make any sound with the nose or larynx during auscultation. Crackles, rhonchi, or wheezes may or may not be apparent with quiet breathing. After the chest has been examined for the quality of breath sounds with normal, quiet breathing, the patient is asked to take several full, slow, deep breaths while the examiner listens over the lung bases posteriorly. The primary purpose of this maneuver is to accentuate crackles. Last, the patient is asked to take in a full, deep breath and then blow it out as hard and fast as possible, a sequence resembling forced expiratory spirometry. The examiner listens over the midback or auscultatory triangle during forced exhalation. The purpose of this maneuver is to bring out wheezes and to assess whether the duration of the expiratory phase is prolonged. The examiner may then return to any sites of abnormality and study them in more detail.

Several techniques listed in texts of physical diagnosis are rarely used. *Egophony* is present when a spoken "e" sound is perceived by the examiner as a nasal, twanging "a" sound. The patient is asked to repeat the letter "e" in a normal voice as the examiner moves the stethoscope over the chest at the area of interest. Partially consolidated lung tissue, as found with pneumonia or atelectasis, may demonstrate egophony. Pleural fluid does not produce egophony. Thus egophony may be helpful in defining a line of demarcation between an area of pneumonia and an adjacent pleural effusion if a thoracentesis is planned (see Fig. 3). *Whispered pectoriloquy* is present when whispered words are transmitted clearly and audibly to the periphery. This finding occurs over sites of consolidation, and is an example of the enhancement of centrally generated sounds by dense tissue rather than air. The patient is asked to whisper a series of numbers, ''one, two, three.'' Over normal lung the examiner hears muffled distant sounds but cannot distinguish the individual words. Over an area of consolidation the whispered words can be heard clearly.

Lung Sounds

A wide variety of normal and pathological sounds can be heard over the chest with auscultation. Normal breath sounds are produced by air moving through large airways and thus are centrally generated sounds. The breath sounds of the respiratory cycle can be heard over the lung periphery in a healthy subject who is breathing quietly at rest. These normal breath sounds consist of the muffled noise of air rushing into the chest with inspiration and silence after the very earliest portion of expiration. This is described as *vesicular breathing*. Auscultation over the trachea demonstrates a harsher sound of air movement, sound is heard throughout expiration as well as inspiration, and the expiratory sound may be louder than inspiration. This is described as *bronchial* or *tubular breathing*. Pathological consolidation, or deep breathing in normal subjects, increases the transmission of centrally generated sounds, and the noise of the respiratory cycle over the periphery becomes bronchial rather than vesicular in quality. Sounds with intermediate characteristics are described as *bronchovesicular*. Breath sounds may be ''distant,'' reduced, or absent over areas of emphysema, pneumothorax, or pleural effusion.

Most abnormal lung sounds are generated near the periphery of the lung or in smaller airways. Crackles (rales, crepitations) are discontinuous, high-pitched sounds that occur almost exclusively during inspiration and sound like cellophane or tissue paper being crumpled. They may be localized over a single site (as with lobar pneumonia), distributed symmetrically at the lung bases (as with pulmonary edema), or present throughout both lungs (as with acute respiratory distress syndrome). These sounds are believed to be generated by small airways snapping open with inspiration or by secretions moving in small airways. The characteristics and implications of crackles are discussed in detail in Chap. 8.

Rhonchi are low-pitched sounds resembling a snore that are generated by secretions vibrating in larger airways. They are heard continuously throughout a respiratory phase, and may occur in both inspiration and/or expiration. A wheeze is a continuous sound caused by turbulent airflow in bronchi narrowed by secretions, edema, and inflammation of the wall, dynamic collapse, or contraction of smooth muscle around the airway. Wheezes are high in pitch with many overtones, creating a musical quality to the sound. Wheezes may be heard in inspiration and/or expiration. A wheeze may be created by localized bronchial compression or by a partially obstructing endobronchial lesion. Stridor is a loud harsh wheeze heard best over the trachea and represents proximal airway constriction or obstruction within the large central airways or the larynx. A coarse sound resembling pieces of saddle leather rubbing together and can sometimes be heard over sites of pleural irritation where the visceral and parietal pleural move against one another with inspiration and/or expiration; this is called a *pleural friction rub*.

CARDIOVASCULAR EXAMINATION FOR RESPIRATORY DISEASE

The close interrelationship of the cardiovascular and the respiratory systems requires particular attention to the findings of the heart examination in evaluating a patient with respiratory complaints. In patients with chronic lung disorders, findings of cor pulmonale indicate the severity of the disorder and can be followed as a measure of the patient's response to therapy. Left ventricular dysfunction and valvular disease, for example, may first present with respiratory symptoms of cough or dyspnea, or precipitate exacerbations in a patient with known chronic lung disease. On the other hand, physical exam evidence of right ventricular (RV) strain may be the only abnormal finding—and an important clue—in a patient who presents with dyspnea from primary pulmonary hypertension. The review of a complete cardiovascular exam is beyond the scope of this chapter. Severe acute or chronic lung disease causes elevation of resistance in the pulmonary vascular bed, a consequent rise in pulmonary artery (PA) pressure in an attempt to maintain flow, and ultimately RV decompensation. Thus, this discussion will focus on the physical findings related to elevated PA pressure and RV failure, the features of cor pulmonale. The interested reader is referred to a review of this topic by NS Hill, listed in the "Suggested Reading," and to Chap. 33. Table 5 summarizes these findings.

Lung disease often makes the cardiovascular examination challenging. Hyperinflation will move the heart away from the chest, muffling sounds and changing the heart's relationship to the surface anatomy of the chest. Abnormal adventitial sounds can obscure the heart sounds. The tachypneic patient may not be able to perform maneuvers or even hold her breath!

Table 5 Cardiovascular Signs of Respiratory Disease

Vital signs
    Pulse (tachycardia, irregular rhythym)
    Blood pressure
    Pulsus paradoxus
Inspection
    Jugular venous distention (pulsations)
    Hepatojugular reflex
Palpation
    Edema (extremities, sacrum)
    Right ventricular parasternal lift (RV heave)
    Peripheral pulses
Auscultation
    Valve closure sounds
        Accentuated S_1 with inspiration
        Accentuated P_2
        Widely split S_2
    Gallop rhythms (S_3, S_4)
    Tricuspid regurgitation
    Pulmonic regurgitation

Inspection

At end expiration, the venous pulsations of the right internal jugular vein provide a direct measure of right atrial filling pressure when the patient is relaxed and the head and chest are elevated to 45 degrees. If these pulsations are not seen, the elevation of the bed can be lowered and a light can be pointed tangentially across the neck to help visualize them. The vertical distance measured from the venous pulsations to the sternal angle of Louis with the addition of 5 cm (the approximate distance of the right atrium below the angle of Louis) is a rough estimate of the right atrial pressure. Normal right atrial pressures are 2–10 mmHg. A hepatojugular reflex may indicate elevated central venous pressure and volume overload. Gentle pressure is applied over the liver with the patient semirecumbent (45 degrees). The jugular vein area is inspected to determine if the vein fills during liver compression.

Palpation

Palpation of the extremities or sacral area can detect peripheral edema—a sign of elevated right atrial pressure, fluid overload, or venous or lymphatic obstruction. Weakness or absence of peripheral pulses is a sign of peripheral vascular disease, an important cause of impaired exercise capacity. Rapid, thready peripheral pulses can be a sign of poor cardiac output from either left or right ventricular failure.

Palpation (or auscultation) of a peripheral pulse while deflating the cuff of a sphygmomanometer can detect an accentuation of the normal variation in systolic pressure during the respiratory cycle. Usually there is a decrease of less than 10 mmHg in the arterial systolic pressure during inspiration as compared with expiration. This is thought to be secondary to increased pooling of blood in the pulmonary vessels and increased venous return to the RV with subsequent interference of left ventricular filling with the fall in intrathoracic pressure during inspiration. Patients with airflow obstruction from asthma or COPD have much greater swings in intrathoracic pressure with an accentuated fall (>10 mmHg) in systolic pressure during inspiration—a finding called *pulsus paradoxus*, or paradoxical pulse, that has been used as an index of the severity of asthma exacerbations. A paradoxical pulse can also be found in patients with pericardial effusions and cardiac tamponade, hypovolemia, and massive pulmonary embolism.

Sustained impulses at the left lower sternal border (the RV area) or a sternal lift (RV heave) are signs of right ventricular dilation. In patients with emphysema, the cardiac impulse may be shifted to the epigastic or xyphoid region by the effects of hyperinflation.

Auscultation

Valve closure sounds emanating from the pulmonary valve are heard best at the second and third left interspace, from the tricuspid valve at the right sternal border, and from the RV at the sternum and lower left sternal border (in the emphysematous patient this may be shifted to the epigastrium).

Right ventricular sounds, in contrast to left ventricular sounds, are usually accentuated on inspiration as blood flow increases to the RV. For example, whereas S_1 normally becomes less prominent during inspiration, the tricuspid component of S_1 can increase or become audible on inspiration in patients with pulmonary hypertension. This respiratory variation can disappear, however, as one or more of the ventricles fail and become unresponsive to changes in intrathoracic pressure. Early systolic ejection clicks can be heard with pulmonary artery stenosis and pulmonary hypertension. If P_2 (heard at the pulmonic area) is louder than A_2 (heard at the aortic area), pulmonary hypertension or a high-flow state (anemia, hyperthyroidism) is suggested. The normal, or physiological splitting of the two components of the second sound is narrower during expiration than with inspiration. With the onset of pulmonary hypertension, this split becomes narrow throughout the respiratory cycle. However, if the RV begins to fail, the split widens during inspiration from the delay in RV emptying. Other causes of a widely split second heart sound include right bundle branch block and an atrial septal defect. Fixed splitting of S_2 usually occurs with atrial septal defect, but has also been reported in massive or chronic thromboembolism.

A right-sided protodiastolic sound (S_3) located at the lower left sternal border that increases with inspiration can be a normal finding in young individuals but in older adults is usually a sign of poor RV compliance. Similarly, a right-sided S_4—heard at the left sternal border; increasing with inspiration—suggests decreased right ventricular compliance from strain or hypertrophy.

Tricuspid regurgitation from right ventricular dilitation or endocarditis is heard as a systolic murmur at the right and left sternal border that usually increases with inspiration unless there is severe right ventricular failure.

Synthesis

The constellation of findings corresponding to right ventricular failure from respiratory diseases depends in part on whether the condition is acute or chronic. The exam findings in patients with acute increases in right ventricular afterload (pulmonary embolism in a previously healthy patient, for example) may include tachycardia, increased venous pressure, prominent jugular A waves, right-sided S_3 and S_4, and a paradoxical pulse. A widely split S_2 and decreasing intensity of P_2 may herald frank right ventricular failure.

In patients with chronic lung disease and persistent increases in pulmonary artery pressures, there is time for the right heart to adapt to the pressure overload. Ejection clicks, an RV heave, and accentuated jugular V waves, and murmurs from tricuspid regurgitation (related to RV dilation) may be found. Peripheral edema, ascites, hepatomegaly, and jaundice are findings of more advanced cor pulmonale.

SYNTHESIS

No part of the physical examination of the thorax stands alone. Inspection, palpation, percussion, and auscultation must be used together and in an integrated fashion in order to fully define and understand the underlying pathology. The examination often must be reiterative: it is not until a few crackles have been noted on auscultation at the right base that percussion is repeated, directed to that site, and detects localized dullness. The examiner must think about the implications of each finding and then use additional tools to expand or confirm the abnormality.

Constellations of physical findings are typical of particular diseases and may be used to suggest a diagnosis. Table 4 lists the patterns found in some common pulmonary diseases. This table is not comprehensive but rather illustrates how findings fit together based on principles of sound transmission. For example, over an area of pneumonia, the increased tactile fremitus, bronchial breathing, and whispered pectoriloquy all result from the enhanced transmission of central sounds caused by lung consolidation. Figures 2 and 3 illustrate diagrammatically the physical signs of a lobar pneumonia and of a pleural effusion. In many instances the physical findings are suggestive but not definitive, and they must be integrated with the respiratory history and confirmed with other objective tests in order to establish a firm diagnosis and define the severity of disease.

SUGGESTED READING

1. Auenbrugger, L. Inventum novum ex percussione thoracis humani, ut signo, abstrusos interni pectoris morbos detegendi. Vienna: Joannis Thomae Trattner, 1761.
2. Burstein HJ, Janicek MJ, Skarin AT. Hypertrophic osteoarthropathy. J Clin Oncol 1997; 15: 2759–2760.
3. Hansen-Flaschen J, Nordberg J. Clubbing and hypertrophic osteoarthropathy. Clin Chest Med 1987; 8:287–298.
4. Hill NS. The cardiac exam in lung disease. Clin Chest Med 1987; 8:273–285.
5. Kanematsu T, Kitaichi M, Nishimura K, Nagai S, Izumi T. Clubbing of the fingers and smooth-muscle proliferation in fibrotic changes in the lung in patients with idiopathic pulmonary fibrosis. Chest 1994; 105:339–342.
6. Laennec RTH. Auscultation mediate, ou traité du diagnostic des maladies des puomons et du coeur, fonde principalement sur ce nouveau moyen d'exploration. Paris: Brosson et Chaude, 1819.
7. Loudon RG, Murphy RLH. State of the art: lung sounds. Am Rev Respir Dis 1984; 130:663–673.
8. Maitre B, Similowski T, Derenne JP. Physical examination of the adult patient with respiratory disease: inspection and palpation. Eur Respir J 1995; 8:1584–1593.
9. Martinez-Lavin M. Hypertrophic osteoarthropathy. Curr Opin Rheumatol 1997; 9:83–86.
10. McGee SR. Percussion and physical diagnosis: separating myth from science. Dis Mon 1995; 41:641–692.
11. Morgan B, Coakley F, Finlay DB, Belton I. Hypertrophic osteoarthropathy in staging skeletal scintigraphy for lung cancer. Clin Radiol 1996; 51:694–697.
12. Piirila P, Sovijarvi AR. Crackles: recording, analysis and clinical significance. Eur Respir J 1995; 8:2139–2148.
13. Sansores RH, Villalba-Caloca J, Ramirez-Venegas A, Salas J, Carrillo G, Chapela R, et al. Reversal of digital clubbing after lung transplantation. Chest 1995; 107:283–285.
14. Sharma OP. Symptoms and signs in pulmonary medicine: old observations and new interpretations. Dis Mon 1995; 41:577–638.
15. Swartz MH. Textbook of Physical Diagnosis. 3rd ed. Philadelphia: Saunders, 1998:248–274.
16. Yernault JC, Bohadana AB. Chest percussion. Eur Respir J 1995; 8:1756–1760.

8

Lung Sounds in Health and Disease

Raymond L.H. Murphy, Jr.
Faulkner Hospital
Lemuel Shattuck Hospital
Tufts University School of Medicine
Boston, Massachusetts

Robert G. Loudon
University of Cincinnati College of Medicine
Cincinnati, Ohio

Physical examination of the chest remains important despite the availability of advanced diagnostic techniques for the management of patients with pulmonary disease. One of the most important reasons for physical examination is to decide whether other testing or therapeutic measures are indicated. This importance varies with the circumstances in which the examination is done: the acutely ill, the chronically ill, or the apparently normal patient. Its importance and urgency also vary with the setting and the suspected illness. For example, physical assessment can be crucial in the detection of upper airway obstruction but is unlikely to be of value in the detection of lung cancer.

This chapter focuses on auscultation of the chest and on the most common conditions found in adults. Before specific conditions are discussed, a review of the fundamentals of the generation of lung sounds and auscultation is presented.

CLASSIFICATION OF LUNG SOUNDS

Respiratory sounds are divided into the normal sounds heard when no respiratory problems exist and the abnormal or adventitious sounds heard in disease. The normal sounds heard over the trachea or large airways have a tubular quality, a sound similar to that of air being blown through a tube, and are relatively louder during expiration than inspiration (see Fig. 1A). Sounds heard over the lung parenchyma at a distance from large airways, called normal breath sounds or vesicular sounds, have a soft murmuring tone (like wind blowing through trees). Normal vesicular breathing is most audible during inspiration and relatively quiet during expiration (see Fig. 1B).

The most common abnormal lung sounds are wheezes, rhonchi, and crackles. *Rales*

(A) NORMAL TRACHEAL   (B) NORMAL VESICULAR

(C) CRACKLES   (D) WHEEZE

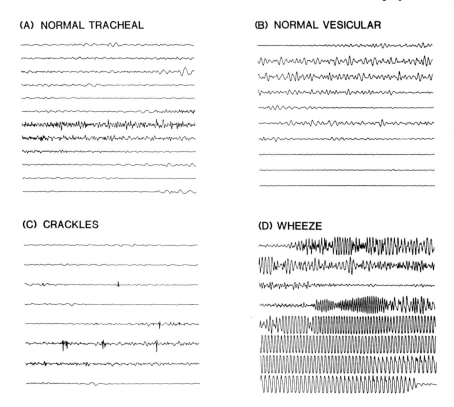

Figure 1 Time-expanded waveforms of lung sounds. The time-intensity plots in this figure are made from tape recordings of lung sounds stored in a computer memory and then visually displayed on a two-dimensional plot, with amplitude or intensity on the *Y* axis and time on the *X* axis. The time axis of the plot is ''expanded,'' or magnified, by playing back slowly from the computer memory. Panels A and B illustrate inspiration and then expiration with normal tracheal and peripheral vesicular sounds. The louder, longer expiratory phase of the tracheal sound is readily recognized, as is the pause between inspiration and expiration. Similarly, the louder inspiratory vesicular sounds are apparent. Crackles (panel C) produce intermittent (''discontinuous'') deflections superimposed on the normal vesicular pattern. Panel D shows a ''continuous'' deflection produced by a wheeze replacing the normal waveform.

or *crepitations* are alternative terms for crackles. Wheezes and rhonchi are classified as ''continuous'' sounds because they last nearly throughout inspiration or expiration, and they are longer than the brief, intermittent explosive ''discontinuous'' sounds called *crackles*. Crackles are usually less than 20 ms in duration, while wheezes and rhonchi usually last longer than 100 ms. Short wheezes (squawks, squeaks) also occur, but careful delineation of the durations of these various sounds has not yet been reported. Wheezes have a musical character or an identifiable pitch. Their acoustic frequency range extends from about 100 Hz to more than 1000 Hz (1 kHz). Rhonchi have a snore-like character and are often associated with airway secretions. They may disappear promptly after coughing in patients with chronic bronchitis. As illustrated in Fig. 1, the various major categories of lung sounds can be distinguished readily in the time-expanded waveform mode, providing objective evidence for classifying lung sounds.

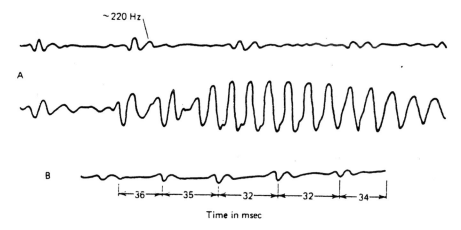

Figure 2 Time-expanded waveform of sections of pleural friction rub. In panel A, the upper section illustrates "discontinuous" sounds; the lower section shows "continuous" sounds associated with a pleural friction rub. In panel B, repeated individual 220-Hz bursts occur at remarkably regular intervals. (From Murphy RLH. Human factors in chest auscultation. In: Human Factors in Health Care. Toronto and London: Lexington Books, 1975: 73–88.)

The most recent International Lung Sound Association classification system divides crackles into categories of "fine" and "coarse." This is a simplification, because by waveform measurement crackles occur with continuous scales of amplitude, duration, initial deflection width, and other features. "Medium" crackles were omitted from the classification because it was not clear that observers could distinguish them reliably from fine or coarse crackles, and their clinical relevance was uncertain. Other experts believe that medium crackles are distinct entities and have specific clinical implications.

There are other sounds that have yet to be added to this classification, including squawks, squeaks, short wheezes, and pleural friction rubs. On waveform analysis, squawks, squeaks, and short wheezes have a sinusoidal pattern and a brief duration (40–80 ms). Squawks were described in bird-fancier's lung, a form of hypersensitivity pneumonitis. They are common in hypersensitivity pneumonitis and in idiopathic pulmonary fibrosis (IPF). They can also be found in pneumonia.

Pleural friction rubs occur with pleural inflammation due to a variety of causes such as infectious pleurisy, pulmonary infarction, or when tumors have extended to the pleural surface. Pleural friction rubs have elements of both a continuous and a discontinuous nature, as shown in Fig. 2. Because objective measurements of sounds are now more readily available and many investigators are now studying lung sounds, it is likely that new entities will be added to this basic scheme.

THE MECHANISMS THAT PRODUCE LUNG SOUNDS

As gas moves through the airways during respiration, vibrations from within the gas or from the walls of the airway are transmitted through the lung tissue to the chest wall. At the chest wall, these vibrations are superimposed on the larger excursions of inspiration and expiration. Due to the remarkable sensitivity of human hearing, a stethoscope allows perception of chest wall vibrations whose amplitude may be 10^{-6} m (10 μm) or less.

The vibrations in the lung that are eventually interpreted as sound can arise from a number of mechanisms. None of these have yet been explained in detail, but there is enough agreement among investigators to allow an outline of the mechanisms for normal and abnormal lung sounds. A summary of these mechanisms is listed in Table 1.

Normal Lung Sounds

Gas flow is laminar in most of the conducting airways of the lung. This smooth flow is replaced by turbulent, swirling, unsteady flow in larger airways. The vibrations of the gas in the large airways are transmitted peripherally to the surface of the chest, and they are also transmitted as airborne sounds centrally toward the mouth. As the sound travels toward the periphery of the lung and thorax, it is progressively filtered and attenuated. Filtering means that components of the sound occurring at different frequencies (or pitches) are transmitted with different efficiencies. The transmission path acts as a "low-pass" filter, preferentially passing sounds below 200 Hz and removing sounds above 200 Hz. This phenomenon is easily demonstrated by listening over the periphery of the lung while a subject speaks; the muffled sounds are hardly intelligible.

Filtering probably accounts for the differences in frequency content between central tracheal or bronchial sounds and the sounds heard over the periphery of the lung (vesicular or distal sounds). Some investigators still argue that sound is generated in the periphery, even though the flow rates are theoretically so low that turbulence is unlikely. The argument for peripheral generation of sound rests largely on the observation that regional differences in the intensity of vesicular sounds at the chest wall are correlated with variations in regional airflow measured with radioactive gas techniques. An alternative explanation for the regional differences in sound is that the turbulent energy in the large airways may be convected with the airflow and that regions with a larger share of the total flow also receive a larger fraction of the airborne sound.

Abnormal Lung Sounds

Bronchial Breathing

The "low-pass" filtering effect is decreased when the transmission path to the surface of the chest is altered by consolidation of the lung parenchyma. With consolidation, the sounds heard over the periphery are bronchial breath sounds, similar to those heard over large airways. Consolidation, as in lobar pneumonia, also alters the transmission of voiced sounds, which are then heard more clearly. This principle is utilized for testing whispered pectoriloquy (see Chap. 7, "Physical Examination").

Adventitious Sounds

Adventitious sounds are generated within the large and small airways and the parenchyma of the lung. They are believed to result from abnormal motion of airway walls or from secretions within the airways during breathing. In contrast, normal sounds result largely from vibrations within the gas itself.

Continuous Sounds

Wheezes and rhonchi are believed to be generated by a regular vibration, or oscillation, of the airway wall at one or more sites in the chest. Likely mechanisms for the production of wheezes include movement of airway secretions and flutter of airway walls. Wheezing

Table 1 Categories and Mechanisms of Lung Sounds[a]

Respiratory Sound	Mechanism	Origin	Acoustics	Relevance
Normal Lung Sounds				
Peripheral lung	Turbulent flow vortices; unknown mechanisms	Central airways (expir); lobar to segmental airways (inspir)	Low-pass filtered noise (<100 to >3000 Hz)	Regional ventilation, airway caliber
Trachea	Turbulent flow impinging on airway walls	Pharynx, larynx, trachea, large airways	Noise with resonances (<100 to >3000 Hz)	Upper airway configuration
Adventitious Sounds				
Wheeze	Airway wall, flutter, vortex, shedding	Central and lower airways	Sinusoid (100 to >1000 Hz, duration >80 ms)	Airway obstruction, flow limitation
Rhonchus	Rupture of fluid films, airway vibrations	Larger airways	Series of rapidly dampened sinusoids (<300 Hz, >100 ms)	Secretions, abnormal airway collapsing
Crackle (rale)	Airway wall stress-relaxation	Central and lower airways	Rapidly dampened wave reflection (duration <20 ms)	Airway closure, secretions

[a] This table lists the major categories of respiratory sounds but does not include friction rubs, squawks, grunting, snoring, or cough. The concepts listed for the mechanisms that generate these sounds are incomplete, unconfirmed, and somewhat theoretical.

is associated clinically with airway narrowing from inflammation, edema, bronchospasm, surrounding fibrosis, intrinsic or extrinsic tumor, or dynamic collapse.

It seems likely that wheezes and rhonchi occur when air passing through a narrowed airway at high velocity produces a decrease in the gas pressure in the airway at the region of constriction. Bernoulli's principle relates the local gas pressure to the local gas flow. As the velocity of the gas increases at the constriction, the pressure decreases. If allowed by the other forces acting on the airway, the airway walls will progressively collapse until there is sufficient resistance and the flow decreases. With decreased flow, the internal pressure increases and the lumen enlarges once more. This oscillation of the wall of the airway between ''almost closed'' and ''almost open'' generates sound and can continue as long as the airflow rate is high enough. Figure 3 illustrates these concepts.

Several theories for the generation of continuous lung sounds have been proposed: turbulence-induced wall resonance, turbulence-induced Helmholtz resonance, acoustically stimulated vortex sound, vortex-induced wall resonance, or fluid dynamic flutter. Equations have been developed to describe these mechanisms. Low-pitched, continuous sounds are frequently encountered in patients who also have sputum production, and the sounds

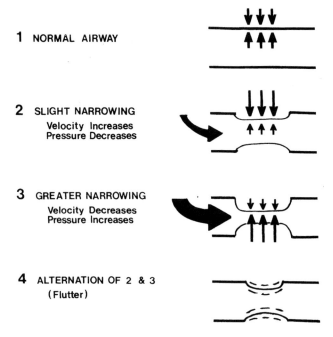

Figure 3 Postulated wheeze mechanism. The stability of the airway wall depends upon a balance between internal air pressure and external forces and on the mechanical characteristics of the airway itself (1). When a narrowing of the lumen occurs, the air velocity must *increase* through the constricted region to maintain a constant mass flow rate. According to Bernoulli's principle, this leads to a decrease in air pressure in the constricted region, thus allowing external compressive forces to further collapse the airway (2). When the lumen has been reduced so much that the flow rate decreases, the process reverses as the pressure inside the airway begins to increase and reopen the lumen. When conditions are right, the airway wall ''flutters'' between open and nearly closed states and produces a continuous sound whose amplitude, pitch, and duration depend on the airflow and mechanical parameters involved (4).

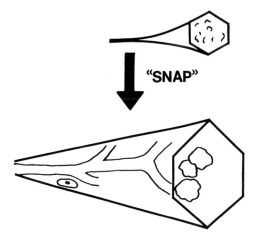

"SNAP"

Figure 4 Postulated mechanisms for crackles. Discontinuous lung sounds (crackles, rales) probably result from more than one physical mechanism. This figure illustrates the concept of an airway remaining closed for a portion of inspiration and then opening suddenly to produce a crackle. The lung downstream of the site of collapse remains underexpanded until upstream air pressure and external fractive forces on the collapsed walls overcome the surface tension of the material on the airway wall. The airway may then open suddenly, allowing a rapid equalization of pressure between the upstream and downstream airspaces. It remains uncertain whether the crackle sound itself results from this air pressure equalization, from the bursting of a film of surface material as the collapsed segment opens, or from a combination of the two sources.

often disappear after coughing and clearance of secretions. Thus, these sounds are probably generated by secretions vibrating in the airstream.

Discontinuous Sounds

Crackles are discrete vibrations that result from the sudden release of energy stored in elastic recoil or surface tension forces within the lung. Forgacs postulated that the sudden opening of collapsed airways is the likely cause of crackles in such conditions as atelectasis or pulmonary fibrosis. It is probably the mechanism for some of the crackles of congestive heart failure (CHF) as well. Dependent portions of the lung tend to collapse because the lung sits on its own weight. According to this theory, crackles occur as closed airways reopen. Some credence for this belief is provided by the observation that when placed in either lateral decubitus position, a patient with CHF will tend to have more crackles on the dependent side. Another mechanism for the production of crackles is related to fluid or secretions in the lung. The coarse, discontinuous sounds occurring in pulmonary edema or other conditions in which fluid is found in the airways are probably caused by rupture of bubbles or disruption of fluid films. Such crackles often occur during both inspiration and expiration. Figure 4 diagrams the mechanisms believed to be responsible for crackles.

ACUTE RESPIRATORY DISORDERS

The evaluation of lung sounds by auscultation and other means of physical assessment often provides characteristic findings in a patient who presents with acute respiratory distress. The term *acute respiratory distress* is used to mean the broad clinical situation in which a patient demonstrates labored breathing, tachypnea, cyanosis, discomfort, and similar signs rather than the specific syndrome of noncardiogenic pulmonary edema, *acute respiratory distress syndrome* (ARDS). Several examples will illustrate typical lung sounds in specific diseases.

Upper Airway Obstruction

Stridor is the characteristic feature of upper airway obstruction. Stridor is a continuous sound heard on auscultation, with or without a stethoscope, that is loudest over the mouth, neck, and upper trachea. It is a monotonous and musical coarse wheeze and may be heard more loudly with inspiration than with expiration. The use of accessory muscles of respiration and retraction of the supraclavicular fossae with inspiration are often observed. Careful inspection of the mouth for evidence of aspiration of food or a foreign body is important. Examination of the neck for masses, scars, and tracheal deviation is also important. The skin should be surveyed for hives, as they may provide a clue to the presence of angioneurotic edema of the glottis, an important cause of upper airway obstruction.

Acute Asthma

Acute exacerbations of bronchial asthma are characterized by inspiratory and expiratory wheezes heard diffusely over the chest. In rare circumstances, the chest can become quiet, presumably because the flow rates are too slow to generate wheezing. This is an ominous finding and only occurs for a brief period in the most severely ill patients prior to either recovery, intubation, or death. These patients begin to wheeze again as they improve and airflow increases. In most patients with severe exacerbations of bronchial asthma, the wheezing is loud and audible at a distance from the patient. The expiratory phase is more prolonged and louder relative to the inspiratory phase.

Exacerbations of Chronic Obstructive Pulmonary Disease

The expiratory phase is also relatively prolonged in exacerbations of chronic obstructive pulmonary disease (COPD). In the absence of a relevant history, it can be difficult to distinguish some patients with exacerbations of bronchial asthma from those with COPD. Fortunately, the history is usually available. Signs of hyperinflation—such as an increased anteroposterior chest diameter, hyperresonnance to percussion, and widening of the costochondral angle—are common to both asthma and COPD. Pursed-lip breathing, emaciation, older age, and hypertrophy of the accessory muscles of respiration provide clues to the presence of COPD.

Acute Bronchitis

Acute bronchitis may be associated with an entirely normal lung examination. Rhonchi are not uncommon and tend to clear after coughing. Wheezing is also quite common. The patient with cough and phlegm production should be asked to cough. Even in the absence of abnormal lung sounds, a loose-sounding or wheezy noise can be detected that is caused by airways disease.

Atelectasis

Atelectasis is commonly associated with fine crackles, probably caused by the opening on inspiration of partially collapsed lung regions. Congestion of the lung tissue leads to increased transmission of sound so that bronchial breathing is also commonly present.

Cardiogenic Pulmonary Edema

Pulmonary edema usually presents with numerous crackles over the chest from the bases to the apices. However, patients with early or mild pulmonary edema do not always have crackles, and careful attention to nonpulmonary findings is important. Cardiac disease signs include jugular venous distention, hepatomegaly, a hepatojugular reflux, peripheral pitting edema, an S_3 or S_4 gallop rhythm, cardiomegaly, or tachycardia (see Chap. 7).

Pneumonia

Severe pneumonia can precipitate respiratory distress. Lobar pneumonia, usually bacterial in origin, demonstrates crackles over the affected region. Dullness to percussion, decreased breath sounds, and bronchial breathing may be present as well. The findings are often variable depending on the severity of the pneumonia and the presence of coexisting illnesses, such as cardiac pulmonary edema or COPD. Viral pneumonia may present with little or no auscultatory abnormalities even when the chest x-ray is diffusely abnormal, or it may be associated with diffuse crackles throughout the lungs.

CHRONIC RESPIRATORY DISORDERS

Asthma

The cardinal feature of bronchial asthma is wheezing. Many asthmatics will have no audible wheezing when they are asymptomatic or their asthma is under good control. Most asthmatics wheeze during exacerbations of their disease, and the wheezing can usually be detected over the entire chest in both respiratory phases in severe cases. The association of wheezing with bronchial asthma is so strong that clinicians need to be reminded that ''all that wheezes is not asthma.'' In particular, early pulmonary edema (''cardiac asthma''), upper airway compression by tumor, or partial airway occlusion by foreign body need to be considered.

As a symptom perceived by the patient, wheezing is very common, being reported by up to 25% of asthma patients in population surveys. Conversely, clinical asthma can occur without wheezing, as can reversible bronchospasm. Auscultation is used widely to guide the outpatient management of patients with bronchial asthma, although objective studies to support this practice are conflicting.

Chronic Bronchitis and Emphysema (COPD)

It is likely that emphysema produces different physical signs than does chronic bronchitis, but most patients present with varying degrees of both processes. Accordingly, the clinician usually encounters a mixture of findings in patients who have both bronchitis and emphysema, the syndrome of chronic obstructive pulmonary disease (COPD, see Chap. 27). The breath sounds are decreased in intensity. Wheezing is common, particularly at end-expiration. It may be brought out by a forced maximum expiratory effort if no wheezing is heard with quiet breathing. Rhonchi are also common and generally clear or change after coughing. Basilar crackles may be present and are usually medium in character, early inspiratory in timing, and few in number. They may be associated with clicking noises at the mouth. COPD patients commonly have an increased anteroposterior chest diameter and widening of the subcostal angle. The sternocleidomastoid muscles may be hypertrophied and tense to palpitation with inspiration. Expiration is prolonged relative to inspiration, and pursed-lip breathing may be used. The percussion note is characteristically hyperresonant.

In the early stages of COPD, physical assessment may be entirely normal except during episodes of exacerbation, when wheezing or rhonchi may be present. A simple bedside technique can be used to detect or assess airflow obstruction. The bell of a stethoscope is placed on the sternal notch at the base of the neck. The patient is asked to take a deep breath in and blow it out as fast as possible. The duration of audible expiration (FET_0) is timed to the nearest half second. If the audible expiratory time is greater than 6 s and airflow continues, then the FEV_1/FVC ratio is less than 0.40. Conversely, if expiration is audible for less than 5 s and airflow stopped, then the FEV_1/FVC ratio is greater than 0.60.

Chronic Diffuse Parenchymal Lung Disease

The presence of crackles may be the first clue that a patient has idiopathic pulmonary fibrosis (IPF) or another chronic diffuse parenchymal lung disease. The number and the distribution of the crackles can be a guide to the severity of IPF and to the response to therapy. The crackles are characteristically fine in character. They are heard initially at the lung bases and are end-inspiratory in timing, but as the disease progresses, they are heard more widely over the entire chest. When heard throughout inspiration, they may have an end-inspiratory accentuation. Squawks and short wheezes have been described frequently in IPF. When crackles are both inspiratory and expiratory, the disease tends to be more severe than when inspiratory crackles alone are heard. In the occupational setting, the presence of fine crackles is useful in detecting and monitoring for interstitial pulmonary fibrosis caused by asbestos.

OBSERVER VARIABILITY

Observer variability in physical assessment of the chest is large, as has been shown in many studies. This variability has been reduced in specific circumstances, as in the detection of occupational lung disease, where observers focused on single findings and had prior agreement on terminology. Possible causes for the variation in auscultatory findings among observers include differences in training, perception, and attention; lack of a common nomenclature; and other problems. In contrast to cardiac sounds, lung sounds can vary considerably over short intervals of time, making bedside teaching more difficult.

COMPUTER-BASED ANALYSIS

The problems with observer variability have stimulated investigators to study computer-based methods of lung sound analysis. These instruments can now be brought to the bed-side or used in the ambulatory setting. Computer-based respiratory sound analysis has been used for quantification of wheezing relative to airflow obstruction and for detection of decreased breath sounds in association with airflow obstruction in the absence of wheezing. It has been used for the detection of sleep apnea. In most subjects undergoing bronchial provocation testing, acoustic changes detected by computer analysis appear one or more challenge dilutions lower than the dose needed to provoke a 20% fall in the FEV_1. This approach may be valuable in children and in adults who are unable to cooperate well in pulmonary function testing.

Computerized analysis can detect and quantify crackles. Time-expanded waveform analysis has been reported to be equivalent to high-resolution computed tomography (HRCT) in the detection of asbestosis. In other studies, objectively measured lung sound intensity correlated closely with regional ventilation as measured by radioactive xenon. Respiratory sound patterns are different in specific diseases, and computerized based analysis may help distinguish the patterns found in some common lung disorders. It is likely that more applications will be found.

CONCLUSIONS

What is the future of physical assessment in general, and the stethoscope in particular? In the acute care setting, clinicians must make important and sometimes life-saving decisions based on physical examination, even when sophisticated medical devices are readily at hand. Clinicians must sometimes undertake immediate therapy based on physical examination and auscultation before diagnostic tests are obtained. Examples include the removal of foreign bodies from the upper airway, providing oxygen to the cyanotic, checking the oxygen supply in oxygen-dependent patients, treating a tension pneumothorax, tapping a large pleural effusion, treating asthma exacerbations with bronchodilators, repositioning a displaced endotracheal tube, patching an open pneumothorax or administering a diuretic to a patient in pulmonary edema. Auscultation can provide important information about chronic diseases, such as asthma or interstitial fibrosis, or in the management of patients with heart failure or COPD. Physical assessment of the chest is likely to remain important despite new technologies. Hopefully, the use of computer-based teaching techniques and tape recordings and the feedback provided by bedside visual acoustic displays will improve the performance of clinicians in this ancient art.

SUGGESTED READING

1. Bettencourt PE, Del Bono EA, Spiegelman D, Hertzmark E, Murphy RLH. Clinical utility of chest auscultation in common pulmonary diseases. Am J Respir Crit Care Med 1994; 150:1291–1297.
2. Gavriely N. Breath Sounds Methodology. Boca Raton, FL: CRC Press, 1995.

3.   Loudon RG, Murphy RLH. State of the art: lung sounds. Am Rev Respir Dis 1984; 130:663–673.

4.   Murphy RLH. A Simplified Introduction to Lung Sounds. Wellesley Hills, MA: Stethophonics, 1977.

5.   Pasterkamp H. Computer assisted learning of chest auscultation: the respiration acoustics laboratory environment. In: Bemmel JH, Zvarova J, eds. Information and Medical Education. New York: Elsevier–North Holland, 1991:244–251.

6.   Pasterkamp H, Kramen SS, Wodicka GR. Respiratory sounds: advances beyond the stethoscope. Am J Respir Crit Care Med 1997; 156:974–987.

9
Pulmonary Function Testing

David A. Kaminsky
University of Vermont College of Medicine
Fletcher Allen Health Care
Burlington, Vermont

INTRODUCTION

What Is Pulmonary Function Testing?

The function of the lungs is to provide effective gas exchange between the environment and the bloodstream. To this end, the lungs must perform the following functions:

1. Move large quantities of air between the atmosphere and the alveolar-capillary membrane, where gas exchange occurs
2. Provide the interface for the interaction of air and blood at the alveolar-capillary membrane
3. Regulate the flow of blood to this interface to allow for gas transport

The ultimate outcome of these functions is adequate oxygenation and carbon dioxide elimination to maintain normal cellular and organ function. Thus, one might expect that an arterial blood gas analysis would be all that is necessary to assess overall lung function. However, because the lungs have a significant functional reserve, normal arterial blood gases might be maintained in the face of severe derangements of other aspects of lung function. In fact, these other derangements, such as limitation to airflow or restriction of lung volume, are more likely responsible for the symptoms of pulmonary disease. Accordingly, these specific aspects of lung function must also be assessed in order to understand the pathophysiology of lung disease.

Considering the three basic functions of the lungs as described above, one can categorize pulmonary function tests (PFTs) into three major groups:

1. Measures of airflow (spirometry) and lung volume
2. Measures of efficiency of gas transfer (diffusion)
3. Measures of efficiency of gas transport (oximetry and exercise studies)

(A fourth area, related to the control of movement of air, is the ventilatory drive mechanism, which is not discussed further here).

This chapter explores each of these areas, with particular attention to spirometry, since this is the most important test of lung function available to the practicing clinician.

A brief survey of more specialized PFTs will also be included in order to familiarize the clinician with additional options for determining lung function. Simple algorithms for obtaining PFTs and interpreting spirometry are provided, and then a number of cases are presented to illustrate key points presented in this chapter.

Before determining physiological abnormality, it is important to define what is meant by *normal*. In pulmonary function testing as in other tests of biological function, there is a wide degree of variation of function among individuals. Thus "normal" becomes somewhat difficult to define. There are three factors to consider in defining normal with regard to PFTs. The first factor is that many PFTs, including spirometry, are dependent upon good patient technique and effort. If a patient simply will not cooperate with testing, then falsely abnormal values may be obtained. The second factor is that various aspects of lung function change normally with age and vary normally with sex and size (with height, but not with weight). For example, one would expect a 25-year-old, 6-ft, 5-in man to have much larger lungs than a 68-year-old, 5-ft, 3-in woman. Therefore, it is usually more meaningful to reference specific functions to their percentage of predicted value rather than to their absolute value.

Finally, the normal range is derived in a statistical sense and is typically defined as any value that falls within 2 standard deviations of the mean, or, likewise, falls within 95% confidence intervals of the mean. Accordingly, roughly 5% of truly normal people will have PFT results outside the published normal range; therefore, the clinical context must always be considered in interpretation. For many PFTs, the normal range based on confidence intervals coincides with test values between 80 and 120% of predicted. However, this range of normal varies from test to test within normal populations; such ranges are shown in Table 1. Given all of these factors, interpreting PFTs can be a real challenge!

Since pulmonary function testing is subject to much biological and individual variation, it is imperative that high-quality, consistent testing be performed. The American Thoracic Society has issued periodic guidelines specifically addressing the technical and

Table 1 Limits of Normal for Common Pulmonary Function Tests

Test	Limits of normal (% predicted)
Peak expiratory flow rate (PEFR)	$\geq 65\%$
Forced vital capacity (FVC)	$\geq 80\%$
Forced expiratory volume in the first second (FEV_1)	$\geq 80\%$
FEV_1/FVC	$\geq 90\%$
Total lung capacity (TLC)	$\geq 80\%$, $\leq 120\%$
Functional residual capacity (FRC)	$\geq 70\%$, $\leq 130\%$
Residual volume (RV)	$\geq 60\%$, $\leq 140\%$
Diffusing capacity of the lung for carbon monoxide (DL_{CO})	$\geq 75\%$, $\leq 125\%$
Maximal inspiratory pressure (MIP)	Male: ≤ -75 cmH$_2$O[a]
	Female: ≤ -50 cmH$_2$O
Maximal expiratory pressure (MEP)	Male: ≥ 100 cmH$_2$O
	Female: ≥ 80 cmH$_2$O

[a] Lower limits of normal based on Clausen JL. Maximal inspiratory and expiratory pressures. In: Clausen JL, ed. Pulmonary Function Testing Guidelines and Controversies. Equipment, Methods and Normal Values. New York: Grune & Stratton, 1984:187–191.

Source: Pennock BE, Cottrell JJ, Rogers RM. Pulmonary function testing: what is "normal"? Arch Intern Med 1983; 143:2123–2127.

performance aspects of spirometry and lung diffusion testing; all equipment and personnel should adhere to these. Therefore, whether pulmonary function testing is performed with a portable spirometer or oximeter in a physician's office or with a full testing system in a specialty lab, strict internal guidelines requiring periodic quality assurance and consistent policies and procedures must be in place. Only then can physicians trust that the values measured on their patients are representative of their patients' actual lung function.

Why Measure Pulmonary Function?

There are a number of reasons to measure pulmonary function (Table 2). The most obvious is that the clinician needs objective information about lung function in order to make a specific diagnosis to explain the common symptoms of cough, shortness of breath, dyspnea, chest pain, or wheezing. Thus, PFTs are used to determine whether or not lung function is normal and, if not, whether a problem with airflow, lung volume, or gas exchange exists. Similarly, if a patient has documented lung disease, PFTs provide a means of objectively following the course of disease—information that is important in determining prognosis and whether treatment is indicated or working. The best example of this is the routine measurement of the forced expiratory volume in the first second (FEV_1) to follow the course of cystic fibrosis, asthma, or chronic obstructive pulmonary disease (COPD).

PFTs also provide objective measures of the effects of treatment for diseases of the lung. For example, in a patient with idiopathic pulmonary fibrosis, it would be important to document improvement or stabilization of lung function while the patient is receiving such potentially toxic medications as prednisone or cyclophosphamide. Likewise, many drugs used for nonpulmonary disorders can have adverse effects on the lungs, and PFTs are useful in documenting the presence of these effects. A classic example is the antiarrhythmic drug amiodarone, which can lead to interstitial fibrosis. Early signs of this toxicity include decrements in the forced vital capacity (FVC) and in the diffusing capacity of the lung for carbon monoxide (DL_{CO}).

Pulmonary function testing is important in determining the risk to patients of surgery of the chest or abdomen. This is especially important in the patient who is about to undergo lung resection surgery: In order to maintain adequate daily function, patients should be predicted to have an FEV_1 of at least 0.8 L remaining following surgery, or 40% of predicted. Similarly, if a patient retains carbon dioxide on routine arterial blood gas analysis ($P_{CO_2} > 45$ mmHg), then the risk of postoperative complications (e.g., prolonged ventilatory support, nosocomial pneumonia) increases. Further discussion on this topic appears in Chap. 45.

Formal disability evaluation from the Social Security Administration also involves

Table 2 Common Indications for Pulmonary
Function Testing

Diagnose lung disease
Follow course of lung disease
Follow effects of treatment for lung disease
Monitor pulmonary side-effects of drugs
Determine preoperative risk
Evaluate disability
Provide disease prognosis

---

measures of pulmonary function, which help define the nature and degree of disability. Similarly, the American Medical Association provides guidelines rating the level of respiratory impairment based on spirometry, DL_{CO}, and maximal oxygen consumption. Pulmonary disability evaluation is also addressed in Chap. 41.

Finally, PFTs provide important information about disease prediction. This is commonly recognized in COPD, where a reduced FEV_1 is associated with an accelerated decline in lung function and an increased risk for the development of bronchogenic carcinoma. Such information can be very important in convincing people to stop smoking. Less well appreciated, however, is the fact that lung function testing is also important in predicting the development of cardiovascular disease as well as overall risk of premature death. For example, analysis of 20 years of follow-up data from the Framingham Study revealed that the FVC ranked high as a predictor of both cardiovascular morbidity and mortality, especially congestive heart failure. The effect of FVC on cardiovascular mortality persisted even after accounting for other cardiovascular risk factors including age, heart rate, blood pressure, cigarette smoking, obesity, cholesterol, and glucose!

SPIROMETRY

The most important measures of pulmonary function obtained in the primary care setting are those derived from simple spirometry. This test involves measuring the volume of air forcibly inspired and expired over time. The common variables FEV_1 and FVC are determined by plotting the expired volume over time (Fig. 1). Additional information is derived from plotting both inspiratory and expiratory flow versus volume, generating a flow-volume loop (Fig. 2). Following an initial period of quiet (tidal) breathing, the patient is instructed to take in a big, deep breath (to total lung capacity, or TLC), and then, without hesitation, to expire the air as hard and as fast as possible until the lungs are empty (at residual volume, or RV). The total volume of air that exits the lung is the FVC. The most important indices of lung function derived from spirometry are the peak expiratory flow rate (PEFR), the FEV_1, the ratio of FEV_1 to FVC, and the flow-volume loop. The forced expiratory flow between 25 and 75% of the vital capacity, or the $FEF_{25-75\%}$, is also commonly reported and interpreted. Each of these indices is considered below.

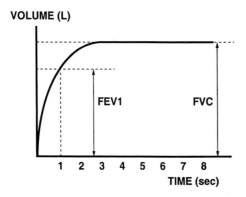

Figure 1   Volume-time curve, obtained as a plot of expired lung volume versus time from a forced expiratory maneuver. The forced expiratory volume in the first second is shown as the FEV_1, and the total amount of air expired is seen as the forced vital capacity (FVC).

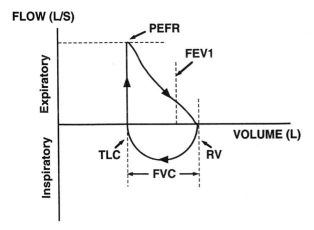

FLOW (L/S)

Figure 2 Flow-volume loop, obtained as a plot of inspired and expired flow versus lung volume during a forced inspiratory and expiratory maneuver. The maneuver begins at residual volume (RV) with an empty lung. Inspiration occurs with negative flow rates until total lung capacity (TLC) is reached; then expiration occurs with the generation of high positive flow rates, culminating in the peak expiratory flow rate (PEFR). Flow rates then diminish as the lung empties back to RV. The FEV_1 is shown along the volume axis.

Peak Expiratory Flow Rate

The most simple index of expiratory flow is the PEFR (Fig. 2). Peak flow normally occurs almost immediately during the FVC maneuver and therefore does not require prolonged expiration. The measurement can be performed on a spirometer (which typically records results in liters per second) or, more commonly, using any of a number of hand-held portable devices (which record results as liters per minute), Fig. 3. However, while the PEFR is simply obtained, the maneuver is very effort- and technique-dependent, making it one of the most variable and poorly reproducible of the expiratory flow indices. As with other PFTs, the range of normal for PEFR varies with age, sex, and height.

Perhaps the most useful function of the PEFR test is the ambulatory monitoring of the asthmatic patient. Since asthma, by definition, is a syndrome of variable airflow limitation, any one measurement of lung function at any given time may or may not be abnormal. By allowing the patient to record lung function with PEFR monitoring over a period of days to weeks, however, the nature of the variability of lung function in asthma can be revealed and documented (Fig. 4). Excessive lability of PEFR is a sign of increasing airways hyperresponsiveness, reflecting a worsening of asthma. When a patient recognizes increasing lability or a consistent reduction in PEFR, which could occur despite no change in symptoms, then the patient should take appropriate measures in order to avoid further clinical deterioration. Typically these measures include prompt communication with the physician, increasing the dosage of medication, or visiting the emergency room. This type of self-directed ambulatory monitoring allows individuals to take a proactive role in their medical care, giving them a greater sense of responsibility and control of their disease.

Forced Expiratory Volume in the First Second

The single most important pulmonary function test derived from spirometry is the FEV_1, or the volume of air expired in the first second of a forced expiratory maneuver from TLC

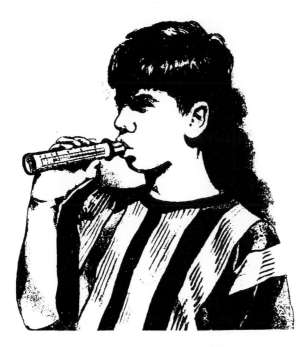

Figure 3 A young boy using his PEFR device. (From the American Lung Association.)

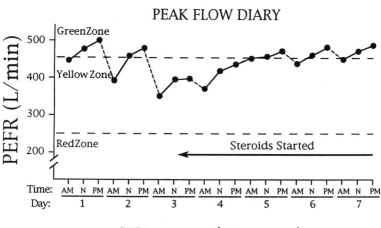

Time (Days)

Figure 4 Peak flow diary. Daily peak expiratory flow rates (PEFR) are plotted three times per day over the course of a week in an asthmatic patient. Notice the fluctuation (lability) in PEFR both within days (typically worse in the morning) and across days. The color zones refer to the levels of individual PEFR performance, as recommended by the National Asthma Education Program (green = 80–100% predicted or previous personal best; yellow = 50–80%; red = <50%). In this case, when the patient noticed persistent PEFRs in the yellow zone, she contacted her physician, who prescribed a course of corticosteroids. In response to therapy, the PEFR improved over the next few days, with less lability. (From Kaminsky DA, Irvin CG. Lung function in asthma. In: Barnes PJ, Grunstein MM, Leff AR, Woolcock AJ, eds. Asthma. New York: Lippincott-Raven, 1997:1277–1300.)

(Fig. 1). Although expressed in units of volume, the FEV_1 is considered to be an indirect measure of airflow, since it reflects the amount of air able to be expired in a fixed amount of time. The normal range of FEV_1 is approximately 80% or more of predicted values, but since the FEV_1 is a portion of the total volume expired (the FVC), it varies with the FVC (see below). Normal aging results in a loss of lung function as assessed by FEV_1, amounting to approximately 20–30 mL/year (Fig. 5). In smokers susceptible to the adverse effects of cigarette smoke, the rate of loss is increased, resulting in an accelerated decline in lung function. This rate of loss correlates with the number of cigarettes smoked per day and amounts to 54 mL/year for a two-pack-a-day smoker. With cessation of smoking, the rate of loss returns to normal; unfortunately, however, the lung function lost to this point cannot be regained. This phenomenon can be used to advantage in smoking cessation strategies. Informing patients that their ''lung age'' is much older than their chronological age may have a powerful motivating effect in convincing them to stop smoking. The ''lung age'' is that age at which the FEV_1 would be within normal limits. Thus, a 50-year-old may have an FEV_1 of 65% predicted for her age, but this same FEV_1 would be normal for an 83-year-old. Such a 50-year-old patient has a lung age of 83 years!

In addition to a normal aging effect, the FEV_1 varies inversely and linearly with the degree of airflow limitation in patients with asthma and COPD. Like other forced expiratory maneuvers, the FEV_1 is dependent on patient effort and requires that the patient perform a truly maximal inspiration followed immediately by a truly maximal expiration. However, the FEV_1 remains the most reproducible of the pulmonary function tests, with a coefficient of variation in normal subjects of 3–5%. The FEV_1 is more sensitive to airflow limitation than the physical examination or patient symptoms.

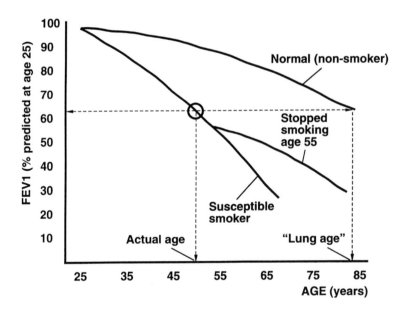

Figure 5 Natural history of lung function as measured by FEV_1. In normals, lung function peaks at approximately age 25 and then decays by 20–30 mL/year. The decay rate is accelerated in smokers but returns to a normal rate if smoking is stopped. The circle and dashed lines show that the FEV_1 of a 50-year-old smoker, corresponding to 65% of predicted for a 25-year-old, would be normal for an 83-year-old, hence giving the smoker a lung age of 83 years. (Adapted from Fletcher C, Peto R. The natural history of chronic airflow obstruction. BMJ 1977; 1:1645–1648.)

Reversibility of airflow obstruction by monitoring of FEV_1 is one of the most important hallmarks of asthma. The criteria established by the American Thoracic Society for demonstrating reversibility are a $\geq$ 12% improvement over baseline FEV_1 (or FVC) *and* a 200-mL absolute improvement. Monitoring the postbronchodilator FEV_1 is very important in following individuals over time, since it represents the "best" value attainable following pharmacological bronchodilatation and therefore minimizes the intrinsic variability of the FEV_1 due to acute (and hence confounding) factors causing bronchospasm during the day of evaluation.

Forced Vital Capacity

The FVC is the total volume exhaled from TLC to RV (Fig. 2). Measuring the FVC is important because it allows correction of flow for lung volume by expressing the FEV_1 as a percentage of the FVC: the ratio of FEV_1/FVC decreases with worsening airflow limitation and is the most sensitive spirometric indicator for the detection of early, mild airflow limitation. In general, a ratio of less than 90% predicted is indicative of airflow limitation. The degree of airflow limitation is then quantified by the percent predicted FEV_1. The differential diagnosis of airflow limitation is derived from considering the possible mechanisms involved in limiting airflow (Table 3).

The FVC is also an indirect measure of lung volume but must be interpreted carefully. The normal range of FVC is approximately 80% or more of predicted. A reduced FVC may be indicative of restrictive lung disease, but the FVC can also be reduced from significant airflow limitation, muscle weakness, or poor effort or technique. Only measurement of lung volumes, concomitant FEV_1, or muscle pressures, respectively, can help sort out this differential.

In restrictive disease, the FEV_1 is usually reduced in roughly the same proportion as the FVC, resulting in a normal (or supranormal) ratio of FEV_1/FVC (Fig. 6). If clinically indicated, measurement of lung volumes is needed to definitively define a restrictive disorder (see "Lung Volumes," below). In airflow limitation, the reduction in FEV_1 exceeds the reduction in FVC (Fig. 7). In this situation, the FVC is reduced because of significant airflow limitation, resulting in air trapping and hyperinflation. Muscle weakness may also reduce the FVC, since the patient may simply not have enough strength to inspire fully

Table 3 Differential Diagnosis of Airflow Limitation

Due to physical obstruction
  Pharyngeal and laryngeal tumors, edema, infection
  Vocal cord dysfunction
  Foreign bodies
  Trachea, large airways: tumors, stenosis, collapse
  Edema, mucus, hyperemia associated with
    bronchitis, bronchiectasis, asthma
  Bronchiolitis (constrictive)
Due to bronchoconstriction
  Bronchitis, asthma
Due to loss of elastic recoil
  Emphysema

FLOW (L/S)

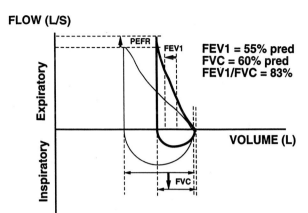

FEV1 = 55% pred
FVC = 60% pred
FEV1/FVC = 83%

Figure 6 Flow-volume loop (bold line) in a restrictive process as compared with normal (light line). Notice that the loop is foreshortened, reflecting the diminished FVC, as well as tall and narrow, reflecting the higher early flow rates (PEFR). Both the FEV_1 and the FVC are reduced roughly in proportion, yielding a normal if not elevated ratio of FEV_1/FVC.

and therefore expire the entire "true" lung volume. Muscle strength can be assessed by measurement of maximal inspiratory and maximal expiratory pressures (MIP and MEP, respectively). To measure MIP, subjects are asked to inhale as hard as they can against a transient occlusion once their lungs are empty (at RV). Likewise, to measure MEP, subjects are asked to exhale as hard as they can against a transient occlusion once their lungs are full (at TLC). Last, the FVC may be reduced if the patient did not make a good effort, either from lack of motivation, inability to understand the directions, or other reasons. This latter problem highlights the importance of having testing performed by highly qualified technologists who are specifically trained to recognize poor effort and coach the patient accordingly.

FLOW (L/S)

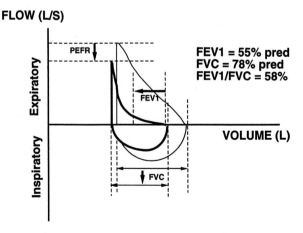

FEV1 = 55% pred
FVC = 78% pred
FEV1/FVC = 58%

Figure 7 Flow-volume loop (bold line) in airflow limitation as compared with normal (light line). The FVC is mildly reduced due to a higher RV, but the FEV_1 is reduced even more, yielding a lower ratio of FEV_1/FVC. PEFR is also reduced.

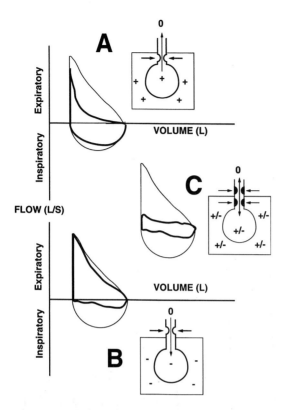

Figure 8   Changes in flow-volume loop shape in variable intrathoracic (A), variable extrathoracic (B), and fixed obstruction (C). The changes in shape are understood by considering the forces involved within the pleural space (depicted by the box) as compared with those within the alveolus and airways (depicted by the circle and tube). In A, net positive pleural pressure during expiration further enhances intrathoracic airway obstruction, as in asthma or bronchitis, to cause reductions in expiratory flow. During inspiration, the obstruction is relieved as pleural forces become negative and act to tether open the airways (hence, the obstruction is variable through the respiratory cycle). In B, net positive atmospheric pressure during inspiration enhances extrathoracic obstruction, as in the case of vocal cord tumors or dysfunction, to cause reductions in inspiratory flow. During expiration, the obstruction is relieved as airway pressures become positive and act to stent open the obstruction. In C, fixed obstruction anywhere within the large airways limits both inspiratory and expiratory flow and does not vary with the respiratory cycle. (From Irvin CG, Corbridge T. Physiologic evaluation of patients for pulmonary rehabilitation. Semin Respir Med 1993; 14:417–429.)

Flow-Volume Loop

A useful measure derived from spirometry is the flow-volume loop, formed by plotting both inspiratory and expiratory flow vs. volume (Fig. 2). The flow-volume loop gives some indication of the degree of effort used in generating it. A good effort is usually manifested as a sharp rise in expiratory flow, showing a distinct peak, followed by a more gradual decay in flow as lung volume is expired. The loop also allows visual pattern recognition of various disease states. In restriction, the loop is foreshortened, reflecting the loss of vital capacity, and narrow and tall, reflecting the enhanced early airflow from increased elastic recoil forces contributing to expiratory flow (Fig. 6). In intrathoracic obstruction, as occurs in asthma or chronic bronchitis, expiratory airflow is limited, resulting in a loop that has a concave expiratory limb (Figs. 7 and 8A). In extrathoracic obstruction, commonly caused by laryngeal tumors, foreign bodies, or vocal cord dysfunction, the loop has a truncated inspiratory limb, usually with preserved expiratory flow (Fig. 8B). Fixed obstruction, occurring anywhere in the large airways and not varying with the respiratory cycle, from such processes as airway tumors, foreign bodies, or stenosis, results in a squared-off flow-volume loop (Fig. 8C). Clinically, it is very important to recognize that extrathoracic obstruction, especially vocal cord dysfunction, commonly masquerades as asthma (see Case 6, below). Vocal cord dysfunction (VCD) is a syndrome manifest by variable extrathoracic obstruction at the level of the vocal cords due to inappropriate closure of the vocal cords during inspiration. Patients are often misdiagnosed as having asthma and present with severe dyspnea, inspiratory wheezing, and stridor. However, up to 50% of VCD patients also have coexistent asthma. A definitive diagnosis of VCD requires laryngoscopy to directly visualize the cords during an attack.

Forced Expiratory Flow

Another common index derived between 25 and 75% of the vital capacity from the FVC maneuver is the $FEF_{25-75\%}$, or the forced expiratory flow between 25 and 75% of the vital capacity. This index was originally thought to be less effort-dependent and more sensitive and specific to obstruction in the small airways than the FEV_1. However, compared with the FEV_1, the $FEF_{25-75\%}$ is more variable, less reproducible, and no more sensitive to airflow limitation. In addition, since the $FEF_{25-75\%}$ calculation relies directly on the FVC, it is highly influenced by changes in lung volume and the shape of the flow-volume loop. For example, as the full vital capacity may not be delivered in severe obstruction, the $FEF_{25-75\%}$, which is based on the FVC, may be falsely elevated and underestimate the degree of airway obstruction. Given these limitations, the $FEF_{25-75\%}$ should not be relied upon in clinical practice to provide any additional useful information.

LUNG VOLUMES

When questions arise regarding whether the lungs are of normal size or are restricted or hyperinflated, direct measurement of lung volume is indicated. Such measurements require more sophisticated equipment and thus are typically made in the pulmonary function laboratory rather than in the office setting. Assessment of changes in lung volumes following bronchodilator treatment may also unmask beneficial changes in airflow not seen by measuring changes in FEV_1 or FVC alone. To measure lung volume, one must first measure FRC. Then, a patient's inspiratory capacity (IC) is determined and added to FRC to yield TLC, and a patient's expiratory reserve volume (ERV) is measured and subtracted from FRC to yield RV (Fig. 9).

Functional Residual Capacity

The boundaries of lung volume are the maximal amount of gas after full inflation (TLC), the minimal amount of gas after full exhalation (RV), and the equilibrium point, or functional residual capacity (FRC), which is the amount of gas at the end of a normal tidal

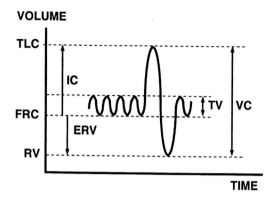

Figure 9 Spirometric tracing of lung volumes and capacities. The subject breathes with normal tidal volumes (TV). End-tidal volume is FRC. Adding the amount of air inspired from FRC until the lung is full (inspiratory capacity, IC) yields TLC, and subtracting the amount of air expired from FRC until the lung is empty (expiratory reserve volume, ERV) yields RV. The total amount of air able to be inspired and expired is the difference between TLC and RV, or the vital capacity (VC).

breath and is determined by the point at which the outward recoil pressure of the relaxed chest wall equals the inward elastic recoil pressure of the lung. FRC is the most reliable and important volume indicator because, unlike TLC and RV, FRC is not dependent on patient effort. A normal FRC is between 70 and 130% of predicted.

One of two methods is usually used to measure FRC. The most common method is the inert gas technique, either helium dilution or nitrogen washout. In the helium dilution technique, the subject quietly breathes the helium gas mixture starting from FRC until an equilibrium concentration of inert gas is established in the exhaled air from the lung. Knowing the initial and final concentrations of inert gas, one can calculate the volume into which it was diluted (FRC) upon reaching equilibrium. In the nitrogen washout technique, the subject quietly breathes pure oxygen starting from FRC to slowly replace the nitrogen that was in the lung at FRC. When the nitrogen has been adequately washed out (no further change in exhaled nitrogen concentration), the total volume of exhaled gas and its nitrogen concentration is measured to derive the quantity of nitrogen exhaled; this amount of nitrogen previously existed in the lung at FRC and was at a concentration of 80%, so FRC can now be calculated. Since the helium dilution and nitrogen washout tests rely on adequate gas mixing and equilibration, these tests may underestimate true FRC in subjects with significant airway obstruction or bullous disease.

The second method is by application of Boyle's law relating pressure and volume using a body plethysmograph (body box). In the most common application of this technique, the thoracic gas volume (TGV) at FRC is determined by having the subject briefly pant against a closed shutter when he or she is at FRC, during which changes in box pressure and mouth pressure are measured. Knowing the pressure-volume characteristics of the box and assuming that mouth pressure during zero flow is equivalent to alveolar pressure, one can calculate the subsequent volume changes in the lung and relate these mathematically to derive the starting volume (FRC). The advantage of determining FRC by the body box method is that it is rapid and reproducible and avoids the underestimation of FRC by the helium dilution technique as described above. It also allows one to simultaneously determine airway resistance (see below). However, many individuals cannot tolerate the panting technique used or the claustrophobia experienced in the body box, and the equipment is bulky and expensive.

Total Lung Capacity and Residual Volume

Once the equilibrium point is measured (FRC), one can then determine TLC and RV. A normal TLC is between 80–120% of predicted; normal RV is 60–140% of predicted. The divisions of lung volume, TLC, FRC, and RV change according to the underlying disease process (Fig. 10). In true lung restriction (Fig. 10A), all lung volumes are reduced and the degree of restriction is qualified according to American Thoracic Society guidelines by the percent reduction in the TLC (see Case 1). The differential diagnosis of such restrictive changes is given in Table 4. In muscle weakness, TLC may be reduced and RV elevated, but FRC is usually maintained in the normal range. This is because both IC and ERV are effort-dependent and therefore may be reduced with muscle weakness (see Case 3). In airflow limitation (Fig. 10B), TLC is usually unchanged but RV and FRC may be elevated, depending upon the degree of airflow limitation. Elevation of FRC in airflow limitation is thought to be predominantly due to air trapping and hyperinflation. With severe airflow limitation, as may occur in emphysema or severe asthma, the lungs may become truly overdistended with elevation of TLC (see Case 2).

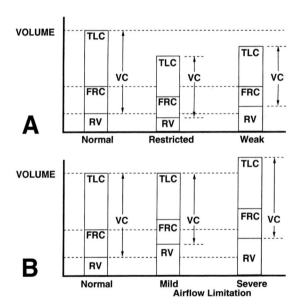

Figure 10 Lung volume changes in processes causing restriction (A) and airflow limitation (B). In true lung restriction, all divisions of lung volume are reduced. In muscle weakness, however, the FRC is normal, but the TLC is reduced and the RV is elevated because of the strength-dependent maneuvers required to reach each of these limits. In mild airflow limitation, FRC and RV may be elevated, resulting in a loss of VC, but TLC is usually unchanged. In severe airflow limitation, the TLC also rises, with the ultimate VC dependent on the relative rise in RV. (From Irvin CG, Corbridge T. Physiologic evaluation of patients for pulmonary rehabilitation. Semin Respir Med 1993; 14: 417–429.)

Table 4 Differential Diagnosis of Lung Restriction

Due to interstitial lung disease[a]
  Interstitial pneumonitis, fibrosis
  Edema
  Granulomatosis
Due to pleural disease
  Pneumothorax, hemothorax, fibrothorax
  Pleural effusion, empyema
Due to chest wall disease
  Kyphoscoliosis
  Extreme obesity
  Ascites, abdominal distention
  Injury
Due to neuromuscular disease
  Any cause (e.g., amyotrophic lateral sclerosis, diaphragmatic injury)

---

[a] Not all interstitial lung diseases are associated with restriction; the following may be associated with preserved lung volumes: lymphangioleiomyomatosis, chronic eosinophilic granuloma, interstitial sarcoidosis, chronic hypersensitivity pneumonitis, tuberous sclerosis, neurofibromatosis.

MEASURES OF GAS EXCHANGE

Diffusing Capacity

The diffusing capacity of the lung is an indirect measure of the ability of the lung to exchange gas at the alveolar-capillary interface. Ideally, one would want to know the diffusing capacity of the lung for oxygen, but it is difficult to measure the partial pressure of oxygen in the pulmonary capillary. Instead, the gas carbon monoxide is used because of its high affinity for hemoglobin and its essentially zero partial pressure in the pulmonary capillary. Although there have been a variety of techniques used to measure the DL_{CO}, only the single-breath technique is widely used.

In the single-breath technique, the subject inhales a single deep breath from RV of a gas mixture containing 0.3% CO, a small quantity of inert gas (such as helium or methane), and the rest air. The subject is instructed to hold his or her breath for 10 s and then to exhale forcefully. The total expired gas is collected, but only the gas coming from the gas exchange area of the lung (the alveolar gas) is analyzed. Knowing the initial and final concentrations of CO and inert gas, one can calculate how much CO was transferred to the alveolar capillaries. A normal DL_{CO} is between 75–125% of predicted. The DL_{CO} can be affected by many variables, including the inhalation and breath-holding times, breath-holding lung volume, size of the alveolar gas sample, and levels of carboxyhemoglobin and hemoglobin. Most of these factors are taken into account using standardized techniques.

The DL_{CO} is expressed both as an absolute number, and also corrected for serum hemoglobin, serum carboxyhemoglobin and the "alveolar volume" (V_A) into which the original test gas was distributed (which should approximate TLC, as the breath is held at TLC). These correcting factors can be extremely important in the final interpretation. The

DL_{CO} will vary directly with the hemoglobin level (increased affinity of CO for the blood) and inversely with the serum carboxyhemoglobin level (decreased affinity due to "back pressure"). Finally, if TLC, and hence V_A, is reduced, as in restrictive lung disease, then the DL_{CO} will be reduced proportionally if the intrinsic diffusing capacity of the lung parenchyma is normal (e.g., as one might expect in a patient with reduced lung volume from prior lung resection surgery). If TLC is normal, however, correction for V_A is not as important, except in the circumstance in which there is substantial gas maldistribution, such as may exist in asthma. Gas maldistribution can be recognized by a lower value of V_A (obtained by a single, 10-breath-hold) compared to TLC (obtained by an equilibrium technique which takes place over minutes, or by body plethysmography) (see Case 2). In this situation, DL_{CO} may be low, but is normal when corrected for V_A (DL_{CO}/V_A), reflecting the poor distribution of the test gas during the testing procedure.

Abnormalities of DL_{CO} may be helpful in distinguishing various disease processes (Fig. 11). Low DL_{CO} and DL_{CO}/V_A are usually due to either abnormalities occurring at the alveolar-capillary interface, such as emphysema, pulmonary vascular disease or interstitial lung disease, or due to severe anemia. Practically speaking, the DL_{CO} is most useful in distinguishing the etiology of airflow limitation. In emphysema, the DL_{CO} will be low, whereas in bronchitis or asthma, it will usually be normal. A high DL_{CO} is usually due to increased hemoglobin available either at the gas exchange interface or free within the alveolus and occurs in a limited number of diseases, such as polycythemia, left-to-right shunt, and alveolar hemorrhage. An elevated DL_{CO} may also be seen in stable, mild asthma, although the reasons for this are less clear.

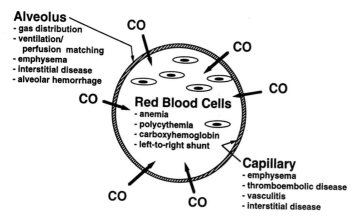

Figure 11   Factors involved in the diffusing capacity of the lung for carbon monoxide (DL_{CO}). Pictured is the alveolar-capillary unit of the lung, with the alveolus on the outside surrounding the pulmonary capillary containing red blood cells. In the alveolar space, abnormalities in the distribution of gas or the matching of ventilation to perfusion will lower the DL_{CO}, as will anatomic disruption or alteration of the alveolar component of the alveolar-capillary membrane (hatched circle), as occurs in emphysema or interstitial lung disease. Free hemoglobin in the alveolar space, as occurs in alveolar hemorrhage, will increase the DL_{CO}. At the level of the capillary, anatomic or functional disruption of the capillary component of the alveolar-capillary membrane will reduce the DL_{CO}, as in emphysema, thromboembolic disease, vasculitis, and interstitial lung disease. Finally, changes in the red blood cell space itself, affecting the capacity for hemoglobin binding of CO or overall CO transport, may either decrease the DL_{CO}, as in anemia or in the presence of carboxyhemoglobin, or increase the DL_{CO}, as in polycythemia or left-to-right shunting.

Although the DL_{CO} is commonly thought to reflect the gas exchange capability of the lung, there is poor correlation between gas exchange during exercise and the DL_{CO}. For this reason, pulse oximetry and full exercise testing are important diagnostic tools.

Pulse Oximetry

The pulse oximeter is a device that measures the percent oxygen saturation of capillary blood. It uses two wavelengths of light to distinguish between the absorption characteristics of oxyhemoglobin and deoxyhemoglobin and thus to calculate the ratio of these two species. The oxygen saturation is then calculated from this ratio, and is normally 95% or greater at sea level. Pulse oximeters are generally accurate to $\pm 4\%$ when the oxygen saturation is above 70%.

Pulse oximeters are highly portable and easy to use and provide valuable information about gas exchange in the ambulatory care setting. They are essential in monitoring those patients on supplemental oxygen therapy and the need for such therapy in all patients with moderate to severe lung disease. In addition, as a diagnostic tool, oximetry during exercise may be the most sensitive indicator of gas exchange, even when the diffusing capacity and resting oxygenation are normal (see Case 7).

However, there are important limitations to the use of pulse oximetry (Table 5). Pulse oximetry only assesses oxygenation expressed as percent saturation but gives no information on P_{O_2}, P_{CO_2}, or any acid-base data. Thus, since saturation is well protected despite a significant decline in P_{O_2}, a low P_{O_2} may be missed if oxygenation is determined only by this method. Likewise, in the intensive care unit setting, the pulse oximeter will read 100% for P_{O_2}'s of both 90 or 490; in such situations where hyperoxia is a concern, direct measurement of P_{O_2} is indicated. In addition, an oximeter cannot be used to assess ventilatory function, which is especially relevant in COPD patients who may retain CO_2 and become acidotic. In both of the above situations, evaluation with arterial blood gases is essential.

Other circumstances must also be recognized during which pulse oximetry may give inaccurate or misleading information. These include the presence of other hemoglobin species (e.g., carboxyhemoglobin, which will yield a falsely high oxygen saturation), low perfusion states (e.g., shock), significant anemia, or excessive external light.

Table 5   Advantages and Disadvantages of Pulse Oximetry

Advantages	Disadvantages
Noninvasive	Unable to monitor P_{CO_2}
Simple	False security (saturation vs. P_{O_2})
Reduce number of ABGs	Inaccurate at saturation <70%
	Limitations: dyshemoglobins (e.g., CO-Hgb, meth-Hg), dyes and pigments (e.g., methylene blue, bilirubin), low perfusion, anemia, increased venous pulsations, external light sources

SPECIAL TESTING

All of the pulmonary function tests discussed above are usually available in any standard PFT lab and are usually sufficient to answer most questions regarding lung function. There are other tests, however, that may provide additional valuable information. Four of these tests—airways resistance, lung compliance, bronchial challenge, and exercise testing—are discussed briefly below.

Airways Resistance

Elevations in airways resistance are usually detected by the resultant decrement in airflow that occurs during forced expiratory maneuvers. However, the measurements of FEV_1 and the FEV_1/FVC ratio are somewhat arbitrary and probably only sensitive to certain types of flow limitation. To increase the sensitivity of detecting abnormalities of airflow, increases in airways resistance can be measured directly. The most common method used clinically is by determining the flow-pressure relationship of the airways at distinct lung volumes, as measured in a body plethysmograph. The normal value for airways resistance (Raw), which includes the upper airway, is approximately 1.5 cmH$_2$O/L/s. However, Raw varies with lung volume in a curvilinear fashion, so a corrected measure, specific conductance (sGaw), is calculated by taking the reciprocal of Raw and then dividing by the volume at which it was measured (usually TGV).

Measurement of sGaw has several advantages. First, it is thought to be more sensitive to induced bronchoconstriction than other measures of airflow. Second, it is measured without forced expiration, eliminating the problems of patient effort, muscle strength, and other mechanical factors. Third, the panting maneuver used during the test opens the vocal cords and therefore allows sGaw to be a better reflection of lower airway (below the cords) caliber. Finally, since 90% of total Raw is in the large, central airways, sGaw may be more sensitive and specific to upper vs. lower airway resistance, allowing some localization of airflow limitation within the bronchial tree.

Lung Compliance

In some clinical circumstances it is unclear whether changes in lung volume are due to intrinsic changes in the elastic properties of the lung tissue or from influences of the chest wall, muscle strength, and other factors. Likewise, it may be unclear whether airflow limitation is predominantly due to increased airways resistance (from bronchoconstriction, airway wall edema, or mucus) or from reduced elastic recoil (as in pure emphysema), which contributes to the driving force for airflow. Since defining the underlying etiology of disease and subsequent therapy may both depend upon these physiological characteristics, it may be useful to measure lung compliance directly.

To measure lung compliance, one must know the change in lung volume for any given change in pressure across the alveolus and the pleural space (the transpulmonary pressure, the driving pressure for effecting changes in lung volume). Lung volume changes are measured with a spirometer, and transpulmonary pressure is estimated by measuring the difference between mouth pressure (which approximates alveolar pressure during conditions of no airflow) and esophageal pressure (which approximates pleural pressure). Esophageal pressure, in turn, is measured by placement of a balloon-tipped catheter into the lower esophagus. Once in place, the patient is instructed to inspire fully to TLC and then slowly expire as the lungs empty in a relaxed fashion. During expiration, a shutter intermittently closes briefly, interrupting airflow and therefore allowing alveolar pressure to be approximated by mouth pressure. This pressure at each level of volume is recorded, and the resulting pressure-volume (PV) data are plotted to determine the static (no-flow) expiratory PV curve of the lungs (Fig. 12).

By convention, lung compliance is determined as the slope of the PV curve at FRC. Increased compliance, usually seen in a curve that is shifted up and to the left, is seen in emphysema, whereas decreased compliance, as seen in a curve shifted down and to the right, is seen in interstitial lung disease. Patients with asthma have curves that usually have normal compliance with a normal shape but are shifted upward, reflecting increased lung volumes. The PV data can also be combined with simultaneously measured flow-volume data to determine the level of resistance occurring in the most peripheral airways of the lung (so-called upstream resistance). These latter data may be useful in distinguishing patients with mixed chronic bronchitis and emphysema, who should be treated with

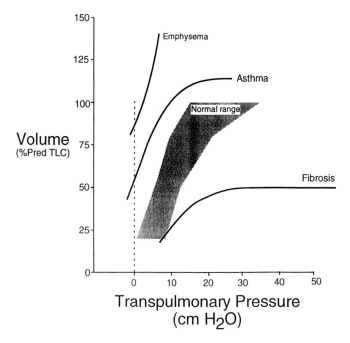

Figure 12 Static pressure-volume curves for the lung for different disorders. In the normal individual (shaded region), lung elastic recoil increases with increasing lung volume in a nonlinear fashion. Processes such as interstitial fibrosis increase lung elastic recoil, shifting the curve down and to the right, with a reduced slope at FRC reflecting diminished compliance. Diseases that decrease elastic recoil, such as emphysema, result in a loss of elastic recoil and a curve shifted up and to the left, with increased compliance. Patients with mild asthma usually have curves shifted upward, due to hyperinflation, but with a normal shape (compliance). (From Corbridge T, Irvin CG. Pathophysiology of chronic obstructive pulmonary disease with emphasis on physiologic and pathologic correlations. In: Casaburi R, Petty T, eds. Principles and Practice of Pulmonary Rehabilitation. Philadelphia: Saunders, 1993: 19.)

bronchodilators and anti-inflammatory agents, from those with pure emphysema, for whom only a more empirical approach to therapy is available.

Bronchial Challenge

Bronchial challenge studies are indicated when a patient gives a clinical history consistent with asthma (or other reactive airways disease) but spirometry is normal and there is no spirometric response to bronchodilator at the time of testing. These normal findings are not inconsistent with the diagnosis of asthma because asthma is a disease not only of variable airflow limitation but also of airways hyperresponsiveness (AHR). The phenomenon of AHR is manifest as an increased sensitivity and response to a stimulus that causes airflow limitation compared to the response in normals. The differential diagnosis of AHR includes not only asthma but also many different diseases in which airway injury or inflammation are present (Table 6). The two most common stimuli used to challenge a subject with possible AHR are methacholine and exercise (Fig. 13).

In a methacholine challenge, increasing doses of the acetylcholine agonist methacholine are administered by inhalation according to a standard protocol. After each level of drug, the FEV_1 is measured and compared with baseline. Subjects with AHR will drop their FEV_1 by 20% or more at a concentration of less than 8 mg/mL. A similar endpoint used in this challenge is a drop of 40% or more in sGaw. People with AHR to methacholine thus demonstrate nonspecific AHR and, in the right clinical setting, fulfill the diagnosis of asthma (see Case 5).

Many subjects with possible asthma will complain of symptoms occurring during or immediately following exercise. In these situations, challenge with exercise can also be performed. This protocol usually involves treadmill or bicycle exercise to a heart rate of 85% predicted maximal heart rate for at least 6 min. A fall in FEV_1 of 15% from baseline following exercise is diagnostic of exercise-induced bronchospasm.

Since bronchial challenge testing is usually performed in patients with suspected asthma, it is important to pay attention to the flow-volume loop during challenge. Progressive truncation of the inspiratory loop during challenge without necessarily any expiratory flow limitation may occur in patients with vocal cord dysfunction (see Case 6) and thus lead to a false-negative result. Other causes of false-negative results are the use of bronchodilating medications prior to challenge, including caffeine and chocolate. False-positive results can occur in patients with transient AHR (Table 6), such as might follow an upper respiratory infection, or if patients simply do not take deep breaths, resulting in low FVCs and hence apparent falls in FEV_1. The latter reason is why it may be helpful to track lung volumes during the challenge and why changes in sGaw (which are corrected for lung volume) are important in assessing the response.

Table 6 Differential Diagnosis of Airway Hyperresponsiveness

Asthma, asthmatic bronchitis
Viral upper respiratory infection
Chemical irritant exposure
Sarcoidosis
Cystic fibrosis
Atopy

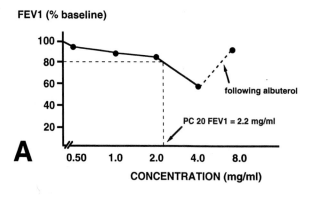

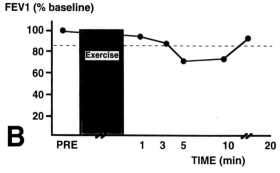

Figure 13   Demonstration of airways hyperresponsiveness (AHR) by methacholine challenge (A) and exercise challenge (B). In a methacholine challenge, changes in FEV_1 relative to baseline are plotted against increasing concentrations of methacholine. If the FEV_1 drops by 20% or more at a dose of less than 8 mg/mL, then the airways are hyperresponsive (compared to normals). The provocative concentration causing the 20% fall in FEV_1 is back-extrapolated (light dashed lines) and termed the PC_{20} FEV_1. Thus, a PC_{20} $FEV_1 < 8$ mg/mL is indicative of AHR. Subjects are given a bronchodilator to reverse the effects of the methacholine (heavy dashed line) following the challenge. In an exercise challenge, AHR is defined by a threshold fall of 15% or more in FEV_1 (dashed horizontal line) following a standard period of exercise. The typical time course of exercise-induced bronchospasm is seen here, with the maximal fall in FEV_1 occurring between 5 and 10 min after the challenge, and the FEV_1 recovering spontaneously over the next 20–30 min.

Exercise Testing

Formal exercise testing, with expired gas and arterial blood gas analysis, can be an invaluable diagnostic tool in determining the cause of exercise limitation. Unlike exercise stress tests performed in the cardiology setting, a symptom-limited, graded exercise challenge test performed in the pulmonary lab will yield additional information about the major physiological functions involved in exercise performance: cardiovascular, ventilatory, and gas exchange.

The protocol for testing usually involves exercising a subject to exhaustion on a treadmill or bicycle ergometer by applying increasing levels of work, usually in 1-min increments. During exercise, measurements are simultaneously made of heat rate, blood pressure, electrocardiogram (ECG), respiratory rate, tidal volume, oxygen consumption, carbon dioxide production, pulse oximetry, and arterial blood gases. From these measurements, indices are derived that relate to the various factors involved in the transport of oxygen and carbon dioxide between the atmosphere and the exercising muscle and mitochondria. The maximal level of work is measured, which determines whether exercise limitation is present. If exercise limitation occurs (less than 80% predicted maximal work rate achieved), then each of the variables related to the cardiovascular, ventilatory, and gas exchange systems can be analyzed to determine the limiting factors. For example, excessive increases in heart rate or blood pressure or the development of ECG abnormalities would suggest problems with the heart or peripheral vascular system. Excessive minute ventilation or ratio of dead space to tidal volume develops during ventilatory dysfunction, and hypoxemia or a rise in the ratio of dead space to tidal volume occurs when there are problems of gas exchange within the pulmonary circulation. Overall, the anaerobic threshold can be measured and can give information about problems with oxygen delivery or utilization or the level of conditioning. With the physiological information derived from exercise testing available, the physician can then pursue the specific underlying cause (e.g., ischemic cardiac disease, restrictive lung disease, or pulmonary vascular disease).

The level of oxygen consumption derived from exercise testing is useful in determining risk from lung resection surgery as well as level of disability in formal disability evaluations. In many cases, exercise testing simply reassures a patient that no functional limitations can be found and that only deconditioning or other psychological factors appear to explain the limited exercise tolerance. Such information can be comforting and can encourage patients to continue to exercise.

SUMMARY

An Algorithmic Approach to Pulmonary Function Test Ordering and Interpretation

Ordering

This chapter has provided the physiological rationale for and outlined the clinical importance of the various common tests of pulmonary function available. Using this information, the following algorithmic approach to determining which PFTs are indicated can be used. First, general pulmonary function should be assessed with two simple tests: spirometry and oximetry. Spirometry will provide the important index of airflow, the FEV_1/FVC ratio, and also a first approximation at lung size, the FVC. The important ambulatory monitoring variable, PEFR, will also be measured, and the flow-volume loop will provide additional information about the nature of airflow limitation. Any concerns about oxygenation at rest or with exercise can easily be addressed with pulse oximetry.

If questions remain, then more sophisticated tests should be performed. If it is unclear whether a patient has airflow limitation, then airways resistance measurements and bronchial challenge testing can be performed. If lung volume restriction is a question, then lung volumes can be measured directly. If muscle strength is a concern, then the MIP and MEP should be measured. The more intrinsic mechanical properties of the lung, such as compliance and upstream resistance, can be assessed by obtaining a PV curve. Last, if gas exchange is compromised, the $D_{L_{CO}}$ may be helpful in sorting out the common diagnoses of emphysema, chronic bronchitis, and interstitial lung disease. Ultimately, full exercise testing can be performed to determine whether exercise limitation is present, and, if so, because of what factors.

Interpretation

Basic rules of interpreting simple PFTs are as follows. Spirometry interpretation is based on the FVC, FEV$_1$, and shape of the flow-volume loop (Fig. 14). The FVC and shape of the flow-volume loop may offer clues as to restriction, muscle weakness, or poor effort. In airflow limitation, the FEV$_1$/FVC ratio determines its presence, and the absolute percent predicted FEV$_1$ points to its degree. Attention to the shape of the flow-volume loop provides additional information about the nature of flow limitation, especially with regard to the extrathoracic upper airway. Lung volume interpretation is mainly based on the TLC, although, because of the effects of muscle strength and effort on determining TLC and RV, FRC may be more important. In evaluating gas exchange abnormalities, resting oxygen saturation by pulse oximetry may be helpful, but a drop in oxygen saturation of greater than 4% with exercise is a more sensitive test. Finally, the DL$_{CO}$, corrected for hemoglobin and lung volume, determines whether gas exchange abnormalities are present, at least at rest.

Perspective

Pulmonary function testing provides important and useful information about the functioning of the lungs, and, in the context of other clinical data, helps characterize the presence of specific pulmonary disease. It offers means not only to diagnose and monitor disease but also to stratify operative risk, determine degree of disability, and predict prognosis.

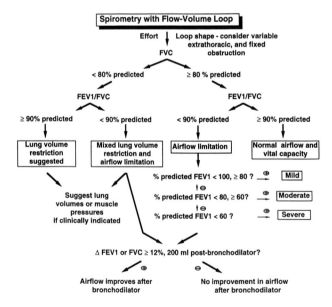

Figure 14   Algorithm to interpret basic spirometry. Interpretation should begin with an assessment of the FVC, keeping in mind patient effort and the shape of the flow-volume loop. A normal FVC means that there is no restrictive process involved, whereas a low FVC is consistent with restriction, muscle weakness, poor effort, or significant airflow limitation. To evaluate these latter possibilities, the FEV$_1$/FVC ratio should be looked at to determine the presence of airflow limitation, and, if present, its severity (based on percent predicted FEV$_1$) and reversibility. Lung volumes and muscle pressures should be obtained to evaluate restriction or muscle weakness.

In some diseases, such as asthma, objective measures of pulmonary function are critically important in assessing disease severity, as patients may have poor perception of their disease. Some argue that a simple measure such as the FEV_1 provides at least as much information as the pulse, blood pressure, respiratory rate, or temperature of a patient, and that especially in a patient who smokes, it should serve as the fifth vital sign.

CASES

Case 1

A 68-year-old man presents with increasing dyspnea on exertion. He has a 20-pack-year history of smoking but quit 30 years ago. He has worked as a firefighter. Physical examination reveals inspiratory crackles at both lung bases, a normal heart, and no digital clubbing. PFTs are obtained:

Spirometry	Measured	%Predicted
FVC (L)	2.48	63
FEV1 (L)	2.15	79
FEV1/FVC (%)	87	126
Lung Volumes		
TLC (L)	3.52	56
FRC (L)	1.56	44
RV (L)	1.07	47
Diffusion		
DLCO (ml/min/mm Hg)	6.36	26
DLCO/VA (ml/min/mm Hg/L)	1.98	50
VA (L)	3.22	51

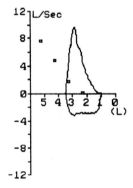

Interpretation

Spirometry shows a low FVC and low FEV_1, with a preserved, indeed elevated, ratio of FEV_1/FVC (dots represent predicted expiratory flow in this and all subsequent cases). These findings alone are consistent with restriction, muscle weakness, or poor effort. However, lung volumes reveal severe lung restriction, with a reduced TLC, FRC, and RV. Diffusion shows a reduced DL_{CO} that does not correct for the low lung volume, indicating an intrinsic loss of diffusing capacity. These results are consistent with an interstitial lung disease, which proved to be idiopathic pulmonary fibrosis on open lung biopsy.

Case 2

A 66-year-old woman presents with increasing dyspnea on exertion. She has a 100-pack-year history of smoking and quit 9 months ago. She has worked as a realtor. Physical examination reveals a cachectic woman, with markedly diminished breath sounds on chest auscultation. PFTs are obtained:

Spirometry	Measured	%Predicted
FVC (L)	2.13	76
FEV1 (L)	0.82	40
FEV1/FVC (%)	38	53
Lung Volumes		
TLC (L)	6.29	136
FRC (L)	4.50	170
RV (L)	4.27	235
Diffusion		
DLCO (ml/min/mm Hg)	7.22	40
DLCO/VA (ml/min/mm Hg/L)	2.08	54
VA (L)	3.48	75

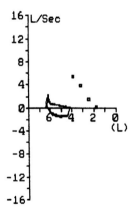

Interpretation

Spirometry shows a reduced FVC and FEV_1, with a greatly reduced ratio of FEV_1/FVC, consistent with mixed lung volume restriction and airflow limitation. There is no response to bronchodilator. To sort out the mixed process, lung volumes were obtained and revealed overdistention, with elevated TLC, FRC, and RV. Together, spirometry and lung volumes are now consistent with either chronic bronchitis, emphysema, or asthma. However, diffusion testing shows a diminished DL_{CO} and DL_{CO}/VA, consistent with disruption of the alveolar-capillary membrane and therefore indicative of emphysema. Notice also that the single breath VA (3.48 L), measured by a 10-s breath-hold, is markedly less than the same lung volume, TLC (6.29 L), measured by an equilibrium technique, revealing significant maldistribution of gas, again consistent with emphysema.

Case 3

A 45-year-old woman with recently diagnosed systemic lupus erythematosis presents with increasing dyspnea on exertion. She is a lifelong nonsmoker and has worked as a nurse. Physical examination of the lungs and heart is unremarkable. PFTs are obtained:

Spirometry	Measured	%Predicted
FVC (L)	1.90	55
FEV1 (L)	1.72	65
FEV1/FVC (%)	91	119
Lung Volumes		
TLC (L)	3.55	69
FRC (L)	2.27	82
RV (L)	1.95	114
IC (L)	1.29	54
ERV (L)	0.32	30
Diffusion		
DLCO (ml/min/mm Hg)	8.04	43
DLCO/VA (ml/min/mm Hg/L)	3.28	82
VA (L)	2.70	53
Muscle Pressures		
MIP (cm H20)	-33	<-50
MEP (cm H20)	31	> 80

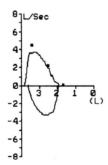

Interpretation

Spirometry shows a reduced FVC and FEV_1 but a normal FEV_1/FVC ratio, consistent with restriction, muscle weakness, or poor effort. Notice that the flow-volume loop lacks a sharp, distinct peak flow, suggestive of muscle weakness or poor effort. Lung volumes reveal a normal FRC and RV but a reduced TLC. Since FRC is effort-independent, this implies that the TLC is low from muscle weakness or poor effort. Indeed, muscle pressure testing shows that the patient has significant muscle weakness (predicted MIP and MEP are given by lower limits of normal), accounting for the low IC and hence

TLC. Likewise, the effort-dependent expiration to RV (ERV) is also low. Diffusion is low, but corrects to normal for lung volume, suggesting that the intrinsic diffusing capacity of the lung is normal. These results are all consistent with the low lung volumes (TLC and FVC) commonly seen in diseases associated with neuromuscular weakness, like lupus.

Case 4

A 20-year-old man presents with chronic cough. He has never smoked or been exposed to any toxic environmental agents. Physical examination is unremarkable. PFTs are obtained:

Spirometry	Measured	%Predicted	Post	(%Δ)
FVC (L)	5.89	101	6.45	+9
FEV1 (L)	3.18	68	4.18	+31
FEV1/FVC (%)	54	68	65	+19
Lung Volumes				
TLC (L)	8.42	111	8.33	-1
FRC (L)	4.82	117	4.60	-4
RV (L)	1.99	112	1.87	-6
Airway Resistance				
sGaw (L/sec/cm H20)	0.08	(0.11-0.40)	0.17	+110
Diffusion				
DLCO (ml/min/mm Hg)	31.40	92		
DLCO/VA (ml/min/mm Hg/L)	3.80	84		
VA (L)	8.26	109		

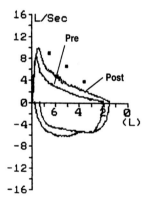

Interpretation

Spirometry shows a normal FVC but a reduced FEV_1 and FEV_1/FVC ratio, consistent with airflow limitation. The FEV_1 improves by 31% following use of a bronchodilator, demonstrating significant reversibility of airflow limitation. Lung volumes are normal but airway conductance is low (predicted value is given by an absolute range), consistent with high airways resistance, and conductance also improves following use of the bronchodilator (a change of +25% or more is considered significant). Diffusion testing is normal. These results are all consistent with the diagnosis of asthma.

Case 5

A 65-year-old woman presents with dyspnea following exercise. She has never smoked. Physical examination is normal. Spirometry shows a normal FVC and FEV_1, with a normal FEV_1/FVC ratio and no response to bronchodilator. Because of the concern that the patient may have asthma, a methacholine challenge test is obtained (Fig. 13A).

Interpretation

As increasing concentrations of methacholine are administered by inhalation, the patient has a gradual decline in FEV_1, eventually reaching and surpassing the 20% threshold for a positive response at a dose less than 8 mg/mL. In this case, the provocative concentration causing a 20% fall in FEV_1 (the PC_{20} FEV_1) was 2.2 mg/mL, indicative of significant airways hyperresponsiveness. In the proper clinical context, this result supports the diagnosis of asthma.

Case 6

A 31-year-old woman presents with episodes of wheezing and shortness of breath; she has been told that she has had asthma since childhood. However, medical therapy has done little to alleviate her symptoms. Spirometry is normal, and there is no response to the use of a bronchodilator. A methacholine challenge test is obtained and is normal, but repeated flow-volume loops during challenge are abnormal.

FLOW (L/sec)

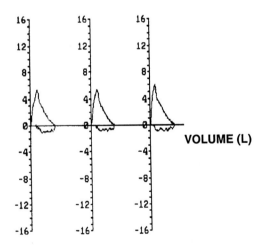

VOLUME (L)

Interpretation

Close inspection of the flow-volume loops reveals consistent truncation of the inspiratory limbs during testing. The larynx was inspected by direct fiberoptic laryngoscopy, revealing significant vocal cord dysfunction. The patient was taken off her asthma medications and treated with voice therapy, with marked improvement in her symptoms.

Case 7

A 68-year-old man presents with increasing dyspnea on exertion. He has a 27-pack-year history of smoking but quit 20 years ago and has worked as a forest ranger. Physical examination is normal. PFTs demonstrated normal spirometry, lung volumes, and diffusion. Exercise oximetry is shown below:

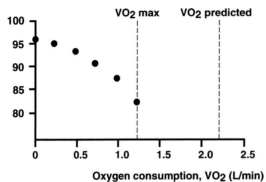

Oxygen saturation (%)

Interpretation

Formal exercise testing confirmed exercise limitation with significant arterial oxygen desaturation, as shown in the figure, as well as low maximal oxygen consumption, an excessive increase in heart rate, and a rise in the ratio of ventilatory dead space to tidal volume. These findings are consistent with pulmonary vascular disease and possible cardiac dysfunction. Further workup with an exercise echocardiogram and pulmonary angiogram revealed the diagnosis of pulmonary hypertension associated with chronic pulmonary thromboembolic disease.

SUGGESTED READING

1. ATS Official Statement. Lung function testing: selection of reference values and interpretative strategies. Am Rev Respir Dis 1991; 144:1202–1218.
2. ATS Official Statement. Single-breath carbon monoxide diffusing capacity (transfer factor). 1995 Update. Am J Respir Crit Care Med 1995; 152:2185–2198.
3. ATS Official Statement. Standardization of spirometry. 1994 Update. Am J Respir Crit Care Med 1995; 152:1107–1136.
4. Crapo RO. Pulmonary-function testing. N Engl J Med 1994; 331:25–30.
5. Enright PL, Lebowitz MD, Cockroft DW. Physiologic measures: pulmonary function tests. Asthma outcome. Am J Respir Crit Care Med 1994; 149:S9–S18.
6. Higgins M, Keller JB, Wagenknecht LE, et al. Pulmonary function and cardiovascular risk factor relationships in black and in white young men and women. The CARDIA Study. Chest 1991; 99:315–322.
7. Kaminsky DA, Irvin CG. Lung function in asthma. In: Barnes PJ, Grunstein MM, Leff AR, Woolcock AJ, eds. Asthma. New York: Lippincott-Raven, 1997:1277–1300.
8. Kannel WB, Hubert H, Lew EA. Vital capacity as a predictor of cardiovascular disease: the Framingham Study. Am Heart J 1983; 105:311–315.
9. Littner MR. Getting the most from your pulmonary function lab. J Respir Dis 1993; 14:1043–1061.
10. Maguire GP, Kleinhenz ME. How—and why—to use spirometry in your office. J Respir Dis 1994; 15:753–772.

11. Newman KB, Dubester SN. Vocal cord dysfunction: masquerader of asthma. Semin Respir Crit Care Med 1994; 15:161–167.
12. Permutt S. Pulmonary function testing and the prevention of pulmonary disease. Chest 1978; 74:608–610.
13. Pratter MR, Irwin RS. The clinical value of pharmacologic bronchoprovocation challenge. Chest 1984; 85:260–265.
14. Wanger J. Pulmonary Function Testing: A Practical Approach. Philadelphia: Williams & Wilkins, 1996.
15. Younes M. Interpretation of clinical exercise testing in respiratory disease. Clin Chest Med 1984; 5:189–206.

10

Principles and Interpretation of the Chest Radiograph

Peter A. Dietrich and Todd Peebles
University of Vermont College of Medicine
Fletcher Allen Health Care
Burlington, Vermont

ROLE OF THE CHEST RADIOGRAPH IN THE EVALUATION OF PATIENTS WITH RESPIRATORY SYMPTOMS

Although many imaging techniques are available to the radiologist in the evaluation of thoracic disease, the chest film remains the mainstay. Conventional posteroanterior (PA) and lateral chest radiographs should be performed as the initial imaging study in all patients with suspected thoracic disease.

Clinical information accompanying the chest film request is most helpful in interpreting the chest radiograph and tailoring the radiographic report. A complete, up-to-date patient problem list should ideally be part of each exam ordered. The ordering physician should also indicate the patient problem(s) for which the film is ordered and the primary clinical differential diagnoses. The radiologist can structure the report around the patient's known problems and specifically include the physician's stated diagnostic considerations as pertinent positives or negatives. As an example of the radiologist using clinical information to reach an impression, a rounded opacity in an older smoker likely represents a malignancy, but in a younger nonsmoker with fever, cough, and purulent sputum, it likely represents a rounded pneumonia.

COMMON RADIOGRAPHIC TECHNIQUES

The routine chest film should be a high-kilovolt technique done on a dedicated chest unit at a 6-ft distance (focal spot to film) using an appropriate grid to clean up scatter radiation. Both PA and left lateral views are routine. The high-kilovolt (peak) requires only a short exposure time, helping to diminish cardiac and respiratory motions and thus allowing sharper margins of the cardiac outline, diaphragms, and pulmonary vessels. Helpful supplemental plain films include lordotic projections, expiratory PA films, and decubitus filming.

Lordotic projections are obtained in the PA or anteroposterior (AP) projection with the x-ray tube angled 15 degrees cephalad. This projection is useful in changing the relative position of the anterior and posterior bony thorax, thus diminishing the summation problem when evaluating possible apical masses. The lordotic projection can also be used to confirm complete collapse of the right middle lobe by positioning this lobe tangent to the x-ray beam if routine projections are inconclusive.

Expiratory PA films are helpful in the detection of pneumothorax and to look for problems of regional air trapping. The increased sensitivity of expiratory films for pneumothorax is due to the increased opacity and decreased volume of the lung after exhalation. This creates a greater differential in radiographic density between the inflated lung and the pleural air.

Decubitus films are useful not only in detecting small effusions, but also in evaluating the compressed underlying lung by moving the fluid away to a new dependent portion of the pleural space. A small pneumothorax can be detected in the nondependent pleural space. The dependent diaphragm moves to a higher position relative to the nondependent diaphragm and, if fluoroscoped in this position, can be observed to move much more than the nondependent one.

Fluoroscopy provides real-time evaluation of diaphragmatic function and can assess for the presence of unilateral diaphragmatic paresis or paralysis. In the evaluation of a nodular opacity seen on only one view, the fluoroscopic observation of the opacity can demonstrate if it represents a pseudonodule caused by an osteophyte, healed rib fracture, or something external to the lung (nipple shadow, skin lesion, or bone island). This examination may obviate the need for computed tomography (CT) or oblique chest films for this determination.

Bedside supine or semiupright filming remains a challenge both in obtaining optimal images and in their interpretation. Filming is done at a 40-in distance, so magnification occurs. A reproducible optimal technique requires daily critique and a bedside record of the factors used.

AN APPROACH TO CHEST FILM INTERPRETATION

The practitioner must use a well-organized approach to chest film interpretation to avoid overlooking important clues.

The first principle in the evaluation of chest films is to obtain any prior films for review before a new film study is obtained. The physician needs to identify and locate any prior chest films that can be used for comparison with the current examination and have them signed into the radiology film library so they are available to the radiologist. Evaluation of the PA upright and left lateral chest begins by placing this baseline comparison exam next to the current study. The frontal and lateral films are then assessed for penetration, rotation, motion, and degree of inspiration. With proper penetration, the intervertebral disk spaces should be faintly visualized through the cardiac outline in the PA view. The rotation of the PA view is best determined by noting the relationship between the medial cortical margins of the clavicular heads and the spinous processes of the thoracic spine. The posterior ribs are almost superimposed on a true lateral view, recognizing that there is almost a 10% magnification of right-sided structures if the body width is 33 cm. Motion will blur vessel margins, simulating pulmonary interstitial disease, so the cardiac margins and sharpness of the diaphragm are examined to determine if the exposure was done at suspended respiration. An appropriately deep inspiration was usually achieved if the apex of the right diaphragm is seen below the tenth posterior rib.

Vessel size should next be examined by comparing the upper, middle, and lower zones of the right and left lungs. The lower-zone vessels should be about twice the diameter of those in the upper zones. If the upper-zone vessels appear to be the same as or larger than vessels in the lower zone, this observation should be confirmed by comparing vessel size on the lateral view in the retrosternal clear space (upper zone) to the retrocardiac vessels (lower zone) (Fig. 1A).

The vessel margins are then evaluated, again by comparing the right and left lungs by zones. Normal vessels are solid cylinders with slightly indistinct margins. If the margins are more indistinct than those in the baseline film and the same filming technique has been used, a significant change may be present. Respiratory and cardiac motion can also blur vessel margins. Conversely, if the margins are too well defined, emphysema is the usual explanation. Emphysema also causes straightening of the vessels and disappearance of side branches of pulmonary vessels.

If vessel margins are indistinct, a common finding is perihilar haze where the summation of many vessels occurs. In addition, the hollow cylinders of bronchi seen end-on near the hila will be thickened (bronchial wall cuffing). These findings should then be compared with those of the baseline chest film. Each costophrenic angle should be examined for the subtle pleural thickening characteristic of laminar effusions, in which the angle remains sharp but is displaced medially by a millimeter or two.

A comparison of diaphragm height with that in the baseline examination will help determine significant interval change. The lung length can be measured from the posterior tubercle of the first rib to the dome of each diaphragm. If the patient has been told to "take in a breath as deeply as you can and hold it," the diaphragm will move consistently to the same level each day as long as there has been no change in the patient's condition.

After review of the lungs as outlined above, has been completed, the interfaces of the lung with the mediastinum should be evaluated. Attention to the mediastinum on the PA view can be divided at the level of the carina. On the lateral view, the image is divided into the retrotracheal, retrosternal, and retrocardiac spaces (Fig. 1A). The retrotracheal lung forms a triangle, whose base formed by the top of the aortic arch and whose apex points upward to the thoracic inlet. This space is bordered anteriorly by the posterior wall of the trachea, posteriorly by the upper thoracic spine, superiorly by the thoracic inlet, and inferiorly by the aortic arch. The relative amount of space in this triangle is estimated. If the space is large (as in thoracic kyphosis), the right apical lung can move behind the trachea and the left apical lung can move over the top of the aortic arch, resulting in a posterior junction line on the PA chest (Fig. 1B). In analyzing this triangle, one needs to visually subtract the scapula summating on the lateral view. No normal opacity should project into this triangle. Lesions can easily hide behind the clavicles and costochondral junction on the PA view but will be observed on the lateral projection in this triangle.

The retrosternal space has been named the *retrosternal clear space*. This space is bordered anteriorly by the sternum, posteriorly by the ascending aorta, superiorly by the brachiocephalic veins, and inferiorly by the anterior heart (right ventricle). Anterior bowing of the sternum will increase this space. If there is available space for the right anterior lung to interface with the left, an anterior junction line will be observed on the PA chest (Fig. 2). This interface is V-shaped superiorly and is an inverted V inferiorly, with a line

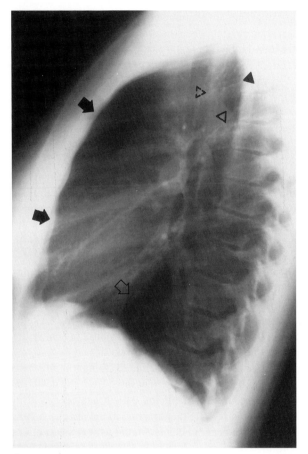

A

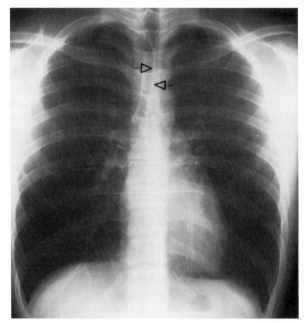

B

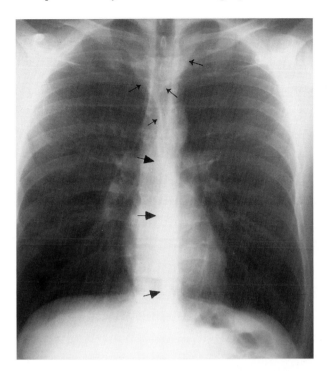

Figure 2   PA view of the chest showing the anterior junction anatomy and line (small arrows) formed by the lungs interfacing in the retrosternal space. The azygoesophageal recess interface (solid arrows) is seen, formed by right lower lobe interfacing with the mediastinum in the retrocardiac space.

in between. Fat may separate the two lungs, producing a parallel band rather than a line. The normal interface should never have a convex outward margin. The retrosternal airspace may be enlarged in patients with emphysema. Cardiac enlargement or mediastinal tumors can encroach on this space.

    The retrocardiac space is bordered anteriorly by the posterior heart (left ventricle and left atrium), posteriorly by the anterior margin of the thoracic spine, and inferiorly by the diaphragm. The available space is increased by the degree of the normal thoracic kyphosis. On the PA view, the medial right lower lobe extends into this space as the azygoesophageal recess (Fig. 2) and the medial right lower lobe extends into this space as the azygoesophageal recess (Fig. 2) and the medial left lower lobe as the preaortic recess. These interfaces on the PA view can be conveniently divided into thirds. The upper

Figure 1   A. Left lateral chest. The retrotracheal triangle outlines the posterior wall of the trachea (broken triangle), anterior wall of the vertebral bodies with the scapula superimposed (solid triangle), and top of the posterior turn of the aorta (open triangle). The retrosternal space is seen beginning posterior to the sternum (solid arrows) and the retrocardiac space beginning at the posterior aspect of the heart (open arrows). B. PA view of the chest showing posterior junction line (open arrows) formed by the lungs interfacing in the retrotracheal triangle.

third relates intimately to the carina, and subcarinal masses may encroach upon this space. The middle third of this interface relates commonly to the left atrium and confluence of pulmonary veins from the lower lobes. This portion of the junction anatomy is frequently gently convex outward toward the right. The inferior third of this interface relates to the distal esophagus and descending aorta. Commonly hiatal hernias are the cause of an altered lower-third interface.

After a review of the available space on the lateral view, each of these three interfaces should be inspected on the PA projection. The carina should be visualized on each PA projection and the mainstem bronchi evaluated for large airway masses; these bronchi serve as points of study of the right and left central pulmonary arteries. The left pulmonary artery always courses over the left-mainstem and upper-lobe bronchus. The right interlobar pulmonary artery is visualized lateral to the bronchus intermedius. Placing one finger on the right main pulmonary artery and another on the left pulmonary artery shows the normal position of the "hilar" vessels, with the right lower than the left in over 90% of normal

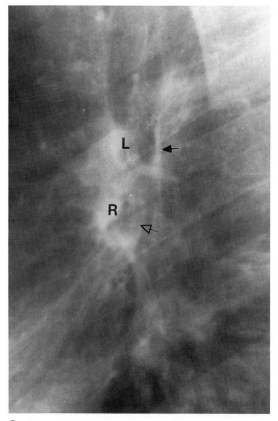

A

Figure 3 Left lateral views of the right and left hila. A. Hila closed, with patient slightly rotated right side posteriorly. B. Hila open, with patient slightly rotated right side forward. Note the position of the right-sided posterior wall bronchus intermedius (solid arrows) in relation to the left upper lobe bronchus, seen end-on (open arrow). The posterior turn of left pulmonary artery is marked L and the right main pulmonary artery adjacent to the bronchus intermedius is marked R.

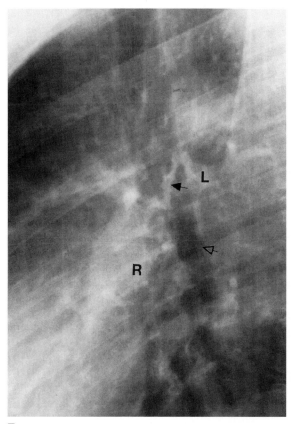

B

individuals. The arching course of the left pulmonary artery (paralleling the more superiorly located aortic arch) is usually observed by finding the black hole of the summating left-mainstem and left-upper-lobe bronchus on the lateral view. The right main pulmonary artery can be located anteriorly and inferiorly by finding the posterior wall of the bronchus intermedius, which runs in a relatively vertical orientation and bisects the end-on left-upper-lobe bronchus on a true lateral view (Fig. 3).

The relationship of the posterior wall of the bronchus intermedius and the black hole of the end-on left-upper-lobe bronchus provides a rapid way of determining differences in degree and direction of rotation of a rotated lateral chest film. If the patient is rotated slightly with the left side forward and right side back, the left pulmonary artery is thrown over the right and the summation results in a ''closed'' position of the major vessels. If the patient is rotated slightly with the right side forward and left side back, the normal separation of the right and left hila is exaggerated and the hila are termed ''open.'' Slight degrees in rotation dramatically change the appearance of the hila on the lateral view and can make comparison to prior lateral films more difficult (Fig. 3). Rotation does allow a separate visualization of each posterior costophrenic sulcus, the most dependent portion of the pleural space. This may allow the detection of small pleural effusions. Determining whether the hila are ''open'' or ''closed'' can become a reliable and rapid way of determining, on the lateral view, which costophrenic sulcus is posteriorly placed if rotation is present. Because of beam divergence, if the ribs are perfectly superimposed on the lateral view, the patient is positioned with the right side slightly forward and the hila are in a minimally open position. If the patient is in a true lateral position, the beam divergence will magnify the right-sided structures and result in slight "closing" of the hila.

If the posterior wall of the bronchus intermedius is observed on the lateral view, its thickness should be compared with that on the baseline chest film. Thickening is usually seen, along with vascular marginal blurring and bronchial wall cuffing. Finding the posterior wall of the bronchus intermedius also allows identification of the interface of the air within the bronchus and the right main pulmonary artery with the middle-lobe bronchus as the inferior continuation of that interface. The confluence of the right-upper-lobe veins overlies the anterior and inferior aspects of the right pulmonary artery and contributes to its size and opacity on the lateral view. The avascular aspect of the composite hilar opacity beneath the right-middle-lobe bronchus on the right and the anterior aspect of the left upper- and lower-lobe junctions is termed the *inferior hilar window*. Enlarged inferior hilar and mediastinal nodes may encroach on this window.

CHEST RADIOGRAPHS IN SELECTED CLINICAL SITUATIONS

Pneumothorax

The manifestation of pneumothorax is variable and depends on multiple factors: the patient's position at the time of radiography, presence of pleural adhesions, pleural fluid or underlying lung disease, and the volume of air in the pleural space. The classical appearance of pneumothorax in the upright position is characterized by a lucent stripe of air outlining the apicolateral portion of lung associated with a thin white visceral pleural line. However, when patients are radiographed in the supine or semiupright position, the distribution of free air in the pleural space is altered and may be more difficult to detect. It is important that ordering clinicians be aware of the various manifestations of pneumothorax.

Left undetected, pneumothorax may progress to potentially life-threatening tension pneumothorax. Radiographic signs suggesting tension pneumothorax include hyperlucency of a hemithorax with contralateral shift of the mediastinum. In nontension pneumothoraces, the mediastinal structures may shift toward the affected side. Depression of the ipsilateral hemidiaphragm is another sign and is almost always present in patients with significant tension. Although these radiographic signs suggest that a pneumothorax may be under tension, the diagnosis must be made on clinical grounds.

When patients are radiographed in the supine or semiupright position, free intrapleural air may accumulate in one or more recognizable regions within the thorax, including the anteromedial, subpulmonic, apicolateral, and posteromedial pleural spaces (Fig. 4). A small pneumothorax will most often manifest itself in the anteromedial pleural space, because this region is the least dependent portion of the chest in a completely supine patient. As the volume of pneumothorax increases, air will gradually accumulate in the subpulmonic recess and then in the apicolateral pleural space. Free intrapleural air accumulating anteromedially above the pulmonary hilus may sharply demarcate superior mediastinal vascular structures (e.g., the azygos vein, superior vena cava, or left subclavian artery) or the anterior junction anatomy. Below the pulmonary hilus, air collecting anteromedially may sharply outline the heart, cardiac fat pads, infracardiac medial hemidiaphragm, infe-

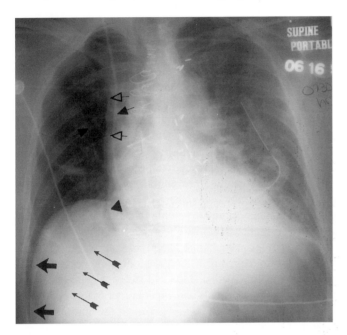

Figure 4 AP supine portable chest radiograph in a postoperative CABG patient with right pneumothorax. Anterior medial pneumothorax causes sharp visualization of the superior vena cava (open arrows) and air separating the right anterior junction of the lung from the anterior mediastinum (closed arrows shows separation). Below the right hilum, a medial pneumothorax outlines the right heart, the cardiac fat pad, and the inframedial hemidiaphragm (solid arrowhead). Pneumothorax accumulating in the subpulmonic recess is seen in the anterior costophrenic sulcus (feathered arrows) running in an oblique inferior course with the horizontal posterior costophrenic sulcus not visualized below this. A right "deep sulcus sign" in the lateral costophrenic sulcus is seen (large solid arrows).

rior vena cava, or anterior costophrenic sulcus. Visualization of a visceral pleural line along the inferior lung surface is direct radiographic evidence of subpulmonic pneumothorax; however, indirect signs of subpulmonic pneumothorax may be more common, including hyperlucency of the left or right upper quadrant, a deep lateral costophrenic sulcus, and visualization of the anterior costophrenic sulcus. The importance of obtaining an adequate radiograph that includes both lateral costophrenic sulci must be emphasized, since a "deep sulcus sign" may be the only evidence of pneumothorax in up to 10% of patients radiographed in supine or semirecumbent position. An apicolateral pneumothorax may be visualized in the supine patient when sufficient air is present in the pleural space to outline the visceral pleura laterally.

The appearance of a visceral pleural line may be mimicked by skin folds, overlying tubing, overlapping ribs, or creases in bed linen. Careful scrutiny of each case is required to avoid misdiagnosis that could lead to unnecessary treatment. Whenever the possibility of pneumothorax is suspected, additional measures must be undertaken to confirm or refute the diagnosis. An expiratory radiograph may be employed to detect pneumothorax. Lateral decubitus radiography with the suspected side up is also a sensitive means of detection. The cross-table lateral radiograph may be employed if the patient is unable to lie in the decubitus position, but it is less sensitive to the presence of pneumothorax because of overlap of the hemithoraces.

Pleural Effusion

The radiographic appearance of pleural fluid is primarily influenced by patient positioning at the time of radiography. In an upright patient, free-flowing effusion of sufficient volume may produce a characteristic meniscus appearance. Intrafissural fluid or loculated collections may simulate mass lesions. Subpulmonic effusions may simulate diaphragmatic elevation. In the supine patient, signs of significant pleural fluid collections may be subtle. The chest radiograph rarely reveals the specific cause or nature of pleural fluid, but some associated findings may help to narrow the range of diagnostic considerations. It is important to be familiar with the various radiographic appearances of pleural effusion to allow detection and plan further diagnostic or therapeutic interventions.

The subpulmonic pleural space is the initial site where pleural fluid collects in an upright individual. Radiographically, this may simulate hemidiaphragmatic elevation, but it can be distinguished by observing several characteristic features. In the frontal projection, the apparent hemidiaphragmatic dome appears more lateral than normal; this finding may be accentuated during expiration. The contour of the pseudodiaphragm is flattened on both sides of the "dome," with a shallow medial slope and steeper lateral slope. On the left side, the distance between the gastric air bubble and upper border of the pseudodiaphragm may be increased. Since this distance normally varies from a few millimeters up to 2 cm, it is helpful to have comparison radiographs present when assessing this sign. Pulmonary vessels normally visible behind the diaphragm may not be seen behind the pseudodiaphragm. This finding may be mimicked by lower-lobe disease or abdominal ascites. On the lateral chest radiograph, the posterior contour of the pseudodiaphragm may appear flattened up to the level of the major fissure, where a small tongue of fluid may occasionally be seen extending into the interlobar fissure. When they are bilateral, subpulmonic effusions may frequently be overlooked.

When the volume of pleural effusion exceeds the capacity of the subpulmonic space, the fluid will collect in the posterior, lateral, and anterior costophrenic angles. A moderate-sized pleural effusion will cause a uniform density, which obscures the hemidiaphragm and the lateral costophrenic sulcus. The upper border creates a hazy meniscus-shaped interface with a higher lateral than medial apex owing to the medial attachment of the pulmonary hilus and inferior pulmonary ligament. The density of pleural fluid may appear greater along the lateral aspect of the chest because the x-ray beam traverses a greater depth of fluid along the lateral hemithorax. Large pleural effusions will obscure the heart border and cause contralateral shift of the mediastinum and airways. Occasionally moderate or large effusions may invert the hemidiaphragm. This occurs more often on the left side, owing to lack of support by the liver, and may be recognized on plain radiographs by noting abnormal inferior displacement of the gastric air bubble or gas within the splenic flexure of the colon. On the right side, this finding is more easily made using CT or ultrasonography.

Free pleural effusion in the supine patient layers posteriorly, rendering it more difficult to detect. The supine chest radiograph has poor sensitivity and specificity in the detection of pleural effusion. Furthermore, the volume of pleural effusion is often underestimated on supine chest radiographs. The most common but least specific sign suggesting pleural effusion on supine radiographs is blunting of the lateral costophrenic angle. Fluid layering posteriorly may cause an increased density over the affected hemithorax; this sign becomes less sensitive in the presence of bilateral effusions because there is no normal side for comparison. An apical cap is a common sign of pleural effusion in the supine patient because the apex is the most dependent portion of the thorax in this position and has a relatively small capacity. The diaphragmatic silhouette may be obscured or appear elevated by pleural effusion. Additional signs include decreased visibility of lower-lobe vessels and accentuation of the minor fissure. While these signs are helpful in the detection of pleural effusion in supine patients, their absence does not exclude a pleural effusion.

Fluid within the minor fissure produces a rounded, sharply demarcated opacity on frontal radiographs, which may simulate a mass or area of consolidation. It appears on a lateral chest radiograph as a lenticular opacity with thin tails of fluid tapering anteriorly and posteriorly within the fissure. The appearance of fluid in the major fissure on frontal radiographs is characterized by a faint, sharp, curvilinear interface that is dense laterally and separated from the mediastinum by a lucent stripe of lung. Fluid accumulation in the inferior portion of the major fissure may simulate middle-lobe atelectasis or consolidation. Findings that support effusion rather than middle-lobe disease are identification of a separate minor fissure and preservation of the right heart border. Lateral films support the diagnosis if the opacity has tapered ends, one or more convex margins, or an anterior margin that contacts the hemidiaphragm.

Loculated pleural fluid collections (i.e., fluid that does not change location with varying patient position) also frequently occur between the lung and the chest wall, diaphragm, or mediastinum. When they are adjacent to the chest wall, loculated collections may be indistinguishable from a pleural-based mass on chest radiographs. When they are viewed in tangent, there may be a dome-like opacity with convex margins toward the lung and smoothly tapered ends. When viewed en face, the margins may be partly sharp and partly indistinct. Further imaging with CT or ultrasonography may be necessary to diagnose a loculated pleural fluid collection.

Additional radiographic evaluation of pleural effusions may include lateral decubitus or semiupright oblique views, ultrasonography, or CT. The lateral decubitus radiograph obtained with the suspected side down may detect as little as 5 mL of freely flowing fluid (Fig. 5). Obtaining radiographs in varying positions is also useful to determine whether pleural fluid is freely flowing or loculated. CT is very helpful in the evaluation of loculated pleural fluid collections, which may simulate a mass lesion on chest radiographs. Loculated collections have a characteristic smoothly marginated lentiform shape with homogeneous attenuation. CT is useful for diagnosis, localization, guidance of intervention, and follow-up of therapy. Additionally, CT may be of limited help in distinguishing transudates from exudates or acute intrapleural hemorrhage.

Ultrasonography may complement the radiological evaluation of pleural effusion in several ways. At the bedside, it may be used to detect effusion in critically ill patients who may be unable to attain proper positioning for chest radiographs. Furthermore, exudates may be distinguished from transudates by demonstrating uniformly echogenic fluid, septations, or complex fluid collections. Combined with plain radiographs, ultrasonography is very accurate in differentiating pleural fluid from solid pleural masses. Finally, ultrasound is a useful modality to guide sampling or percutaneous drainage of pleural fluid collections (see Chap. 17).

Patients with Dyspnea and Cough

The symptoms of dyspnea and cough require a careful examination of the chest radiograph for abnormalities of both the pulmonary parenchyma and airways. Heart size and pulmonary vascularity are reviewed for evidence of congestive heart failure. Parenchymal opaci-

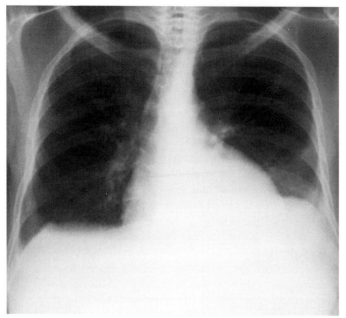

A

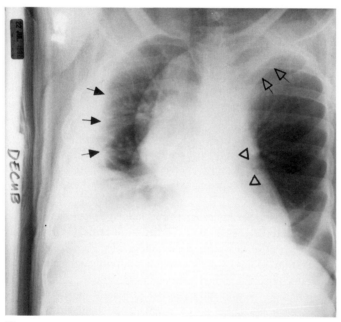

B

Figure 5   Bilateral free-flowing subpulmonic effusions. A. PA view showing lateral doming of the diaphragms. B. Right lateral decubitus view showing right effusion moving laterally (solid arrows outline interface between inflated lung and fluid) and left larger effusion moving against the left mediastinum, displacing the apical lung laterally (open arrows), and preaortic recess of lung (open arrowheads). C. Left lateral decubitus radiograph showing right effusion moving laterally (solid arrows outline interface between inflated lung and fluid) and right smaller effusion moving against the right mediastinum, displacing apical lung laterally (open arrows), medial left lung now inflates (open arrowheads).

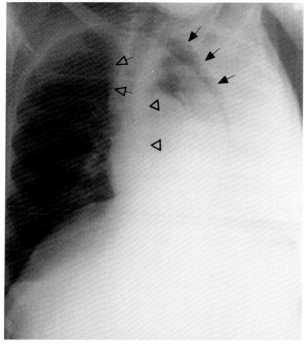

C

ties, such as consolidations from pneumonia or infarctions from emboli, are sought. Although the plain-film findings of emphysema and accompanying chronic bronchitis are subtle, advanced parenchymal changes can be observed. Secondary findings of low, flat diaphragms, increased AP diameter, and bowing of the sternum may be present in advanced pulmonary emphysema. Interstitial lung diseases can be manifest as reticular or reticulonodular patterns on chest radiographs. When an interstitial process is detected, it is important to note the distribution of the infiltrate and any associated adenopathy or pleural effusion as well as to evaluate the lung volumes. Prior radiographs and correlation with pertinent clinical history is helpful in determining the etiology of interstitial lung disease. Often, however, the chest radiograph findings are nonspecific and further workup with high-resolution CT of the chest is necessary. This may reveal findings that allow a specific diagnosis without invasive testing (see Chap. 11).

If the lung parenchyma is normal, the central airway and major bronchi are examined for subtle findings such as bronchial wall thickening or central airway masses. As with any new film, subtle new findings are more easily detected when the current film is compared with a film from an earlier study.

Diffuse Parenchymal Disease

Subtle changes in diffuse parenchymal disease can sometimes be more quickly assessed on the chest film than on CT. An optimal chest film done the same day as the chest CT is complementary and useful in reviewing subsequent chest films. The diaphragm's height is a good measure of lung compliance on an upright full inspiratory effort in a cooperative patient. However, changes in technique from film to film make the assessment of change difficult. Comparing an upright in-department chest film with a portable AP supine film on the same patient remains a formidable challenge. Accurate assessment of changes in a diffuse lung opacity requires a consistent technique. Although CT does not suffer from the obvious problems of summation that are inherent in the chest film, the chest film gives a one-look overview that is rapid and at times conclusive. Using the patient's prior films increases one's ability to pick up subtle changes not obvious on any one current study.

Lung Mass

In patients who present with a lung nodule or mass, it is first necessary to establish that the finding is real and not an artifact. This may be as simple as confirming the finding on standard PA and lateral views or may require additional workup with shallow (5- to 10-degree) oblique views, lead markers on skin lesions or nipples, a lordotic projection, or fluoroscopy. If the lesion is determined to be in an intrapulmonary location, the next step is a comparison with any prior radiographs to assess interval growth. Any interval growth of a lesion raises the possibility of a malignancy and warrants further investigation with chest CT to better characterize the lesion. Lesions that show no interval change in size over 2 year are almost always benign (see Chap. 20).

The plain radiographic features of a peripherally located mass that suggest malignancy include lobulated or spiculated margins, a peripheral notch or umbilication, cavitation, and size greater than 3 cm. Superior sulcus (Pancoast) tumors may present as apical pleural thickening. Any asymmetry greater than 5 mm in apical pleural thickening should raise the suspicion of malignancy. An apical lordotic view may be helpful in evaluating lesions in the lung apex. Clearly plain film features such as associated rib or vertebral body destruction or a chest wall soft tissue mass should be further evaluated with CT or magnetic resonance imaging (MRI).

Features of a centrally located lung mass that suggest malignancy include associated lobar atelectasis, chronic or recurrent pneumonia, ipsilateral hilar or mediastinal adenopathy, or increased hilar density. The Golden "S" sign is a classic radiographic appearance due to a central mass that causes right-upper-lobe atelectasis and bulging of the inferomedial portion of the minor fissure, creating a reverse S contour. The presence of any feature suggesting malignancy should trigger further evaluation with CT or MRI.

The presence of a benign pattern of calcification within a lesion could be sufficient to end a workup. The detection of calcification within a lesion may be difficult on standard high-kilovolt chest radiographs; better characterization of calcifications may be obtained using targeted low-kilovolt plain radiographs or thin-section CT. Identifying benign patterns such as uniform diffuse calcification, laminated, central, or "popcorn-like" allows a high degree of certainty that the lesion is benign.

Further evaluation of a lung mass using CT is standard and provides further characterization of the lesion, serves to detect additional lesions that may not be visualized on the chest radiograph, and is useful for cancer staging. MRI evaluation complements CT by providing multiplanar capability; it is useful in evaluating possible brachial plexus extension by apical lung neoplasms (see Chap. 32).

The Opacified Hemithorax

Opacification of a hemithorax may be a striking radiographic finding. Obtaining prior chest radiographs for comparison may aid in determinating the cause (e.g., prior pleural effusion that progressed, prior neoplasm that required pneumonectomy). It is helpful to provide the interpreting radiologist with relevant clinical information regarding the character, onset, duration of symptoms, and any relevant prior medical conditions. The majority of cases that present with unilateral diffuse lung opacity are caused by a handful of diagnoses including pulmonary edema, pneumonia, aspiration, radiation pneumonitis, or lymphangiitic tumor spread. The congenital causes of hemithorax opacification are beyond the scope of this text and are not discussed.

Assessing the shift in mediastinal structures relative to the affected hemithorax may aid in the evaluation of an opaque hemithorax. Pleural effusion may be associated with a midline mediastinum or may be large enough to shift the mediastinal structures toward the contralateral hemithorax. If a small or medium-sized effusion is present, it may cause a uniform veiling density with apical pleural capping on the affected side when the patient is radiographed in the supine position. Decubitus or upright radiographs will confirm the presence of an effusion if the fluid flows freely.

The mediastinal structures may remain midline in cases of unilateral pulmonary consolidation; air bronchograms may also be observed. Unilateral consolidation may be the result of pneumonia, aspiration, unilateral pulmonary edema, or radiation pneumonitis. Rarely, mesothelioma may cause encasement of the lung and prevent contralateral shift of the mediastinal structures.

When a hemithorax is completely opacified with ipsilateral mediastinal shift, unilateral complete lung atelectasis is the most likely etiology. Atelectasis of an entire lung may be the result of an endobronchial lesion, bronchial wall abnormality, or extrinsic compression of a mainstem bronchus. The clinical presentation and prior medical history help determine the cause of unilateral lung atelectasis. Ipsilateral shift of the mediastinal structures also occurs in postpneumonectomy patients. The hemithorax becomes uniformly dense after lung resection and the contralateral lung hyperexpands in a compensatory manner. Signs of a prior thoracotomy (clips and staples) may be evident on the affected side. Ipsilateral shift of the mediastinum may also occur in cases of unilateral lymphangiitic carcinomatosis. The involved lung may demonstrate coarse reticular or nodular opacities. Hilar or mediastinal adenopathy may also be present.

LIMITATIONS OF THE CHEST FILM

Even with an optimal PA and lateral chest film, pattern recognition is a difficult task because the films are summation images. The lateral view largely summates left-sided structures on the right. The PA view allows comparison of the right to the left lung, but the chest wall and bony thorax overlie much of the lung tissue. This summation problem is largely circumvented by high-resolution chest CT. Technical factors such as large patient size, large focal-spot size, respiratory motion, and cardiac motion all limit our ability to recognize patterns on plain films. Because of problems in resolution, significant pulmonary disease can hide in the normal or near-normal chest film.

On the other hand, a good-quality PA and lateral chest film allows the pulmonary physician to look at the whole thorax at one point in time, allowing rapid comparison with prior exams to reveal subtle changes. A chest film taken on the same day as a high-resolution CT serves as a powerful combined test to evaluate the lung and mediastinal anatomy, which can then be correlated with patient symptoms. This radiological pathological correlation will result in more accurate plain-film interpretations in subsequent films.

SUGGESTED READING

1. Glossary of terms for thoracic radiology: recommendations of the nomenclature committee of the Fleischner Society. Am J Roentgenol 1984; 143:509.
2. Moskowitz PS, Griscom NT. The medical pneumothorax. Radiology 1976; 120:143–147.
3. Müller NL. Imaging of the pleura. Radiology 1993; 186:297–309.
4. Proto, AV. Spectman JM. The left lateral radiograph of the chest. Med Radiogr Photogr 1980; 56:38–63.
5. Proto, AV, Spectman JM. The left lateral radiograph of the chest. Med Radiogr Photogr 1979; 55:30–74.
6. Raasch BN, Carsky EW, Lane EJ, O'Callaghan JP, Heitzman ER. Pleural effusions: explanation of some typical appearances. Am J Roentgenol 1982; 139:899–904.
7. Reed, JC. Chest Radiology: Plain Film Patterns and Differential Diagnoses. 4th ed. St. Louis: Mosby–Year Book, 1997.
8. Tocino IM. Pneumothorax in the supine patient: radiographic anatomy. Radiographics 1985; 5:557–588.

11
Computed Tomography

Kevin K. Matsuba and Jeffrey S. Klein
University of Vermont College of Medicine
Fletcher Allen Health Care
Burlington, Vermont

GENERAL UTILITY OF COMPUTED TOMOGRAPHY OF THE CHEST

Computed tomography (CT) of the chest has proven useful for a variety of indications (Table 1). Although standard protocols suffice for the majority of chest CT examinations, it is important to recognize that the scan must often be tailored to the individual patient so that the appropriate acquisition parameters are utilized and useful information is obtained. In addition, proper communication with the radiologist, either by providing detailed history and pertinent physiological data on the radiological requisition or by telephone,

Table 1 Indications and Technique for Chest CT Examinations

Indication	Technique
1. Staging of lung cancer	Contrast-enhanced 5- to 7-mm helical scans from apex through liver
2. Detection of metastatic disease	Contrast-enhanced 5- to 7-mm helical scans from apex to base
3. Evaluation of complex pleuroparenchymal infection (abscess, empyema)	Contrast-enhanced 7- to 10-mm helical scans from apex to base
4. Detection/characterization of chronic infiltrative lung disease/bronchiectasis	High resolution 1-mm scans every 10 mm with expiratory scans
5. Solitary pulmonary nodule	Noncontrast 1-mm helical scans through nodule with densitometry
6. Detection of pulmonary emboli	Contrast-enhanced 3-mm helical scans from arch to lower lobe for 12-cm distance
7. Aortic disease (aneurysm, dissection)	Nonenhanced helical scans apex to base to detect intramural blood, then enhanced helical scans from apex to aortic bifurcation
8. Rule out tracheobronchial lesion (hemoptysis)	Noncontrast 3-mm helical scans from thoracic inlet to proximal lower lobe segmental bronchi

169

Table 2 Indications for HRCT of the Lungs

1. Detection of disease in patients with normal chest radiographs and clinical/functional suspicion of infiltrative disease/emphysema
2. Specific characterization of lung disease in patients with nonspecific radiographic and clinical findings
3. Preoperative localization for choosing site of transbronchial/open lung biopsy
4. Determining the degree of disease activity in patients with diffuse infiltrative lung disease
5. Assessing reponse to therapy or progression of underlying disease
6. Determining the presence and extent of bronchiectasis

is an essential part of the consultative process and optimizes the quality of the CT interpretation.

The standard chest CT examination (''staging'' chest CT) is used for determining the extent of disease in patients with bronchogenic carcinoma. Contrast-enhanced scans are obtained from the lung apex through the inferior edge of the liver to assess for mediastinal nodal, hepatic, and adrenal metastases. The detection of pulmonary or mediastinal nodal metastases from extrathoracic malignancy is assessed with a more limited contrast-enhanced examination that extends only through the lung bases. Similarly, the evaluation of complex parenchymal and pleural inflammatory disease requires contrast-enhanced scans to help distinguish infected pleural fluid collections from abscess formation.

Patients with diffuse parenchymal lung disease or with clinical or functional evidence of interstitial disease are best evaluated with nonhelical high-resolution CT (HRCT) (Table 2).

The use of helical scanners capable of providing rapid imaging during the phase of maximal contrast enhancement allows for the accurate assessment of pulmonary vascular and aortic disease. A dedicated helical acquisition for the evaluation of pulmonary embolism is performed through the midthorax with a rapid injection of contrast at high flow rates (i.e., 3–5 mL/s vs. 2 mL/s for routine chest CT) and thin collimation (3–5 mm) to optimize the detection of small intraluminal thromboemboli. The evaluation of acute aortic dissection or intramural hematoma requires precontrast scans to detect clotted intramural blood followed by contrast-enhanced scans to assess for intimal flaps, false lumina, and aortic ulceration or aneurysm formation.

In the patient with hemoptysis, the central airways are examined by obtaining 3-mm collimated helical scans through the tracheobronchial tree, which is then supplemented by HRCT to evaluate for the presence of bronchiectasis. The axial images can be reconstructed in a two- or three-dimensional format to aid in bronchoscopic localization of endoluminal lesions.

SPECIFIC DIAGNOSTIC PROBLEMS

Solitary Pulmonary Nodule

The advantages of CT examination of a solitary pulmonary nodule (SPN) include superior density discrimination and depiction of the margins of the nodule. Helical CT scans through a SPN obtained as a volume of information during a single breath-hold accurately detects calcium or fat within the lesion (Fig. 1). Additionally, the increased sensitivity of helical CT of the lungs in the detection of small lung nodules occasionally demonstrates the presence of multiple nodules, thus changing the diagnostic considerations.

CT Characteristics of a SPN

Size and Growth Rate.   The larger the SPN, the greater the likelihood of malignancy. SPNs exceeding 3 cm in diameter (arbitrarily defined as masses) have a high likelihood of malignancy; therefore densitometry is not performed for these lesions. Another important consideration in evaluating a SPN is its change in size from prior CT studies. When radiological follow-up of a SPN is chosen as an alternative to an invasive diagnostic procedure, a limited thin-section CT studies of the nodule are performed at 3-month intervals for 6 months, then every 6 months for a total of 2 years. A nodule that shows either no growth or an increase in diameter of less than 25% on follow-up CT over a 2-year period is considered benign.

Margins.   In general, a nodule demonstrating smooth contours on thin-section CT is likely to be benign. Therefore, in patients with a low likelihood of lung cancer, a small (< 1 cm) smooth nodule lacking calcification on CT can be followed by CT to confirm stability of the lesion. This option is particularly useful for lesions inaccessible to transthoracic needle biopsy or thoracoscopic resection.

There are several appearances of pulmonary nodules that suggest specific disease processes. The presence of small satellite nodules at the periphery of a SPN as seen on thin-section CT is highly suggestive of granulomatous infection. The presence of a rim of low attenuation surrounding a SPN in a neutropenic immunocompromised patient has been termed the *CT halo sign* and is highly suggestive of invasive pulmonary aspergillosis. Alternatively, a SPN with lobulated or spiculated margins on thin-section CT is highly suspicious for malignancy and requires further evaluation.

Density.   The presence and pattern of calcification within a SPN as demonstrated by thin-section CT is the most useful characteristic in distinguishing benign from malignant lesions. The presence of diffuse, central, concentric, or popcorn-like calcification is indicative of a benign lesion, most often a granuloma or hamartoma (Table 3; Fig. 2). However, the absence of visible calcification on CT does not exclude the presence of microscopic calcification and requires nodule densitometry for definitive analysis. With this technique, the CT attenuation value of each pixel [expressed in Hounsfield units (HU), with 0 HU = water] making up the central portion of the nodule is determined on a thin-section, noncontrast CT study and a mean attenuation value generated. Assuming that the nodule is smooth and < 3 cm in diameter, benign calcification is said to exist if at least 10% of the pixels making up the cross-sectional area of the nodule measure greater than 200 HU and are distributed in a benign pattern.

The presence of fat indicates a benign lesion, either a hamartoma or exogenous lipoid pneumonia. Additional CT characteristics of a hamartoma include a diameter < 2.5 cm., smooth margins, and the presence of ''popcorn'' calcification.

CT occasionally demonstrates the presence of gas within a SPN. Branching tubular or cystic lucencies within a SPN, particularly in lesions with lobulated or irregular margins, are most suggestive of an adenocarcinoma. Central necrosis or cavitation is a nonspecific finding that may be seen with inflammatory lesions, infarcts, or neoplasms.

Despite detailed evaluation of SPNs with thin-section CT, the majority of studies fail to detect benign calcium or fat. These lesions will require a definitive tissue diagnosis,

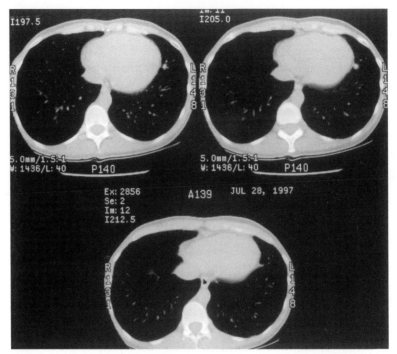

A

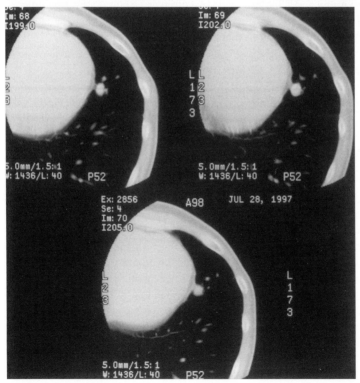

B

Table 3 Patterns of
Calcification Within SPN on CT

1. Diffuse
2. Central nidus
3. Popcorn-like
4. Laminar/concentric
5. Stippled
6. Eccentric

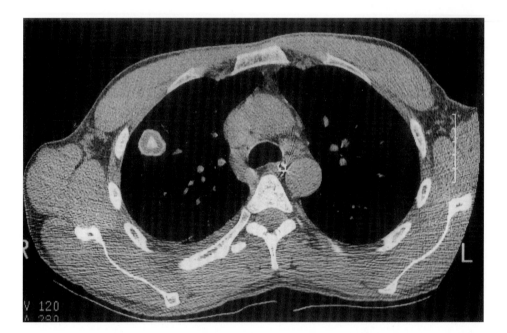

Figure 2 Benign calcification on thin-section CT. CT scan with 1-mm collimation shows concentric calcification indicative of a healed granuloma.

Figure 1 Helical CT for calcium detection in a SPN. A. Single breath-hold helical CT acquisition with 5-mm collimation through a lingular nodule does not show definite calcification. B. The same acquisition reconstructed with scans through the center of the nodule shows peripheral laminar calcification, probably within an old granuloma due to *Histoplasma*.

which can be achieved by bronchoscopy, transthoracic needle biopsy, video-assisted thoracoscopic surgery (VATS), or thoracotomy.

Staging of Lung Cancer

The accurate staging of lung cancer guides appropriate therapeutic approaches to the disease and provides a prognosis for patients who have unresectable disease. The anatomic staging of patients with bronchogenic carcinoma is based on a TNM classification, which includes the location and morphological characteristics of the primary tumor (T), the presence or absence of hilar or mediastinal nodal metastases (N), and the presence or absence of distant metastases (M) (Table 4).

The key distinction in the staging of lung cancer is between resectable disease (stages I–IIIa) and unresectable disease (stages IIIb and IV).

Primary Tumor (T)

A primary tumor is classified T4 if there is mediastinal invasion with involvement of the heart, great vessels, trachea, esophagus, vertebral body, or carina or there is a malignant pleural effusion. Tumors locally invading the chest wall—including the superior pulmonary sulcus, diaphragm, mediastinal pleural, pericardium, or proximal main bronchus—are considered resectable by some surgeons and are classified as T3 lesions.

Chest Wall Invasion (T3).   Direct invasion of the pleura and chest wall by a peripheral bronchogenic carcinoma may or may not indicate that the tumor is unresectable. For example, superior sulcus (Pancoast) tumors were once considered unresectable when extrapulmonary invasion was present. However, local irradiation followed by en bloc resection of the tumor and adjacent chest wall have resulted in 5-year survival rates of up to 30%.

The CT diagnosis of chest wall invasion is problematic. CT findings that may indicate chest wall invasion include the presence of obtuse angles at the point of contact between tumor and pleura, contact between tumor and the pleural surface exceeding 3 cm, pleural thickening adjacent to the mass, and increased density of extrapleural fat. Surprisingly, none of these findings has proved to be of great value in making this diagnosis with an overall accuracy of approximately 40–70%. Although the presence of a gross

Table 4 International Staging
System for Lung Cancer

Resectable	
Stage Ia	= T1,N0,M0
Stage Ib	T2,N0,M0
Stage IIa	= T1,N1,M0
	T2,N1,M0
Stage IIb	T3,N0,M0
Stage IIIa	T3,N1,M0
	T1-3,N2,M0
Unresectable	
Stage IIIb	= **T4**,anyN,M0
	AnyT,**N3**,M0
Stage IV	= AnyT,anyN,**M1**

soft tissue mass or rib destruction is specific for chest wall invasion, these findings are insensitive. In patients with superior sulcus tumors, magnetic resonance imaging (MRI) is the optimal modality to evaluate the local extent of disease.

Mediastinal Invasion.   In patients with lung cancer, contiguous invasion of the tumor into the mediastinum with involvement of the heart, great vessels, trachea, or esophagus precludes resection (Fig. 3). Localized invasion of the mediastinal pleura or pericardium does not prevent resection, although extensive invasion of mediastinal fat usually does.

As with the diagnosis of chest wall invasion, CT demonstration of a mass contiguous with or producing thickening of the mediastinal pleura does not necessarily indicate mediastinal extension or unresectability. However, a significant mediastinal mass contiguous with a lung tumor that results in compression of mediastinal vessels or esophagus or replacement of mediastinal fat by soft tissue density strongly suggest invasion. Other findings that may suggest mediastinal invasion include (1) obliteration of the fat plane normally seen adjacent to the descending aorta or other mediastinal vessels, (2) tumor contacting more than one-quarter of the circumference of the aortic wall, or (3) tumor contacting more than 3 cm of the mediastinum. If none of these findings is present, the tumor is likely resectable, even though 29% of resectable lesions lacking any of these findings are still found to invade the mediastinum locally. However, the presence of any of these findings is not particularly helpful in identifying invasive tumors.

Pleural Effusion.   Conventional radiographs, including decubitus films, are suffi-

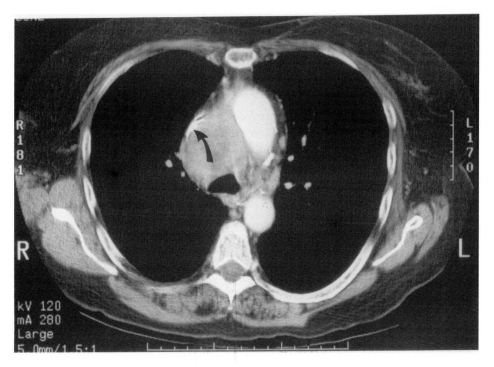

Figure 3   T4 bronchogenic carcinoma due to mediastinal invasion. Enhanced CT at the level of the aortic arch shows a large mediastinal mass replacing mediastinal fat and distorting the superior vena cava (arrow). CT-guided transthoracic biopsy revealed large-cell carcinoma of lung.

cient for the detection of pleural effusion in patients with lung cancer and lead to diagnostic thoracentesis and/or pleural biopsy. The presence of pleural thickening or pleural nodularity on CT is suggestive of pleural malignancy but requires cytologic or histological confirmation.

Proximal Airway Involvement. In some cases, conventional radiographs or CT can demonstrate the relationship of a proximal tumor mass to the main bronchus, carina, or trachea; but as a rule, bronchoscopy is more accurate in this regard. At bronchoscopy, minimal mucosal involvement by tumor can be diagnosed, while only discrete intraluminal masses are visible on CT or radiographs. Bronchoscopic confirmation of an apparent carinal or tracheal tumor is usually necessary unless the CT findings are gross.

Mediastinal Nodal Involvement (N)

Ipsilateral mediastinal or subcarinal node metastases are classified N2 and are considered potentially resectable. Contralateral hilar, mediastinal, and supraclavicular or scalene nodal metastases are considered N3 and are unresectable.

The accuracy of CT in detecting mediastinal nodal metastases from bronchogenic carcinoma depends upon the lymph node diameter arbitrarily chosen to distinguish normal from abnormal. The use of a large node diameter to distinguish benign from malignant nodes on CT increases specificity but decreases sensitivity in detecting metastases. Alternatively, the use of a small node diameter increases sensitivity and decreases specificity. A greatest node diameter of 1 cm is often used and provides acceptable accuracy without sacrificing sensitivity.

When the mediastinum is carefully explored surgically and all nodes are submitted for histological study (total nodal sampling), the sensitivity of CT found in experimental studies is lower than when the mediastinum is evaluated only by mediastinoscopy or palpation at surgery. With total nodal sampling, metastases in normal-sized nodes will be detected. In a study correlating the results of preoperative CT with total lymph node sampling, the sensitivity for mediastinal nodal metastases on a per-patient basis was 64%, with a specificity of 62%.

Approximately 60–70% of patients with no enlarged mediastinal nodes (nodes < 1 cm in greatest or least diameter) on CT will be free of nodal metastases at surgery. In such patients, thoracotomy without prior mediastinoscopy may be appropriate, with a mediastinal node exploration conducted at surgery. Alternatively, patients with enlarged mediastinal lymph nodes on CT have nodal metastases in 60% of cases (Fig. 4). Patients with enlarged nodes who have intranodal metastases may be considered resectable by some surgeons if the nodes are not contralateral, numerous, or "bulky." Most surgeons will perform mediastinoscopy in patients with enlarged mediastinal nodes seen on CT.

Despite these difficulties, most authors consider CT to be helpful in staging for mediastinal lymph node metastases. Although not highly accurate in nodal staging, CT can provide valuable information in guiding therapy and directing invasive diagnostic procedures, particularly mediastinoscopy.

Distant Metastases (M)

Each patient with proven lung cancer should be carefully evaluated for the presence of metastatic disease (M1). Common sites of extrathoracic spread in patients with lung cancer include lymph nodes, liver, adrenal gland, bone, brain, and the opposite lung.

Imaging studies used to evaluate patients for metastatic disease include radionuclide bone scanning with technetium 99m–methylene diphosphonate, contrast-enhanced brain

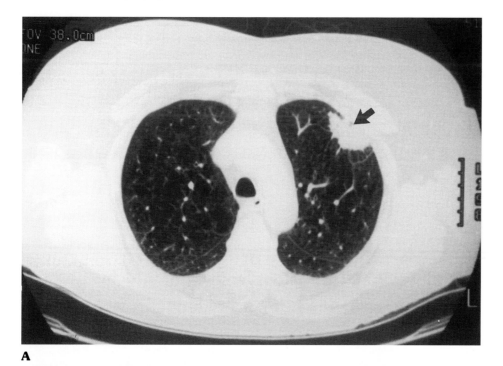

A

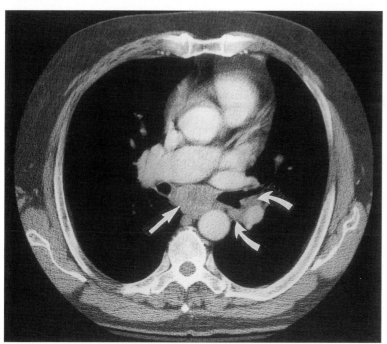

B

Figure 4 N2 nodes on CT. A. CT scan displayed at lung window settings demonstrates an irregular lingular nodule (arrow) representing a non-small-cell carcinoma. B. Same scan displayed at mediastinal window settings reveals enlarged left hilar (curved arrows) and subcarinal (straight arrow) lymph nodes. CT-guided biopsy of the subcarinal lymph node mass confirmed nodal metastases.

and abdominal CT, MRI, and ultrasound. MRI of the brain is usually reserved for patients with equivocal contrast CT studies or with iodine allergy. If tissue confirmation of metastatic disease is necessary, this is obtained via CT- or ultrasound-guided fine-needle aspiration biopsy.

CT scans of the chest performed for the staging of lung cancer should include imaging of the liver and adrenal glands to detect upper abdominal metastases. The presence of fat within an adrenal mass, detected when an unenhanced CT shows the density of the lesion to be less than 18 HU, is highly specific for an adrenal adenoma and warrants no further evaluation.

Pulmonary Embolism

The ability to scan a large volume of the chest in a single acquisition during maximal arterial enhancement with helical CT has led to the evaluation of this technique in the detection of pulmonary emboli. Pulmonary emboli are recognized on helical CT as partial or complete low attenuation filling defects within the opacified artery (Fig. 5). Preliminary studies comparing helical and electron beam CT pulmonary angiography with conventional angiography have found a sensitivity for central (i.e., main, lobar, or segmental) pulmonary emboli of 86–100%, with few false-positive examinations. However, the precise role of helical CT in the evaluation of suspected pulmonary embolism awaits further clinical studies.

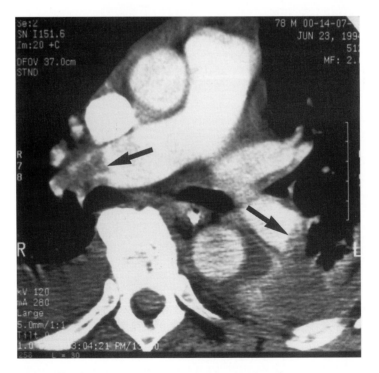

Figure 5   Pulmonary embolism on helical CT. CT pulmonary angiogram in a patient with chest pain and dyspnea shows right and left lobar pulmonary emboli (arrows).

Diffuse Parenchymal Disease

Chest radiographs are of limited utility in patients with known or suspected diffuse lung disease. Since the development of HRCT nearly 15 years ago, clinical studies have demonstrated its superiority in the detection and characterization of diffuse parenchymal lung disease. The technique is most useful in patients with normal or nonspecific clinical, functional, or radiographic findings of chronic infiltrative lung disease (Fig. 6).

Normal Anatomy

The accurate interpretation of an HRCT of the lung requires a knowledge of the normal appearance of the secondary pulmonary lobule, bronchi, blood vessels, interlobar fissures, and pulmonary parenchyma. The secondary pulmonary lobule is defined as a unit of lung supplied by three to five terminal bronchioles that is separated from adjacent lobules by interlobular septa. These connective tissue septa contain branches of the pulmonary veins and lymphatics. The secondary pulmonary lobule is supplied by a centrilobular pulmonary arteriole and preterminal bronchiole. In normal patients, the centrilobular artery appears as a dot-like or Y-shaped structure that is seen approximately 1 cm from the pleural surface (Fig. 7). The centrilobular bronchiole is normally invisible unless the wall is thickened or the lumen is dilated, thereby producing a V- or Y-shaped opacity.

Within the central lung, the bronchi and pulmonary arteries course together in a connective tissue sheath, termed the axial or bronchovascular interstitium, that extends

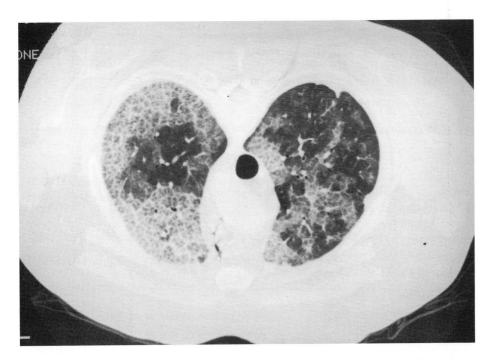

Figure 6 Pulmonary alveolar proteinosis. Prone HRCT through the upper lobes shows a patchy ground-glass pattern of parenchymal disease. Note the thickened interstitial lines within the areas of ground glass. This combination of ground-glass and interstitial lines has been termed ''crazy paving'' and is characteristic of pulmonary alveolar proteinosis. Following therapeutic whole-lung lavage, there was dramatic clinical and radiographic improvement.

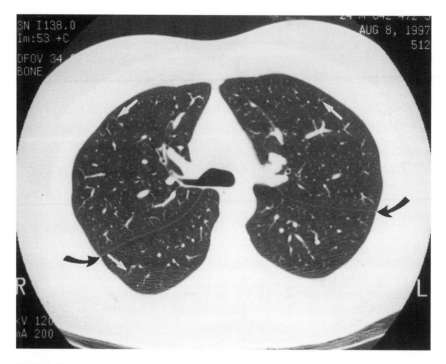

Figure 7 Normal HRCT lung anatomy. An HRCT midlung scan shows peripheral centrilobular arterioles (straight arrows) visible to within 1 cm of the pleura. Note the visibility of the interlobar fissures (curved arrows) as curvilinear structures and the normal smooth interface between lung and pleura.

from the mediastinum to the lung periphery where it merges with the parenchymal or alveolar interstitium. The interface between the bronchoarterial bundle and the surrounding lung is normally sharp and smooth on HRCT. As they travel peripherally, both structures taper slightly; at any given level, the diameter of the bronchus is no greater than that of the accompanying artery. The pulmonary veins run in a separate connective tissue sheath and are distinguished from the pulmonary arteries by their horizontal course and lack of constant relationship to the airways.

The interlobar fissures appear as a thin, smooth curvilinear lines on HRCT (Fig. 7). Similarly, the interface between the lung and the mediastinal and costal pleura is smooth, interrupted only by the oblique fissures. The normal pulmonary parenchyma has a uniform dark gray appearance with a gravity-dependent increase in attenuation.

HRCT Findings of Diffuse Lung Disease

Reticular or Linear Pattern.   A reticular pattern identified on HRCT results from thickening of the bronchovascular (axial), intralobular (parenchymal), and interlobular (peripheral) interstitium. Thickening of the interlobular septa with distortion of the lobule produces a honeycomb pattern which is easily recognized on HRCT in patients with end-stage pulmonary fibrosis (Fig. 8). Parenchymal bands are linear scars 2–5 cm in length that extend to the pleural surface and may contribute to a reticular pattern on HRCT. These opacities are seen in patients with idiopathic pulmonary fibrosis, asbestosis, sarcoidosis, silicosis, and tuberculosis.

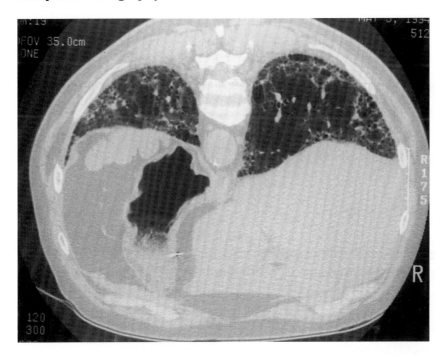

Figure 8 Reticulation/honeycombing in UIP. Prone HRCT through the lung bases in a patient with biopsy-proven UIP shows subpleural honeycombing, representing end-stage pulmonary fibrosis.

Linear interstitial disease results from thickening of the interlobular septa. Common causes of a linear interstitial pattern on HRCT include lymphangitic carcinomatosis, in which there is infiltration by malignant cells producing lymphatic distention and interstitial fibrosis (Fig. 9), and interstitial pulmonary edema.

Within the secondary pulmonary lobule, intralobular lines can result from diseases affecting the core structures, including the centrilobular arteriole, bronchiole, or peribronchovascular interstitium. Thickening of the core structures usually results from dilatation and inspissation within small airways, which appear on HRCT as thickened centrilobular dots, lines, or Y-shaped branching opacities. Prominent intralobular lines that radiate from the core structures peripherally toward the interlobular septa are caused by fibrosis of the peribronchovascular interstitium and are seen in asbestosis and idiopathic pulmonary fibrosis.

Nodular Pattern. A nodular pattern may be a feature of either interstitial or airspace disease. In general, small, sharply defined nodules 2–10 mm in diameter represent interstitial nodules and reflect either granulomatous or metastatic disease. Nodules 6–10 mm in diameter that are poorly marginated represent airspace nodules and are typically seen within the center of secondary pulmonary lobules.

In patients with interstitial nodules, the distribution of nodules within the lungs and particularly within the interstitial compartments provides important clues to the diagnosis. For example, the presence of nodules in a peribronchovascular and subpleural (peripheral interstitial) distribution is highly suggestive of sarcoidosis (Fig. 10), Langerhans cell histiocytosis, silicosis, or lymphangitic spread of tumor. Silicosis and sarcoidosis have an upper

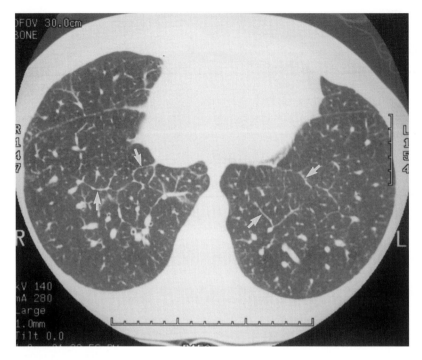

Figure 9 Lymphangitic carcinomatosis. HRCT through the lower lobes shows scattered thickening of interlobular septae (arrows), representing lymphangitic carcinomatosis due to adenocarcinoma of the pancreas. The diagnosis was confirmed by transbronchial lung biopsy.

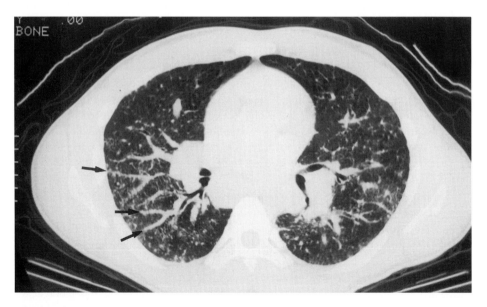

Figure 10 Sarcoidosis. In a 32-year-old man with shortness of breath, an HRCT through the hilar region shows marked nodular thickening along vessels (arrows) and bronchi and in the subpleural regions. Note the presence of bilateral hilar enlargement due to lymphadenopathy.

lobe predilection, while hematogenous metastases and miliary granulomatous infections—including tuberculosis, histoplasmosis, and coccidioidomycosis—have a uniform distribution within the lungs without predilection for any of the interstitial compartments.

Ground-Glass or Airspace Pattern.   A ground-glass pattern of parenchymal disease reflects either thickening of the alveolar wall or incomplete or nonuniform filling of the airspaces within the lung. The presence of ground-glass opacification as the predominant finding on HRCT suggests an active parenchymal process (i.e., edema, inflammation, or accumulation of intraalveolar protein) (Fig. 6) that is potentially reversible with the appropriate therapy.

Two patterns of ground-glass opacification are typically seen on HRCT. When the ground-glass opacities appear as low-attenuation, ill-defined centrilobular nodules, this represents airspace disease affecting the peribronchiolar alveoli. The differential considerations for centrilobular ground-glass opacities include bronchiolitis [e.g., respiratory bronchiolitis, bronchiolitis obliterans organizing pneumonia (BOOP), infectious bronchiolitis], subacute hypersensitivity pneumonitis (Fig. 11), pulmonary edema, and pulmonary histiocytosis.

More commonly, ground-glass opacification appears as scattered regions of uniformly increased attenuation that are sharply demarcated from adjacent normal areas of lung and contain visible bronchi and vessels. Since the histological processes producing ground-glass attenuation on HRCT are diverse, the conditions resulting in ground-glass

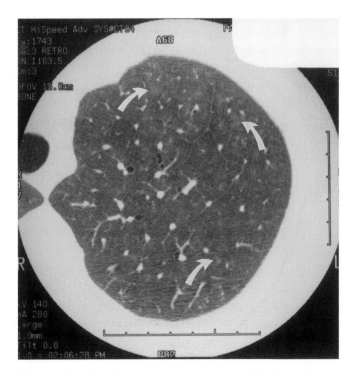

Figure 11 Centrilobular nodules in subacute HP. Magnified view of the left upper lobe on an HRCT in a 57-year-old woman shows ill-defined centrilobular nodules (arrows). A diagnosis of bird fancier's lung was made on basis of clinical and radiological findings in this patient, who was living with two doves in her home.

attenuation include both interstitial and airspace disorders. This pattern may be seen in the active inflammatory phase of usual interstitial pneumonitis, desquamative interstitial pneumonitis, subacute hypersensitivity pneumonitis, pulmonary edema, *Pneumocystis carinii* pneumonia (Fig. 12), diffuse pulmonary hemorrhage, alveolar proteinosis, bronchiolitis obliterans organizing pneumonia, and acute interstitial pneumonia (Hamman-Rich syndrome).

Airspace opacification on HRCT appears as consolidated lung containing air bronchograms that coalesces in areas of severe involvement, producing a lobar or segmental distribution with obscuration of vessels. Diseases that produce chronic airspace opacification on HRCT include alveolar proteinosis, bronchioloalveolar cell carcinoma, lymphoma, BOOP, and lipoid pneumonia.

Discrete Low-Attenuation Lesions.   Emphysema is identified as sharply marginated regions of low attenuation lacking definable walls. In centrilobular emphysema, the lucencies on HRCT are seen within the central portion of the secondary pulmonary lobule with a predilection for the upper lobe (Fig. 12). Bullae are thin-walled cystic spaces exceeding 1 cm in diameter with a predilection for the apical lung regions. Although they are most often seen in patients with generalized emphysema, bullae may be an isolated finding and can result in recurrent spontaneous pneumothorax.

Lung cysts or cystic airspaces are arbitrarily defined as discrete air-containing lesions marginated by thin (1- to 3-mm) walls. Diseases characterized by predominantly

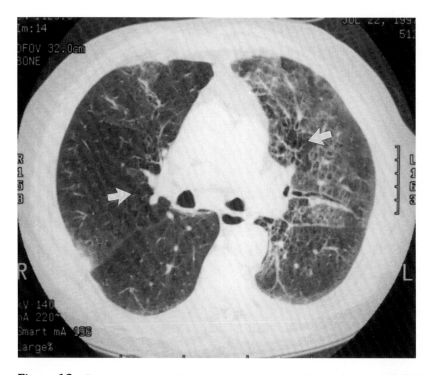

Figure 12   *Pneumocystis carinii* pneumonia in a patient with emphysema. HRCT in a 67-year-old man with chronic lymphocytic leukemia and progressive shortness of breath shows bilateral areas of ground-glass opacification. Note the presence of bilateral regions of centrilobular emphysema (arrows). *Pneumocystis carinii* was recovered from bronchoalveolar lavage.

cystic lesions include Langerhans cell histiocytosis (Fig. 13), lymphangioleiomyomatosis (LAM) and tuberous sclerosis, and end-stage pulmonary fibrosis. Honeycomb cysts are airspaces ranging from several millimeters to 2 cm in diameter and represent bands of fibrous tissue surrounding dilated alveolar ducts and bronchioles (Fig. 8).

Specific Diseases

Emphysema.   The three main subtypes of emphysema are well depicted on HRCT. Centrilobular emphysema has an upper-lung-zone predominance and is seen as abnormal areas of decreased attenuation lacking definable walls surrounding the centrilobular arteriole and bronchiole. With severe disease, the areas of parenchymal destruction become confluent and are indistinguishable from panlobular emphysema (Fig. 12). Panlobular emphysema involves uniform destruction of the entire secondary pulmonary lobule, resulting in widespread areas of low attenuation on HRCT with a concomitant decrease in the number and size of pulmonary vessels in the affected regions. The disease has a predominantly lower lobe distribution. The third type of emphysema is paraseptal emphysema, which can be associated with centrilobular emphysema or is an isolated finding in young adults. On HRCT, the lucencies in paraseptal emphysema are most evident in the subpleural portions of the lung apices adjacent to interlobular septa.

Langerhans Cell Histiocytosis (Eosinophilic Granuloma) of Lung.   Pulmonary histiocytosis is an idiopathic disease characterized histologically by the presence of peribronchial granulomatous nodules containing histiocytes and eosinophils that progresses to peribronchiolar fibrosis and cyst formation. The findings on HRCT depend on the stage of

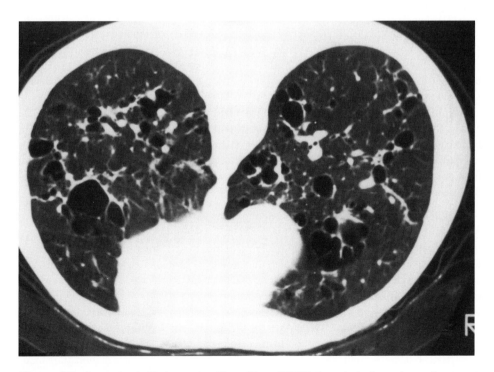

Figure 13   Langerhan's histiocytosis of lung. Prone HRCT through the lower lungs shows scattered clusters of thin-walled cysts characteristic of histiocytosis of lung.

disease at time of diagnosis. Early disease is characterized by centrilobular nodules with a predominant distribution in the upper and midlung zones. Occasionally, larger nodules will show central lucencies, which represent dilated bronchiolar lumina. In the later stages of disease, small, thin-walled cystic airspaces, often with unusual shapes, can be seen to replace the nodules (Fig. 13).

Lymphangioleiomyomatosis.   Lymphangioleiomyomatosis (LAM) is a rare disease resulting from the progressive abnormal proliferation of spindle cells in the pulmonary interstitium and lymphatics. HRCT of LAM demonstrates innumerable thin-walled lung cysts with intervening normal parenchyma. In contrast to the cysts seen in pulmonary histiocytosis, the cysts tend to be uniformly distributed throughout the lung without zonal predilection.

Usual and Desquamative Interstitial Pneumonitis/Idiopathic Pulmonary Fibrosis. Usual interstitial pneumonitis and desquamative interstitial pneumonitis represent two ends of the spectrum of chronic interstitial pneumonitis. HRCT findings in idiopathic pulmonary fibrosis (IPF) vary with the stage of disease and from one area of the lung to another. In the active, inflammatory stage of desquamative interstitial pneumonitis (DIP), intraalveolar inflammatory cells cause airspace opacification that appears on HRCT as ground-glass opacity. As the disease progresses usual interstitial pneumonitis (UIP), the findings of intralobular and interlobular interstitial thickening predominate on HRCT (Fig. 8). This results in a fine reticular pattern with irregular interfaces between the lung and pulmonary vessels, bronchi, and pleural surfaces, which progresses to honeycombing and traction bronchiectasis in the peripheral portions of the lower lobes.

Hypersensitivity Pneumonitis.   Hypersensitivity pneumonitis (HP) or extrinsic allergic alveolitis results from an allergic reaction to a variety of inhaled organic antigens. The HRCT findings of HP vary with the stage of disease. The acute stage follows heavy antigenic exposure and results in the filling of alveolar spaces with leukocytes. HRCT performed during the acute phase typically shows patchy airspace opacification. In the subacute stage of disease, which follows recurrent or low-level antigen exposure, HRCT shows diffuse ground-glass opacity and ill-defined centrilobular nodules (Fig. 11). The chronic stage of HP develops months to years after the initial exposure and is characterized by interstitial fibrosis. HRCT performed in chronic HP shows intralobular and interlobular interstitial lines, irregular interfaces, visible intralobular bronchioles, honeycombing, and traction bronchiectasis. The distribution of fibrosis is patchy, with no specific zonal predominance.

Sarcoidosis.   Sarcoidosis is a systemic disorder characterized by the presence of noncaseating granulomas. The characteristic HRCT finding in sarcoidosis is the presence of small, well-defined nodules <1 cm in diameter distributed along the peribronchovascular and subpleural interstitium. Nodular thickening of bronchial walls and vessels and subpleural nodules are seen in an upper-lobe and perihilar distribution (Fig. 10). Conglomerate masses of granulomatous tissue may develop in the perihilar regions. Fibrosis in the form of intralobular and interlobular lines, ground-glass opacity, and honeycombing may be seen in advanced disease. When severe fibrosis results in bronchiectasis or bullae, HRCT can be useful in the detection of mycetomas.

HRCT scans through the mediastinum in patients with sarcoidosis demonstrate bilaterally symmetrical hilar and paratracheal lymphadenopathy. In addition, HRCT often demonstrates enlargement of anterior mediastinal, subcarinal, internal mammary, and periesophageal nodes, which is not well seen on chest radiographs. Lymph node calcification may be identified and is occasionally peripheral or "eggshell" in distribution.

Bronchiolitis Obliterans Organizing Pneumonia (Cryptogenic Organizing Pneumonia). Bronchiolitis obliterans organizing pneumonia (BOOP) is a pathological entity characterized by the widespread presence of granulation tissue within the lumens of bronchioles, with patchy areas of adjacent organizing pneumonia. The HRCT appearance of BOOP is bilateral, patchy airspace or ground-glass opacity, often in combination (Fig. 14). In most cases a subpleural or peribronchovascular distribution of disease is present. Small, ill-defined peribronchiolar nodules (1–10 mm in diameter), representing localized areas of organizing pneumonia, can also be seen. Bronchial wall thickening and dilatation may be seen in regions of extensive disease.

Respiratory Bronchiolitis-Associated Interstitial Lung Disease. Respiratory bronchiolitis–associated interstitial lung disease represents a nonspecific inflammatory reaction of the lung to cigarette smoke, with macrophages seen within respiratory bronchioles and adjacent alveolar ducts and alveoli. The findings on HRCT reflect the alveolar wall thickening and inflammation, with bilateral ground-glass opacity seen in a patchy distribution.

Pneumocystis carinii Pneumonia. *Pneumocystis carinii* pneumonia (PCP) is a common infection in immunocompromised patients. HRCT in the early phase of PCP shows bilateral areas of perihilar ground-glass opacity (Fig. 12). In patients with more extensive parenchymal inflammation, areas of dense airspace consolidation are seen. During the resolving phase of pneumonia, reticular opacities are seen, representing thickening of the interlobular septa and intralobular lines as a result of the organization of intra-

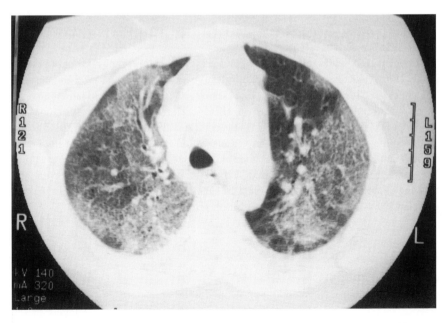

Figure 14 Bronchiolitis obliterans organizing pneumonia. HRCT in a 57-year-old woman shows bilateral ground-glass and airspace opacification. Diagnosis of BOOP was made on open lung biopsy.

alveolar exudate. Thin-walled cysts are frequently identified on HRCT within the upper lung zones in patients with PCP and can result in spontaneous pneumothorax.

Airways Disease

Bronchiectasis

CT has all but eliminated the need for contrast bronchography in the evaluation of bronchiectasis. The use of thin-section CT scans obtained at 10-mm intervals has an accuracy exceeding 95% in the detection of bronchiectasis. Cylindrical bronchiectasis appears either as multiple, dilated thick-walled circular lucencies when scanned in cross section or as parallel linear opacities or "tram tracks" when scanned along their length. Cystic bronchiectasis is easily recognized as clusters of rounded lucencies often containing air/fluid levels; this appearance has been likened to a cluster of grapes. Varicose bronchiectasis cannot be differentiated from cylindrical bronchiectasis unless sectioned longitudinally in the midlung regions, where the pattern of dilatation simulates the contour of a caterpillar or string of beads.

Small Airways Disease

HRCT is a sensitive indicator of small airways disease. There are both direct and indirect findings that may be evident on HRCT and allow detection of this process. The direct sign of small airways disease is centrilobular opacities, which represent diseased preterminal bronchioles. These are seen on HRCT as sharply defined or ground-glass nodules or Y- or V-shaped tubular branching opacities centrally situated within the secondary pulmonary lobule.

   The indirect signs of small airways disease result from expiratory air trapping and are most easily seen on HRCT. Those portions of lung most severely affected by small airways disease are poorly ventilated and perfused and appear relatively hyperlucent adjacent to areas of normal lung. This results in an appearance on HRCT termed *mosaic attenuation*, which is virtually indistinguishable from the changes seen in primary pulmonary arterial occlusive disease. Furthermore, infiltrative processes such as PCP and desquamative interstitial pneumonitis, which produce patchy ground-glass opacification, also result in a mosaic attenuation appearance on HRCT. The use of both inspiratory and expiratory HRCT scans helps distinguish between these various disorders (Fig. 15). In a patient with mosaic attenuation, attenuated vessels within the lucent regions of lung indicate that the lucent regions are abnormal due to decreased perfusion. This finding allows distinction from ground-glass opacification, where the caliber of vessels in normal and abnormal lung is comparable. The presence of small airways disease is confirmed on expiratory HRCT by noting air trapping within the hyperlucent regions.

Pleural Disease

Normal Pleural Anatomy on CT

Normally the visceral and parietal pleural layers are too thin to be visible on either conventional or HRCT of the chest. Only pathological thickening of the pleural layers or the presence of pleural effusion render the pleura visible on CT. Pleural thickening is most easily recognized on CT as a uniform band of soft tissue internal to the inner cortex of a rib.

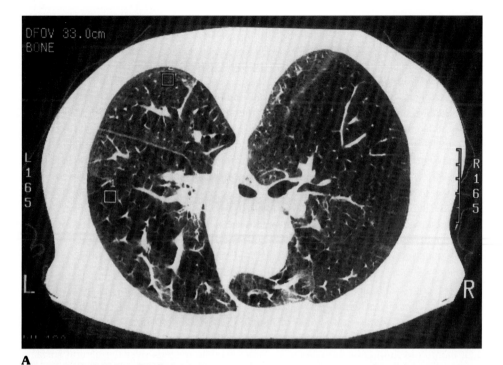

A

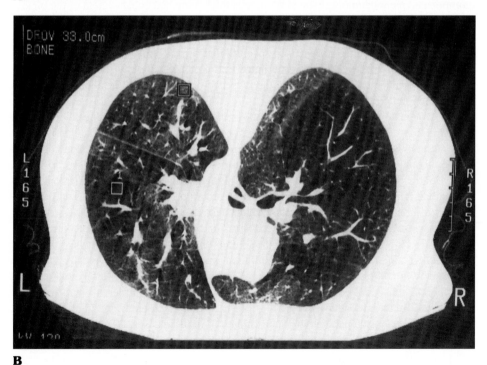

B

Figure 15 Inspiratory/expiratory HRCT in small airways disease. Paired inspiratory (A) and expiratory (B) HRCT scans at the level of the tracheal carina demonstrate a mosaic attenuation pattern that remains constant following expiration. This represents small airways disease with expiratory air trapping due to constrictive bronchiolitis (idiopathic bronchiolitis obliterans).

CT Appearance of Pleural Effusion

On axial CT scans, pleural fluid layers posteriorly with a characteristic meniscoid appearance and an attenuation value of 0–20 Hounsfield units (HU). Ultrasound is particularly useful in detecting free-flowing pleural effusions and distinguishing pleural from peritoneal collections. Since it is portable and relatively inexpensive, it should be used liberally, particularly if a diagnostic thoracentesis or therapeutic drainage is considered.

CT is commonly utilized to detect and localize loculated pleural fluid collections. The characteristic finding is a sharply marginated lenticular mass of fluid attenuation conforming to the concavity of the chest wall and forming obtuse angles at its edges. Loculated pleural effusions typically compress and displace the subjacent lung. Fluid loculated within the leaves of visceral pleura in an interlobar fissure results in an elliptical opacity oriented along the length of the fissure. These loculated collections of pleural fluid are termed *pseudotumors* and are most often seen within the minor fissure on frontal radiographs in patients with congestive heart failure. Multiple fluid locules can mimic pleural metastases or malignant mesothelioma radiographically; CT or ultrasound can confirm the fluid characteristics of these pleural ''masses.''

Infection.   The most common indication for CT of the pleura is in the evaluation of a parapneumonic effusion. The CT appearance of a parapneumonic effusion depends upon the stage of disease at the time of imaging. An uncomplicated parapneumonic effusion is often indistinguishable from a transudative effusion and appears as a gravity-dependent meniscoid fluid collection. As a fibrinous exudate extends over the pleural surfaces (complicated parapneumonic effusion), there is thickening and enhancement of the pleura, most easily seen on contrast-enhanced CT. In fact, the CT demonstration of thickened pleural layers separated by fluid is specific for an exudative pleural effusion, although it is not specific for infection and may be seen in other pleural inflammatory conditions and malignant pleural disease. It should be noted that although CT may show an apparently simple, homogeneous fluid collection, the presence of intrapleural fibrinous septations is significantly underestimated by CT and is more easily appreciated on ultrasound (Fig. 16). As the parapneumonic effusion progresses, visceral-to-parietal pleural adhesions result in the formation of fluid locules on CT. This appears as an elliptical fluid collection seen most commonly within the posterior and inferior pleural space. The collection conforms to and maintains a broad area of contact with the chest wall.

Contrast-enhanced chest CT is most useful in making the distinction between empyema and peripheral lung abscess. Lung abscesses are round, fluid-filled masses with irregular margins that form acute angles with the adjacent chest wall. Since abscesses represent necrotic parenchyma, there is minimal compression of the adjacent lung. In contrast, empyemas are elliptical fluid collections that create obtuse angles with the chest wall and displace and compress adjacent lung. While the wall of an abscess is typically thick and enhances with contrast, the inflamed pleural layers encompassing an empyema are thin and smooth, enhancing homogeneously, and producing the ''split pleura'' sign, which is helpful in differential diagnosis (Fig. 17). The detection of an empyema may be difficult when there is extensive parenchymal consolidation. In these cases, CT and ultrasound are useful in detecting parapneumonic fluid collections and guiding diagnostic thoracentesis and pleural drainage.

Neoplasm.   Pleural effusion may be seen with benign or malignant intrathoracic tumors. The tumors most commonly associated with pleural effusion are lung carcinoma, breast carcinoma, pelvic tumors, gastric carcinoma, and lymphoma. Pleural fluid formation

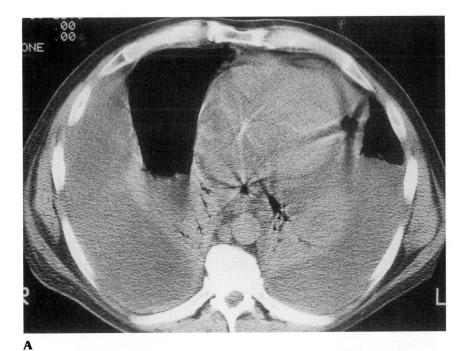

A

B

Figure 16 Parapneumonic effusion: CT vs. ultrasound. A. A CT scan in a patient with bilateral pneumonia shows large bilateral pleural effusions that appear unilocular and meniscoid in appearance. B. Ultrasound performed prior to diagnostic thoracentesis reveals multiple curvilinear septations (arrows) indicating a complicated, organizing collection. Thoracentesis yielded only 10 mL of serosanguinous fluid.

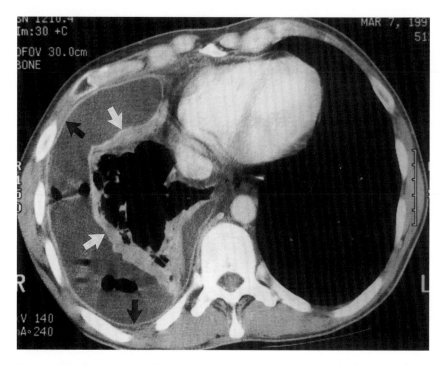

Figure 17 Empyema on CT. Contrast-enhanced CT through the lower chest in a patient with pneumonia and large right pleural collection on chest radiograph demonstrates a loculated pleural fluid collection marginated by enhancing visceral (white arrow) and parietal (black arrow) pleural layers indicative of an empyema. Air bubbles reflect recent thoracentesis. This collection required open drainage and decortication.

may result from pleural involvement by tumor or from lymphatic obstruction anywhere from the parietal pleura to the mediastinal nodes. The effusions are exudative and may be bloody. The demonstration of malignant cells on cytological examination of pleural fluid obtained at thoracentesis is necessary for the diagnosis of a malignant effusion. Closed or thoracoscopically guided biopsy is reserved for patients with negative cytological examination.

Clues to the presence of a malignant pleural effusion on CT include pleural thickening, mediastinal or hilar lymph node enlargement or mass, or solitary or multiple parenchymal nodules. In patients with pleural thickening, features that strongly suggest malignant pleural disease include pleural thickness exceeding 1 cm, lobulated pleural thickening, and circumferential thickening with involvement of the mediastinal pleural surface. CT is useful in demonstrating pleural masses or underlying parenchymal lesions in those with large effusions and opaque hemithoraces on chest radiographs.

Focal Pleural Disease

Localized Pleural Thickening.   Localized pleural thickening from fibrosis is usually the end result of peripheral parenchymal and pleural inflammatory disease, with pneumonia the most common cause (Table 5). Additional causes include pulmonary embolism with infarction, asbestos exposure, trauma, prior chemical pleurodesis, and drug-related pleural disease. Focal areas of pleural fibrosis are best appreciated on conventional and

Table 5 Differential Diagnosis of Pleural Masses

Focal mass
   Loculated effusion
   Lipoma arising from subpleural fat
   Localized fibrous tumor of pleura (formerly benign
     mesothelioma)
Mutiple masses/lobulated pleural thickening
   Multiloculated effusion (empyema, neoplasm, hemothorax)
   Metastatic pleural disease
   Malignant pleural mesothelioma

---

high-resolution CT scans and are distinguished from deposits of subpleural fat by their CT density. Apical pleural thickening, particularly if new, asymmetrical, or accompanied by symptoms suspicious for Pancoast's syndrome, requires CT or MRI examination, often with needle biopsy to exclude a superior sulcus tumor.

    Pleural Calcification. Pleural calcification is most often unilateral and involves the visceral pleura. It is usually the result of prior hemothorax or empyema (e.g., tuberculous), although pleural thickening of any cause may calcify. Visceral pleural calcification from pleural hemorrhage or infection are indistinguishable radiographically. Asbestos exposure can cause bilateral calcified parietal pleural plaques (Fig. 18). CT is particularly useful in detecting pleural calcification.

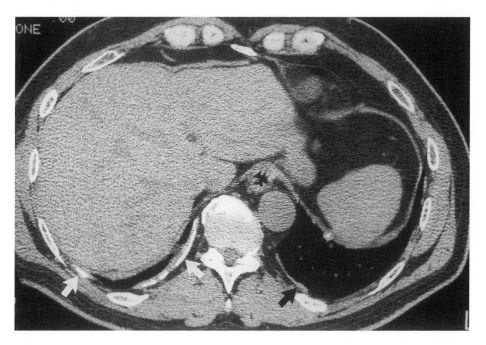

Figure 18 Pleural plaques. HRCT at the lung bases shows calcified (white arrow) and non-calcified (black arrow) pleural plaques indicative of previous asbestos exposure.

Mass.   Focal pleural masses are usually benign neoplasms such as fibrous tumors and lipomas, although loculated pleural fluid can mimic a pleural mass radiographically. Lipomas of the thorax may arise in the chest wall or subpleural fat, the latter producing a pleural mass. Homogeneous fatty attenuation on CT scan (-30 to -100 HU) is diagnostic. Localized fibrous tumors are rare benign pleural neoplasms. They appear as well-defined, spherical, or oblong masses that arise from the visceral pleura in 80% of cases. The CT appearance of a localized fibrous tumor is that of a sharply marginated homogeneous soft tissue mass of variable size. The larger the lesion, the more difficult it is to discern the pleural origin of the mass and the more likely some necrosis will be seen on CT.

Diffuse Pleural Disease

Fibrothorax.   Diffuse pleural fibrosis (fibrothorax) most commonly results from the resolution of an exudative pleural effusion, (including asbestos-related effusions), empyema, or hemothorax (Table 5). The fibrothorax can encompass the entire lung and produce entrapment. When pleural fibrosis results in a restrictive ventilatory defect, pleurectomy (decortication) may be necessary to restore function to the underlying lung.

HRCT is more sensitive than conventional radiographs in the detection of pleural thickening. The diminished volume of the affected hemithorax seen with extensive fibrothorax is more easily appreciated on axial CT images than on frontal radiographs. HRCT provides an unimpeded view of the underlying lung in patients with diffuse pleural thickening, allowing detection of associated interstitial pulmonary fibrosis.

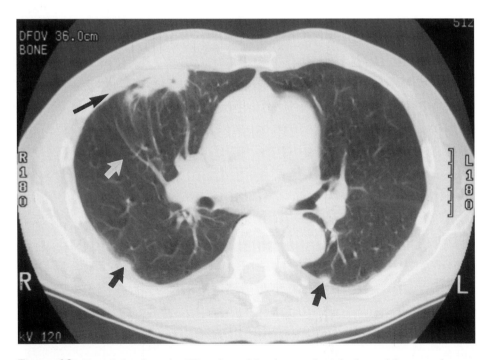

Figure 19   Rounded atelectasis. CT performed for the question of a lower lobe mass shows an oval opacity within the subpleural aspect of the middle lobe contacting a large pleural plaque (large black arrow). Note the presence of a ''comet tail'' of vessels and bronchi curving toward the mass from the hilum and the associated anterior displacement of the oblique fissure (white arrow), indicating volume loss. Additional pleural plaques are visible posteriorly (short black arrows).

Pleural Malignancy.   Metastatic disease to the pleura commonly causes irregular or lobulated pleural thickening, usually in association with a pleural effusion. The malignant tumors with a propensity to metastasize to the pleura include adenocarcinomas of the lung, breast, ovary, kidney, and gastrointestinal tract and invasive thymomas. Malignant mesothelioma is seen almost exclusively in asbestos-exposed individuals.

Contrast-enhanced CT can distinguish solid pleural masses from loculated pleural fluid, and can show discrete pleural masses or thickening in those with large effusions. In contrast to benign pleural thickening, malignant pleural disease is more likely when CT shows pleural thickening that is circumferential and nodular, greater than 1 cm in thickness, or involves the mediastinal pleura. Mesothelioma is radiographically indistinguishable from metastatic pleural disease. Chest wall invasion by pleural tumor, seen as rib destruction or soft tissue infiltration of the subcutaneous fat and musculature, is better appreciated on CT than on plain films.

Asbestos-Related Pleural Disease

Pleural Plaques.   CT and HRCT are highly sensitive in detecting calcified and noncalcified pleural plaques in asbestos-exposed individuals and distinguishes plaques and diffuse pleural fibrosis from subpleural fat deposits (Fig. 18).

Pleural Effusion.   The diagnosis of a benign asbestos pleural effusion is one of exclusion and requires the exclusion of tuberculosis or pleural malignancy (i.e., mesothelioma or metastatic adenocarcinoma). There are no distinguishing CT features of asbestos-related effusions, although pleural thickening may be seen.

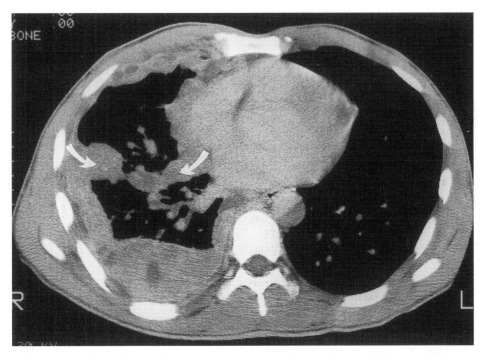

Figure 20 Malignant mesothelioma. CT scan through the lower lungs demonstrates marked nodular circumferential soft tissue thickening of the pleura with extension into the oblique fissure (curved arrows). Closed pleural biopsy revealed malignant mesothelioma.

Diffuse Pleural Thickening.   Diffuse pleural thickening or fibrosis may follow asbestos pleural effusion or result from the confluence of pleural plaques. HRCT is useful for determining the extent of pleural thickening, involvement of the interlobar fissures, and detecting underlying fibrosis or emphysema. Diffuse pleural fibrosis can result in symptomatic restrictive lung disease requiring pleural decortication.

Rounded Atelectasis.   A subset of patients with resolving exudative pleural effusions from asbestos exposure may develop an unusual form of lung collapse, termed *rounded atelectasis*, due to the development of intrapleural fibrinous adhesions that prevent normal lung reexpansion. CT and HRCT show typical findings of an enhancing round or oval mass adjacent to a thickened pleural surface with bronchi and vessels entering the central aspect of the lesion (''comet tail'' appearance) (Fig. 19). The volume loss in the affected lung is depicted on CT as displacement of the oblique fissure. While patients with typical CT findings can be followed conservatively, those lacking the classic findings should be considered for lung biopsy.

Malignant Mesothelioma.   CT is the imaging modality of choice in the evaluation of malignant mesothelioma and depicts the extent of pleural involvement and invasion of the chest wall and mediastinum (Fig. 20). Diaphragmatic invasion by tumor can be assessed by coronal reconstructions of helical CT scans and is important in those considered for curative resection.

SUGGESTED READING

1. Aquino SL, Webb WR, Gushiken BJ. Pleural exudates and transudates: diagnosis with contrast-enhanced CT. Radiology 1994; 192:803–808.
2. Glazer HS, Kaiser LR, Anderson DJ, Molina PL, Emami B, Roper LL, Sagel SS. Indeterminate mediastinal invasion in bronchogenic carcinoma: CT evaluation. Radiology 1989; 173:37–42.
3. Grenier P, Maurice F, Musset D, Menu Y, Nahum H. Bronchiectasis: assessment by thin-section CT. Radiology 1986; 161:95–99.
4. Grenier P, Valeyre D, Cluzel P, Brauner MW, Lenoir S, Chastang C. Chronic diffuse interstitial lung disease. Diagnostic value of chest radiography and high-resolution CT. Radiology 1991; 179:123–132.
5. Kuhlman JE. Complex disease of the pleural space: the 10 questions most frequently asked of the radiologist—new approaches to their answers with CT and MR imaging. Radiographics 1997; 17:1043–1050.
6. Leung AN, Muller NL, Millere RR. CT in the differential diagnosis of diffuse pleural disease. AJR 1990; 154:487–492.
7. Lynch DA. Imaging of small airways disease. Clin Chest Med 1993; 14:623–634.
8. Mathiesen JR, Mayo JR, Staples CA, Muller NL. Chronic diffuse infiltrative lung disease: comparison of diagnostic accuracy of CT and chest radiography. Radiology 1989; 171:111–116.
9. McLoud TC, Bourgouin PM, Greenberg RW, Kosivic JP, Templeton PA, Shepard JO, Moore EH, Wain JC, Mathisen OJ, Grillo MC. Bronchogenic carcinoma: analysis of staging in the mediastinum with CT by correlative lymph node mapping and sampling. Radiology 1992; 182:319–323.
10. Muller NL. Imaging of the pleura. Radiology 1993; 186:297–309.
11. Remy-Jardin M, Remy J, Wattinne L, Giraud F. Central pulmonary thromboembolism: diagnosis with spiral volumetric CT with the single breath-hold technique—comparison with pulmonary angiography. Radiology 1992; 185:381–387.

12. Siegelman SS, Zerhouni EA, Leo FP, Khouri NF, Stitik FP. Solitary pulmonary nodules. CT assessment. AJR 1980; 135:1–13.
13. Webb WR. Radiologic evaluation of the solitary pulmonary nodule. AJR 1990; 154:701–708.
14. Webb WR, Gatsonis C, Zerthouni EA, Heelan RT, Glazer GM, Francis IR, McNeil BJ. CT and MR imaging in staging non-small cell bronchogenic carcinoma: report of the Radiologic Diagnostic Oncology Group. Radiology 1991; 178:705–713.
15. Webb WR, Muller NL, Naidich DP. Standardized terms for high resolution lung CT: a proposed glossary. J Thorac Imaging 1993; 8:167–175.
16. Zerhouni EA, Stitik FP, Siegelman SS, Naioich DP, Sagel SS, Proto AV, Muhm JR, Walsh JW, Martinez LR, Heelan RT, Brantly P, Bozeman RE, Disantis OJ, Ettenger N, McCauley D, Augmenbaugh GL, Brown LR, Miller WE, Litt AW, Leo FP, Fishman EK, Knouri NF. CT of the pulmonary nodule: a cooperative study. Radiology 1986; 160:319–327.

12

Bronchoscopy in Diagnosis and Management of Pulmonary Diseases

Michael Unger

Thomas Jefferson University
Jefferson Medical College
Fox Chase Cancer Center
Philadelphia, Pennsylvania

OVERVIEW

While few primary care physicians perform bronchoscopy, they see many patients who require bronchoscopic procedures for either diagnostic or therapeutic indications. This chapter provides the referring physician with information on the different classifications of bronchoscopy, the indications for diagnostic bronchoscopy, the expanding list of bronchoscopic interventions, and complications of the procedure.

Tracheobronchial evaluation was first utilized as a method to remove foreign bodies from the airways. In 1887, Gustav Killian reported the first in vivo observation of the trachobronchial tree while evaluating a patient who had aspirated a piece of pork bone into the right mainstem bronchus. He subsequently removed the foreign body using an esophagoscope. Increasing interest in this field, combined with rapid technological progress, permitted direct visualization of the trachea and bronchi via a rigid metal tube—the rigid bronchoscope. This eventually led to the development of a new field and specialization in bronchoesophagology. Leading this progress was the school established by Chevalier Jackson in Philadelphia. In 1967, Shigeto Ikeda developed the clinical use of a flexible bronchoscope using fiberoptic technology. This led to the current wide use of bronchoscopy for both clinical and investigational purposes.

The recent development of various noninvasive imaging technologies, such as three-dimensional computed tomography reconstruction (''virtual'' bronchoscopy), has not reduced the value of bronchoscopy, which permits not only visualization but also acquisition of diagnostic specimens. Aliquots of bronchial washings or lavage fluid can be processed in various laboratories, including those dedicated to microbiology, cytopathology, immunology, histochemistry, and genetics. Larger collections of cells can be obtained with bronchial brushes from specific areas of the tracheobronchial tree and processed by the previously mentioned techniques (see Chap. 13, on diagnostic sampling of lung tissues and cells). Specimens of endobronchial and pulmonary parenchymal tissue for histological examination can be obtained with a variety of sharp-edged cup biopsy devices passed through the lumen of the bronchoscope. For more peripheral tissue collection, specially designed curettes can be used. Transbronchial needle aspiration and core biopsy can sample tissue from hilar or mediastinal masses and lymph nodes. Finally, there has been continuing development of interventional techniques for airway obstruction, endobronchial tumors, and foreign bodies.

CLASSIFICATION OF BRONCHOSCOPY

Bronchoscopic procedures can be classified into two general types: those performed through a rigid metal tube and those performed with flexible instruments. Each has its advantages and disadvantages. In certain situations, they are used at the same time. Flexible bronchoscopes can be passed via the rigid bronchoscope to visualize distal airways while still maintaining the excellent control of the airway that the rigid scope affords.

Rigid Bronchoscopy

The first six decades of bronchoscopy were restricted by available technology to the use of rigid metal tubes. Rigid bronchoscopies are performed in the operating room, usually under general anesthesia. There are several obvious advantages to this technique:

> Large-bore rigid tubes facilitate suctioning and control of the central airways. With special attachments, mechanical ventilation can be provided through the tube during the procedure (Figs. 1 and 2).

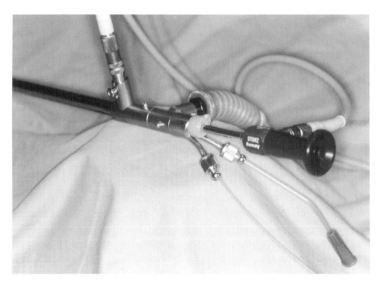

Figure 1 Proximal end of the rigid bronchoscope. The optical telescope is inserted into the rigid metal tube of the bronchoscope. The side connector for mechanical ventilation, the laser light guide, and suction tube are also attached.

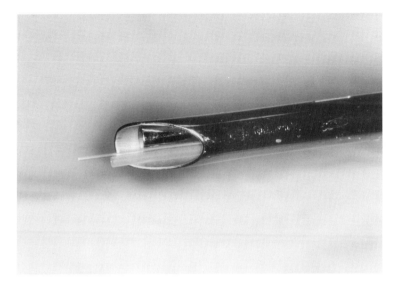

Figure 2 Distal tip of the rigid bronchoscope containing the telescope, laser-light guide, and suction channel.

With the addition of high-quality telescopes, these instruments provide excellent optics.

Rigidity of the metal scope permits selective application of pressure to the tracheo-bronchial tree to achieve tamponade of a bleeding source and easier control of hemorrhage.

The large lumens of the metal tubes permit faster debulking of tumors and removal of secretions, debris, or blood clots. The large lumen also facilitates the placement of various stenting and other interventional devices described below.

The disadvantages of rigid bronchoscopy are not negligible:

Because of certain requirements, rigid bronchoscopy is usually done under general anesthesia, with its associated complications. Operating room facilities add to the complexity and overall cost of the procedure.

Lack of flexibility of these instruments results in limited access to certain areas, particularly the segments of both upper lobes, and is also associated with a higher risk of trauma to lips, teeth, gums and upper airways.

Rigid bronchoscopy cannot be performed in patients with cervical spine injury or those who are unable to have their neck hyperextended.

Flexible Bronchoscopy

The advent of fiberoptic bronchoscopes drastically changed diagnostic and interventional bronchoscopic procedures (Fig. 3). Recently, the development of electronic transmission of the image from a charge-couple device at the tip of the bronchoscope (''videochip bronchoscope'') has improved image resolution and provided excellent photographic documentation. Flexible bronchoscopes include a separate instrumentation channel through which secretions and bronchial washings or bronchoalveolar lavage (BAL) specimens can

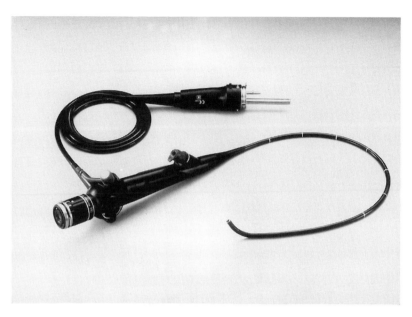

Figure 3 Fiberoptic bronchoscope (Olympus USA). The distal tip of the bronchoscope is partially flexed. The viewing lens and suction control button are visible at the proximal end of the instrument.

be aspirated and collected. Alternatively, the same channels may serve as conduits for the introduction of diagnostic brushes, biopsy devices, and transbronchial needles capable of collecting cytological or histological specimens (Fig. 4).

Flexible bronchoscopes offer a number of advantages:

> The small size of flexible bronchoscopes permits the passage of the scope through not only the mouth but also the nasal passages. This can also be accomplished with less risk of trauma to the upper airways and vocal cords.
>
> Fiberoptic bronchoscopies can be performed with local anesthesia and conscious sedation in a bronchoscopic suite or even at the bedside. These instruments can also be used in patients who are intubated and mechanically ventilated in the intensive care unit (ICU) or operating room.
>
> The flexibility and size of various flexible bronchoscopic instruments permit their use in neonatal and pediatric patients.
>
> The flexible bronchoscope provides visualization of more peripheral airways, including upper lobe segments, allowing acquisition of specimens of bronchial washings, lavage fluid, brushings, and tissue biopsies from these areas.
>
> In contrast with the rigid technique, there is no need for neck hyperextension to perform the procedure.

There are also significant disadvantages with the use of these instruments:

> Flexible bronchoscopes have relatively small instrumentation channels with limited ability to suction and remove secretions, endobronchial debris, or blood clots.
>
> The fiberoptic and video bronchoscopes are fragile instruments, and hence more costly to maintain.
>
> Because of their more complex structure and the use of various synthetic materials,

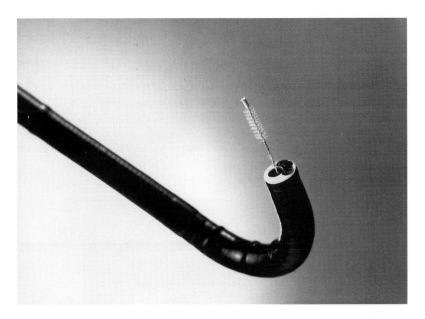

Figure 4 Distal tip of the fiberoptic bronchoscope. The tip is flexed and the cytology brush protrudes from the working channel. The light bundles and optic viewing bundle are seen adjacent to the channel.

there is the risk of microbiological colonization and transmission to subsequent patients if cleaning and maintenance are inadequate.

The decision of which type of bronchoscopy to perform is determined primarily by the patient's disease and comorbidities, though operator availability, skill, and experience are also factors. Most diagnostic bronchoscopies can be performed with flexible instruments unless there are copious secretions or significant hemorrhage that require the rigid bronchoscope's advantages of suctioning and airway control. Complex interventional bronchoscopic procedures have usually been performed via a rigid bronchoscope. However, laser-light guides, cryotherapy, electrocautery devices, dilatation balloons, and stenting devices have been adapted for the flexible bronchoscope, expanding the interventional role of these instruments.

INDICATIONS FOR DIAGNOSTIC BRONCHOSCOPY

Arbitrarily and for didactic reasons, the indications for diagnostic bronchoscopy can be divided into two categories: patients with abnormalities on chest radiographs and those with respiratory signs or symptoms who do not have chest radiographic changes. Table 1 is a summarization of indications for bronchoscopy.

Bronchoscopy in Patients with Abnormal Radiographic Findings

Malignancy

Persistent pulmonary infiltrates and densities that do not respond to therapy or observation may justify diagnostic bronchoscopy in an attempt to differentiate between malignant

Table 1 Indications for Bronchoscopy

Diagnostic bronchoscopy
  Abnormal radiograph
    Suspected malignancy
    Infection
    Diffuse parenchymal and interstitial infiltrates
    Chest trauma
  Normal radiograph
    Hemoptysis
    Localized wheezing or stridor
    Chronic cough
    Abnormal sputum cytology
Therapeutic bronchoscopy
  Removal of foreign body
  Removal of secretions
  Ablation of proximal endobronchial tumor
  Placement of airway stents

and benign processes. Malignant processes will include, first and above all, primary lung carcinomas of various types. Except for those patients presenting with oncological emergencies that demand immediate therapy [superior vena cava (SVC) syndrome or upper airway obstruction], it is essential to secure appropriate tissue diagnosis prior to initiation of chemotherapy or radiation therapy, given their attendant adverse effects. Bronchoscopic airway evaluation and transbronchoscopic needle aspiration of mediastinal lymphadenopathy may also help establish the TNM stage of the tumor (see Chap. 32). The importance of precise pathological staging of carcinomas for planning of therapeutic interventions cannot be overemphasized. Therapeutic decisions should not be made based solely upon clinical or radiographic staging. In many cases, the judicious use of transbronchial biopsy of lymph nodes with specially designed needles will obviate more complicated surgical procedures. With mastering of the technique, cytological aspirations and needle core biopsy from lymph nodes adjacent to the trachea, carina, or selected bronchi can be used for flow cytometry as well as for routine cytohistopathological studies and special stainings.

In the case of an endoscopically visible lesion or tumor, precise diagnosis will be secured in over 90% of the cases. When the lesions are more peripheral and not directly seen via the scope, acquisition of diagnostic specimens improves with fluoroscopic guidance. Bronchial brushes, forceps, and needle biopsies can be guided fluoroscopically toward these lesions while minimizing the risk of pneumothorax. The sensitivity of bronchoscopy with peripheral lesions depends on the size of the mass. Lesions larger than 2 cm can be adequately sampled 60% of the time by bronchoscopy; peripheral lesions smaller than 2 cm are better approached with radiographically guided transthoracic needle aspiration (see Chaps. 11 and 20).

Infection

Immunocompromised patients presenting with fever, productive cough, and pulmonary infiltrates may be treated initially with empirical therapy for bacterial infection. However, if there is further radiographic extension of disease and/or the patient does not respond to empirical treatment, bronchoscopy should be performed with BAL, brushing, and, if not contraindicated, biopsy. BAL is performed by advancing the bronchoscope distally until it is wedged in a airway subsegment, at which point aliquots of saline are sequentially instilled and then aspirated. Bronchoscopy with BAL has become the technique of choice for the diagnosis of opportunistic, mycobacterial, and other infections in both immunocompromised and immunocompetent patients from whom sputum is not obtainable.

There is still controversy as to the use of bronchoscopy either with BAL or with protected specimen brushes (PSB) for the diagnosis of nosocomial pneumonia in patients on mechanical ventilation. There has been good correlation between results obtained by BAL and PSB, so there is no justification for performing both procedures in the same patient for determination of bacterial pathogens. Provided that there is an adequate return, BAL offers sampling from a larger portion of the lung in a less costly manner than PSB.

Diffuse Parenchymal and Interstitial Infiltrates

Persistent pulmonary infiltrates, lymphadenopathy, or other parenchymal changes justify bronchoscopic evaluation and collection of specimens. Bronchoscopic biopsy established itself as one of the most reliable diagnostic techniques for sarcoidosis and lymphangitic carcinomatosis, with minimal morbidity and good sensitivity and specificity. Its specificity and sensitivity, however, are inferior to those of open or thoracoscopic lung biopsy for other interstitial lung diseases. Sampling of the alveolar lining fluid and resident cellular population by BAL for research purposes has led to important insights into disease pathophysiology. BAL can be diagnostic for pulmonary alveolar proteinosis, primary or secondary pulmonary malignancies, lymphangitic spread of carcinomas, eosinophilic pneumonia, and histiocytosis X. However, BAL has not yet been demonstrated to be useful for guiding therapy in patients with idiopathic pulmonary fibrosis, documented sarcoidosis, or hypersensitivity pneumonitis (see Chaps. 28 and 29).

Trauma

Chest trauma can result in injuries to the tracheobronchial tree. In this setting, bronchoscopy plays an important part in emergency management. Several publications have documented the usefulness of this procedure in early diagnosis of severe injury and some even recommend it routinely in cases of major thoracic trauma. The bronchoscopic procedure should be performed by an experienced bronchoscopist as the lesions are not always readily evident. Only rarely are traumatic fistulae or ruptures visible. They can, however, masquerade as blood clots, heaped up mucosa, edema, or lacerations of mucosa.

Bronchoscopy in Patients Without Obvious Radiographic Findings

Bronchoscopy may be indicated in patients presenting with various symptomatologies or medical histories even in the absence of radiographic abnormalities.

Hemoptysis

Patients presenting with hemoptysis can have a wide variety of disorders, reviewed in Chap. 21. In many of these patients, bronchoscopy is indicated to identify the site of bleeding and to evaluate for potential causes—endobronchial malignancies, bronchiectasis, and broncholithiasis (erosion into the airway of calcified mediastinal lymph nodes). In cases of massive hemoptysis, rigid bronchoscopy will be the instrument of choice to facilitate rapid removal of large amounts of blood while simultaneously providing ventilation. Bronchoscopically guided insertion of balloon catheters or endotracheal tubes can provide temporary control of the bleeding until more definitive procedures can be performed.

Localized Wheezing

The physical examination finding of localized wheeze or stridor can be secondary to significant narrowing of an airway. The differential diagnosis includes postintubation tracheal injuries, stenosis at the site of a previous bronchial anastomosis, benign or malignant endobronchial tumors, destruction of cartilaginous rings, focal extrinsic compression of the airways, an aspirated foreign body, or acute inhalation injury (toxic fumes).

Chronic Cough

The vast majority of patients with the predominant symptom of a persistent cough who have a normal or unchanged chest radiograph will have cough secondary to asthma, postnasal drip, gastroesophageal reflux, chronic bronchitis, or the use of certain medications (e.g., angiotensin-converting enzyme inhibitors) (see Chap. 15). The yield of bronchoscopy in unselected patients with this problem is quite low. However, if the more common causes of chronic cough are eliminated, bronchoscopy is definitely indicated to evaluate for aspirated foreign bodies, endobronchial tumors, or other endobronchial abnormalities.

Positive Sputum Cytology

Patients with sputum cytology positive for malignancy, even in the absence of obvious radiographic changes, require diagnostic bronchoscopy to evaluate for endobronchial lesions. A technique called the lung imaging fluorescence endoscopy (LIFE) system recently approved by the FDA is not yet widely available; however, it improves the sensitivity of standard bronchoscopy by using a helium-cadmium laser as a light source. In response to illumination with this light, normal bronchial mucosa emits green fluorescence. Abnormal or suspicious-for-malignancy areas lose this natural green fluorescence but maintain red fluorescence. Even small areas of brownish red discoloration (1 to 2 mm in diameter) can then be detected and biopsied for diagnosis, enhancing the rate of detection of premalignant lesions (severe dysplasia), early carcinoma in situ, or minimally invasive lung cancer. Patients with positive findings for malignant or premalignant lesions may benefit from various early interventions with chemoprevention, photodynamic therapy, laser therapy, electrocautery, local endobronchial irradiation, or local excision. This new bronchoscopic technique may also improve our understanding of the natural history of lung cancer, which still remains very rudimentary.

THERAPEUTIC INTERVENTIONAL BRONCHOSCOPY

The rigid and flexible instruments can be used not only for visual observation and acquisition of information but are also powerfuls tool for therapeutic interventions.

Removal of Foreign Bodies and Secretions

Inadvertent inhalation of foreign bodies seems to occur most frequently at the extremes of the life span—in children and the elderly. In children, the optimal approach for removal of these objects is via the rigid scope. In adults, flexible bronchoscopy with the use of various ingenious accessory instruments—grasping forceps, retrieval mechanical baskets, and magnets—can be successful, avoiding the complications of general anesthesia.

Urgent flexible bronchoscopy is required to suction out inspissated secretions in patients who are in respiratory distress or who have severe refractory hypoxemia from lobar or whole-lung atelectasis. In otherwise stable patients, atelectasis from secretions often responds to aggressive pulmonary toilet (chest percussion, incentive spirometry, cough, and bronchodilators), with bronchoscopy reserved for those patients who do not improve within 24 h. In patients supported by mechanical ventilation, clearance of pulmonary secretions is impaired but can be managed with appropriate respiratory and nursing care. Unfortunately, bronchoscopy is still abused and overused in this situation.

Bronchoscopic Management of Proximal Endobronchial Tumors

Unresectable endobronchial tumors can cause dyspnea, bleeding, cough, and obstructive pneumonitis. A variety of endoscopic techniques have been used to treat endobronchial tumors, including laser therapy, cryotherapy, electrocautery, and brachytherapy. Bronchoscopic laser therapy via either rigid or flexible bronchoscopy is useful and very effective in cases of obstruction by fungating endoluminal masses, either benign or malignant. The more proximal the mass, the more critical it is from a physiological standpoint and the more likely it is that there will be a rewarding relief of symptoms with successful interventions. Because of its superb coagulating characteristics and vaporization capabilities, the Nd:YAG (neodymium aluminum garnet) laser has become the instrument of choice in treating highly vascular endobronchial tumors. The primary aim is to produce coagulation and devascularization of the tumor, which then permits debulking and subsequent enlargement or reestablishment of the airway lumen. Argon, copper, or gold pumped lasers emit an optimal wavelength for activation of photosensitizers and are used for photodynamic therapy of small, minimally invasive carcinomas.

Attempts have been made to achieve similar results with cryotherapy and bronchoscopic electrocoagulation. The initial cost of the instrumentation for these procedures is less, but there is much less local control of the depth of penetration and an expanded risk of perforation or bleeding. For the electrocautery procedures, specially insulated flexible bronchoscopes have to be used to avoid electric leak or arcing, which can be dangerous to both the patient and the operator.

Brachytherapy is the delivery of radiation therapy from a ionizing radiation source placed within or near the tumor. It is most often used in patients with recurrent bronchogenic carcinoma who have failed external-beam irradiation. While a number of ionizing radiation sources have been used, the most frequently applied is iridium 192 (^{192}Ir). The bronchoscopist carefully measures the distance to the tumor and precisely inserts an afterloading catheter into the airway lumen, with the distal end beyond the visible tumor. The afterloading catheter is then left in the airway lumen after removal of the bronchoscope and the high dose rate (HDR) radiation source is introduced by a remote, computer-controlled afterloading machine while the patient remains in a radiation-protected room. When high dose rates are used, the short-duration treatments are fractionated at 1 week intervals and the patients require three different bronchoscopies. The number of procedures can be limited to one bronchoscopy when intermediate or low dose rates are used. The cost of these procedures is also significantly reduced then, since no special afterloading equipment is required. While 80% of patients will have symptomatic improvement with brachytherapy, fatal hemorrhage from either complications of the procedure or tumor progression has been reported in up to 12% of these patients.

Management of Tracheobronchial Obstruction with Airway Stents

Placement of an endobronchial or tracheal prosthesis for airway obstruction was attempted in the early stages of interventional bronchoscopy. However, the results with the rubber or metal devices were disappointing. The development of silicone material permitted the construction of much more acceptable stents. Some of these also combine various metal scaffolding and others consist of a metal base covered with polyurethane or polyvinyl. The fact that we now have access to a large variety of these stents proves that none of them is ideal or useful in all situations.

The "dedicated stent" developed by J. F. Dumont is the most frequently and widely used prosthesis. These cylindrical silicone stents are produced in various diameters and lengths, including a Y-shaped prosthesis designed to fit into the lower trachea over the carina with extensions to both mainstem bronchi. To minimize the possibility of displacement, the external wall of these stents is irregular and contains multiple anchoring studs. As useful as these stents are, they also have several disadvantages. The thickness of their wall, which is necessary to provide adequate counterpressure to the area of stenosis, reduces the internal lumen, contributing to increased airflow resistance. The longer the segment of silicone, the more surface area for adhesion of secretions, promoting plugging of airways. Among the most noticeable complications, however, is displacement and migration of the stents themselves. Insertion of these stents and most other preformed prostheses requires the use of rigid scopes with or without specifically designed stent introducers. Another drawback of this technique is in its placement, which is done blindly, without simultaneous visual observation.

The self-expanding stents (Wallstent, Ultraflex) overcome some of these disadvantages. They can be introduced and deployed under continuous visual observation with flexible bronchoscopes. Their biggest problem lies in the inability or extreme difficulty of removing them after inappropriate deployment. They also produce more mechanical problems than the softer silicone stents, and they can promote the formation of severe granular tissue reactions.

Mechanical dilatation can improve endoluminal narrowing from concentric stenosis. This can be achieved either by introducing progressively larger rigid scopes or by inflating high-pressure balloons. This technique should be evaluated and chosen judiciously to avoid the potential complication of bronchial rupture. In general, the relief of symptoms, although immediate, is transitory, since in most cases the primary cause is not addressed. To a certain degree, the rate of recurrence can be modulated with the use of anti-inflammatory medications. In cases of posttraumatic stenosis involving a short segment of the trachea, radial cuts using the Nd:YAG laser can provide more durable results. Long bottleneck type stenoses, however, respond poorly to this and most other endoluminal bronchoscopic procedures.

COMPLICATIONS

Although the overall morbidity and mortality of bronchoscopic procedures are acceptably low, there are potential complications that can be related to the patient, the anesthesia, and the procedure itself.

Patient-Related Complications and Their Prevention

The potential benefits of the diagnostic and therapeutic procedure should outweigh the potential risks. Bronchoscopy in patients who have preexisting ventilatory insufficiency or hypoxemia may initiate a cascade of respiratory, cardiovascular, and neurological disasters. Invasive acquisition of tissue specimens or aggressive therapy should be withheld in patients with thrombocytopenia, other clotting defects, or uremia or those who are receiving therapeutic anticoagulation or medications affecting platelet function. Rigid bronchoscopy should not be attempted in patients for whom cervical hyperextension could be dangerous.

Appropriate preparation prior to the procedure as well as monitoring during and after bronchoscopy are crucial. Anticoagulants or any other medication that could increase the bleeding potential should be withheld prior to the procedure. Aspirin should be discontinued, if possible, for 5–7 days. Patients should remain fasting for at least 6 h prior to bronchoscopy to avoid the risk of aspiration pneumonia. Recently published recommendations of the American Heart Association and the excellent review of the subject provide straightforward guidelines for antibiotic prophylaxis before bronchoscopy. Every patient should have a well-established intravenous access for additional sedatives, anesthetics, or other medications required for reversal of oversedation, resuscitation, or other complications. All patients should have continuous electrocardiographic and oximetry monitoring, and intermittent blood pressure and respiratory rate measurements. Supplemental oxygen is administered and adjusted to maintain oxygen saturation above 90–92%.

Complications of Anesthesia

Either general or topical anesthesia is applicable for all the bronchoscopic techniques. The most frequently used local anesthetic is lidocaine. Systemic anticholinergic medications decrease the quantity of airway secretions and limit vasovagal reactions, bradycardia, and bronchospasm. In many circumstances, conscious sedation with intravenous anxiolytics and cough suppressants can make the procedure much more comfortable for the patient and the physician.

The potential complications of general anesthesia are self-evident. Local anesthetic problems, in conjunction with conscious sedation, are also not negligible. The potential toxicity of lidocaine includes seizures, arrhythmias, and methemoglobinemia. Early recognition of methemoglobinemia can be lifesaving, and it is imperative that methylene blue be available in every endoscopic procedure room, as this complication is not responsive to supplemental oxygen. Sedatives can cause hypoventilation and apnea. It should be remembered that oximetry does not provide sensitive information about ventilation and carbon dioxide level in patients undergoing bronchoscopy.

Complications Related to Bronchoscopic Procedures

Bronchoscopic procedure–related complications include injuries of the upper and lower airways, severe bleeding from injury to a bronchial artery, and bleeding due to perforation of a major mediastinal pulmonary vessel. Vigorous suctioning or flooding of airways with lavage fluid can cause further oxygen desaturation. Peripheral biopsy or manipulations without fluoroscopic guidance increase the risk of pneumothorax, particularly in patients with substantial emphysema or other destructive parenchymal diseases. Bleeding and bronchial perforations have been reported as complications of all modalities of interventional bronchoscopy.

Among other potential complications of bronchoscopy, fever has occured in 10–20% of cases, often associated with performance of BAL. The pathogenesis of the elevated temperature (around 38° C) is not clear, but its clinical significance is low. In the majority of cases, the febrile episode will resolve spontaneously or with the use of an antipyretic for 24 h.

Several studies have confirmed that proper cleaning and disinfection of bronchoscopes with glutaraldehyde is adequate to prevent transmission of HIV and other pathogens. Thorough cleaning of all the components of the scopes first with detergent and water and then with complete immersion in 2% glutaraldehyde for at least 20 min provide optimal results. Hence, strict adherence to these recommendations obviates the need for separate scopes for patients with documented or suspected HIV infection.

SUMMARY

In well-trained hands and with application of appropriate precautions as well as adherence to criteria for indications and contraindications, the morbidity and mortality of bronchoscopy are very low. This makes it an invaluable technique in diagnosis and management of many pulmonary diseases.

SUGGESTED READING

1. Becker H. Flexible versus rigid bronchoscopic placement of tracheobronchial prostheses (stent): pro flexible bronchoscopy. J Bronchol 1995; 2:252–256.
2. Cortese DA. Rigid versus flexible bronchoscopy in laser bronchoscopy: pro rigid bronchoscopic laser application. J Bronchol 1994; 1:72–75.
3. Dumon JF, Cavaliere S, Diaz-Jimenez JP, Vergnon JM, Venuta F, dumon MC, Kovitz KL. Seven-year experience with the Dumon prosthesis. J Bronchol 1996; 3:6–10.
4. Edell ES, Cortese DA. Photodynamic therapy in management of early superficial squamous cell carcinoma as an alternative to surgical resection. Chest 1992; 102:1319–1322.
5. Griffin JJ, Meduri GU. New approaches to the diagnosis of nosocomial pneumonia. Med Clin North Am 1994; 78:1091–1122.
6. Homasson JP. Bronchoscopic cryotherapy. J Bronchol 1995; 2:45–53.
7. Prakash UBS, Cortese DA. Tracheobronchial foreign bodies. In: Prakash UBS, ed. Bronchoscopy. New York: Raven, 1994:253–277.
8. Kirkpatrick MB, Middleton RM. Bronchoscopic diagnosis of bacterial pneumonia: protected specimen brush versus bronchoalveolar lavage: pro protected brush. J Bronchol 1997; 4:255–259.
9. Lam S, MacAulay C, LeRiche JC, Profio AE, Palcic B. Detection of dysplasia and carcinoma in situ by lung imaging fluorescence endoscope (LIFE) device. J Thorac Cardiovas Surg 1993; 105:1035–1040.
10. Lin MC, Lin HC, Lan RS, Tsao TCY, Tsai YH, Chuang ML, Huand CC. Emergent flexible bronchoscopy for evaluation of acute chest trauma. J Bronchol 1995; 2:188–191.
11. Meduri GU. Diagnosis and differential diagnosis of ventilator-associated pneumonia. Clin Chest Med 1995; 16:61–93.

12. Prakash UBS, Offord KP, Stubbs SE. Bronchoscopy in North America: the AACP survey. Chest 1991; 100:1668–1675.
13. Prakash UBS. Prophylactic antibacterial therapy for bronchoscopy: indications. J Bronchol 1997; 4:281–285.
14. Shure D. Transbronchial biopsy and needle aspiration. Chest 1989; 95:1130–1138.
15. Unger M. Rigid versus flexible bronchoscopy in laser bronchoscopy: pro flexible bronchoscopic laser application. J Bronchol 1994; 1:69–71.
16. Wang KP, Gonullu U, Baker R. Bronchoscopy needle aspiration versus transthoracic needle aspiration in the diagnosis of pulmonary lesions. J Bronchol 1994; 1:199–204.

13

Diagnostic Sampling of Lung Tissues and Cells

Kevin O. Leslie, Louis A. Lanza, Richard A. Helmers, and Thomas V. Colby
Mayo Graduate School of Medicine
Mayo Clinic Hospital
Scottsdale, Arizona

INTRODUCTION

A limited number of diagnostic sampling techniques are available for the study of lung tissues and cells. The rationale and approach for each depends on the given clinical circumstances, and the radiographic findings, and the pathological conditions being considered. A multidisciplinary approach assures the most cost-effective and accurate results. Communication and discussion between pulmonologist, radiologist, pathologist, and thoracic surgeon before sampling is advisable in most cases but absolutely required in others (e.g., open-lung biopsy). In this chapter, we review commonly used sampling procedures and guide the reader through effective specimen handling necessary to achieve diagnostic results (Table 1).

SPECIMENS FROM BRONCHOSCOPY

Endobronchial Biopsy

Diseases intrinsic to the large airways, endobronchial tumors, and metastatic disease involving the airway lymphovascular network are best approached by endobronchial biopsy. The cup forceps is commonly employed and produces a 2- to 3-mm fragment of bronchial mucosa, including variable amounts of submucosa, muscular wall, and cartilage. The specimen should be removed from the forceps with a sterile needle and placed directly into fixative solution or culture medium. If this is not feasible, a Telfa pad with sterile saline is a reasonable intermediary prior to transfer into fixative solution. For routine hematoxylin and eosin–stained sections viewed by light microscopy, standard fixation is accomplished using 10% neutral buffered formalin (4% formaldehyde). In some laboratories, nonaldehyde fixatives (usually alcohol-based) have replaced formalin for safety and disposal cost issues, so it may be important to know where the biopsy will be interpreted. Other specialty fixatives may be used depending on the preference of the local pathology department (e.g., methacarn, mercurial fixatives). When in doubt, 10% formalin may be used to fix the

Table 1   Handling of Lung Tissue and Fluid Specimens

Specimen	Optimum Handling
Endobronchial biopsy Transbronchial biopsy	Remove specimen from biopsy forceps with sterile needle. Place directly into culture medium or fixative (10% formalin).
Bronchial brushing Bronchial washing	Brush can be directly applied to slides followed by fixation. Washings should be split for processing (cytology, chemistry, microbiology, cell count, others).
Bronchoalveolar lavage	Lavage specimens are handled the same as brush/wash specimens but represent greater volumes.
Transbronchial needle aspiration	Direct application to glass slides with or without immediate fixation (check with lab). Alternately, discharge into carrier medium.
Thoracentesis	Split fluid for analysis in lab.
Closed pleural biopsy	Remove specimen from forceps with sterile needle. Place directly into culture medium or fixative (10% fixative).
Transthoracic needle aspiration	Direct application to glass slides with or without immediate fixation (check with lab). Alternately, discharge into carrier medium.
Transthoracic needle biopsy	Remove specimen from forceps with sterile needle. Place directly into culture medium or fixative (10% fixative).
Open (wedge) biopsy	Always with clinicoradiological and surgical consultation. Fresh biopsy sent to pathology for intraoperative consultation. Pathologist or surgeon may take sample for cultures. Touch imprints are useful for direct visualization of organisms. Agitation of specimen in fixative solution or injection helps reduce compression artifacts.

specimen. If the biopsy must be transferred (nonsterile) from one container of solution to another before processing in the histology laboratory, a disposable polystyrene plastic pipette is used, cut off to produce a large-bore opening. With this method, the biopsy is aspirated and discharged without the potential for crushing. For microbiological evaluation, biopsies should be transferred directly into carrying medium (obtained in advance from the laboratory), using sterile technique. As discussed elsewhere in this text, the number of biopsies required for accurate assessment may depend somewhat on the potential diseases being considered. Nevertheless, more is always better from the perspective of pathological diagnosis, given that all endoscopic biopsies represent limited sampling by their nature.

Transbronchial Biopsy

Diseases involving the alveolar parenchyma can be sampled by transbronchial biopsy. The Machida crocodile forceps (as well as cup forceps instruments) produce quite reasonable samples of lung parenchyma using the transbronchial biopsy method. Here, the forceps is positioned closed in a distal airway, retracted slightly, and then advanced into the peripheral lung with the jaws open, forcing the bronchiolar wall and peribronchiolar lung parenchyma into the mouth of the device before it is closed. Closing the forceps at end-exhalation may facilitate this. The biopsy specimens appear ''fluffy,'' with delicately ragged edges. These should be handled as described above for the endobronchial biopsy.

Bronchial Brushings

Like the endobronchial biopsy, bronchial brushings and washings are best for sampling disease processes intrinsic to the larger airways and endobronchial tumors. A fine, bristled conical brush is used to sample mucosal lesions. The brush is rubbed against the airway surface to collect cells forcibly into the bristles. Once removed from the patient, the brush may be smeared directly onto slides, which are then fixed immediately by immersion in 95% ethanol for staining with the Papanicolaou method. If the Wright-Giemsa method is preferred by the cytology department, then the slides can be allowed to air-dry. It is important to check with the lab. Cytopathologists trained in one modality of preparation (e.g., alcohol-fixed) may be uncomfortable with the other (e.g., air-dried), since each produces special artifacts. An alternative is to place the brush into a small vial of saline, followed by vigorous agitation. With this technique, cells are released into the saline and can be processed by a variety of means before or after fixation, including Millipore filtration and cytocentrifuge application directly onto slides.

Bronchial Washings and Bronchoalveolar Lavage

These two techniques are useful for sampling cells from a larger area of lung than is achieved by brushing or biopsy. The bronchial wash consists of local airway secretions and saline used during the bronchoscopy procedure that are aspirated to obtain a sample of locally shed or dislodged cells. The bronchoalveolar lavage (BAL) permits the study of cells associated with the most peripheral airways and alveoli. The lavage procedure is performed by instilling multiple aliquots of relatively large volumes of sterile saline (20–50 mL) with the flexible bronchoscope wedged into a segmental airway. The instilled fluid is allowed a variable dwell time and is then aspirated or allowed to flow by gravity into syringe or flask, respectively. Normal BAL fluid contains primarily macrophages and a few inflammatory cells. Noncellular elements include surfactant, mucus, and small quantities of serum proteins, including albumin, immunoglobulins, and enzymes. The clinical utility of BAL in interstitial lung disease is somewhat controversial; as a research tool, it is extremely valuable as a method to obtain alveolar material. Clinically, BAL is most widely used for the diagnosis of pulmonary infection, particularly in the immuno-compromised host.

Once BAL fluid is retrieved, decisions must be made regarding processing. For example, in a patient with a complex inflammatory disease picture, a lavage might require a differential cell count on a centrifuged sediment specimen (fresh by the operator or the lab), chemical analysis (fresh to the lab), microbiological cultures (fresh to the lab), and complete cytological analysis (fresh preferred; refrigerate if processing must be delayed), electron microscopy (fixation in equal amount of 3% glutaraldehyde), and flow cytometric analysis (fresh to the lab). Some cytology laboratories prefer fixed bronchial wash specimens using an equal volume of either Saccomanno's fixative (2% carbowax in 50% ethyl alcohol) or 50% (sometimes 70%) ethyl alcohol.

Transbronchial Needle Aspiration

This technique, popularized by Wang and colleagues in 1978 for the diagnosis of right paratracheal tumors, has gained wider utility in the diagnosis and staging of lung cancer. The aspiration is intended to yield a small quantity of homogenized cellular material (approximately the needle volume). The syringe attached to the needle may be filled with 1–2 mL of sterile saline or used dry. If saline is used, the combined saline and aspirated material is flushed directly into 95% ethyl alcohol or sent directly to the cytology department for processing. If a dry syringe is used, once the needle and syringe have been removed from the bronchoscope, the needle is removed, air is drawn into the syringe barrel, the needle (with specimen inside) is replaced on the syringe, and the air is jetted through the needle directly onto a glass microscope slide. The jetted material can be immersion-fixed immediately as is or smeared out (with a technique similar to making blood films on slides) and then immediately immersed in 95% ethyl alcohol.

SPECIMENS FROM TRANSTHORACIC NEEDLE BIOPSY AND ASPIRATION

Thoracentesis

It is important to check with the laboratory that will be performing the fluid analysis before beginning the procedure, since many have specific handling protocols for body fluids. Because a number of specific types of analysis will be performed on a typical pleural fluid, the fresh, unfixed specimen is split for processing. After normal laboratory business hours, the collected fluid can be placed in a specimen refrigerator without fixative for processing the next day. Aliquots are distributed in the laboratory for chemical analysis (e.g., glucose, LDH, amylase), evaluation of constituent inflammatory cells, microbiological studies as appropriate, and cytological evaluation for malignancy.

For cytological evaluation, a large, fresh, unfixed aliquot is optimal (more than 50 mL is preferred in order to achieve sufficient numbers of cells). Refrigerated storage for 24 h has minimal effect on the constituent cells when infection is of low probability. If the fluid is infected, bacterial by-products may lead to cellular damage with prolonged unfixed storage. If a specimen must be fixed, an equal volume of at least 50% ethyl alcohol (the exact concentration is not critical) can be added to the fluid (for cytological evaluation only). In the cytology laboratory, an air-dried or fixed smear from a small aliquot of centrifuged sediment can be stained and directly visualized for selection of the best preparation strategy.

Closed Pleural Biopsy

Inflammatory, infectious, and neoplastic diseases of the pleura can be diagnosed by pleural biopsy. The three most commonly used pleural needle biopsy devices (Cope, Abrams, and Tru-Cut) all produce very small tissue specimens. These biopsies should be handled just like the bronchoscopic and transbronchial biopsy specimens.

Transthoracic Fine-Needle Aspiration and Biopsy of the Lung

Diagnosis by transthoracic needle aspiration was first performed over a century ago, but recent advances in needle technology have permitted widespread, safe use of this technique for the diagnosis of neoplasms and infections in the lung. The procedure is always performed under radiographic guidance and samples are similar in amount to those achieved by transbronchial needle aspiration. It has become common practice to have assistance from a cytotechnologist or pathologist, who makes immediate slide preparations for evaluating specimen adequacy. Such assistance can reduce patient callbacks and rescheduling problems but requires coordination with the cytopathology laboratory. Recent variations on this procedure include the Rotax needle biopsy device, which produces a fine spiral core of tissue (especially useful in lung tissue) and the Biopty gun device, which has a side cutting port for retrieving a fine core of tissue. Since these techniques may produce solid tissue cores, these specimens should be either sent fresh to the laboratory for microbiological studies and/or fixed in 10% neutral buffered formalin for routine histological processing. Transthoracic cutting needle or drill biopsies are not commonly used in North America.

SPECIMENS FROM THORACOSCOPY AND THORACOTOMY

The most common lung specimen received from surgical procedures in which the chest is opened in limited fashion is the wedge biopsy of lung. The open-lung biopsy is useful for the evaluation of a wide variety of diseases in the lung, ranging from infection (e.g., *Coccidioides*) to autoimmune disease (e.g., Wegener's granulomatosis) to neoplasm (e.g., bronchogenic carcinoma). The selection of method for this procedure depends on a number of factors, including operator preference, experience, and equipment availability. The video-assisted thoracoscopic (VATS) method has gained in popularity recently, presumably based on speed of patient recovery. Proponents of the VATS biopsy claim shorter hospital stays and decreased morbidity as compared with open thoracotomy biopsy, but we are unaware of any randomized prospective trial data to support this opinion unequivocally. In our experience, the differences between limited thoracotomy and VATS biopsy procedures are more related to cost (higher for VATS) and specimen quality (slightly more artifacts for VATS). We do find that access to widely separated lung segments is actually better using the thoracoscope, and access to targeted segments, in general, is better with this technique. On this same theme of targeted segments, for the open lung biopsy to be useful in the evaluation of inflammatory lung disease, it is essential for the radiologist, chest physician, and thoracic surgeon to communicate with each other. Random biopsy for disease restricted to a specific anatomic location by radiographs may be nondiagnostic. In the best scenario, the surgeon combines his or her best surgical judgment with any specific characteristics of the disease in question in selecting areas for biopsy. For example, patients with usual interstitial pneumonia (UIP) may have dramatic fibrosis with honeycombing at the bases peripherally, but an additional, less involved area, will make the diagnosis more definitive.

The biopsy is performed at the lung periphery adjacent to a fissure, using a linear stapling and cutting device with 3.5-mm staples. All lung segments can be reached using thoracoscopic techniques. For microbiological studies, the specimen should be sampled with sterile technique and a portion thereof (or additional piece) can be sent directly to the microbiology laboratory. In some institutions, all of the specimens are sent directly to the pathologist after removal, and sterile samples are taken during processing for frozen-section analysis. The specimen should be handled carefully during all prefixation procedures such as microbiological sampling and frozen section, since the unfixed lung can be distorted and compressed, producing undesirable artifacts.

Once a sample has been fixed and processed, it is too late to make cytological preparations. Cytological smears and touch imprints are very useful for immediate special stains for organisms and the evaluation of lymphoproliferative disease. They are easy to perform, can be fixed or air-dried, and can be discarded later if they are not required.

Intraoperative frozen-section analysis of lung tissue is a useful routine, even if only to guide specimen processing. Freezing air-filled lung tissue poses special problems. First, the unfixed tissue is easily compressed, especially after it has been sliced into a 3- to 5-mm slab for freezing. Compression results in artifactual atelectasis and can make interpretation difficult. To avoid this, the pathologist may choose to use a 22- to 25-gauge needle on a 5-mL syringe filled with saline or a dilute solution of saline and embedding compound, which is gently injected into the sectioned portion of the biopsy to be frozen. Even at 3- to 5-mm thickness, the alveolar parenchyma will fill with fluid and, upon freezing, provide a stable matrix for producing thin sections for intraoperative microscopic evaluation.

Once intraoperative consultation has been completed, the remaining specimen should be fixed in 10% neutral buffered formalin (or another fixative of choice). To do this, several methods have been recommended. First, vigorously shaking the specimen in a container of fixative works well but may not decompress areas of atelectasis. Second, a small volume of carbonated water can be added to the fixative to assist in reexpansion. Finally, some pathologists prefer to inflate their samples with fixative using a needle and syringe. To do this, a small needle (22–25 gauge), small syringe (5 mL), and very gentle pressure should be used. The needle is inserted through the pleura at several locations with the specimen floating in a container of fixative. The specimen is well perfused when the lung floats at the fixative surface rather than above it (it usually will not sink completely). After a few hours of additional immersion, the biopsy can be sectioned easily and safely at 5-mm intervals for histological processing.

In conclusion, communication between pulmonologist, radiologist, surgeon, and pathologist enhances all facets of lung tissue sampling. The certainty and accuracy of diagnosis for any of the techniques presented here can only be improved by this multidisciplinary approach.

SUGGESTED READING

Transbronchial Biopsy

1. Anderson H. Transbronchial lung biopsy for diffuse pulmonary diseases: results in 939 patients. Chest 1978; 73:734–736.
2. Cazzadori A, Di Perri G, Todeschini G, Luzzati R, Boschiero L, Perona G, Concia E. Transbronchial biopsy in the diagnosis of pulmonary infiltrates in immunocompromised patients. Chest 1995; 107:101.
3. Kvale PA. Bronchoscopic biopsies and bronchoalveolar lavage. Chest Surg Clin North Am 1996; 6:205.
4. Katzenstein A-LA, Askin FB. Interpretation and significance of pathologic findings in transbronchial lung biopsy. Am J Surg Pathol 1980; 4:223–234.
5. Phillips MJ, Knight RK, Green M. Fiberoptic bronchoscopy and diagnosis of pulmonary lesions in lymphoma and leukemia. Thorax 1980; 35:19–25.
6. Prakash UBS, Offord KP, Stubbs SE. Bronchoscopy in North America: the ACCP Survey. Chest 1991; 100:1668–1675.
7. Shure D. Transbronchial biopsy and needle aspiration. Chest 1989; 95:1130.
8. Wall CP, Gaensler EA, Carrington CB, Hayes JA. Comparison of transbronchial and open lung biopsies in chronic infiltrative lung diseases. Am Rev Respir Dis 1981; 123:280–285.

Biopsy—Thoracoscopic and Open

1. Brody A, Craighead J. Preparation of human lung biopsy specimens by perfusion-fixation. Am Rev Respir Dis 1975; 112:645.
2. Churg A. An inflation procedure for open lung biopsies. Am J Surg Pathol 1983; 7:69–71.
3. Churg A. Lung biopsy: handling and diagnostic limitations. In: Thurlbeck WM, ed. Pathology of the Lung. Stuttgart: Thieme, 1988:67–78.
4. Ferguson MK. Thoracoscopy for diagnosis of diffuse lung disease. Ann Thorac Surg 1993; 56:694.
5. Gaensler EA, Carrington CB. Open lung biopsy for chronic diffuse infiltrative lung disease: clinical, roentgenographic and physiological correlations in 502 patients. Ann Thorac Surg 1980; 30:411–426.
6. Hazelrigg SR, Nunchuck SK, Landreneau RJ, Mack MJ, Naunheim KS, Seifert PE, Auer JE. Cost analysis for thoracoscopy: thoracoscopic wedge resection. Ann Thorac Surg 1993; 56: 633.
7. Jaffee JP, Maki DG. Lung biopsy in immunocompromised patients: one institution's experience and an approach to management of pulmonary disease in the compromised host. Cancer (Philadelphia) 1981; 48:1144–1153.
8. Kadokura M, Colby TV, Myers JL, Allen MS, Deschamps C, Trastek VF, Pairolero PC. Pathologic comparison of video-assisted thoracic surgical lung biopsy with traditional open lung biopsy. J Thorac Cardiovasc Surg 1995; 109:494.
9. McKenna RJ, Jr, Mountain CF, McMurtry MJ. Open lung biopsy in immunocompromised patients. Chest 1984; 86:671–674.
10. Miller RR, Nelems B, Muller NL, Evans KG, Ostrow DN. Lingular and right middle lobe biopsy in the assessment of diffuse lung disease. Ann Thorac Surg 1987; 44:269–272.
11. Molin LJ, Steinberg JB, Lanza LA. VATS increases costs in patients undergoing lung biopsy for interstitial lung disease. Ann Thorac Surg 1994; 58:1595.
12. Ray JF III, Lawton BR, Myers WO, Toyama WM, Reyes CN, Emanuel DA, Burns JL, Pederson DP, Dovenbarger WV, Wenzl FJ, Sautter RD. Open pulmonary biopsy: 19 years experience with 416 consecutive operations. Chest 1976; 69:43–47.
13. Shah RM, Spirn PW, Salazar AM, Steiner RM, Cohn HE, Wechsler RJ. Role of thoracoscopy and preoperative localization procedures in the diagnosis and management of pulmonary pathology. Semin Ultrasound CT MR 1995; 16:371.
14. Toledo-Pereyra LH, DeMeester TR, Kinealey A, MacMahon H, Churg A, Golomb H. The benefits of open lung biopsy in patients with previous nondiagnostic transbronchial lung biopsy: a guide to appropriate therapy. Chest 1980; 77:647–650.
15. Warner D, Warner M, Divertie M. Open lung biopsy in patients with diffuse pulmonary infiltrates and acute respiratory failure. Am Rev Respir Dis 1988; 137:90.

Transbronchial and Percutaneous Needle Aspiration and Biopsy

1. Austin JH, Cohen MB. Value of having a cytopathologist present during percutaneous fine-needle aspiration biopsy of lung: report of 55 cancer patients and metaanalysis of the literature. AJR 1993; 160:175.
2. Berquist T, Bailey P, Cortese D, Miller W. Transthoracic needle biopsy: accuracy and complications in relation to location and type of lesion. Mayo Clin Proc 1980; 55:475.
3. Boiselle PM, Shepard JA, Mark EJ, Szyfelbein WM, Fan CM, Slanetz PJ, Trotman-Dickenson B, Halpern EF, McLoud TC. Routine addition of an automated biopsy device to fine-needle aspiration of the lung: a prospective assessment. AJR 1997; 169:661.
4. Crosby JH, Hager B, Hoeg K. Transthoracic fine-needle aspiration: experience in a cancer center. Cancer 1985; 56:2504.

5. Dijkman JH, Van der Meer JWM, Bakker W, Wever AM, Van der Broek PJ. Transpleural lung biopsy by the thoracoscopic route in patients with diffuse interstitial pulmonary disease. Chest 1982; 82:76.
6. Hsu WH, Chiang CD, Hus JY, Kwan PC, Chen CL, Chen CY. Ultrasound-guided fine-needle aspiration biopsy of lung cancers. J Clin Ultrasound 1996; 24:225.
7. Jeffrey PB. Fine-needle aspiration of the lung. Pathology 1996; 4:439.
8. Mitruka S, Landreneau RJ, Mack MJ, Fetterman LS, Gammie J, Bartley S, Sutherland SR, Bowers CM, Keenan RJ, Ferson PF, et al. Diagnosing the indeterminate pulmonary nodule: percutaneous biopsy versus thoracoscopy. Surgery 1995; 118:676.
9. O'Reilly PE, Brueckner J, Silverman JF. Value of ancillary studies in fine needle aspiration cytology of the lung. Acta Cytol 1994; 38:144.
10. Saleh H, Masood S. Value of ancillary studies in fine-needle aspiration biopsy. Diagn Cytopathol 1995; 13:310.
11. Santambrogio L, Nosotti M, Bellaviti N, Pavoni G, Radice F, Caputo V. CT-guided fine-needle aspiration cytology of solitary pulmonary nodules: a prospective, randomized study of immediate cytologic evaluation. Chest 1997; 112:423.
12. Wang KP, Marsh BR, Summer WR, Perry PB, Erozan YS, Baker RR. Transbronchial aspiration for the diagnosis of lung cancer. Chest 1981; 80:48–50.
13. Weissberg D, Kaufman M. Diagnostic and therapeutic pleuroscopy: experience with 127 patients. Chest 1980; 78:732.
14. Zavala D, Bedell G. Percutaneous lung biopsy with a cutting needle. An analysis of 40 cases and comparison with other biopsy techniques. Am Rev Respir Dis 1972; 106:186.

Lavage

1. Crystal RG, Reynolds HY, Kalica AR. Bronchoalveolar lavage: the report of an international conference. Chest 1986; 90:122.
2. Daniele RP, Elias JA, Epstain PE, Rossman MD. Bronchoalveolar lavage: role in the pathogenesis, diagnosis, and management of interstitial lung disease. Ann Intern Med 1985; 102:93.
3. Martin WJ, 2d, Smith TF, Sanderson DR, Brutinel WM, Cockerill FR 3d, Douglas WW. Role of bronchoalveolar lavage in the assessment of opportunistic pulmonary infections: utility and complications. Mayo Clin Proc 1987; 62:549.
4. Poletti V, Romagna M, Gasponi A, Baruzzi G, Allen KA. Bronchoalveolar lavage in the diagnosis of low-grade, MALT type, B-cell lymphoma in the lung. Monaldi Arch Chest Dis 1995; 50:191.

14
Dyspnea

Donald A. Mahler
Dartmouth Medical School
Dartmouth–Hitchcock Medical Center
Lebanon, New Hampshire

Roberto Mejia
National Institute of Respiratory Diseases
Mexico City, Mexico

INTRODUCTION

Breathing difficulty is a common medical problem. The initial part of this chapter considers the related questions "What is dyspnea?" and "What causes dyspnea?" The three types of dyspnea based on the temporal features (acute onset, development with specific body positions, and chronic nature) are described. Guidelines are presented to help the health care provider apply information obtained from the medical history and physical examination so as to select appropriate tests to diagnose the cause of dyspnea. Diagnostic testing directed at the most likely cause of dyspnea is recommended, rather than a "shotgun" approach.

Once a diagnosis has been made, therapy should be directed toward the underlying pathophysiology in an effort to relieve or at least reduce the severity and distress of breathlessness. Specific treatments for the major respiratory diseases are recommended in various chapters of this book. However, if dyspnea remains a problem for the individual patient, additional strategies are available. These include physical (exercise reconditioning and inspiratory muscle training), psychological (cognitive-behavioral strategies), pharmacological (anxiolytics and opiates), and surgical (bullectomy and lung volume reduction surgery) modalities that can and hopefully will provide some relief of breathlessness.

WHAT IS DYSPNEA? WHAT CAUSES DYSPNEA?

Dyspnea, or breathlessness, is a subjective experience of breathing difficulty. Before the individual with dyspnea decides to seek medical attention, he or she must first recognize that the experience originates in the respiratory system (as a sensation) and then must perceive the sensation as being abnormal (as a symptom). Often, the person mistakenly sees exertional breathlessness as a result of "getting older" or "being out of shape." This may, unfortunately, delay a diagnosis and thereby limit potential therapeutic benefit.

Table 1 Descriptors of Breathlessness by Cluster and Disease Conditions

Cluster	COPD n = 56	Asthma n = 56	ILD n = 37	CHF n = 17	CF n = 9	DECOND n = 8	NM n = 6
Work/effort	X	X	X	X	X	X	X
Suffocating				X			
Exhalation		X			X		
Tight		X		X			X
Inhalation							
Shallow						X	X
Rapid			X			X	
Breathing more						X	
Heavy					X		
Air hunger							

Abbreviations: COPD, chronic obstructive pulmonary disease; ILD, interstitial lung disease; CHF, congestive heart failure; CF, cystic fibrosis; DECOND, deconditioning; NM, neuromuscular disease.

Specific clusters represent one or more of the three most common descriptors selected by patients with a particular diagnosis to describe their "uncomfortable awareness of breathing." Most, but not all, patients reported the descriptors that were used to derive the clusters. "Suffocating," "shallow," and "air hunger" were not selected frequently enough by patients with any of the seven diseases and probably represent experiences in other conditions or situations.

Source: Reproduced from Mahler DA, Harver A, Lentine T, et al. Descriptors of breathlessness in cardiorespiratory disease. Am J Respir Crit Care Med 1996; 154:1361.

When questioned carefully, patients with different cardiorespiratory disorders frequently describe distinct qualities of breathing difficulty (Table 1). As each of the seven diagnoses was associated with a unique set of descriptors, it is likely that these different experiences relate to the pathophysiology of the specific condition. For example, patients with chronic obstructive pulmonary disease (COPD) typically reported that ''My breathing requires effort,'' and ''It is hard to breathe.'' When patients with COPD perform even trivial physical tasks, they develop dynamic hyperinflation (i.e., they breathe at a higher lung volume) in order to increase expiratory airflow. One consequence of hyperinflation is an increase in the elastic recoil of the lung. This adaptation places an added load on the diaphragm, which is also functionally weakened due to shortening of the vertical muscle fibers. These alterations presumably contribute to the ''work and effort'' of the respiratory muscles during physical activities in patients with COPD. The cluster ''work/effort'' characterized all seven diseases reported in Table 1. This finding, along with the observation that patients identified that dyspnea was experienced more frequently during inspiration rather than during expiration, supports the concept that respiratory muscles are important in the experience of dyspnea.

Those with asthma frequently report that ''My chest feels tight,'' in addition to the work/effort of breathing. The tight feeling is most likely due to activation of receptors in large airways during acute bronchoconstriction. Cystic fibrosis, another disease in which acute airway constriction may occur, was the only other condition associated with chest tightness. Patients with interstitial lung disease (ILD) indicated that rapid breathing characterized their breathlessness; this is consistent with the expected pattern of breathing resulting from an increased elastic load due to the diffuse infiltrative process. Patients with neuromuscular disease noted that the terms *rapid* and *inhalation* characterized their sensation of breathlessness in addition to *work/effort*. These descriptions are likely the result of respiratory muscle weakness, as inspiration requires the active contraction of the diaphragm and other inspiratory muscles, whereas expiration is passive, owing to the elastic recoil of the lung. The descriptors *suffocating, shallow*, and *air hunger* were not selected frequently enough by patients with any of the seven diagnoses studied and therefore probably represent breathlessness experienced in other conditions or situations. These examples illustrate that the physician should inquire about the qualities of a patient's breathlessness, as such information may enable him or her to identify the ''most likely'' cause of dyspnea.

In addition, many patients with respiratory disease experience hypoxemia and/or hypercapnia. These alterations in arterial blood gases can stimulate peripheral and central chemoreceptors, respectively, and thereby increase ventilation. This enhanced ''drive to breathe'' is commonly associated with the sense of breathlessness. Similarly, metabolic acidosis, which develops during high-intensity exercise, is a stimulus of the central chemoreceptor area in the medulla, which contributes to exercise hyperpnea; this may be perceived as unpleasant breathing by some healthy individuals.

TYPES OF DYSPNEA

One approach to classify dyspnea is to consider the temporal features. *Acute dyspnea* is the immediate or sudden onset of breathing difficulty. *Positional dyspnea* refers to the development of breathlessness in a specific body position. *Chronic dyspnea* can be defined by the presence of breathlessness for at least 1 month. Although certain conditions can have both acute and chronic presentations, such as asthma or pulmonary embolism, the

Table 2   Characteristics of Dyspnea to Be
Considered

Onset
Descriptive qualities
Frequency
Intensity
Duration
Triggers
Provoking activities
Associated respiratory symptoms
   (cough, sputum, wheezing, orthopnea,
   paroxysmal nocturnal dyspnea, chest pain)
Strategies or actions that provide relief

classification of dyspnea based on the onset and/or duration can provide a framework within which clinicians can consider certain diseases and prioritize diagnostic testing. Various characteristics of dyspnea should be considered regardless of the type (Table 2).

ACUTE DYSPNEA

The acute onset of breathlessness, immediate or within hours, is usually an urgent or emergent medical problem that requires prompt evaluation and treatment. It may represent the major manifestation of a life-threatening illness or injury that can be accompanied by a ''feeling of impending doom.'' Generally, there are only a limited number of conditions that cause acute dyspnea (Table 3). Congestive heart failure (26%), asthma (25%), and COPD (15%) accounted for the three leading causes of acute dyspnea in the emergency department of one community hospital.

There are several important *initial* questions that the physician can ask the patient who has a sudden onset of breathlessness.

When did your breathing difficulty start? Most patients are able to provide a specific
time or duration.
What were you doing at the onset of dyspnea? A recent insect bite or sting, exposure
to an aeroallergen or airborne irritant, ingestion of foods or medication, etc.,
may cause laryngeal edema or bronchospasm. An injury or accident can lead
to upper airway or chest trauma. Prolonged travel, recent hospitalization, or
immobilization can predispose to thrombophlebitis and pulmonary embolism.
Do you have any medical illnesses? As examples, a history of asthma may suggest
acute bronchospasm or an allergic reaction; a history of COPD or cystic fibrosis may relate to an acute exacerbation of the underlying disease and may also
be a risk factor for a pneumothorax; difficulty breathing after eating raises
concern about food aspiration into the upper airway or proximal tracheobronchial tree; and a history of psychiatric illness or recent emotional stress might
suggest possible hyperventilation syndrome.
Are you having chest pain? If so, where is it located? Substernal chest pain/heavi-
ness is commonly observed in patients who have ischemic heart disease or

Table 3 Causes of Acute Dyspnea

Cause	Types of Chest Pain	Major Physical Findings
Airway obstruction		
Upper airway		Inspiratory stridor, especially over the neck
Bronchoconstriction	"Tightness"	Expiratory wheezing, prolonged expiratory phase
Alveolar hemorrhage		Inspiratory crackles
Hyperventilation	"Discomfort"	Normal chest exam
Inhalation injury		Site of injury depends on water solubility of toxin and intensity of exposure
Pneumonia	Lateral chest if parietal pleura involved	Unilateral inspiratory crackles, ? consolidation
Pneumothorax	Upper chest	↓ Intensity of breath sounds, possible shift of trachea
Pulmonary edema	Substernal, sharp	
Cardiac		Diffuse bilateral crackles, S3
Noncardiac		Diffuse bilateral crackles
Pulmonary embolism	Lateral chest	Variable
Trauma	At site of injury	Chest wall tenderness, ↓ intensity of breath sounds

have experienced a myocardial infarction. Chest "tightness" is frequently reported by patients with acute bronchoconstriction due to either asthma or cystic fibrosis. Pain in the upper chest area may occur with spontaneous pneumothorax, while pain in the lateral chest is more likely due to trauma, pneumonia, or pulmonary embolism. Chest "discomfort" may occur with the hyperventilation syndrome.

The responses to these initial questions should enable the physician to narrow the differential diagnosis to one or two probable causes for acute dyspnea. The physical examination may or may not provide confirmation of the presumptive diagnosis. *A 12-lead electrocardiogram (ECG), a chest radiograph (CXR), and oximetry should probably be obtained as initial tests in most if not all patients with acute dyspnea.* The purpose of the ECG is to detect an arrhythmia or to demonstrate ischemia. A chest radiograph may show hyperinflation (consistent with obstructive airway disease), pulmonary infiltrates (due to alveolar hemorrhage, pneumonia, or pulmonary embolism), pneumothorax, pulmonary edema, or evidence of chest trauma. Oximetry will provide a quick estimate of oxygenation and overall severity of disease. A normal or increased oxygen saturation should suggest acute hyperventilation syndrome.

An astute clinician must understand the different possible diseases in order to decide which patient will require more specialized diagnostic testing.

POSITIONAL DYSPNEA

The effect of body position on the experience of dyspnea is more common than health care providers generally appreciate. It is important to ask patients whether lying down (orthopnea), lying on one side (trepopnea), or sitting upright (platypnea) causes or increases breathlessness. If so, postural changes most likely alter lung mechanics and/or gas exchange and thereby contribute to dyspnea.

Orthopnea (dyspnea in the supine position) is the most common type of positional dyspnea. Although there are numerous causes or orthopnea (Table 4), congestive heart failure (CHF) and COPD are the two most frequent etiologies. In patients with left ventricular dysfunction, redistribution of fluid from the lower extremities can increase central blood volume, which may present an excessive preload on the left ventricle; this can elevate left ventricular end-diastolic pressure and pulmonary capillary hydrostatic pressures, leading to edema. Typically, orthopnea develops within minutes to hours after a patient with CHF lies supine, depending on the severity of left ventricular dysfunction.

In patients with COPD, the mechanical changes that occur normally in the supine position (the positive pressure in the abdomen "pushes up" the diaphragm and there is a decrease in lung volume) may compromise diaphragmatic function and increase ventilatory work. For those who have reduced respiratory muscle function, these alterations may cause breathlessness. Hypoxemia may also develop in the supine position and contribute to dyspnea. By sitting upright, the individual can reduce the abdominal "load" and utilize gravity to assist in diaphragm function.

Other less common causes of orthopnea include neuromuscular disease with weakness of the respiratory muscles, conditions of abdominal "loading" (e.g., obesity, pregnancy, and ascites), and compression of the tracheobronchial tree (e.g., anterior mediastinal mass and thoracic aortic aneurysm).

Trepopnea (dyspnea in one lateral position but not in the other) is usually due to unilateral chest disease, such as pneumonia, pleural effusions, or obstruction of the proximal airway. The most likely mechanism is positional mismatching of ventilation to perfusion leading to hypoxemia.

Platypnea (dyspnea in the upright position relieved by lying supine) is an unusual complaint (Table 4). Orthodeoxia (arterial oxygen desaturation in the upright position and improved by recumbency) typically occurs in association with platypnea. Although differ-

Table 4   Causes of Positional Dyspnea

Orthopnea (dyspnea in the supine position)
   Left ventricular failure
   Pericarditis
   Obstructive airway disease
   Respiratory muscle weakness/dysfunction
   Obesity
   Pregnancy
   Ascites
   Anterior mediastinal mass
   Thoracic aortic aneurysm
   Tracheomalacia
Platypnea (dyspnea in the upright position and relieved by lying supine)
   Intracardiac shunts (e.g., atrial septal defect)
   Vascular lung shunts
      Congenital (e.g., pulmonary arteriovenous malformations)
      Acquired (e.g., vascular dilatations in cirrhosis)
   Parenchymal lung shunts

ent mechanisms may contribute to platypnea-orthodeoxia, a right-to-left shunt in the heart and vascular lung shunts are the common causes. A right-to-left shunt across a persistent foramen ovale has been observed in some patients after pneumonectomy. Platypnea can develop more than 1 month after resection. As the incidence of a patent foramen ovale is 15–20% in the general population and the incidence of bronchogenic carcinoma has been increasing, platypnea-orthodeoxia may likely also increase after a pneumonectomy for resection of lung cancer.

The diagnosis of positional dyspnea requires a complete medical history and physical examination. A 12-lead ECG, CXR, oximetry, *and spirometry* are appropriate screening tests. *When are additional tests indicated?* For orthopnea, respiratory muscle weakness should be considered when the most common causes of orthopnea, CHF and COPD, are not evident. Spirometry may show a restrictive pattern with reduced values for forced vital capacity (FVC) and forced expiratory volume in 1 s (FEV$_1$) but a normal FEV$_1$/FVC ratio. To diagnose respiratory muscle weakness, inspiratory (PI$_{max}$) and expiratory (PE$_{max}$) mouth pressures should be obtained. The other causes of orthopnea (see Table 4) are usually evident on examination and/or chest radiograph. For platypnea, an unusual complaint, the physician must accept the symptom "as real." An initial evaluation should be oximetry measured in the upright and supine positions. The finding of desaturation in the upright position compared with the supine position, which is opposite to the expected normal change, indicates orthodeoxia. Additional diagnostic testing is then indicated based on concomitant findings. If an intracardiac shunt is suspected, tilt-table contrast two-dimensional echocardiography is indicated. If pulmonary arteriovenous malformations are suspected, dynamic computed tomography should be ordered.

CHRONIC DYSPNEA

In one study of 85 patients seen in a pulmonary outpatient clinic with a chief complaint of breathlessness, four disorders—asthma, COPD, interstitial lung disease, and cardiac disease—accounted for two-thirds of the cases. In another study of 72 patients referred for "unexplained dyspnea," the primary causes were pulmonary disease (36%), hyperventilation (19%), and cardiac disease (14%). From these experiences it is apparent that most but not all patients with chronic disease, or disease present for at least 1 month, will have a recognizable cause and that the disease spectrum is broad.

A comprehensive history is the starting point to evaluate the problem of chronic dyspnea. It is imperative to differentiate whether "an awareness of breathing" is normal and appropriate, particularly with vigorous activities, or whether "unpleasant or labored" breathing is a manifestation of an illness. This consideration should include the patient's age, comparison with peers, daily or usual activities, overall fitness, and any other medical problem. The physician should inquire about various characteristics of dyspnea (Table 2). As patients usually reduce activities to minimize breathing difficulty, it is important, in order to assess the impact of the individual's dyspnea on his or her functional status, to ask the patient "What are your daily activities?" and "What activities have you stopped doing?" Additional information about social history (cigarette smoking, occupation, current or previous inhalational exposures, hobbies, etc.) is essential.

The physical examination should include the neck, thorax, lungs, heart, and extremities. Selected abnormal findings are described in the respective chapters on specific diseases.

Using information obtained from the medical history and physical examination, the physician should be able to categorize the possible etiologies for chronic dyspnea into suspected cardiac disease, suspected respiratory disease, or unexplained (i.e., no real clues as to the cause) chronic dyspnea. For example, any two of the following is highly predictive of airflow limitation: 70 or more pack-years of cigarette smoking, decreased breath sounds, or history of COPD. The cognitive process whereby the physician integrates available data is based on knowledge and experience. The purpose of developing a ''working hypothesis'' to identify the probable cause of dyspnea is to focus diagnostic testing rather than using a ''shotgun'' approach. More specific approaches for suspected cardiac and respiratory diseases are covered in other sections of this volume.

If the cause of dyspnea *remains unclear* after the history and physical examination, then spirometry and diffusing capacity, a CXR, a resting 12-lead ECG, and oximetry are recommended as initial screening tests. A low diffusing capacity with all other screening tests being normal raises the possibility of anemia or pulmonary vascular disease. A complete blood count should then be obtained to measure the hemoglobin level. An echocardiogram is a good initial test to investigate for pulmonary hypertension. If the results of these tests are normal (i.e., the cause of the patient's dyspnea is not obvious based on the screening tests), then anxiety/hyperventilation, deconditioning, and mild respiratory muscle weakness are the likely etiologies. Next, PI_{max} and PE_{max} should be measured to evaluate for respiratory muscle weakness. If respiratory muscle strength is normal, then a cardiopulmonary exercise test (CPEX) should be performed. The purpose of the CPEX is to simulate the patient's experience of breathlessness and to identify psychogenic dyspnea or deconditioning. Psychogenic dyspnea can be confirmed by inconsistent and fluctuating levels of ventilation during exercise, an irregular pattern of breathing, and elevated levels of ventilation relative to metabolism. Deconditioning can be diagnosed by a decreased maximal oxygen consumption but normal cardiorespiratory exercise responses.

Patients who experience dyspnea due to a chronic respiratory condition generally report an increase in the severity over time. Although the person may assume that greater breathlessness is due to progression of disease, it is important for the physician to repeat physiological testing, including oximetry or arterial blood gases, in order to determine whether there has been a measurable deterioration in lung function. If there has been little or no change in pulmonary function tests, then deconditioning and/or weight gain are likely explanations for progressive dyspnea.

TREATMENT STRATEGIES

1.   Treat the underlying disease. The first objective in relieving dyspnea is to treat the underlying disease. Specific therapy directed at the pathophysiology of the condition is described in the various chapters of this book.

2.   Assess for oxygen therapy. Once optimal medical therapy has been provided and the patient remains breathless, the physician should evaluate whether the patient might benefit from supplemental oxygen. Specific criteria have been established for prescription of supplemental oxygen (see Chap. 22). Selected patients may benefit from oxygen therapy for relief of dyspnea even when an arterial oxygen tension is $\geq$ 60 mmHg. An objective method should be used to evaluate the use of oxygen in such individuals. One approach is to measure exercise endurance and the intensity of dyspnea during submaximal treadmill walking while breathing supplemental oxygen and again while breathing room air at the

same flow rate with the patient "blinded" to the therapy. An improvement in exercise capacity and a corresponding reduction in the severity of dyspnea indicate a benefit. Presumably, supplemental oxygen would diminish stimulation of the peripheral chemoreceptor and thus decrease the chemical "drive to breathe."

   3.   Upper and lower extremity exercise training. Most patients with chronic dyspnea are severely deconditioned due to the downward spiral of dyspnea → sedentary lifestyle → deconditioning. Therefore, many of these patients will benefit from a structured exercise training program. Specific guidelines for comprehensive pulmonary rehabilitation are provided in Chap. 27.

   Several randomizd controlled studies have demonstrated that patients with COPD can perform higher levels of work with a reduced sensation of breathing difficulty after exercise training. Improvements in dyspnea after a reconditioning program have been attributed to concomitant increases in expiratory airflow or respiratory muscle strength, a reduction in the ventilatory demand as mediated by physiological training responses or enhanced mechanical efficiency, and a tolerance of or desensitization to dyspnea.

Inspiratory Muscle Training

Respiratory muscle weakness may develop as part of the general deconditioning process that occurs with reduced physical activities in many patients with a chronic respiratory disease. The rationale for inspiratory muscle training is that increasing the strength and/or endurance of the diaphragm as well as other respiratory muscles may contribute to reduced breathlessness.

   Measurement of PI_{max} and PE_{max} (see Chap. 9) is the first step to assess whether there is respiratory muscle weakness. If so, inspiratory resistance training using an inspiratory threshold loading device may be prescribed at an initial intensity of 30–40% of PI_{max} for 30 min per day with a respiratory frequency of 12 to 15 breaths per minute. As with any training program, a minimum of 4–6 weeks may be required to observe a training response. Several randomized controlled trials have demonstrated increases in respiratory muscle strength and corresponding reductions in dyspnea in patients with COPD *when* inspiratory flow or pressure has been controlled and *when* appropriate instruments have been used to measure breathlessness. Some pulmonary rehabilitation programs incorporate inspiratory muscle training in addition to upper and lower extremity exercises.

Cognitive-Behavioral Strategies

Although coping and behavioral interventions to relieve dyspnea are frequently incorporated as part of a comprehensive pulmonary rehabilitation program, these approaches may be taught and used separately. Usually, a nurse or respiratory therapist discusses these strategies as part of an educational session and then encourages application during exercise training or at another time when the patient experiences breathlessness. Distraction strategies involve willful dissociation from a noxious physical sensation or from one's own reaction to it; active dissociation can increase physical tolerance and attenuate both physiological arousal and psychological distress. Distraction techniques include relaxation, biofeedback, music, hypnosis, guided imagery, and self-talk.

   Attention strategies may be more appropriate and helpful for patients with long-term or chronic breathlessness. Because dyspnea can be a constant problem for some patients, it may be necessary for these individuals to focus or concentrate on their breathing rather than try to dissociate from the symptom. By recording the intensity and timing of dyspnea, the patient may recognize certain ''triggers'' or patterns that may be avoided. Self-care includes having a specific plan to deal with severe breathlessness, such as ''breathing stations,'' pacing certain activities, pursed-lips breathing, appropriate use of metered-dose inhalers, etc. Another attention technique involves graduated levels of dyspnea (i.e., gradual increases in breathing difficulty, as might be experienced with exercise or inspiratory muscle training) in an attempt to desensitize the individual to the severity of breathing distress.

Surgical Options

Patients, usually with COPD, may develop large bulla(e) that can compress adjacent lung tissue. In many of these patients, the severity of dyspnea may be disproportionate to the degree of airflow obstruction. A bulla may cause anatomic (chest wall and diaphragm) and physiological (altered mechanics of breathing and hypoxemia) changes. Selection criteria for surgical resection include a bulla that occupies at least one-third of the hemithorax and radiographic evidence by computed tomography of compression of adjacent parenchyma. Resection (preferably by a thorascopic approach) would be expected to allow compressed lung to expand and to reduce the effects of hyperventilation by allowing the diaphragm to assume a more normal position.

Several observational and some controlled studies have reported that lung volume reduction surgery (resection of ~20% of emphysematous lung tissue typically in the apices) improves lung function and reduces dyspnea. Presently, the National Heart, Lung, and Blood Institute and the Health Care Finance Agency is sponsoring a 7-year, multicenter, randomized trial comparing lung volume reduction surgery preceded by pulmonary rehabilitation versus pulmonary rehabilitation alone to examine selection criteria and efficacy of this surgical procedure.

Diaphragmatic plication (surgical stabilization) has been used in selected patients with unilateral diaphragmatic paralysis and coexistent lung disease for relief of breathlessness. A paralyzed hemidiaphragm undergoes a paradoxical upward displacement on inspiration as a result of negative intrathoracic pressure from the normal hemidiaphragm. In those with underlying respiratory disease, this process may increase the work of breathing and lead to breathlessness. Surgical plication of the paralyzed diaphragm has been shown to increase lung function, with a corresponding decrease in exertional dyspnea.

Pharmacological Options

Many patients with advanced lung disease experience anxiety and/or depression. Although randomized clinical trials of various anxiolytic and antidepressant medications have not shown consistent benefits, none of these studies selected patients with chronic lung disease and coexisting anxiety or depression. Experience with individual patients in whom anxiety and/or depression are major problems sometimes reveals dramatic relief of distressful breathing with appropriate treatment. Therefore, a trial of an anxiolytic medication is indicated in patients with anxiety complicating their respiratory disease. Similarly, an antidepressant medication should be tried in such patients with signs or symptoms of depression.

The use of opiate medications to relieve dyspnea is an often neglected modality for the care of patients with severe, near-terminal lung disease. ''Control of dyspnea'' for patients with respiratory disease may be considered analogous to the widely accepted "control of pain" for those with cancer. Opiate medications may reduce the sensation of breathlessness by decreasing ventilation, decreasing responsiveness to hypoxemia and hypercapnia, and/or altering the process of the "dyspnea signal" in the central nervous system. Inhaled, oral, subcutaneous, or intravenous opiate medications (e.g., morphine or one of its derivatives) may be tried in patients with severe, disabling dyspnea who are terminally ill. A low dose should be prescribed initially and then titrated to achieve symptomatic benefit. With such an approach, published reports indicate that relief of dyspnea can be achieved without necessarily causing major decreases in respiratory rate or oxygen saturation. Sedation is considered a common but acceptable side effect of systemic opiate use based on a "compassionate approach" to minimize the distress of breathing as part of end-of-life care.

SUMMARY

Dyspnea is a complex respiratory sensation that can be modified by physiological and psychological factors. The diagnosis of dyspnea can be enhanced by the appreciation that breathlessness encompasses different qualities based on the pathology of the disease. The categorization of dyspnea into acute, positional, and chronic types is helpful to establish a differential diagnosis for possible causes. Focused diagnostic testing is recommended in a sequential order to minimize cost. If the cause of chronic dyspnea is unclear or unexplained, spirometry and measurement of diffusing capacity, a chest radiograph, a resting 12-lead ECG, and oximetry are recommended as initial screening tests. Cardiopulmonary exercise testing may be helpful to diagnose deconditioning and psychogenic dyspnea and to distinguish respiratory from cardiac limitations.

The initial strategy to relieve breathlessness is to treat the underlying disease. Next, the patient should be evaluated for supplemental oxygen therapy. Exercise training can provide substantial benefits for reducing dyspnea and is considered the major component of pulmonary rehabilitation. Inspiratory muscle training may be considered in patients with respiratory muscle weakness as part of a comprehensive exercise training program or as a separate modality. Coping and behavioral strategies should be reviewed with symptomatic individuals and practiced in a supervised, supportive environment. Various surgical options are available for selected problems. Anxiolytic medications, antidepressants, and opiates may also be prescribed for selected patients.

SUGGESTED READING

1. Bruera E, MacEachern T, Ripamonti C, Hanson J. Subcutaneous morphine for dyspnea in cancer patients. Ann Intern Med 1993; 119:906–907.
2. Carrieri-Kohlman V, Douglas MK, Gormley J, Stulbarg MS. Desensitization and guided mastery: Treatment approaches for the management of dyspnea. Heart Lung 1993; 22:226–2234.
3. Cooper JD, Trulock EP, Triantafillou AN, Patterson GA, Pohl MS, Deloney PA, Sundaresan RS, Roper CL. Bilateral pneumonectomy (volume reduction) for chronic obstructive lung disease. J Thorac Cardiovasc Surg 1995; 109:106–119.
4. Kohlman-Carrieri V, Janson-Bjerklie S. Coping and self-care strategies. In: Mahler DA, ed. Dyspnea. Mt. Kisco, NY: Futura, 1990:201–230.

5. Lisboa C, Munoz V, Beroiza T, Leiva A, Cruz E. Inspiratory muscle training in chronic airflow limitation: comparison of two differnt training loads with a threshold device. Eur Respir J 1994; 7:1266–1274.

6. Mahler DA, ed. Dyspnea. New York: Marcel Dekker, 1998.

7. Mahler DA, Harver A, Lentine T, Scott JA, Beck K,Schwartzstein RM. Descriptors of breathlessness in cardiorespiratory disease. Am J Respir Crit Care Med 1996; 154:1357–1363.

8. Mahler DA, Horowitz MH. Clinical evaluation of exertional dyspnea. Clin Chest Med 1994; 15:259–269.

9. Manning HL, Harver A, Mahler DA. Dyspnea in the elderly. In: Mahler DA, ed. Pulmonary Disease in the Elderly Patient. New York: Marcel Dekker, 1993:81–111.

10. Martinez FJ, Stanopoulos I, Acero R, Becker FS, Pickering R, Beamis JF. Graded comprehensive cardiopulmonary exercise testing in the evaluation of dyspnea unexplained by routine evaluation. Chest 1994; 105:168–174.

11. Pratter MR, Curley FJ, Dubois J, Irwin RS. Cause and evaluation of chronic dyspnea in a pulmonary disease clinic. Arch Intern Med 1989; 149:2277–2282.

12. Sassi-Dambron DE, Eakin EG, Ries AL, Kaplan RM. Treatment of dyspnea in COPD: a controlled clinical trial of dyspnea management strategies. Chest 1995; 107:724–729.

13. Teramoto S, Fukuchi Y, Nagase T, Matsuse T, Shindo G, Orimo H. Quantitative assessment of dyspnea during exercise before and after bullectomy for giant bullae. Chest 1992; 102: 1362–1366.

14. Weiser PC, Mahler DA, Ryan KP, Hill KL, Greenspon LW. Dyspnea: symptom assessment and management. In: JE Hodgkin, GL Connors, CW Bell, eds. Pulmonary Rehabilitation: Guidelines to Success, 2d ed. Philadelphia: Lippincott, 1993:478–511.

15. Meek PM, Schwartzstein RM, Adams L, Altose MD, Breslin EH, Carrieri-Kohlman V, Gift A, Hanley MV, Harver A, Jones PW, Killian K, Knebel A, Lareau SC, Mahler DA, O'Donnell D, Steele B, Stuhlbarg M, Titler M. Dyspnea: mechanisms, assessment, and management: A consensus statement. Am J Respir Crit Care Med 1999; 159:321–340.

15

Management of Cough

Richard S. Irwin and J. Mark Madison
University of Massachusetts Medical School
UMass Memorial Health Care
Worcester, Massachusetts

INTRODUCTION

The modern era of managing cough began in the late 1970s. In 1977, a systematic manner of evaluating patients with chronic cough was first proposed. It was an anatomic, diagnostic approach. At its core was the evaluation by history, physical examination, and laboratory tests of the anatomy of the afferent limb of the cough reflex, schematically depicted in Fig. 1. This approach was conceived after a review of animal histological data, case reports of clinical observations in humans, and a few prospective epidemiological studies. From this review, it was reasoned that cough could be caused by a multiplicity of diseases in a variety of anatomic locations and that extrapulmonary as well as pulmonary diseases needed to be routinely considered as potential causes.

In 1981, the duration of cough was proposed as the criterion for prospectively evaluating the usefulness of the anatomic diagnostic protocol. A duration of more than 3 weeks was chosen as the definition of chronic cough to separate out most patients who had the transient, self-limited acute cough of the common cold from those with other, more persistently troublesome conditions. It was in this same year that the validity of the anatomic diagnostic approach to evaluating chronic cough was first prospectively established. Subsequently, because there have been patients with respiratory tract infections more severe than the common cold who have complained of cough for longer than 3 weeks and had it spontaneously disappear within 8 weeks, a chronic cough has been variously defined in the literature as one that has been persistently troublesome for more than 3–8 weeks.

Since the end of the 1970s, a great deal has been learned about the management of cough. In reviewing this information, a series of questions are posed and answered below.

WHAT DOES COUGH MEAN TO THE PHYSICIAN?

Cough is an important defense mechanism that helps clear excessive secretions and foreign material from the airways; it is also the most common symptom for which adult patients seek medical attention from primary care physicians in the United States. Additionally,

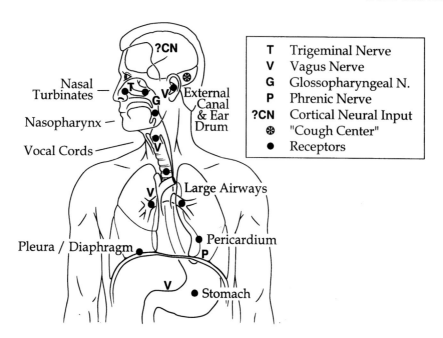

Figure 1 Schematic representation of the anatomy of the cough reflex. This sketch was derived primarily from clinical material and may not be anatomically correct. For instance, in the upper respiratory tract, cough receptors have been identified only in the hypopharynx, and there are no experimental data showing that the trigeminal nerve subserves the cough reflex. Moreover, while the sketch is clinically useful, there are experimental physiological data suggesting that involuntary coughing is entirely a vagal phenomenon. (From Irwin RS, Rosen MJ, Braman SS. Cough: a comprehensive review. Arch Intern Med 1977; 137:1186–1191. Copyright 1977, American Medical Association.)

referrals of patients with persistently troublesome chronic cough have been shown to account for up to 38% of a pulmonologist's outpatient practice.

WHY DO PATIENTS WITH COUGH SEEK MEDICAL ATTENTION SO FREQUENTLY?

They do so because cough can substantially and significantly affect their quality of life in multiple adverse ways.

During vigorous coughing, intrathoracic pressures up to 300 mmHg, expiratory velocities up to 28,000 cm/s or 500 mph (i.e., 85% of the speed of sound), and energies from 1 to 25 J may be generated. While the pressures, velocities, and energies of these magnitudes allow coughing to be an effective means of clearing the airways and providing cardiopulmonary resuscitation, they can also cause a variety of cardiovascular, central nervous system, gastrointestinal, genitourinary, and respiratory complications. While such physical complications have been significantly associated with health-related dysfunction in patients with chronic cough, the health-related dysfunction has been shown to be more commonly psychosocial in nature.

Since the health-related dysfunction associated with chronic cough significantly improves with successful treatment of the cough, and since chronic cough can be successfully treated in the great majority of patients who adhere to appropriate specific therapy, it is not appropriate to minimize a patient's complaint of chronic cough or to advise him or her to "live with it." In taking a history, physicians should specifically note psychosocial as well as physical complications. Failure to address the patient's concern about embarrassment, sense of exhaustion, and impact on social interactions may lead the dissatisfied patient to seek referral to other physicians. Since the literature has shown that successful specific therapy may require a minimum of three physician visits, psychosocial concerns related to chronic cough may need to be addressed if patients are to achieve maximal benefit.

WHAT HAS BEEN LEARNED ABOUT THE WORKUP OF CHRONIC, PERSISTENT COUGH?

From numerous studies performed in adults in university and community hospital settings and in children in a tertiary care setting, we have learned a great deal. These studies have primarily been performed in immunocompetent patients. Key points include the following:

Utilizing the systematic, anatomic diagnostic protocol initially established in 1981 and then modified in 1990, the cause of chronic cough has been determined from 88–100% of the time, leading to "specific therapy" and to success rates between 84 and 98%. Lower rates of success have been reported when protocols have been used other than those that have consistently been shown to be effective.

Chronic cough is often due to the simultaneous effects of more than one condition. A single cause has been found from 38–82% of the time, multiple causes from 18–62%. Cough with multiple causes has been due to three diseases up to 42% of the time.

While most smokers have a cough, they have not been the group of patients who most commonly seek medical attention complaining of cough.

Postnasal drip syndrome (PNDS), asthma, and gastroesophageal reflux disease (GERD) are the three most common causes of chronic cough in children above the age of 1, adults of all ages, and the elderly.

Chronic cough is found to be due to four common disorders in up to 94% of adults in prospective studies: PNDS, asthma, GERD, and chronic bronchitis (Fig. 2).

Cough in immunocompetent adults has been shown in prospective studies to be due to PNDS, asthma, and/or GERD at least 99% of the time in nonsmoking patients who are not taking an angiotensin-converting enzyme (ACE) inhibitor and who have normal or nearly normal and stable chest roentgenograms.

Cough can be the sole presenting manifestation of asthma and GERD up to 57% and 75% of the time, respectively. Nonspecific pharmacological bronchoprovocation challenge testing [e.g., methacholine inhalational challenge (MIC)] and 24-h esophageal pH monitoring have been singularly useful in diagnosing these patients.

Unless the chest roentgenogram is abnormal—an uncommon occurrence (no more than 7%)—flexible bronchoscopy will have a very low diagnostic utility (ap-

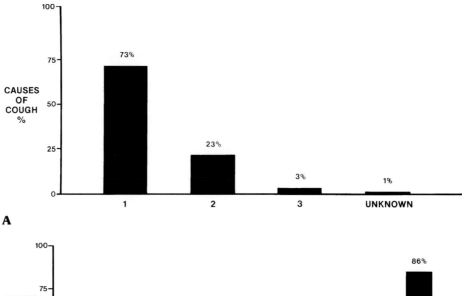

A

B

Figure 2 Representative causes of chronic cough in adults. A. The cause of chronic cough was prospectively determined in 99% of patients; it was due to a single cause in 73% and multiple causes in 26%. B. The spectrum and frequency of the 131 causes. (PND, postnasal drip syndrome; GERD, gastroesophageal reflux disease; bronch, bronchitis; bronchiect, bronchiectasis; misc, miscellaneous.) The miscellaneous conditions included bronchogenic carcinoma in 2 patients, left ventricular failure in 1; stage 3 pulmonary sarcoidosis in 1, angiotensin-converting enzyme inhibitor–induced cough in 1, and aspiration from a Zenker's diverticulum in 1. (From Irwin RS, Curley FJ, French CL. Chronic cough: the spectrum and frequency of causes, key components of the diagnostic evaluation, and outcome of specific therapy. Am Rev Respir Dis 1990; 141:640–647.)

proximately 4%). When bronchoscopy has been diagnostic, it has almost always been when the chest roentgenogram was abnormal and suggested the presence of a neoplastic or inflammatory lung disease.

The principal strength of the anatomic diagnostic protocol is in ruling out suspected possibilities (Table 1). The principal limitation is that a positive test cannot necessarily be relied upon to establish the diagnosis, and a positive test has not consistently been able to predict a favorable response to "specific therapy." For example, when a MIC is negative, asthma is essentially ruled out

Table 1 Testing Characteristics of Anatomic Diagnostic Protocol

Test	Sens	Spec	PPV	NPV
Chest x-ray	100%	54–76%	36–38%	100%
Sinus x-ray	97–100%	75–79%	57–81%	95–100%
Methachol IC	100%	67–71%	60–88%	100%
Barium esoph	48–92%	42–76%	30–63%	63–93%
Esophageal PM	<100%	66–100%	89–100%	<100%
Bronchoscopy	100%	50–92%	50–89%	100%

Abbreviations: Sens, sensitivity; spec, specificity; PPV, positive predictive value; NPV, negative predictive value; methachol IC, methacholine inhalational challenge; esoph, esophagography; esophageal PM, esophageal pH monitoring for 24 h.

as a cause of cough. An exception is the patient who may have occupational asthma in its earliest stage. However, in this occupational setting, longitudinal studies have shown that the test will become positive as the exposure continues. On the other hand, MIC can be falsely positive for predicting that asthma is causing the patient's cough (i.e., the cough does not respond to asthma therapy but does respond to specific therapy for another condition). Therefore, it must be appreciated that a positive test by itself, without a favorable response to therapy, is not diagnostic of asthma as the cause of cough.

A carefully taken history—with detailed questioning of the character, timing, or complications of chronic cough—is not likely to be helpful in diagnosing the cause of cough. For instance, PNDS, asthma, and GERD are the three most common causes of chronic cough irrespective of patient-reported quantity of daily sputum production. Moreover, a paroxysmal cough is not predictive of asthma as the cause, a barking or honking cough is not predictive of psychogenic cough, and a nocturnal cough is not predictive of GERD.

WHAT PROTOCOLS ARE RECOMMENDED FOR EVALUATING COUGH?

Guidelines for Evaluating Chronic Cough in Immunocompetent Patients

The following systemic diagnostic approach has been validated in immunocompetent patients with chronic cough (Fig. 3).

1. Review the patient's history and perform a physical examination concentrating on the anatomy of the afferent limb of the cough reflex (Fig. 1) and specifically the most common causes of chronic cough (Fig. 2).

2. Second, order a chest roentgenogram in nearly all patients. It is extremely useful for initially ranking differential diagnostic possibilities and directing laboratory testing. For example, a normal roentgenogram or one that shows nothing more than an abnormality consistent with an old, stable, and unrelated process makes PNDS, asthma, and/or GERD likely and bronchogenic carcinoma or sarcoidosis unlikely. Chest roentgenograms do not have to be routinely ordered before beginning therapy for presumed PNDS in young nonsmokers or in pregnant women.

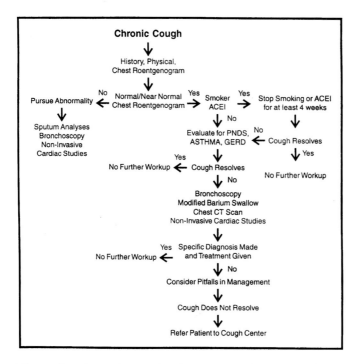

Figure 3 Diagnostic algorithm for managing chronic cough. ACEI, angiotensin-converting enzyme inhibitor; PNDS, postnasal drip syndrome; GERD, gastroesophageal reflux disease. (From Irwin RS. Cough. In: Irwin RS, Curley FJ, Grossman RF, eds. Diagnosis and Treatment of Symptoms of the Respiratory Tract. Armonk, NY: Futura, 1997: 22.)

3. It is advisable to withhold ordering of additional laboratory studies in present smokers with normal chest roentgenograms or patients taking an ACE inhibitor until the response to cessation of smoking or discontinuation of the drug for 4 weeks can be assessed. Cough due to these etiologies should substantially improve or disappear during this period of abstinence.

4. Depending on the results of the initial evaluation, smoking cessation, or discontinuation of the ACEI inhibitor, the following may be obtained:

> Sinus roentgenograms and allergy evaluation
> Spirometry pre- and postbronchodilator or MIC
> Barium esophagography and/or 24-h esophageal pH monitoring
> Sputum for microbiology and/or cytology
> Flexible bronchoscopy
> Computed tomography of the chest
> Modified barium swallow
> Noninvasive cardiac studies

Sinus roentgenograms and allergy evaluation are utilized to determine the possible causes of PNDS; spirometry pre- and postbronchodilator or MIC to investigate asthma; and barium esophagography or esophageal pH monitoring for GERD. While barium esophagography is a much less sensitive and specific test than 24-h esophageal pH monitoring, it may occasionally be singularly helpful in diagnosing GERD as the cause of cough. It has been able to reveal reflux to the thoracic inlet at a time when refluxate from the stomach had pH values similar to those of the normal esophagus, precluding its detection in the esophageal pH tracings. It is important to emphasize that diagnostic testing for GERD is recommended only in patients who do not have prominent upper gastrointestinal symptoms of GERD (i.e., "silent" GERD). It is not indicated in patients with cough who complain at least weekly of sour taste in the mouth, regurgitation, or heartburn, since the frequency of these symptoms is itself indicative of GERD. If the chest roentgenogram is normal or nearly normal, the order of tests is as listed above. On the other hand, if the chest roentgenogram is abnormal (e.g., a central mass is seen), sputum studies and bronchoscopy should be ordered first. In patients with risk factors for aspiration due to pharyngeal dysfunction, a modified barium swallow may be helpful. Chest computed tomography may be used to assess for bronchiectasis not suggested by routine chest roentgenograms. Unless the clinical evaluation or chest roentgenogram suggests a cardiac cause, noninvasive cardiac studies should be ordered last.

  5. The cause(s) of cough may be determined by observing which specific therapy eliminates cough as a complaint. If the evaluation suggests more than one possible cause, therapies should be initiated in the same sequence that the abnormalities were discovered. Since cough can be due to more than one condition, therapy that appears to be partially successful should not be stopped but rather added to sequentially.

Guidelines for Evaluating Chronic Cough in Immunocompromised Patients

While a systematic diagnostic approach for evaluating chronic cough in immunocompromised (e.g., HIV-positive) patients has not been validated, guidelines similar to those for immunocompetent patients are likely to be helpful. The major modification to the algorithm shown in Fig. 3 is the assessment of gas exchange during exercise by oximetry and blood CD4+ lymphocyte counts in the setting of a normal chest roentgenogram. If oxygen saturation with exercise does not fall below 90% or if the blood CD+ counts are greater than $0.200 \times 10^9/L$, it is unlikely that a clinically significant opportunistic lung infection in HIV-positive patients is present and evaluation for such can be withheld initially.

Guidelines for Evaluating Acute Cough

A clinical approach is recommended for evaluating acute cough; it consists of history, physical examination, and the estimated frequency of conditions. The most prevalent causes are the common cold, acute bacterial sinusitis, pertussis, exacerbation of chronic bronchitis, allergic rhinitis, and environmental irritant rhinitis. Less common causes include asthma, congestive heart failure, pneumonia, aspiration syndromes, and pulmonary embolism.

WHAT IS THE ROLE OF EMPIRIC THERAPY IN DIAGNOSING THE CAUSE OF CHRONIC COUGH?

The role of empiric therapy in diagnosing the cause of chronic cough has not been rigorously studied. Nevertheless, it is reasonable to consider when PNDS, asthma, and/or

GERD are likely possibilities and MIC, sinus imaging studies, and prolonged esophageal pH monitoring cannot be performed.

The principles recommended for empirically diagnosing and treating cough due to PNDS, asthma, and GERD are summarized in Table 2. The setting in which one or more of these three conditions are extremely likely is when the patient has the following clinical profile:

Complains of cough for at least 3 weeks duration
Is a nonsmoker
Is not taking an ACE inhibitor
Has a normal or nearly normal chest roentgenogram

Guidelines for Empirically Diagnosing and Treating PNDS

1. *Consider that PNDS is likely to be present*. PNDS is likely to be present when (1) the patient has the clinical profile described above; (2) the patient describes the sensation of having something drip down into the throat, nasal discharge, and/or the need to frequently clear the throat; (3) friends and/or relatives notice that the patient frequently clears his or her throat; (4) physical examination of the nasopharynges and oropharynges reveals mucoid or mucopurulent secretions and/or a cobblestone appearance of the mucosa.

2. *Consider the differential diagnosis of PNDS*. Conditions to consider include allergic rhinitis, nonallergic rhinitis, postinfectious rhinitis, drug-induced rhinitis, vasomotor rhinitis, environmental irritant rhinitis, and chronic sinusitis.

3. *In choosing initial therapy, consider the etiology of the PNDS and treat accordingly*. If allergic rhinitis, environmental irritant rhinitis, or drug-induced rhinitis is deemed operative, encourage avoidance of environmental irritants and allergens, cessation of ACE inhibitors. Before treating the other conditions, consider whether benign prostatic hypertrophy, glaucoma, or systemic hypertension is present. If these are not obvious concerns, begin therapy with a first-generation H_1 antagonist decongestant combination and reassess

Table 2 Recommended Principles for Empirically Diagnosing and Treating Chronic Cough Due to PNDS, Asthma, and GERD

1. Identify patients likely to have these conditions.
2. Add treatment for one condition at a time and always start with PNDS, since it is the single most common cause.
3. Do not stop therapy that appears to be partially successful; rather, add to it sequentially.
4. Use treatment regimens that have been shown to be useful.
5. Do not use systemic corticosteroids because:
   Cough due to asthma will likely get better with other asthma therapy.
   Asthma may be misdiagnosed if cough goes away.
6. Do not assume that these conditions have been definitively ruled out if the therapy, no matter how intensive, is not successful. For instance, GERD may not respond to maximal medical therapy but only to surgery.

Abbreviations: PNDS, postnasal drip syndrome; GERD, gastroesophageal reflux disease.

in 1 week. The first-generation H_1 antagonist is recommended as the first choice since it is more likely to be helpful in all the conditions mentioned above than the newer, relatively nonsedating H_1 antagonists. These newer agents have been shown to work only when the PNDS is histamine-mediated. It is quite likely that these newer agents have failed in non-histamine-mediated conditions, such as the common cold, when the older, potentially more sedating H_1 antagonists have succeeded, because the newer drugs possess relatively little if any anticholinergic activity. If benign prostatic hypertrophy, glaucoma, or systemic hypertension are concerns, consider using intranasal ipratropium and/or intranasal cortico-steroids. Unless there is strong clinical evidence that sinusitis is present (e.g., nasal puru-lence) antibiotics can be withheld initially.

4. *When there is no response in 1 week, consider sinusitis.* At this time, order imaging studies of the sinuses rather than empirically treating with antibiotics and treat according to the results. Multiple prospective studies have shown that four-view sinus roentgenograms are very helpful in ruling out sinusitis as a cause of chronic cough (Table 1). If the roentgenograms show nothing more than 5 mm of mucosal thickening in any sinus, sinusitis is essentially ruled out as a cause of PNDS 95–100% of the time. Sinus CT scans are not recommended routinely, since their role in diagnosing sinusitis as a cause of cough has not been assessed and they are more expensive. In treating chronic sinusitis, antibiotics should be directed against *Haemophilus influenzae*, *Streptococcus pneumoniae*, and upper respiratory tract anaerobes. The antibiotic plus a first-generation antihistamine decongestant oral medication should be given for at least 3 weeks and a decongestant nasal spray for a maximum of 5 days.

Guidelines for Empirically Diagnosing and Treating Asthma

1. *Consider that asthma is likely to be present.* Asthma should be suspected when (1) the patient has the clinical profile described above; (2) the patient complains of episodic wheezing, shortness of breath, plus cough and is heard to be wheezing on physical exami-nation; or (3) the patient complains only of cough in the absence of wheezing and cough has not been eliminated with treatment for PNDS.

2. *In choosing initial therapy, determine whether or not inhaled therapy provokes coughing.* Uncomplicated cough-variant asthma is likely to respond initially to all asthma medications including theophylline, oral beta$_2$ agonists, inhaled beta$_2$ agonists, and inhaled corticosteroids, inhaled nedocromil, and systemic corticosteroids. Randomized controlled clinical trials have shown that cough will begin to improve within 1 week with an inhaled beta$_2$ agonist and disappear with inhaled corticosteroids within 6–8 weeks. Therefore, begin treatment with an inhaled beta$_2$ agonist plus either an inhaled corticosteroid or in-haled nedocromil. If these agents provoke patients to cough in clinic even after changing formulations and using spacer devices, oral beta$_2$ agonists may be used. Therapy for PNDS should continue if it has been partially successful.

3. *Reassess in 1 week and then 6–8 weeks.* If cough is better after initial therapy, try again to institute inhaled therapy. If this is tolerated and cough is not better after 6–8 weeks, asthma is not likely to be present and further testing is not likely to be helpful. If inhaled medications still provoke coughing, then perform a MIC; if it is positive, pre-scribe only systemic corticosteroids.

Guidelines for Empirically Diagnosing and Treating GERD

1. *Consider that GERD is likely to be present.* GERD should be suspected when (1) the patient has the clinical profile described above, (2) the patient frequently complains at least weekly of heartburn or a sour taste in his or her mouth, or (3) the patient only complains of cough that has not improved with therapy for PNDS and asthma.

2. *In choosing medical therapy, consider initially giving maximal rather than submaximal therapy.* This recommendation is made because maximal therapy for GERD may take 2–3 months before it starts to work and 5–6 months to be successful. In addition, GERD may fail to respond to maximal medical therapy. Maximal medical therapy includes the following: (1) a high-protein, low-fat (e.g., 45 g per day) antireflux diet that eliminates beverages and foods that are acidic and have a tendency to relax the lower esophageal sphincter; (2) acid suppression; (3) prokinetic agent; (4) continuing treatment for PNDS and asthma if partially successful; (5) treating obstructive sleep apnea; (6) eliminating, when possible, medications for comorbid conditions that may be making GERD worse (e.g., progesterone, calcium channel antagonists, theophylline).

3. *Reassess in 1–3 months.* If cough is no better by 3 months, further diagnostic testing (e.g., 24-h esophageal pH monitoring) will be necessary to determine whether GERD is still present. If maximally treated GERD is still the likely cause of cough but has failed maximal therapy, then antireflux surgery should be considered.

Perspective

If patients with chronic cough are managed empirically according to the principles and guidelines presented, it is likely that the great majority will get better. If cough does not improve or go away, one *can* be reasonably certain that PNDS due to a condition other than sinusitis or asthma has been ruled out. If cough does not improve or go away, one *cannot* be certain that PNDS due to sinusitis or GERD have been ruled out. Whether management with empiric therapy will be shown to be more cost-effective than management with diagnostic testing is not clear. The authors speculate that doing some initial diagnostic testing routinely (e.g., MIC) will prove to be best.

WHAT HAS BEEN LEARNED ABOUT THE TREATMENT OF CHRONIC, PERSISTENT COUGH?

A great deal has been learned from numerous published studies in immunocompetent adults:

> The treatment of cough can be divided into two main categories: (1) antitussive therapy that controls, prevents, or eliminates cough and (2) protussive therapy that makes cough more effective.
> Antitussive therapy can be either specific or nonspecific. Specific therapy is directed at the etiology or operant pathophysiological mechanism responsible for cough. It is the only therapy that has a chance of being definitive. Nonspecific therapy is directed at the symptom; it is indicated when specific therapy cannot be given or does not work (e.g., inoperable lung cancer).
> Following utilization of a systematic, anatomic diagnostic protocol, specific therapy

for chronic cough has been reported to have a success rate between 84 and 98%. Therefore, because of the high probability of being able to determine the specific cause(s) of cough and of prescribing specific therapy that can be successful, there is a limited role for nonspecific antitussive therapy.

Protussive therapy is indicated when cough performs a useful function and needs to be encouraged (e.g., bronchiectasis). However, there are no data demonstrating convincingly that any protussive pharmacological agent leads to improved clinical outcomes.

Specific Antitussive Therapy

Specific therapy for the most common causes of chronic cough (Fig. 2B) is stressed in this chapter.

1. *PNDS, asthma, GERD*. Recommendations for treatment have already been discussed in the sections concerning empirically diagnosing and treating these conditions.

2. *Chronic bronchitis*. Specific therapy for cough due to chronic bronchitis is removal of the environmental irritant, such as cigarette smoke. Cough has been shown to disappear or markedly decrease in 94% of patients with smoking cessation. When it disappeared, it did so within 4 weeks 54% of the time.

3. *Bronchiectasis*. Cough due to exacerbations of bronchiectasis has been treated successfully with mucociliary stimulants such as theophylline and/or beta$_2$ agonists, chest physiotherapy and postural drainage, and intermittent courses of antibiotics directed against *H. influenzae, S. pneumoniae*, and upper respiratory tract anaerobes. If initial therapy is unsuccessful, the coverage may need to be expanded to include antibiotics against facultative gram-negative enteric rods and *Staphylococcus aureus*. It sometimes becomes necessary to extend antibiotic coverage for 3 weeks or longer and to evaluate the patient for a comorbid condition (e.g., endobronchial obstructing lesion, an aspiration syndrome) that predisposes him or her to frequent exacerbations.

4. *Cough induced by an ACE inhibitor*. While sulindac, nifedipine, indomethacin, and inhaled cromolyn have been shown to mitigate cough in some patients, withdrawal of all ACE inhibitors is the most consistently effective manner of definitively treating this cough. Switching from one ACE inhibitor to another will usually not be beneficial, since cough is a class effect of these drugs. Losartan, an angiotensin II receptor antagonist, can be used as an alternative drug to ACE inhibitors. It appears to effectively block the renin-angiotensin-aldosterone system by a mechanism other than ACE inhibition and it is not associated with an increased incidence of cough.

5. *Postinfectious cough*. By definition, this cough comes on following an upper or lower respiratory tract infection and lasts no more than 8 weeks. Some authors have advocated prescribing a 2- to 3-week course of systemic corticosteroids for those patients whose coughs are particularly troublesome. However, since the majority of patients with chronic cough from a variety of causes, when asked, provide a history suggesting that their chronic cough began after a respiratory infection, we believe that the diagnosis of postinfectious cough should be one of exclusion and made only when other causes such as PNDS, asthma, and GERD have been ruled out. It follows that we would recommend systemic corticosteroids only when these other conditions are shown not to be present. In the case of presumed *pertussis*, treatment with a macrolide antibiotic for the sick individual and prophylaxis for exposed persons has been shown to be effective in decreasing

the severity and transmission of the disease to others if therapy is begun within the first 8 days of the infection.

6. *Miscellaneous diseases.* When cough has been due to irritation of the eardrum by a hair, it will go away when the hair is removed. When it is due to an exposed endobronchial suture, it will disappear when the suture is removed. The cough due to pneumonia will respond to an appropriately prescribed antibiotic; pulmonary embolism, to intravenous anticoagulation; resectable bronchogenic carcinoma, to surgery; sarcoidosis, to systemic corticosteroids; and left ventricular failure with atrial fibrillation, to digitalis and diuretics.

Nonspecific Antitussive Therapy

In the relatively small group of patients with chronic cough in whom nonspecific antitussive therapy is indicated, dextromethorphan and codeine appear to be the most suitable choices. Ipratropium bromide aerosol may be helpful in patients with chronic bronchitis.

WHAT ARE THE COMMON PITFALLS IN MANAGING PATIENTS WITH CHRONIC COUGH?

If a patient continues to complain of persistently troublesome cough even after an extensive evaluation, it is recommended that the clinician resist the temptation to diagnose psychogenic cough. Even in patients with bizarre personalities, psychogenic cough is a rare condition. Rather, consider the following pitfalls in management:

Assuming that a positive MIC, all by itself, is diagnostic of asthma as the cause of cough

Not considering that inhaled medications prescribed for cough due to asthma may be making the cough worse;

Assuming that all H_1 antagonists are equal and that the newer, relatively nonsedating H_1-antagonists will effectively treat the postnasal drip of non-histamine-mediated conditions

Not considering that more than one condition is simultaneously contributing to the cough

Failing to consider the most common causes of cough in the presence of other seemingly "obvious" culprits (e.g., chronic interstitial pneumonia)

Not appreciating that "silent" GERD can be the cause of cough; that it may take up to 2 to 3 months of treatment before the cough starts to improve and up to 5 or 6 months before the cough disappears

Not appreciating the importance of prolonged esophageal pH monitoring in diagnosing GERD as the cause of cough and failing to understand how to interpret the study (e.g., conventional indices of reflux may be misleadingly normal)

Not appreciating that patients with cough due to GERD may fail to improve with the most intensive medical therapy and that the adequacy of the treatment regimen (and/or need for surgery) can be assessed by performing 24-h esophageal pH monitoring while the patient continues to take medical therapy

SUGGESTED READING

1. Corrao WM, Braman SS, Irwin RS. Chronic cough as the sole presenting manifestation of bronchial asthma. N Engl J Med 1979; 300:633–637.
2. Curley FJ, Irwin RS, Pratter MR, Stivers DH, Doern GV, Vernaglia PA, Larken AB, Baker SP. Cough and the common cold. Am Rev Respir Dis 1988; 138:305–311.
3. Irwin RS, Cough. In: Irwin RS, Curley FJ, Grossman RF, eds. Diagnosis and Treatment of Symptoms of the Respiratory Tract. Mt. Kisco, NY: Futura, 1997:1–54.
4. Irwin RS, Corrao WM, Pratter MR. Chronic persistent cough in the adult: the spectrum and frequency of causes and successful outcome of specific therapy. Am Rev Respir Dis 1981; 123:413–417.
5. Irwin RS, Curley FJ, Bennett FM. Appropriate use of antitussives and protussives: a practical review. Drugs 1993; 46:80–91.
6. Irwin RS, Curley FJ, French CL: Chronic cough: the spectrum and frequency of causes, key components of the diagnostic evaluation, and outcome of specific therapy. Am Rev Respir Dis 1990; 141:640–647.
7. Irwin RS, French CL, Curley FJ, Zawacki JK, Bennett FM. Chronic cough due to gastroesophageal reflux: clinical, diagnostic, and pathogenetic aspects. Chest 1993; 104:1511–1517.
8. Irwin RS, French CL, Smyrnios NA, Curley FJ. Interpretation of positive results of a methacholine inhalation challenge and 1 week of inhaled bronchodilator use in diagnosing and treating cough-variant asthma. Arch Intern Med 1997; 157:1981–1987.
9. Irwin RS, Pratter MR, Holland PS, Corwin RW, Hughes JP. Postnasal drip causes cough and is associated with reversible upper airway obstruction. Chest 1984; 85:346–352.
10. Irwin RS, Rosen JM, Braman SS. Cough: a comprehensive review. Arch Intern Med 1977; 137:1186–1191.
11. Irwin RS, Zawacki JK, Curley FJ, French CL, Hoffman PJ. Chronic cough as the sole presenting manifestation of gastroesophageal reflux. Am Rev Respir Dis 1989; 140:1294–1300.
12. Lacourciere Y, Brunner H, Irwin RS, Karlberg BE, Ramsay LE, Snavely DB, Dobbins TW, Faison EP, Nelson EB, and the Losartan Cough Study Group: effects of modulators of the renin-angiotensin-aldosterone system on cough. J Hypertens 1994; 12:1387–1393.
13. Mello CJ, Irwin RS, Curley FJ. The predictive values of the character, timing, and complications of chronic cough in diagnosing its cause. Arch Intern Med 1996; 156:997–1003.
14. Smyrnios NA, Irwin RS, Curley FJ. Chronic cough with a history of excessive mucus production: the spectrum and frequency of causes, key components of the diagnostic evaluation, and outcome of specific therapy. Chest 1995; 108:991–997.

16

Chronic Rhinitis and Sinusitis

Sidney S. Braman

Brown University School of Medicine
Providence, Rhode Island

ANATOMY AND PHYSIOLOGY OF THE NOSE AND PARANASAL SINUSES

Anatomic Considerations

Anatomically, the nose and sinuses are usually described as two separate and distinct structures. In fact, both the structure and the function of these two areas have many similarities and it is, therefore, helpful to consider the two as one unit. The epithelium of the nose and paranasal sinuses is continuous, and most offending agents—such as viruses, air pollutants, and aeroallergens—result in consequences simultaneously in both regions, even when symptoms predominate in one or the other. For instance, viruses of the common cold cause nasal symptoms such as sneezing, watery discharge, and nasal obstruction. Computed tomography (CT) scans of the paranasal sinuses in such patients also commonly show fluid and mucosal thickening in these structures. These abnormalities resolve with resolution of the cold symptoms. While it is conventional and clinically useful to discuss rhinitis and sinusitis as separate entities, it is helpful to remember that, in fact, the pathological state may be one of rhinosinusitis and that treatment of both may be necessary to effect complete cure.

The anatomic areas of the nose include the anterior nares, vestibule, nasal passages, posterior nares, and nasopharynx. The anterior nares (nostrils) mark the beginning of the double nasal airway. The external nose is made up of bone and cartilage. It surrounds the nasal vestibule, which is lined by facial skin and hair and extends to the ciliated mucosa at the anterior ends of the turbinates. The two nasal passages extend posteriorly on both sides of the nasal septum to the end of the nasal turbinates. The three turbinates—inferior, middle, and superior—occupy much of the nasal cavity. Their mucosal lining is highly vascular and has an abundance of mucous glands. During normal nasal breathing, most of the airstream is directed toward the floor of the nasal cavity and therefore is in contact with the inferior turbinates. Only with vigorous sniffing is the airflow directed to superior regions of the nasal passages. Since the olfactory epithelium occupies the superior portions of the nasal passages and sends branches of the olfactory nerves through the cribriform plate above, sniffing augments the ability to smell. At the posterior nares, the nasal septum ends and the nasopharynx begins. The nasopharynx marks a transition to squamous epithelium. The eustachian tubes enter the nasopharynx on its lateral walls and the adenoid tissue is located on the roof of the nasopharynx. The paranasal sinuses are called the maxillary, frontal, sphenoid, and ethmoid sinuses. They are a group of airspaces that surround the nasal cavity laterally and anteriorly and normally are in constant communication with it through small openings, called ostia, of 2–6 mm in diameter. Each ostium is connected to the nasal cavity by a small tubular passage, called the infundibulum, which is approximately 6 mm in length and 3 mm in diameter. Mucus and other fluids are transported through the infundibulum and into the nose by ciliary action. The sphenoid and posterior ethmoid sinuses drain into the nasal cavity through the superior meatus, which lies above the superior turbinate. The maxillary and anterior ethmoids drain through the middle meatus, which lies between the inferior and middle turbinates. The sinuses are lined by ciliated mucus-secreting epithelium. Ciliary function is essential for clearance, since maxillary sinus drainage is uphill.

Physiological Functions

The width of the airstream through the turbinates is narrow, and—if one considers the whole cross-sectional area of each level of the respiratory system, from nose to alveoli— the narrowest point is just anterior to the inferior turbinate. The nose, in fact, accounts for up to two-thirds of the total respiratory resistance. Despite the fact that nasal breathing as compared with mouth breathing doubles the resistance to breathing we prefer to breath through our noses. A small exchange of air occurs in the paranasal sinuses with each change in intranasal pressure. A number of factors affect nasal resistance, including normal cyclical variations in vascular congestion oscillating from one side of the nose to the other, posture, exercise, and cold air. In addition, pathological conditions can increase nasal resistance. This occurs in response to noxious air pollutants, aeroallergens, infectious organisms, and certain pharmacological agents.

The principal function of the nose is to warm, humidify, and filter inspired air. It is the first line of defense against infectious and noxious agents. The nasal vasculature that is within the nasal septum and turbinates is of an erectile nature similar to that of the genitalia. Blood flow to the mucosa is regulated by constriction and dilation of small arteries, arterioles, and arteriovenous anastomoses. These are called the nasal resistance vessels. In addition, there are large venous sinusoids within the mucosa. These are the capacitance vessels with erectile properties. The sudden changes in vascular capacitance allow for an efficient exchange of heat and humidity to properly condition the inspired air. The airstream through the nose is subjected to rapid changes in direction and velocity and causes considerable turbulence in flow. This helps mixing and conditioning of the air and causes particles that are suspended in the inspired air to impact on the nasal mucosa, where they can be transported posteriorly to the nasopharynx by mucociliary clearance mechanisms.

The nose is a highly effective filter. Vibrissae in the nasal vestibule are capable of removing most of the particles in the inspired air that are 15 μm in diameter and larger. A large proportion of the particles small enough to enter the nose are trapped within the nasal secretions. Very small particles of an aerodynamic size less than 2 μm may pass through the nose into the lungs and be immediately exhaled without deposition. Some particles in the range of 4 μm and less, including droplet nuclei carrying infectious organisms, do impact on the tracheobronchial tree or even deeper into the lung. Once trapped in the nose, particles are cleared by the nasal secretions through the beating action of cilia. While there is wide individual variation in the rate of nasal mucociliary transport, it has been estimated to proceed at an average rate of 6 mm/s. Transport is increased during exercise and decreased during sleep. Dehydration also diminishes mucociliary clearance. Hot drinks and soups have been shown to increase clearance. Once particles are deposited into the pharynx, they are effectively swallowed.

Nasal mucus contains immunoglobulins, primarily IgA, and other antibacterial proteins such as lysozyme and lactoferrin, which are capable of affording some protection against microorganisms. Unlike the respiratory tract below the larynx, which harbors no microorganisms, the upper airways, including the nasal passages, are always colonized with bacteria despite these protective mechanisms and the highly effective mucociliary transport system. In addition to normal respiratory flora such as corynebacteria and alpha-hemolytic streptococci, nasal swab cultures may reveal *Staphylococcus aureus*, beta-hemolytic streptococci, pneumococci, and *Haemophilus influenzae*. Under normal conditions, the paranasal sinuses, which communicate with the nasal cavity, are sterile. The mechanisms that maintain sterility are not fully understood. Mucociliary clearance and components of the immune system are undoubtedly important. In addition, it has been discovered that antibacterial concentrations of nitric oxide are present in the sinuses.

Nervous System Control

The neural innervation of the nose controls nasal blood flow, regulates nasal secretions, and subserves a number of protective reflexes that protect the lower airway from irritants. The sensory nerves include the olfactory nerve and branches of the trigeminal nerve, which serve the mechanical, tactile, and nociceptive functions of the nose. The trigeminal nerve, therefore, receives the sensations of touch, hot, cold, pain, and itch and responds to chemical irritants such as ammonia and sulfur dioxide. Nerves from the sympathetic and parasympathetic nervous system regulate vasomotor function and secretion. The classic neurotransmitters of the postganglionic autonomic nerves are acetylcholine and norepinephrine. There is evidence that nonadrenergic, noncholinergic neuropeptide-containing nerves participate in the regulation of nasal blood flow and glandular secretions. These regulatory neurotransmitters lie along the neural axon of predominantly small, nonmyelinated C fibers and diffuse locally to receptors on target cells. When stimulated, they are capable of causing a widespread injury response and produce glandular secretion and alterations in blood flow in both resistance and capacitance vessels. The neurotransmitters involved in these reactions include calcitonin gene–related polypeptide and various tachykinins such as substance P, neurokinin A, and neuropeptide K.

Nasal Reflexes

There are two types of nasal reflexes: those that are initiated by stimulation of the nasal mucosa and those that arise from elsewhere in the body and reflexly involve the nose. The most common and well known of the former group is the sneeze reflex. This protective reflex occurs following stimulation of the nasal mucosa by a variety of substances including irritant chemicals, aeroallergens, and histamine. Sneezing can also be initiated by direct nerve stimulation of branches of the trigeminal nerve, exposure to bright light, and skin cooling. Sneezing involves a forceful exhalation against a closed glottis after a deep inspiration. The reflex often begins with a paresthetic nasal sensation and is followed by lacrimation and rhinorrhea.

Another important protective reflex is called the rhinosinobronchial reflex. It has also been called the diving reflex because in its classic form it involves immersion of the head into cold water, which results in sudden apnea. Other reflex effects include laryngospasm, bronchospasm, systemic vasoconstriction, and bradycardia. This reflex is generally triggered by stimulation of the nasal mucosa by smoke, dust, chemicals, and other irritants. This reflex, therefore, links the upper and lower airways through a trigeminal afferent–vagal efferent neural arc. It has been postulated that asthma can be exacerbated in patients with inflammation of the nose and sinuses through stimulation of this reflex. This concept is not new and actually dominated medical thinking from the early Christian era until the seventeenth century. Upper and lower airway symptoms were considered to have one common cause, and a common treatment for lung diseases such as asthma was to purge the nostrils to relieve the breathing passages. There has been a considerable revival of attention in this century to the understanding of this reflex. In both animal and human experimentation, there is evidence to suggest that it is an important reflex. Spraying crystalline silica particles in the nose results in an increase in lower airway resistance. This can be blocked by atropine and by cooling of the vagus nerve. In one study, subjects with tic douloureux who had undergone unilateral transection of the second branch of the trigeminal nerve for symptomatic relief were subjected to the nasal silica dust challenge. Challenge on the neurally intact side caused mucosal burning and reflex bronchoconstriction. The denervated side failed to produce either local or reflex symptoms. Other studies, however, failed to demonstrate significant changes in airway resistance when the nose strongly reacted to the local instillation of histamine or to aeroallergens in previously sensitized individuals. The importance of this reflex in the pathogenesis of lower airway disease is not defined.

Another important reflex is the nasocardiac reflex. Nasal stimulation causes reflex bradycardia, a decrease in the cardiac output, and vasoconstriction. There are reports of extreme responses to this reflex, which have resulted in severe arrhythmia and even death. It is possible that this reflex contributes to the sudden death that has been described in those seeking a ''high'' after sniffing glue and cleaning fluid. Reflexes that arise in other parts of the body and affect the nose most often involve a sudden change in nasal resistance due to congestion in the capacitance vessels. This occurs after assuming the supine position, on the ipsilateral side in the lateral decubitus position, and on the ipsilateral side after placing a crutch under the axilla. This later reflex, called the crutch reflex, occurs over 80% of the time when tried. Exercise reflexly causes a drop in nasal airway resistance and cold air in the nose causes rhinorrhea and nasal congestion. Cooling of the extremities causes an increase in nasal resistance. Finally, there is the bronchonasal reflex: stimulation of the lower airways with nebulized distilled water can cause reflex nasal congestion. While this reflex can be elicited in normal individuals, it is more consistently seen in subjects with allergic rhinitis. This suggests that there is a critical threshold of nasal disease that is necessary before the nose will respond to such stimuli.

SYMPTOMS OF RHINITIS AND SINUSITIS

Inflammation of the nose causes a variety of symptoms, including sneezing paroxysms, itching, nasal obstruction, loss of smell, rhinorrhea, and occasionally—with severe irritation and ulceration of the nasal mucosa—bleeding. Sneezing is induced by both allergic and nonallergic inflammation and by direct stimulation of trigeminal nerve endings. Chemical mediators such as histamine, which can be released by mast cells and basophils residing in the nasal mucosa, can cause pruritus. Nasal obstruction can be caused by a pre-existing bony deformity, a large amount of viscid secretions and, most importantly, mucosal swelling. Mucosal swelling results from interstitial edema fluid and from vascular engorgement in the capacitance vessels.

Bilateral loss of smell can be caused by a number of systemic diseases and by local diseases of the nose and sinuses. Examples of systemic diseases include neurological diseases like multiple sclerosis, Parkinson's disease, and head trauma as well as metabolic disorders such as diabetes mellitus, hypothyroidism, Cushing's syndrome, and pseudohypoparathyroidism. Anosmia can also be associated with cystic fibrosis, acute viral hepatitis, hepatic cirrhosis, chronic renal failure, sarcoidosis, zinc deficiency, toxin exposures, and certain drugs. Local diseases that can cause bilateral loss of smell include infectious and noninfectious rhinitis, sinusitis, nasal polyposis, Sjögren's syndrome, adenoid hypertrophy, and viral infections. Inflammatory nasal disease and postviral disease are the most common causes of bilateral loss of smell. Unilateral anosmia is a rare phenomenon and may be due to unilateral nasal inflammatory disease; it can also be a sign of frontal lobe tumor.

Rhinorrhea is a recurrent or chronic watery nasal drainage. Nasal secretions are composed of a complex mixture of substances including secretions from the seromucous glands and goblet cells, capillary fluid transudate, sloughed nasal mucosal cells, and cellular debris from nasal inflammatory cells. In some patients inflammation is the cause, either infectious or noninfectious; this can be detected by the presence of inflammatory cells on nasal biopsy and the presence of vasoactive mediators in the nasal discharge. In other patients there is no sign of inflammation and it is believed that the rhinorrhea is caused by dysfunction of the autonomic nervous system, a condition that has been called vasomotor rhinitis. This, of course, is a misnomer, since the suffix *itis* usually implies inflammation. A clear fluid running from the nose in a patient who has recently suffered trauma should suggest the diagnosis of cerebrospinal fluid rhinorrhea. This may occur as a result of a fracture of the cribriform plate; the fluid is at times mixed with blood that does not clot. Rhinorrhea with a very high level of glucose (greater than 30 mg/dL) approximating that of the cerebrospinal fluid (40–80 mL/dL) would tend to support the diagnosis of cerebrospinal fluid rhinorrhea.

The nasal examination can be accomplished with the use of a nasal speculum. If significant nasal obstruction is present, it is advisable to repeat the examination after the use of a topical decongestant, such as 1% phenylephrine. In allergic rhinitis the mucosa is pale or bluish, boggy and swollen. In nonallergic rhinitis, it has often been described as being deep red in color and boggy. Swollen turbinates, nasal polyps and bony abnormalities should be noted.

While sinusitis can be defined as inflammation of one of the sinus cavities, in practical use the term refers to an infection in the sinuses. This usually results from inflammation of the nose, which causes obstruction of the sinus ostia and a secondary infection. Symptoms that are seen in sinusitis are fever, malaise, purulent nasal discharge, facial pain, headache, either productive or nonproductive cough, nasal congestion, poor response to nasal decongestants, maxillary toothache, painful mastication, and hyposmia. Structural defects of the nasal cavity—such as polyps, septal deviation, tumors, and foreign bodies (especially in children)—should be looked for on physical examination because they may cause sinus ostium obstruction and acute or recurrent sinusitis. Physical findings of sinusitis include the presence of purulent secretions coming from the middle meatus, tenderness to palpation over the sinuses, tenderness of the maxillary teeth elicited by tapping them, and the failure to transilluminate through the maxillary sinus cavity. The accuracy of these individual symptoms and signs for the diagnosis of sinusitis is poor. However, used in combination, they can be quite helpful. Three symptoms (maxillary toothache, poor response to decongestants, and a history of colored nasal discharge) and two signs (purulent nasal secretions and abnormal transillumination) are the best predictors of sinusitis. When none are present, sinusitis can be ruled out.

EPIDEMIOLOGY OF RHINITIS AND SINUSITIS

Since characteristic symptoms of rhinitis may occur in normals, it is difficult to obtain precise and accurate epidemiological statistics. In addition, most information comes from self- or physician-reported disease. Furthermore, the allergic status is not always known. A number of studies have shown that the prevalence of rhinitis has been increasing in developing countries. This may be explained by the rise in atopic sensitization that has also been observed. One recent community-based study from London showed that the prevalence of all kinds of rhinitis was 24%; among these individuals, 3% had seasonal symptoms alone, of which 78% were atopic; 13% had perennial symptoms alone, of which 50% were atopic; and 8% had perennial rhinitis with seasonal flare-ups. Nasal blockage was more common in patients with perennial symptoms, and pruritus of the eyes was more common with seasonal symptoms. Wheezing occurred more in those who were atopic (39%) as opposed to those who were nonatopic (18%). The prevalence of allergic rhinitis is lowest below age 5 and rapidly reaches a peak in adolescence and early adulthood. Data on long-term follow-up is scant. One study of children showed that hay fever was reported at age 23 in 52% of patients who had hay fever at age 7. Asthma or wheezing commonly develop in patients with rhinitis. The prevalence is higher in those with allergic as opposed to nonallergic rhinitis. The reported prevalence of asthma in hay fever patients is between 13 and 38%. This compares to 5–8% in the general population. Conversely, the prevalence of hay fever in asthmatics is between 28 and 50%, as opposed to 10–20% in the general population. The prevalence of eczema in hay fever patients is also higher than in the general population.

Why allergic rhinitis is a risk factor for asthma is not known. Initially, it was postulated that infected secretions from the upper airway were being aspirated into the bronchi and were causing asthma. There is no proof for this and aspiration in other conditions does not cause asthma. The rhinobronchial reflex has been implicated, but this is unlikely, since the reflex is quite weak. Could there be a systemic absorption of inflammatory mediators that produces bronchial inflammation? When the nose is blocked, do more aeroallergens get bypassed into the lungs and cause allergic sensitization? Answers to these questions regarding the pathogenesis of asthma in allergic rhinitis might prove useful.

The incidence of sinusitis is quite high if you consider that nearly every common cold is, in reality, a viral rhinosinusitis. A small portion of colds turn into bacterial sinusitis. This has been reported to occur in approximately 0.5–2% of cases. Other risk factors for bacterial sinusitis are allergy, swimming, nasal polyps, foreign bodies, tumors, and immune deficiency states.

CHRONIC RHINITIS

When the physician is faced with chronic or recurring symptoms of nasal obstruction, rhinorrhea, nasal itching and sneezing, a diagnosis of rhinitis is made. A number of classifications for rhinitis have been proposed to assist in its diagnosis and treatment. But because rhinitis symptoms have a number of causes, some of which are not inflammatory at all, and because it is not always easy to determine the etiology and pathogenesis of the patient's symptoms, the term *rhinopathy* was suggested to describe the various afflictions of the nose. Table 1 offers a practical guide for distinguishing the various chronic diseases of the nose. Table 2 lists treatment options for rhinitis.

Acute Viral Rhinitis

Viral rhinitis is caused by the many different kinds of cold viruses, including rhinovirus, coronavirus, respiratory syncytial virus, parainfluenza virus, adenovirus, and influenza virus. Evidence suggests that the infection begins in the adenoidal area and spreads to the nose. The virus attaches to the ciliated epithelia by binding to an intercellular adhesion

Table 1 Classification of Rhinitis

Infectious
  Viral
  Bacterial
  Fungal
  Atrophic rhinitis
Allergic
  Seasonal
  Perennial
Nonallergic
  NARES syndrome
  Vasomotor rhinitis
Drug-induced
  Rhinitis medicamentosa
  Antihypertensives
  Estrogens
Disease-related rhinitis
  Endocrine/hormonal
    Hypothyroidism
    Pregnancy
  Granulomatous rhinitis
    Wegener's granulomatosis
    Midline granuloma
    Sarcoidosis
  Autoimmune disease
    Sjögren's disease
    Relapsing polychondritis
    Lupus erythematosus
  Dyskinetic cilia syndrome
    Kartagener's syndrome

Table 2 Treatment of Allergic Rhinitis

Treatment	Examples	Effectiveness	Disadvantages
Nonpharmacologic	Avoidance of allergens High-efficiency air filters Saline irrigation Humidification	May give short-term relief	Avoidance not always possible; humidification does not treat allergic reactions
First-generation antihistamines	Chlorpheniramine Diphenylhydramine Clemastine Brompheniramine	Prevents sneezing, itching, and rhinorrhea but not nasal blockage	Sedation, impaired cognition, anticholinergic activity, paradoxical CNS stimulation
Second-generation antihistamines	Loratadine Astemizole Cetirizine Azalastine	Fewer anticholingeric effects No sedation Topical nasal spray available	Some agents prolong QT interval, cause arrhythmia (terfenidine, astemizole)
Nasal decongestants	Pseudoephedrine Phenylpropanolamine Phenylephrine Oxymetazoline	Relieve nasal congestion and rhinorrhea but not itching or sneezing	Tachycardia, insomnia, increased blood pressure, urinary obstruction, rhinitis medicamentosa with topical abuse
Inhaled corticosteroids	Beclomethasone Flunisolide Triamcinolone Budesonide Fluticasone	Best drug to control all rhinitis symptoms Useful for nasal polyps Safe and effective	Few disadvantages; possibly local nasal irritation
Inhaled antihistamines	Azelastine	Useful for rhinorrhea, sneezing, eye itching	Bitter taste; occasional somnolence
Anticholinergic	Ipratropium	Useful for rhinorrhea	No effect on sneezing or itching; occasional local nasal irritation
Allergen immunotherapy	Desensitization to cat, dust mite, ragweed, tree, and grass mold allergies	Effective in patients who cannot avoid allergens or with poor pharmacological response	Anaphylaxis

molecule ICAM-1 receptor. Viral replication proceeds, with maximum viral shedding on days two and three. Symptoms usually persist for 3 to 7 days. However, symptoms of cough, throat clearing, postnasal drip, and nasal discharge frequently persist 2 or more weeks after onset. Since the average preschool child experiences 6–10 colds per year and the average adult has 2–4 per year, the effect may seem more like a chronic or recurring condition. Smokers, especially, are more likely to develop upper respiratory viral infections; when they do, they are more likely to develop symptoms after the infection. Stress is another risk factor that increases susceptibility to colds. Typically, viral rhinitis is associated with a clear, watery nasal discharge due to the elaboration of inflammatory mediators. Kinins, prostaglandins, histamine, interleukins-1, -6, and -8, and tumor necrosis factor have all been implicated in the pathogenesis of the common cold. The nasal secretions may become cloudy because of the presence of white blood cells and desquamated columnar epithelial cells. Most colds, however, are not associated with a significant degree of tissue necrosis and epithelial damage. Other nasal symptoms are sneezing and nasal obstruction. Fever, scratchy or sore throat, and nonproductive cough are also typical. The common cold is usually a benign, self-limited infection. Occasionally complications such as bacterial sinusitis, otitis media, and exacerbation of asthma or chronic obstructive lung disease occur.

Bacterial and Other Infectious Rhinitis

Acute bacterial rhinitis can occur spontaneously or as a consequence of viral rhinitis. Bacterial superinfection occurs after viral infection because the virus damages the mucociliary transport system. Cigarette smoke and mucosal drying have the same effect. The mucosa is swollen, red, tender, and coated with purulent secretions. Symptoms include nasal obstruction, purulent nasal secretions, facial pain, nasal crusting, and often fever. Usual organisms include *Streptococcus pneumoniae, Staphylococcus aureus, Haemophilus influenzae*, and group A beta-hemolytic streptococci.

Primary atrophic rhinitis is a chronic, progressive nasal disease accompanied by nasal cultures growing *Klebsiella ozaenae*. It occurs in elderly patients and is predominantly seen in less developed countries. This disease is characterized by nasal mucosal atrophy, resorption of underlying bone, and formation of thick nasal crusting with a characteristic fetid odor. It can occur in previously healthy people or can be seen in those with previous nasal disruption because of nose and sinus surgery, tuberculosis, and syphilis. Symptoms of nasal congestion, constant bad smell (ozena), and headache are present. Sinusitis is a frequent complication. While the etiology of primary atrophic rhinitis is considered to be infectious, the presence of organisms may represent contamination of a previously damaged mucosa. In addition *K. ozaenae* produces a ciliostatic effect by creating intraciliary adherence that leads to poor mucociliary clearance. Antibiotic therapy is usually successful in controlling the rhinitis and accompanying sinusitis.

Other infectious causes of rhinitis are seen particularly in those living in lower socioeconomic conditions and who are poorly nourished. The gram-negative organism *Klebsiella rhinoscleromatis* causes a foul-smelling, purulent rhinorrhea and progressive growth of granulomatous nodules that may result in progressive enlargement of the nostrils and upper lip. In *Mycobacterium tuberculosis* infection of the nose, the granulomatous inflammation causes ulceration of the nasal septum and turbinates which results in pain, nasal obstruction, and bloody nasal discharge. *Mycobacterium leprae* can also cause nasal discharge, crusting, bleeding, and nasal obstruction. As well, congenital and acquired syphilis may have nasal manifestations. In congenital syphilis, there is a purulent nasal discharge and fissures are seen around the anterior nares. In acquired syphilis, the nose can be infected after primary infection at other sites. Progressive destruction of the nasal skeleton by gumma can lead to the saddle deformity of the dorsum of the nose and destruction of the nasal septum. Fungal infection of the nose usually involves the sinuses and is seen in patients with underlying immunodeficiency and debilitation. The symptoms are nonspecific and include nasal discharge and nasal obstruction.

Allergic Rhinitis

Allergic rhinitis is an IgE-mediated inflammatory process of the nose that affects between 25 and 30 million Americans. This number actually underestimates the magnitude of this disease, as it represents only those who report their illness to a doctor. It may be seasonal and is often referred to as hay fever or pollinosis. More commonly, it is called perennial when the offending aeroallergens are present in the environment throughout the year. While there in no universal definition for perennial rhinitis, most experts feel that for this diagnosis to apply, symptoms should be present for at least 9 months of the year. Symptoms of sneezing, itching, rhinorrhea, and nasal blockage occur when offending pollens and molds are inhaled into the nose by susceptible individuals. They are often accompanied by ocular symptoms such as itching and tearing. The presence of other allergically mediated diseases such as atopic eczema or asthma or a positive family history of atopy all point to an allergic etiology.

Allergic inflammation is a complex reaction involving eosinophils, mast cells, basophils, T cells and neutrophils. When the allergens come into contact with the respiratory mucosa in susceptible individuals, they cause the formation of specific IgE antibodies. Antigen contact with either mast cells or basophils bearing specific IgE against the inhaled allergen leads to degranulation and release of preformed mediators such as histamine or to newly synthesized mediators such as prostaglandins and leukotrienes. This causes both an immediate, rapid reaction and a sustained, delayed reaction beginning from 3–24 h after the immediate reaction. The basophil is responsible for the late-phase reaction and the mediators are the same as in the earlier phase except for prostaglandin D_2, which is not produced by the basophil.

The tissue reaction in the nose is due to increased vascular permeability, tissue edema, vasodilatation, increased mucus production, and stimulation of nerve endings. Chemotactic factors attract eosinophils, basophils, and neutrophils into the nasal tissue. An essential mechanism of allergic inflammation seems to be the expression of endothelial adhesion molecules that control the attachment and migration of these leukocytes. The late-phase reactions produce obstruction and are caused by cellular infiltration. They are probably the cause of chronic rhinitis symptoms and are more difficult to treat. The amount of antigen required to induce an allergic response in the nose is less during the allergy season than out of season. This phenomenon is called priming and is related to the presence of neutrophils at the site of inflammation. The presence of eosinophilia, however, is most suggestive of an allergic reaction. While not diagnostic, the finding of 10% or more eosinophils on a nasal smear can be helpful in detecting the allergic reaction and is especially predictive of a good therapeutic response to corticosteroids. It can also distinguish allergic rhinitis from infectious rhinitis, which is characterized by neutrophils on smear.

Skin testing with suspected aeroallergens can be used to confirm specific IgE-mediated reactions and can be useful when coupled with the clinical history. Positive responses have correlated well with nasal allergic challenges. Standardized extracts of the suspected allergens can be administered with the skin-prick test; a wheal-and-flare reaction, which occurs after 15–20 min, is considered positive when the control reaction with saline is negative. Intradermal testing can be used when the prick tests are negative or equivocal. In vitro blood tests are available to measure the total quantity of IgE and specific IgE antibodies to common allergens. The radioallergosorbent (RAST) test is most commonly used to detect specific IgE antibodies. These blood tests are not necessary when skin testing can be done.

Seasonal allergic rhinitis is caused by inhaled pollens; trees in the springtime and grasses and weeds commonly in the summer and fall. Perennial rhinitis is most commonly caused by indoor allergens such as dust mites, molds, cockroaches, and animal dander. Common indoor fungi are *Aspergillus* and *Penicillium*. Their growth is promoted by elevated humidity. Information regarding the local pollen seasons can be extremely helpful for the treating physician even in patients with perennial allergic rhinitis, since many patients respond to a number of offending agents and experience perennial complaints with seasonal exacerbations. For instance, the ragweed season in many areas of the United States begins in mid-August and continues until the first frost. Most trees—such as birch, oak and alder—pollinate in the spring and early summer. Important exceptions are the mountain cedar, which begins in the winter, and the elm, which has a spring season in the North and a summer season in the South. Symptoms in sensitized patients are typically most intense during a defined season in which the aeroallergens are most abundant in the outdoor air. Ingested food antigens to which the patient is sensitive rarely produce isolated symptoms of rhinitis. More commonly, such allergic reactions are associated with other symptoms such as urticaria, facial or lip swelling, swelling of the tongue, and bronchospasm. As a rule, rhinitis symptoms after food ingestion is not caused by an allergic reaction but rather by vasodilatation from substances such as beer, wine, and other alcoholic drinks.

Nonallergic Rhinitis

Nonallergic rhinitis with eosinophilia syndrome (NARES) is a chronic nasal disease that is identical to perennial rhinitis except that allergy skin testing and IgE levels are normal. Symptoms include profuse watery rhinorrhea, sneezing, nasal itching, and nasal obstruction. During symptomatic periods, nasal smears show an abundance of eosinophils, even as high as 20–25%. The cause of this syndrome remains obscure and the prevalence in the general population is not known.

Vasomotor rhinitis is another form of nonallergic perennial rhinitis that causes symptoms of nasal obstruction and watery nasal drainage. Itching and sneezing are less common. There are no eosinophils on nasal smears and signs of atopy, such as positive skin testing, are absent. The etiology of the rhinitis is unknown, but as the name implies, there is thought to be an abnormality in the neural efferent innervation of the nasal mucosa. Symptoms are provoked by nonspecific irritants such as tobacco smoke, cold air, spicy foods, changes in humidity, odors, bright lights, and emotional stress. A copious watery rhinorrhea immediately following the ingestion of spicy foods has been called gustatory rhinitis.

The irritants that provoke vasomotor rhinitis are believed to stimulate the parasympathetic nervous system in an exaggerated way, thereby causing vasodilatation, nasal congestion, and excessive seromucous secretions. Anticholinergic agents given by nasal spray can block muscarinic receptors and offer symptomatic relief. Inhaled topical corticosteroids are not particularly effective in vasomotor rhinitis, as would be expected in a noninflammatory condition.

Drug-Induced Rhinitis

Rhinitis medicamentosa is caused by the prolonged use of topical alpha-adrenergic decongestant sprays. The use of such sprays for a week or more causes a rebound nasal congestion upon withdrawal. The patient then requires the decongestant again, often more frequently because of tachyphylaxis, in order to maintain nasal patency. This leads to an inflammatory hypertrophy of the nasal turbinates and an intense red color of the mucosa.

Drug-induced rhinitis can also be caused by a number of other agents taken either orally or topically. Cocaine, a recreational drug sniffed into the nose, can cause intense vasoconstriction and similar changes to the alpha-adrenergic agents. Nasal congestion and rhinorrhea are typical symptoms and, with intense, prolonged use, nasal perforation can result. A number of antihypertensives can cause rhinitis symptoms, including the central adrenergic blockers (methyldopa and clonidine); postganglionic blockers (reserpine and guanethedine); vasodilators (hydralazine); beta blockers (nadolol and labetalol); alpha blockers (prazosin and terazosin) and diuretics (thiazide and amiloride). Aspirin and nonsteroidal anti-inflammatory drugs can cause rhinorrhea, and oral contraceptives and conjugated estrogens can cause congestion and rhinorrhea. Drugs containing iodides that have been prescribed for expectoration can cause nasal stuffiness.

Dyskinetic Cilia Syndrome

Viruses associated with the common cold inhibit ciliary movement. Restoration of normal mucociliary clearance occurs between 2–6 weeks after the viral infection. The dyskinetic cilia syndrome is a genetic disorder whose molecular lesion produces defective ciliary function. This results in chronic rhinitis, sinusitis, bronchitis, and—after recurrent infections of the lung—bronchiectasis. Ultrastructural abnormalities of the cilia can be detected on nasal or bronchial biopsy and on spermatozoa. A subset of the immotile cilia syndrome is Kartagener's syndrome, which is the triad of bronchiectasis, sinusitis, and situs inversus (see Chap. 5, on host defense mechanisms of the lung).

Nasal Mastocytosis

This disease causes symptoms of rhinorrhea and nasal blockage without pruritus. The nasal mucosa contains large numbers of mast cells and few eosinophils. Typical signs of atopy are absent in these patients.

Rhinitis Associated with Systemic Disease

Endocrine Disorders

Hypothyroidism can produce an extremely boggy nasal mucosa with white turbinates in as many as 40% of patients. Complaints of excessive nasal discharge, recurrent "colds," and nasal stuffiness are even more common. Other signs of thyroid hormone deficiency suggest the diagnosis. During pregnancy and menstruation, the nasal mucosa becomes hyperemic and swollen in some women. Symptoms typical of vasomotor rhinitis that may occur during pregnancy are often difficult to treat and may not abate at the termination of pregnancy. Rhinitis has also been described in uremia and diabetes.

Malignancy

Superior vena caval syndrome may present with considerable nasal stuffiness in addition to the other typical symptoms of periorbital erythema and edema, progressive facial swelling, and headaches. Early in the course, symptoms may mimic an allergic upper respiratory syndrome and the patient may be referred for an allergic workup. This could delay the correct diagnosis, which usually is a malignant thoracic neoplasm. Tumors of the sinuses and nasopharynx may present with symptoms of nasal blockage or those resembling vasomotor rhinitis. Prolonged occupational exposure to chemicals such as nickel chromate and formaldehyde can result in carcinoma of upper airway structures.

Granulomatous Rhinitis

Systemic immunological diseases associated with granulomatous infiltration of tissues include Wegener's granulomatosis, sarcoidosis, and midline granuloma. Wegener's granulomatosis is a systemic necrotizing granulomatous disease associated with vasculitis. It affects the upper and lower respiratory tract, yet some patients present with symptoms of either the upper or lower tract and have no systemic involvement. The disease was initially called "rhinogenic granulomatosis" by Wegener. The upper airway is involved in 72% of patients with Wegener's granulomatosis and the most common symptom is nasal obstruction with the finding of nasal crusting. A serosanguinous discharge is frequently present and a deep central facial pain is experienced. A saddle deformity of the nose may result from destruction of nasal cartilage. The ears and sinuses are also commonly involved. Often confused with Wegener's granulomatosis is midline granuloma, a disease of unknown cause that is associated with progressive, localized destruction of the nose, paranasal sinuses, and palate. Nasal manifestations of sarcoidosis are uncommon and include mucosal hypertrophy, mucosal yellowish and bluish plaques, a solitary nasopharyngeal mass, saddle-nose deformity, and septal perforation.

Systemic Inflammatory Diseases

Other nongranulomatous systemic inflammatory diseases can also cause rhinitis symptoms. Relapsing polychondritis is a rare autoimmune, recurrent inflammatory disease of all cartilage. It may lead to saddle-nose deformity. Sjögren's syndrome causes a general dryness of mucosae, particularly dryness, crusting, and atrophy of the nasal mucosa. Systemic lupus erythematosus can cause petichiae, purpura and ulcerations of the mucosa. Behçet's disease causes apthous ulcers in the upper airways, digestive tract, and genitalia. Churg-Strauss syndrome comprises systemic vasculitis, asthma, tissue eosinophilia, and nasal polyposis. The vasculitis and mucosal ulcerations can lead to septal perforations and saddle-nose deformity.

NASAL POLYPOSIS

Nasal polyps are smooth, gelatinous, round, freely movable, semitranslucent outgrowths of the nasal mucosa. They usually arise from the surfaces of the middle turbinates or ostia of the ethmoid or maxillary sinuses. Most commonly they are found in the middle meatus, extending to the nasal cavity. Most patients who develop nasal polyps have a long-standing history of perennial rhinitis. The polyps may be unilateral or bilateral; when they occlude the nasal cavity, the voice commonly becomes nasal. Other symptoms include hampered breathing, especially at night, when snoring becomes problematic. Anosmia frequently occurs and loss of taste follows. Nasal polyps have an intact ciliated epithelium like normal nasal mucosa. The polyps, however, are infiltrated with inflammatory cells, including eosinophils, mast cells, plasma cells, and lymphocytes.

The etiology of nasal polyps is unknown; atopy and infection have been proposed. The prevalence of atopy, however, is no more common in patients with polyps than in the general population. Nasal polyps are most commonly found in nonatopic asthmatic patients over 40 years of age. The overall frequency in this group is about 7%; it is even higher in asthmatics with severe steroid dependence and in those with aspirin intolerance. The frequency may be as high as one in three patients. There is also evidence that patients with nasal polyps and no history of asthma show evidence of bronchial hyperreactivity in the pulmonary testing laboratory. The long-term incidence of asthma is greater in this group than in the general population. Chronic infection may be important in the pathogenesis of asthma in some patients, but it is not a universal finding. Polyps are seen in patients with cystic fibrosis and dyskinetic cilia syndrome without chronic infection. It is likely that there is no single etiology for nasal polyps but rather that they are the result of intense mucosal swelling from multiple causes.

The treatment of nasal polyposis should initially be medical, with surgical intervention reserved as a last resort. Intranasal topical corticosteroids are capable of reducing the size of the polyps and can prevent recurrence after surgery. Side effects are few and consist of local irritation and possibly bleeding from mucosal dryness. In severe cases, treatment with oral corticosteroids is necessary for brief periods of time. The suggested dose is 30 mg of prednisone for 7 days followed by a tapered dose for another 10–20 days. Topical corticosteroids should be given concomitantly and antibiotics should be used for complicating sinus infection. When infection cannot be cleared with this therapy or other obstructive symptoms persist, surgical management may be necessary to restore nasal patency. Polyps may be removed with a snare, but in more severe cases endoscopic sinus surgery is employed. In patients who require recurrent polypectomy, intranasal or transantral ethmoidectomy should be performed.

LUNG FUNCTION IN ALLERGIC RHINITIS

A number of studies have shown abnormalities in lower airway function in nonasthmatic patients with allergic rhinitis despite the absence of lower respiratory tract symptoms. There is evidence for abnormalities in both central and peripheral airway function in such patients. Further evidence suggests that there may be a seasonal variation in lung function. Airflow obstruction may be found during the symptomatic pollen season. This may spontaneously improve out of season. The airways of some patients with allergic rhinitis are more responsive to bronchoconstricting agents such as histamine and methacholine than are normal subjects. In some studies, as many as 50% of patients with allergic rhinitis show evidence of bronchial hyperresponsiveness. Some studies have shown that individuals in this group may be more likely to develop asthma in future years. Unlike the abnormalities in atopic asthma, the lower airway findings of airflow obstruction and bronchial hyperresponsiveness in allergic rhinitis are mild and not of the magnitude that causes pulmonary symptoms.

NASAL HYPERREACTIVITY

Just as the asthmatic's airway is many times more reactive when nonspecific stimuli are inhaled into the lungs, patients with all types of rhinitis will demonstrate nasal hyperreactivity. The nose has an exaggerated response to a variety of stimuli, including those encountered in everyday life, like dust, fumes, cold air, perfumes, and other strong odors. This response is particularly exaggerated in the rhinitis patient after a viral respiratory illness, and this reaction may last for weeks or months after the viral shedding has stopped. The nose of such rhinitis patients responds with an excessive production of nasal secretions and with mucosal swelling and nasal blockage. The cause of nasal hyperreactivity in patients with infectious, allergic, and nonallergic rhinitis is not known. Just as with vasomotor rhinitis, a neural imbalance theory has been proposed. It is probable that some modulation of afferent impulses occurs, possibly coupled with increased sensitivity of the nerve endings.

NASAL DISEASE AND OBSTRUCTIVE SLEEP APNEA

Patients with excessive daytime sleepiness are often found to have abnormal sleep patterns at night and are sleep-deprived. The most common cause of this disorder is the obstructive sleep apnea syndrome, a condition characterized by excessive snoring and repetitive apneic or hypopneic episodes due to collapsed segments in the upper airway during sleep. This prevents adequate time in the deeper stages of sleep (see Chap. 31). The primary site of obstruction in this syndrome is believed to be in the oropharyngeal-hypopharyngeal region. A few studies have implicated the nasopharyngeal region. Ultrafast magnetic resonance imaging to visualize the upper airway in sleep has shown that in as many as 1 out of 10 patients, the nasopharynx is the primary site of collapse.

Nasal inflammation has been observed in patients with obstructive sleep apnea despite the absence of symptoms. Inflammatory mediators and cells are both abnormally present, but the significance of this is not clear. By inducing nasal obstruction with artificial packing in healthy individuals and in those with sleep apnea, the number of apneic episodes during sleep can be increased. Similarly, during symptomatic ragweed season, the number of apneas per hour of sleep and the duration of the apneas is significantly increased. Despite this, lowering nasal resistance with nasal decongestants and intranasal stents has not been shown to improve obstructive sleep apnea. It is likely that partial or complete nasal obstruction has a minor influence on the pathogenesis of sleep apnea.

ACUTE AND CHRONIC SINUSITIS

Pathogenesis of Sinusitis

The major precipitating event that causes acute and chronic sinusitis is viral rhinitis. Sinus abnormalities are seen in 9 out of 10 patients with the common cold. Computed tomography (CT) has revealed that the most prominent abnormality of the sinuses is mucosal thickening. Its irregular appearance on the walls of the sinus cavities and the presence of gaseous bubbles within this thickening has suggested that it is a highly viscous substance that is adherent to the floor, sides, and roof of the sinus cavities. During a cold virus outbreak, CT has shown that the infundibulum is occluded in 77% of patients. Mucociliary clearance is markedly abnormal during a cold virus infection. This, coupled with the excess amount and thickening of the mucous blanket and the infundibular and osteomeatal obstruction from mucosal edema, collectively predispose to bacterial colonization. The specific factors that lead to bacterial invasion of the sinuses are unknown. Sneezing, coughing, and nose blowing may be factors, as they create pressure differentials that favor sinus invasion. Once bacteria enter an obstructed sinus, growth factors favor exuberant bacterial growth.

Acute Sinusitis

It is often difficult to determine whether the patient has an acute viral or bacterial sinusitis. Most signs and symptoms and even the sinus roentgenogram are not that specific, and unless sinus cavity cultures are collected without nasal contamination, they are not useful. The ''gold standard'' for microbial diagnosis is sinus cavity puncture and aspiration. This technique, while not painful if done by an experienced operator, is not suitable for routine clinical use. CT has a very high sensitivity for detecting sinusitis and has, in many centers, supplanted the routine x-ray examination. A positive air-fluid level with a flat meniscus suggesting thin fluid suggests a high likelihood of bacterial infection. CT is not necessary for the diagnosis of the routine case of acute, community-acquired sinusitis. The diagnosis is usually made on clinical grounds. The most common scenario is a typical viral upper respiratory infection that does not result in a typical resolution of symptoms in a week. If symptoms of fever, facial pain, nasal discharge, and nasal obstruction are still present after 10 days, there is a high likelihood of bacterial sinus infection and treatment should be begun. Sometimes symptoms of an antecedent typical viral upper respiratory infection are absent and the patient presents with the classic features of sinusitis, such as fever, facial pain, tenderness, erythema, or swelling. Empirical antibiotics are necessary in this setting too. Nosocomial sinusitis occurs most commonly in the intensive care unit setting. Prolonged nasotracheal intubation is an important risk factor. Sinusitis can be the cause of occult fever and sepsis in the hospitalized patient.

The bacteriology of acute community-acquired sinusitis is listed in Table 3. *Streptococcus pneumoniae* and *H. influenzae* account for a combined percentage of over 50% of cases. Most sinusitis due to anaerobic bacteria involves multiple organisms and arise from infection in the premolar teeth. Only about 60% of sinus aspirates will yield a positive culture for bacteria. It is possible that viral, *Mycoplasma pneumoniae*, or *Chlamydia pneumoniae* infections are the cause in culture-negative cases.

With the proper antibiotic and given in the proper dosage, therapy for 10 days can cure over 90% of acute sinus infections. The emergence recently of resistant organisms to commonly used antibiotics has been alarming. Examples include penicillin and methacillin resistance for *Staphylococcus aureus* and resistance to beta-lactam agents by *H. influenzae* and *Mycobacterium catarrhalis*. The most serious problem, however, has been the emergence of multiply resistant strains of *S. pneumoniae*. Recommendations for the treatment of acute bacterial sinusitis have accordingly changed in recent years. Drugs that have proven effective include such agents as amoxicillin clavulanate and cefuroxime axetil. They should especially be considered in areas with high antimicrobial resistance patterns. Oral decongestants and topical corticosteroids may be useful, especially if there is an allergic component to the rhinitis.

Table 3 Bacteriology of Sinusitis

Common pathogens
  Streptococcus pneumoniae
  Haemophilus influenzae
Less common pathogens
  Other streptococcal species
  Moraxella catarrhalis
  Staphylococcus aureus
  Mixed anaerobic infection
Pathogens following sinus surgery
  Staphylococcus aureus
  Pseudomonas aeruginosa
Pathogens in compromised hosts
  Staphylococcus aureus
  Pseudomonas aeruginosa
  Haemophilus influenzae
  Streptococcus pneumoniae
Nosocomial sinusitis
  Staphylococcus aureus
  Pseudomonas aeruginosa
  Acinetobacter baumanni
  Enterobacteriaceae

Chronic Sinusitis

Chronic sinusitis is defined as persistent inflammation of the sinuses at least 4 weeks after initiating appropriate therapy. The sinuses are characterized by inflammatory thickening and polypoid changes of the mucosa. Marked tissue eosinophilia is present. Whether bacterial infection is important in the pathogenesis of chronic sinusitis is not established. In patients who fail medical therapy with antibiotics, corticosteroids, and decongestants and, when indicated, allergen control, surgery should be considered. Surgery is also indicated in sinus disease for large obstructing polyps, a suspicion of tumor, mucocele or pyocele, fungal sinusitis and when the sinusitis is complicated by brain abscess, meningitis, cavernous sinus thrombosis, or subdural empyema.

SUGGESTED READING

1. Bert F, Lambert-Zechovsky N. Microbiology of nosocomial sinusitis in intensive care unit patients. J Infect 1995; 31:5–8.
2. Braman SS. Lung function in allergic rhinitis. In: Settipane GA, ed. Rhinitis, 2d ed. Providence, RI: Oceanside Publications, 1991.
3. Del Borgo C, Del Forno A, Ottaviani F, Fantoni M. Sinusitis in HIV-infected patients. J Chemother 1997; 9:83–88.
4. Giannoni CM, Stewart MG, Alford EL. Intracranial complications of sinusitis. Laryngoscope 1997; 107:863–867.
5. Holmberg K, Karlsson G. Nasal polyps: medical or surgical management? Clin Exp Allergy 1996; 26:23–30.

6. Iwen PC, Rupp ME, Hinrichs SH. Invasive mold sinusitis: 17 cases in immunocompromised patients and review of the literature. Clin Infect Dis 1997; 24:1178–1184.

7. Kaliner MA, Osguthorpe JD, Fireman P, Anon J, Georgitis J, Davis ML, Naclerio R, Kennedy D. Sinusitis: bench to bedside—current findings, future directions. Otolaryngol Head Neck Surg 1997; 116:S1–S20.

8. Kirkpatrick GL. The common cold. Primary Care 1996; 23:657–675.

9. Knight A. The differential diagnosis of rhinorrhea. J Allergy Clin Immunol 1995; 95:1080–1083.

10. Kupferberg SB, Bent JP, Kuhn FA. Prognosis for allergic fungal sinusitis. Otolaryngol Head Neck Surg 1997; 117:35–41.

11. Kushida CA, Guilleminault C, Clerk AA, Dement WC. Nasal obstruction and obstructive sleep apnea: a review. Allergy Asthma Proc 1997; 18:69–71.

12. Meltzer EL. An overview of current pharmacotherapy in perennial rhinitis. J Allergy Clin Immunol 1995; 95:1097–1110.

13. Poole MD. Antimicrobial therapy for sinusitis. Otolaryngol Clin North Am 1997; 30:331–339.

14. Tan RA, Siegel SC. Diagnosis and management of seasonal and perennial allergic rhinitis. Compr Ther 1996; 22:363–374.

15. Williams JW, Simel DL. Does this patient have sinusitis? Diagnosing acute sinusitis by history and physical examination. JAMA 1993; 270:1242–1246.

17

Pleural Effusion and Pneumothorax

Patrick A. Dowling
University of Wisconsin
Madison, Wisconsin

Veena B. Antony
Indiana University School of Medicine
Indianapolis, Indiana

INTRODUCTION

Pleural diseases, most commonly pleural effusions and pneumothoraces, account for as many as 40% of all pulmonary consultations in clinical practice. Pleural diseases can be secondary manifestations of other underlying disease states—for example, parapneumonic effusion with pneumonia or secondary spontaneous pneumothorax with emphysema. Likewise, the pleura can be the primary site of disease, as with mesothelioma. Various conditions involving the pleura are potentially life-threatening emergencies, such as tension pneumothorax and empyema. Although much is known about the clinical patterns of pleural diseases, surprisingly little is understood about their pathogenesis. In this chapter, we emphasize the clinical patterns of pleural diseases, their diagnosis, and their treatment, touching briefly on the pathophysiology and rationale for our approach.

PLEURAL EFFUSION

Clinical Presentation

Patients with pleural effusion may present asymptomatically or with a variety of symptoms such as pleuritic chest pain (due to inflammation of the parietal pleura), nonproductive cough (resulting from pleural inflammation or compression of the underlying lung), and dyspnea, which is frequently disproportionate to the amount of fluid present. Characteristic physical findings include diminished tactile fremitus, decreased thoracic excursion on the affected side, and diminished breath sounds. Typically, the chest is dull to percussion in the location of the effusion. Bronchophony, or accentuated breath sounds, may be noted at the superior border of the effusion along with egophany and whispered pectoriloquy. A pleural friction rub is sometimes noted.

Pathophysiology

Normally, the pleural space is 10 to 20 μm in diameter, positioned between the parietal and visceral pleura. Each pleural surface consists of a mesothelial cell monolayer overlying a layer of connective tissue. The blood supply to the parietal and visceral pleura from the systemic circulation allows for the normal flow of fluid down hydrostatic and oncotic pressure gradients into the pleural space according to Starling's law. Stoma are present in the parietal pleura, which allows the mesothelial cells to become continuous with lymphatic endothelial cells and permits normal physiological flow of fluid from the pleural space to the draining lymphatics. The capacity for lymphatic clearance of fluid is 20- to 30-fold greater than the usual rate of fluid influx. Normally, pleural fluid has a low protein concentration, usually less than 1.5 g/dL, and a cell count on the order of 1500 cells per microliter with a monocyte predominance.

Fluid accumulates in the pleural space, with alternations in membrane permeability, microvascular pressure gradients, and lymphatic drainage. Mechanisms for pleural fluid accumulation (Table 1) include an increase in hydrostatic pressure in the microvasculature (as seen in congestive heart failure), the leak of increased pulmonary interstitial fluid across the visceral pleura, a decrease in microvascular oncotic pressure (as seen in malnutrition with hypoalbuminemia), a decrease in pleural pressure (as seen in atelectasis), an increase in microvascular permeability (as seen with inflammation), impairment of lymphatic drainage (as seen with lymphatic obstruction by tumor cells), and movement of fluid from the peritoneum through the diaphragm (as seen with ascites). When the rate of fluid entry exceeds the capacity of lymphatic clearance, a pleural effusion results.

Radiographic Manifestations

Chest Radiography

The hallmark of the presence of a pleural effusion on the standard upright posteroanterior chest radiograph is blunting of the costophrenic angle. Typically, this implies the presence of 175–500 mL of pleural fluid. Additional signs include meniscus formation at the lateral

Table 1 Postulated Mechanisms for Pleural Fluid Accumulation

Increased production
Changes in microvasculature
Increased hydrostatic pressure
Decreased oncotic pressure
Increased permeability
Increased leak of interstitial fluid across visceral pleura
Decreased pleural pressure
Transdiaphragmatic movement of ascitic fluid
Decreased clearance
Impaired lymphatic drainage

rib margin and obliteration of the posterior costophrenic angle, obscuring the diaphragm on the lateral chest radiograph. Bilateral decubitus radiographs help to quantify effusion size. Fluid that exceeds 10 mm in diameter from the inside margin of the rib to the outside margin of the lung is amenable to thoracentesis. Decubitus films also determine the nature of the effusion—free-flowing or loculated—and allow evaluation of the underlying lung parenchyma.

Subpulmonic effusions can distort the contour or position of the hemidiaphragm without blunting the costophrenic angle. Diaphragmatic flattening, ipsilateral hemidiaphragm elevation, lateral displacement of the dome of the diaphragm, or widening of the gap between the left hemidiaphragm and gastric bubble to greater than 2 cm are clues to the presence of a subpulmonic effusion.

Various other findings on the chest radiograph can provide additional information in evaluation of the effusion. Fluid accumulation in the minor fissure can result in the appearance of a pseudotumor. Usually, the mediastinum shifts to the contralateral side away from a pleural effusion. Shifting toward the ipsilateral side implies a fixed mediastinum (by fibrosis or malignant infiltration), underlying pulmonary pathology (such as bronchial obstruction by tumor), or trapped lung (as in mesothelioma). Effusions without parenchymal pulmonary abnormalities are more likely to be either transudates or due to tuberculosis, pancreatitis, viral pleurisy, malignancy, collagen vascular disease (lupus or rheumatoid pleuritis), or pulmonary embolism. Bilateral effusions are typically associated with congestive heart failure. When seen with a normal cardiac silhouette, bilateral effusions can be due to malignancy, collagen vascular disease, esophageal rupture, nephrotic syndrome, or cirrhosis.

Ultrasound and Computed Tomography

Additional radiographic modalities are useful in the evaluation of pleural disease. Ultrasound localizes fluid loculations and provides imaging guidance for difficult thoracenteses. It is superior to computed tomography (CT) for distinguishing pleural fluid collections from pleural masses and thickening. CT is particularly useful to distinguish pleural from parenchymal abnormalities. Likewise, CT is helpful to evaluate the status of the underlying lung parenchyma for consolidation, mass, or lymphadenopathy.

Diagnostic Procedures

Thoracentesis

Diagnostic thoracentesis is performed to evaluate the etiology of a new pleural effusion and to look for complications of a parapneumonic effusion in the appropriate clinical context (for example, persistent fever with increasing effusion size). A 35- to 50-mL sample is sufficient for a thorough diagnostic evaluation. Patients with typical clinical features of congestive heart failure who have bilateral effusions can be safely observed without thoracentesis; however, any atypical feature, such as fever or pleurisy, justifies fluid evaluation. Watchful waiting of a parapneumonic effusion for 24 h or more is not advisable. In fact, delaying thoracentesis has been shown to lengthen hospital stay and increase costs. Clinical experience advocates performing initial thoracentesis at the time a new effusion is noted. Therapeutic thoracentesis is performed for the relief of dyspnea.

A bleeding diathesis is a contraindication to the procedure; however, thoracentesis is routinely performed safely when the International Normalized Ratio (INR) is less than 2.0 and the partial thromboplastin time (PTT) is less than twice the upper limit of normal.

Local cutaneous diseases such as pyoderma gangrenosum or herpes zoster are relative contraindications to the procedure.

Potential complications are numerous, but serious complications are rare. Pneumothorax occurs in up to 10% of patients, but only 2% require chest tube thoracostomy. Pneumothorax is less common when the procedure is performed by an experienced operator and when ultrasound guidance is utilized. Chest pain at the thoracentesis site is common and occurs in 20% of patients. Cough can occur; when it is severe and excessive, cough may necessitate termination of the procedure. Other potential complications include hypoxemia, vasovagal reaction, intercostal artery laceration (resulting in hemothorax), infection, and subdiaphragmatic placement (with hepatic, splenic, or renal laceration). Reexpansion pulmonary edema is reported to occur when volumes exceeding 1500 mL are rapidly withdrawn. Of note, larger volumes have been withdrawn without complications by maintaining pleural pressures greater than -20 cmH_2O.

Bedside thoracentesis is typically performed when more than 10 mm of free-flowing fluid is present on a lateral decubitus film. Ultrasound guidance is best reserved for sampling difficult loculated effusions or when technical difficulties—for example, a "dry tap"—have previously been encountered.

Pleural Biopsy

Pleural biopsy is usually performed as a next step, following thoracentesis, in the evaluation of an undiagnosed exudative effusion. It is especially helpful in the evaluation of lymphocytic exudates, most commonly due to tuberculosis and malignancy. The diagnostic yield in cytology-negative malignant effusions is approximately 60%. For tuberculous effusions, biopsy specimens reveal granulomas in 50–80% of cases and culture mycobacteria in 75%.

Contraindications to the procedure include coagulopathy, tenuous respiratory status, empyema, an uncooperative patient, dermatological disease, or the absence of pleural fluid. Risks of the procedure are similar to those of thoracentesis, with noted increases in incidence of pneumothorax (up to 15%), bleeding (less than 1%), and vasovagal reactions (1–5%). Another potential complication is tumor studding of the biopsy tract in the appropriate clinical setting.

Thoracoscopy

Some 10–25% of effusions remain undiagnosed after thoracentesis, fluid cytological analysis, and blind pleural biopsy. Medical thoracoscopy, performed by a pulmonologist utilizing local anesthesia and conscious sedation, has a diagnostic yield of 80–90%. For diagnosis of tuberculous and malignant disease, the sensitivity approaches 95%. Thoracoscopy allows for direct visualized biopsy sampling of the pleural surfaces. Although more invasive than thoracentesis or pleural biopsy, it has superior diagnostic and therapeutic capabilities, especially for the management of malignancy. Pleural metastases more commonly involve the visceral pleura and are usually positioned in the lower half of the thorax. Thus, the location of disease is difficult to access by blind pleural biopsy but is readily visualized by thoracoscopy. Therapeutic pleurodesis with talc insufflation can also be undertaken simultaneously.

Contraindications to thoracoscopy include trapped lung, uncontrollable cough, coagulopathy, severe hypoxemia, and severe cardiac disease. Complications encountered include postprocedure fever (15%), prolonged air leak (2–5%), hypoxemia (<2%), bleeding (1%), infection (<1%), metastatic studding of the access tract, and death (0.1%).

Fluid Analysis: Transudate vs. Exudate

Historically, the differential diagnosis of the origin of pleural effusions has relied upon the concepts of transudate and exudate (Table 2). Classically, transudative effusions occur without alterations in capillary permeability. Exudates are a result of increased capillary leak or diminished lymphatic clearance. Initially proposed in 1972, Light's criteria classify an exudate as any fluid with one of the following characteristics:

> Fluid/serum protein ratio > 0.5
> Fluid/serum lactate dehydrogenase (LDH) ratio > 0.6
> Absolute LDH $> 2/3$ upper limit of normal

A transudate meets none of these criteria. This classification scheme has a sensitivity and specificity of 98 and 82% respectively. A recent metanalysis confirms the use of the cutoff points for LDH and protein ratios used in Light's criteria but modifies the fluid LDH cutoff to 45% of the upper limit of normal. The analysis suggests that other test combinations have similar diagnostic accuracy to Light's criteria, specifically:

> Fluid LDH > 0.45 upper limit of normal
> Fluid cholesterol > 45 mg/dL

> Fluid protein > 2.9 g/dL
> Fluid LDH > 0.45 upper limit of normal
> Fluid cholesterol > 45 g/dL

No particular test combination is diagnostically superior. A strategy employing pleural fluid testing without serum testing has clear-cut cost savings and convenience benefits with equivalent diagnostic accuracy. A confounding factor encountered with the diagnostic separation of transudates and exudates is seen in diuretic-treated congestive heart failure, where the fluid protein can be elevated to the range of 3 to 4 g/dL. Fluid cholesterol has proven to be extremely helpful in classifying such effusions.

Common Tests

Common tests routinely performed on all effusions (Table 3) include protein, LDH, glucose, pH, cholesterol, and cell count with differential. Additional studies performed for exudative effusions include Gram stain and culture, KOH preparation and fungal culture, AFB smear and culture, and cytology. In the appropriate clinical context, additional studies may be useful including rheumatoid factor, antinuclear antibody (ANA), adenosine deaminase (ADA), amylase, triglycerides, and complement studies.

Test Interpretation

Insight can be gained by gross examination of the fluid. Bloody fluid in the absence of trauma implies neoplastic or pulmonary embolism etiologies. White fluid is usually associated with chylothorax, elevated levels of cholesterol, or empyema. Chocolate brown–colored, anchovy paste–consistency fluid is seen with transdiaphragmatic rupture of an amebic liver abscess. Black fluid is attributed to *Aspergillus* infection. Yellow-green fluid is described with rheumatoid pleural effusions. Viscous effusions are associated with the presence of pus (empyema) or hyaluronic acid (seen with mesothelioma). A fetid smell is associated with anaerobic infection, and an ammonia scent is associated with urinothorax.

A few drops of blood in a traumatic thoracentesis can turn the fluid sanguinous. Fresh traumatic effusions will clot. Because the fluid is defibrinated, old (hours to weeks)

Table 2   Causes of Pleural Effusions

Transudates

Congestive heart failure
Cirrhosis/ascites
Hypoalbuminemia
Peritoneal dialysis
Nephrotic syndrome
Urinothorax

Superior vena caval obstruction
Myxedema
Pulmonary embolism
Malignancy (secondary to atelectasis)
Atelectasis

Exudates

Infectious disease
  Parapneumonic
  Empyema
  Tuberculous
  Fungal infections
    Aspergillosis
    Blastomycosis
    Coccidioidomycosis
    Cryptococcosis
    Histoplasmosis
  Viral infections
  Actinomycosis
  Nocardiosis
  Parasitic infections
    Paragonimiasis
    Amebiasis
    Echinococcosis
Gastrointestinal disease
  Hepatitis
  Pancreatitis
  Pancreatic pseudocyst
  Abscess (subdiaphragmatic, intraabdominal, hepatic,
    splenic)
  Esophageal perforation
  Abdominal surgery
  Postsclerotherapy
  Enteral tube feeding misadventure
Collagen vascular disease
  Rheumatoid arthritis
  Systemic lupus erythematosus
  Wegener's granulomatosis
  Sjögren's syndrome
  Churg-Strauss vasculitis
  Familial Mediterranean fever
  Mixed connective tissue disease
  Immunoblastic lymphadenopathy

Malignancy
  Metastatic carcinoma
  Lymphoma
  Mesothelioma
Lymphatic disease
  Chylothorax
  Yellow nail syndrome
  Lymphangiomyomatosis
Other
  Pulmonary embolism
  Postcardiac injury syndrome
  Sarcoidosis
  Benign asbestos pleural effusion
  Uremia
  Meigs' syndrome
  Radiation therapy
  Central venous line malposition
  Trapped lung
  Ovarian hyperstimulation syn-
    drome
  Postpartum
  Postthoracotomy
  Hemothorax
  Chylothorax
Drugs
  Nitrofurantoin
  Amiodarone
  Drug-induced lupus
  Dantrolene
  Methysergide
  Procarbazine
  Bromocriptine
  Minoxidil
  Bleomycin
  Methotrexate
  Mitomycin

Table 3 Common Pleural
Fluid Tests

All effusions
Protein
Lactate dehydrogenase
pH
Cholesterol
Cell count with differential
Exudative effusions
Gram stain and culture
KOH preparation
Fungal culture
AFB smear and culture
Cytology

hemorrhagic effusions should not clot. Elevation of the red blood cell (RBC) count to greater than $100,000/mm^3$ is seen with trauma, neoplasm, pulmonary embolism or infarction, benign asbestos pleural effusion, and the postcardiac injury syndrome. When the hematocrit exceeds 50% of the blood value, hemothorax is diagnosed and chest tube thoracostomy should be considered.

The absolute white blood cell (WBC) count is usually of limited value. Transudative effusions typically have an absolute count below $1000/mm^3$ with a monocyte predominance. Chronic exudative effusions, such as malignant and tuberculous effusions, usually have a cell count in the range of $5000/mm^3$. A cell count greater than $10,000/mm^3$ implies a significant degree of inflammation.

The WBC differential can provide clues toward or away from various diagnoses. Acute processes are usually neutrophil-predominant. Lymphocyte-predominance implies tuberculous or malignant effusions in 94% of cases. Monocyte predominance is seen with any of the transudates as well as with the chronic exudative effusions. Eosinophilia (> 10%) implies the presence of blood (hemothorax, pulmonary embolism, or infarction) or air (pneumothorax, prior thoracentesis) in the pleural space. It is also seen with parasitic and fungal infections, drug-induced effusions, benign asbestos pleural effusion, and Churg-Strauss vasculitis. It is relatively rare with tuberculosis and extremely uncommon with malignant effusions. The presence of mesothelial cells is distinctly uncommon in tuberculous pleuritis. Basophilia (>10%) implies leukemic involvement of the pleura, and the presence of many plasma cells implies pleural involvement by multiple myeloma.

Besides their utility in separating transudates from exudates, specific routine tests provide additional insight for the diagnosis, management, and course of various pleural diseases. Fluid protein can be elevated in as many as 20% of patients with congestive heart failure usually associated with diuresis. When markedly elevated (greater than 7 g/dL), this implies a paraproteinemia such as Waldenstrom's macroglobulinemia or multiple myeloma. The fluid LDH reflects the degree of inflammation; when rising on serial thoracentesis, it implies progressive inflammation. The pleural fluid glucose is usually equivalent to the serum value. When it is less than 60 mg/dL or less than 50% of the serum value, this implies diminished transport into the pleural fluid or increased consumption by bacteria, malignant cells, or neutrophils. The differential diagnosis should focus on rheumatoid effusion, empyema, parapneumonic effusion, malignant effusion, tuberculous effusion, lupus pleuritis, and esophageal rupture. Marked depression in the fluid glucose (0–30 mg/dL) is seen in rheumatoid effusions, empyema, and rarely in bulky tumor involvement of the pleura. Pleural fluid pH normally exceeds that of blood due to active bicarbonate transport into the pleural space. A pH below 7.3 is seen in esophageal rupture (100%), empyema (95%), tuberculous effusion (20%), rheumatoid effusion (85%), lupus pleuritis (20%), malignant effusion (30%), and systemic acidosis. In parapneumonic effusions, falling pH serves as a marker for complications necessitating chest tube placement. In malignant effusions, a low pH (<7.3) is associated with shorter survival (2 compared with 10 months), increased diagnostic yield for cytology and pleural biopsy, and poor response to conventional sclerotherapy.

Less common tests can likewise be of value. In the evaluation of autoimmune diseases, the initial presentation of disease, although uncommon, may be limited to the pleura. A rheumatoid factor > 1:320 or fluid-to-serum ratio > 1 suggests rheumatoid pleural effusion. An ANA > 1:160 or fluid to serum ratio > 1 likewise suggests lupus pleuritis. Complement levels are low in both these disorders. Visualization of LE cells is considered diagnostic for lupus. Pleural fluid amylase is normally low. When it is greater than the serum value or upper limit of normal, this implies one of the following disorders: pancreatitis, pancreatic pseudocyst, esophageal rupture, ruptured ectopic pregnancy, or malignancy (elevated in 10–14%). Elevated triglycerides (>110 mg/dL) are seen with chylous effusions. Adenosine deaminase (ADA) levels greater than 50 IU/L have been seen in tuberculous, rheumatoid, empyema, and lymphoma effusions.

Transudative Effusions

Congestive Heart Failure

Congestive heart failure (CHF) is the most common cause of all pleural effusions. Likewise, effusions are common with heart failure occurring in 60–70% of patients. The location is most commonly bilateral (73–88%), followed by right-sided (8–19%) and left-sided (4–9%). Some 25% of patients with unilateral effusions clinically attributable to CHF have concomitant pneumonia or pulmonary embolism.

The presence of pleural effusions in heart failure is specifically related to left ventricular dysfunction. As expected, the pulmonary capillary wedge pressure is significantly greater in heart failure patients with effusions than in those without. Effusions are not seen in patients with isolated right ventricular dysfunction or pulmonary hypertension. As pressure in the alveolar capillaries rises in heart failure, interstitial edema ensues. This edema fluid traverses across the visceral pleura and into the pleural space. The influence of elevated systemic venous pressure on lymphatic clearance has been postulated to play a confounding role in fluid development.

Clinically, pleural effusions in patients with CHF usually accompany other signs and symptoms associated with CHF. These include dyspnea on exertion, paroxysmal nocturnal dyspnea, orthopnea, peripheral edema, jugular venous distension, pulmonary rales, and an S3 gallop.

Chemical analysis of the fluid typically reveals a transudate. Long-standing effusions from heart failure and acute diuresis can result in a rise in fluid protein and/or LDH, as previously noted.

Patients with bilateral effusions and the accompanying physical findings of left ventricular dysfunction can safely be observed without thoracentesis and fluid evaluation.

However, failure of the effusion to respond to intensive heart failure management should prompt evaluation by thoracentesis. Size discrepancy between sides of an effusion and unilateral positioning are indications for thoracentesis among CHF patients. Likewise, associated pleuritic chest pain or fever, uncommon in heart failure, should prompt fluid evaluation. Finally, in the clinical setting of CHF, the finding of bilateral effusions without concomitant cardiomegaly should incite thoracentesis, as only 4% of these cases are due to CHF alone.

Therapy for the effusion in these cases is aimed at treatment of the underlying disorder. For patients with refractory effusions, pleuroperitoneal shunting and pleurodesis may be utilized.

Cirrhosis

Pleural effusions occur in 6% of patients with cirrhosis and ascites. Effusions solely associated with cirrhosis and hypoalbuminemia without the presence of ascites are distinctly uncommon ($<$1%). Such effusions are usually large and most commonly right-sided (67%). Left-sided and bilateral effusions are seen less commonly (16 and 17%, respectively). The proposed mechanism for fluid accumulation is the flow of fluid across diaphragmatic defects into the lower-pressure pleural space. Thoracentesis is recommended to confirm the diagnosis. Of note, the fluid present in the pleural space can become infected without concomitant spontaneous bacterial peritonitis. Antibiotic therapy in this specific instance is usually sufficient without the need for chest tube thoracostomy. The therapeutic approach to the patient with a pleural effusion due to liver disease is aimed at treatment of the underlying disorder with sodium restriction, furosemide, and spironolactone administration. In patients with refractory effusions despite intensive medical management, peritoneal to jugular venous shunting, pleurodesis, and thoracotomy with repair of diaphragmatic leaks may also be utilized.

Other Causes

Other less common causes of transudative effusions include peritoneal dialysis, nephrotic syndrome, superior vena caval (SVC) obstruction, urinothorax, myxedema, and pulmonary embolism.

Some 2–10% of patients being treated with continuous ambulatory peritoneal dialysis (CAPD) develop pleural effusions. In this instance, the effusion is usually right-sided (90%), occurs within 30 days of starting peritoneal dialysis (50%), has a protein $<$ 1 g/dL, a low LDH, and a glucose value between that of the dialysate and serum. The mechanism is similar to that seen with hepatic hydrothorax. Treatment options include a change to hemodialysis, small-volume increased-frequency peritoneal dialysis, pleurodesis, and surgical closure of the pleuroperitoneal diaphragmatic defects.

Patients with nephrotic syndrome (20%) are prone to the development of pleural effusions. These effusions are most commonly bilateral and subpulmonic. The mechanism is most likely due to diminished plasma oncotic pressure. Of note, patients with nephrotic syndrome are at increased risk for pulmonary embolism, which occurs in 22%.

Obstruction of the superior vena cava (SVC) has rarely been associated with pleural fluid accumulation. An important diagnostic consideration includes pleural metastatic involvement by malignancy.

Urine in the pleural space—urinothorax—arises from retroperitoneal passage associated with ureteral obstruction. The pleural fluid characteristically has a low pH, low glucose, ratio of fluid to serum creatinine $>$ 1, and ammonia smell. In these cases, the effusion usually resolves spontaneously with relief of the underlying obstruction.

Pleural effusions among patients with myxedema occur in 25–50% of cases and can be transudative or exudative in nature. However, only 3% of these are without a concomitant disease process that can explain the source of the effusion.

Finally, it is noteworthy that 20% of patients with pulmonary embolism and pleural effusion will have a transudative rather than an exudative effusion.

Exudative Effusions

Infectious Causes

Parapneumonic Effusions and Empyema.   Parapneumonic effusions are those that are associated with bacterial pneumonia or lung abscess. They are the most common cause of exudative effusions in the United States. In fact, 40% of pneumonia cases have an associated pleural effusion. Characteristically, uncomplicated parapneumonic effusions have a pH > 7.30, glucose > 60 mg/dL, and LDH < 1000 IU/L. The fluid leukocyte count usually exceeds 10,000/mm^3. When antibiotic therapy is begun at this stage, the effusion should resolve spontaneously.

Uncomplicated parapneumonic effusions fall at one end of the spectrum of disease, which includes complicated parapneumonic effusions and empyema. In pneumonia, parenchymal infection results in neutrophil attachment to the pulmonary capillary endothelium. This leads to endothelial cell injury and an increase in capillary permeability. As permeability rises, interstitial fluid increases. Subsequently, fluid seeps across the visceral pleura and into the pleural space. This is the exudative stage of parapneumonic effusions. The fluid at this stage is characterized by a neutrophil predominance, an elevated protein, and a normal pH and glucose.

Without treatment, the process progresses to the fibrinopurulent stage. This is characterized by a further influx of neutrophils and protein, including clotting factors. There is an associated loss of the normal fibrinolytic activity in the pleural space by inflammatory injury. Cellular debris accumulates. Eventually, the fluid will become infected as bacterial entry ensues. LDH levels rise and fluid pH and glucose fall. The decline in fluid glucose is thought to be due to a net increase in cellular glycolysis from bacterial metabolism and neutrophil phagocytosis. The activity of the clotting factors turns the fluid into a gelatinous coagulum, which provides a meshwork for fibroblast proliferation and fibrin deposition. As a result, there is membrane formation and the effusion becomes loculated.

The final stage is characterized by organization. Fibroblasts grow from both pleural surfaces into the exudative fluid, eventually encasing the lung and creating the so-called pleural peel.

Clinically, fever, pleuritic chest pain, and rigors may be present in acute infections. With subacute presentations, patients may have weight loss, anemia, and a peripheral blood leukocytosis. The clinical presentation of an uncomplicated parapneumonic effusion may be identical to that of empyema. Hence, the examination of pleural fluid is of critical importance. Mortality from empyema in the elderly or in those with a severe underlying illness approaches 40–70%. As can be expected, in the young and healthy, mortality is significantly lower and on the order of 2–15%.

Empyema is defined as the presence of pus in the pleural space, bacteria on a fluid Gram stain, or bacterial growth from fluid culture. It clearly warrants immediate drainage. Consensus regarding criteria to define a complicated parapneumonic effusion is lacking. There is general agreement that, in the absence of any criteria defining empyema, a pleural fluid pH < 7.0, glucose < 40 mg/dL, and LDH > 1000 IU/L constitutes a complicated parapneumonic effusion. Antibiotics alone will be insufficient treatment, and drainage with a large-bore (28 Fr or greater) chest tube is necessary. Some authors advocate drainage of such effusions at pH levels below 7.10 or 7.20. Of note, some of these patients with abnormal fluid chemistries will resolve their effusions with antibiotic treatment alone. On the other hand, delayed chest tube drainage has been associated with a fivefold rise in mortality. Generally, patients who fall in the border zone between uncomplicated and complicated parapneumonic effusions should have serial thoracentesis at 12–24 h with worsening indices indicative of the need for chest tube thoracostomy. Watchful waiting should be carefully weighed against the potential for increased morbidity and mortality.

Empyema arises from a contiguous parenchymal source in the manner described in a majority of cases. Other potential etiologies include as a postoperative complication of thoracic surgery, thoracentesis, or chest tube placement; posttraumatic injury; infection of a sterile effusion; or from contiguous extension of an extrapulmonary source of infection. The microbiology of empyema focuses on anaerobes such as *Bacteroides, Fusobacterium, Peptostreptococcus* species, *Staphylococcus aureus*, gram-negative aerobes, and *Streptococcus pneumoniae*. Anaerobic infections are more common among patients with alcoholism, gingivitis, and those prone to unconsciousness (seizure, stroke, etc.).

Inadequate drainage, insufficient response to drainage, or the progressive development of loculations should prompt aggressive management with early imaging and intervention. Management options include thrombolytic therapy, additional chest tube placement, or surgical intervention. Intrapleural installation of thrombolytics such as streptokinase (250,000 U in 100 mL normal saline) or urokinase (100,000 U in 100 mL normal saline) daily for 10–14 days has been associated with improved drainage and successful lysis of fibrinous loculations. There is little risk of any effect on systemic coagulation parameters; however, use of streptokinase has been associated with a specific immunoglobulin G antistreptokinase antibody response, which persists for as long as 4 years. Additional chest tube placement and radiography-guided percutaneous ''pigtail'' catheter placement have been reported to carry a 60–90% success rate. Generally, many authors advocate surgical intervention when multiple loculated fluid collections are present. Nonsurgical therapy has a 27% success rate in this population, whereas surgical methods have a 93% success rate.

Surgical options include decortication and open drainage. Decortication is the process by which the fibrous tissue and empyema are removed from the visceral pleura. It can be accomplished by video-assisted thoracic surgery (VATS) but may necessitate full thoracotomy. Decortication carries a 95% success rate without a substantial change in mortality and with minimal increases in morbidity in selected patients. When the patient is unable to tolerate decortication, open drainage procedures are undertaken. In one approach, ribs are resected with insertion of short, large-bore empyema tubes for irrigation and drainage. The tubes are left open and the wound is dressed with an ostomy bag to collect draining fluid. Another method is the Eloesser flap procedure, which consists of the creation of an open drainage tract by placement of a skin and muscle flap to line the tract between the pleural space and surface of the chest wall after rib resection. Both open drainage procedures have been associated with complete healing within a 6-month period.

Tuberculous Effusions. Tuberculous pleural effusions are relatively rare, comprising approximately 1000 cases annually in the United States. Typically, tuberculous effusion presents as an acute illness (60%) characterized by cough (92%), pleuritic chest pain (75%), and fever (86%). Patients may have other associated symptoms including sweats, chills, dyspnea, weakness, and weight loss. Symptom onset may also occur insidiously. Tuberculous involvement of the pleura is thought to arise from the rupture of acaseous subpleural focus of infection which sets off a delayed hypersensitivity response. PPD skin test is reportedly negative in one-third of patients; however, most convert to PPD-positive status when retested at 4 to 6 weeks unless there is evidence of underlying immunosuppression. Radiographic manifestations range from effusions with infiltrates to those without.

Examination of the fluid reveals a lymphocyte-predominant exudate. When the differential exceeds 90% lymphocytes, the likelihood of tuberculous effusion is increased. Mesothelial cells and eosinophils are uncommon. Fluid pH and glucose may be low in as many as 20% of cases. LDH is usually mildly elevated to the 700 IU/L range. The fluid protein is usually greater than 5 g/dL. An elevated ADA is suggestive of tuberculosis, but the specificity of this test is questionable. Overall, fluid acid-fast (AFB) smear and culture are relatively poor detectors of disease. The combination of biopsy and fluid cultures with biopsy histology yields the diagnosis in 90% of cases.

Untreated tuberculous effusions will spontaneously resolve over 3–6 months. However, in 65% of cases, active tuberculosis will recur within 5 years. Therefore, the goals of treatment are to relieve symptoms, to prevent subsequent active tuberculous disease, and to prevent development of fibrothorax. Standard antituberculous therapy is given for 6 months. Serial thoracentesis has not been demonstrated to improve outcome as measured by pulmonary function, pleural thickening, or symptomatology. Historically, steroid therapy was reported to hasten resolution of symptoms and of the effusion and to prevent pleural fibrosis. A recent double-blinded, placebo-controlled, randomized clinical trial found no difference between steroid-treated and untreated groups for resolution of subjective symptoms, pleural thickening, or restrictive ventilatory abnormalities. Rarely, tuberculous effusions are complicated by tuberculous empyema or bronchopleural fistula formation, both of which necessitate chest tube thoracostomy.

Pleural effusions have also been described in 5% of patients with atypical mycobacterial disease due to *Mycobacterium kansasii* or *Mycobacterium avium-intracellulare*. Such effusions are usually small to moderate in size and one characteristically lymphocytic exudates. Isolated pleural involvement without other evidence of disease is distinctly uncommon, and an alternative cause should be sought.

Other Causes—Fungal, Viral, and Parasitic Diseases.   A variety of other infectious diseases can result in pleural effusions, including fungal and viral infections, *Actinomycetes* infections, and parasitic infestations.

Aspergillosis

Pleural effusions due to *Aspergillus* species are predominantly due to *Aspergillus fumigatus*. Pleural involvement is seen in a variety of circumstances: as a complication of thoracic surgery (lobectomy or pneumonectomy) with an associated bronchopleural fistula, following artificial pneumothorax as a treatment for tuberculosis, in an immunocompromised host with disseminated aspergillosis, and in association with allergic bronchopulmonary aspergillosis (ABPA). The fluid may be black in appearance as a result of the presence of black-pigmented spores and may contain calcium oxalate crystals. Culture of *Aspergillus* from the pleural fluid confirms the diagnosis. Serum *Aspergillus* precipitins are usually positive in these instances, but their significance has been questioned. Treatment involves surgical resection of the infected pleura accompanied by systemic antifungal therapy with parenteral amphotericin B. Debilitated patients who are unlikely to tolerate thoracotomy may benefit from chest tube placement and local daily irrigation of the pleural space with 25 mg amphotericin B along with systemic therapy.

Blastomycosis

Patients with pleural involvement with *Blastomyces dermatitidis*, seen in 10% of cases, usually present with cough, fever, pleuritic chest pain, and a pulmonary infiltrate. Erythema nodosum may be seen as an associated finding. The fluid is typically a neutrophilic or lymphocytic exudate. Fluid smears and culture may demonstrate broad-based budding yeast forms. Pleural biopsy reveals noncaseating granulomas. Treatment is reserved for chronic or disseminated disease and utilizes oral itraconazole or intravenous amphotericin. A normal host should need no specific therapy, and the pleural effusion should resolve without treatment.

Coccidioidomycosis

Endemic to the southwestern United States, *Coccidioides immitis* infection is accompanied by pleural involvement in 7% of cases with primary disease. The typical presentation includes fever and pleuritic chest pain. Over half of patients have concomitant pulmonary radiographic infiltrates and half of patients have an associated erythema nodosum or erythema multiforme. Chronic cavitary pulmonary disease acutely ruptures into the pleural space and results in an associated hydropneumothorax in 1–5% of cases. Such patients become acutely ill, with the rapid onset of signs of systemic toxicity and sepsis. The pleural effusion is typically a small, left-sided exudate with lymphocytic predominance. Fluid eosinophilia is distinctly uncommon, while peripheral eosinophilia is seen in up to one-third of patients. Diagnosis is made rarely by positive fluid smear. Fluid and biopsy culture and serum complement fixation titers greater than 1:16 are more commonly diagnostic.

Cryptococcosis

Some 25% of patients with pulmonary infection with *Cryptococcus neoformans* will have an associated pleural effusion. They may present with pleuritic chest pain or be asymptomatic. Pleural involvement is usually associated with an underlying immunosuppressive illness or therapy. The effusion is typically unilateral and a lymphocytic exudate. Fluid culture is positive in less than 50% of cases. Pleural biopsy culture is frequently necessary to confirm the diagnosis. Normal hosts without evidence of dissemination should resolve their effusion over a period of weeks without the need for antifungal therapy. Intravenous amphotericin B and 5-flucytosine are reserved for immunocompromised hosts; those with evidence of disseminated disease, such as the presence of cryptococcal antigen in the serum or cerebrospinal fluid; and patients who have a progressive increase in size of the effusion over time.

Histoplasmosis

Histoplasma capsulatum is a fungus endemic to the Mississippi and Ohio River valleys. Pleural effusion is uncommon and occurs in less than 1% of cases. Typically, the effusion is ipsilateral to the parenchymal infiltrate and is characteristically a lymphocytic exudate. Its presentation is usually that of a subacute illness with a low-grade fever and pleuritic chest pain. The organism can be cultured from fluid, sputum, and biopsy materials. Additional studies of benefit include complement fixation titers greater than 1:16 and the presence of an H band on fungal gel immunodiffusion. Classically, the effusion will resolve spontaneously over a period of weeks without specific therapy.

Actinomycetes

Classically grouped with fungal infections because of their clinical presentation, infections due to the actinomyces bacteria include actinomycosis and nocardiosis. *Actinomyces israelii* is an endogenous gram-positive anaerobe found in infected gingiva, tonsils, and dental abscesses. Some 75% of pulmonary infections involve the pleura, usually by direct extension from the pulmonary parenchyma or from mediastinal involvement due to esophageal disease. The effusion presents as a neutrophil- or lymphocyte-predominant exudate. Identification of organisms in the pleural fluid or of characteristic sulfur granules comprising a conglomeration of the filamentous organisms with clubbed peripheral radiations is diagnostic for disease. However, the presence of actinomyces in sputum or bronchoalveolar lavage fluid without evidence of invasive disease carries no clinical significance. Characteristically, the radiographic manifestations of parenchymal consolidation, pleural effusion, and periosteal rib proliferation are indicative of the disease. Treatment is with chest tube drainage and long-term high-dose penicillin.

Effusions may occur with the partially acid-fast aerobic organism *Nocardia asteroides*. They are found in 15 to 50% of patients with pulmonary nocardiosis and are usually associated with a clinical picture of disseminated disease. Associated symptoms include purulent sputum production, shortness of breath, pleuritic chest pain, hemoptysis, anorexia, and weight loss. The organism is slow-growing and may require up to 2 weeks for identification. Contrary to actinomycosis, the demonstration of *Nocardia* is diagnostic. Primary treatment includes sulfonamide antibiotics.

Viral Infections

Numerous viral infections have been associated with pleural effusions. Effusions are usually small in size and accompany parenchymal infiltrates. Of note, viral pleurisy without radiographic infiltrates has been shown to produce pleural effusions. Viral agents implicated in pleural effusion formation include Hepatitis A, B, and C, Epstein Barr virus (EBV), Respiratory Syncytial virus (RSV), Influenza, Adenovirus, Measles, Cytomegalovirus, Herpes Simplex virus, Hantavirus, and Lassa Fever virus. Effusions typically resolve with time.

Q Fever

10% of cases of Q fever, the rickettsial disease due to Coxiella burnetii infection, have an associated pleural effusion.

Amebiasis

Parasitic infestation with Entamoeba histolytica can result in pleural effusions. Transdiaphragmatic rupture of an amebic liver abscess will result in an acute illness which can rapidly progress to the systemic inflammatory response syndrome (SIRS). Such effusions are classically described as anchovy paste or chocolate brown in appearance. More commonly, diaphragmatic irritation from an underlying abscess results in a right-sided sympathetic effusion. In addition to microscopic analysis, gel diffusion and hemagglutination serology are positive in greater than 98% of cases. Treatment is with Metronidazole and possibly Dihydroemetine. A ruptured abscess should be treated with large bore chest tube drainage.

Paragonimiasis

Endemic to Southeast Asia, effusions due to *Paragonimus westermani*, the lung fluke, can be seen in Indochinese immigrants. Some 48% of infected patients have pleural effusions, and half of these have associated radiographic infiltrates. The disease typically presents as a subacute to chronic illness. Analysis of the fluid reveals a pH < 7.10, glucose < 10 mg/dL, LDH > 1000 IU/L, and an eosinophilia. This constellation of parameters is seen in only one other condition—Churg-Strauss vasculitis. Complement fixation antibody titers greater than 1:64 are highly suggestive of the disease. Demonstration of parasite eggs is diagnostic, but they are rarely found in effusion fluid. Treatment is with the antiparasitic agent praziquantel.

Echinococcosis

Echinococcus granulosus, the dog or wolf tapeworm, can produce pleural effusion by transdiaphragmatic rupture of a liver or splenic hydatid cyst, rupture of a pulmonary hydatid cyst, involvement of the pleura by a primary pleural cyst, and by diaphragmatic irritation resulting in a sympathetic effusion. Fortunately, less than 5% of hydatid cysts rupture. When rupture occurs, it usually presents as an acute illness with shock. Demonstration in pleural fluid of the classic scolices with hooklets is diagnostic. Treatment involves thoracotomy with closure of any fistula, cyst excision, and systemic antiparasitic therapy with mebendazole or albendazole.

Malignancy

Some 40% of exudative pleural effusions are due to malignancy. Malignant effusions are the most common cause of exudates in the elderly. When found, they imply a poor prognosis with a limited survival. Malignant effusions usually represent metastatic disease and are most commonly due to lung or breast cancer (30% and 25%, respectively). Of patients with bronchogenic carcinoma, 15% will develop pleural effusions, with the greatest portion associated with adenocarcinoma. Breast cancer is the leading cause of malignant effusions among women. As many as 50% of women with disseminated breast cancer will have an associated pleural effusion. In breast cancer, the effusion typically represents disseminated or recurrent disease. Lymphoma is responsible for 20% of malignant effusions: 16% of Hodgkin's disease patients and the majority of patients with non-Hodgkin's lymphoma will have pleural effusions. Lymphoma and mesothelioma-associated effusions are discussed separately. The remaining malignant effusions are associated with ovarian cancer, gastric cancer, tumor from an unknown primary site, other gastrointestinal cancers, other urogenital neoplasms, and melanoma. As many as 50% of effusions in patients with malignancies are due to reasons other than direct tumor involvement of the pleura, the so-called paramalignant effusions. Mechanisms for these effusions include reduced pleural pressures associated with bronchial obstruction, parapneumonic effusions from postobstructive pneumonia, hypoalbuminemia associated with malnutrition or cachexia, pulmonary embolism, or sequelae of radiation or chemotherapy. In lung cancer, such ''paramalignant effusions'' do not imply metastatic or class T4 disease and may be excluded as a staging element according to the 1997 American Joint Committee on Cancer (AJCC) guidelines. Thus, correct diagnosis of the cause of pleural effusions in malignancy is of critical importance.

Direct tumor involvement affects the visceral pleura in 100% and the parietal pleura in 60% of cases. With lung cancer, the effusion is typically located ipsilateral to the primary disease site. With the other malignancies, there is no side predilection for the effu-

Table 4   Treatment Options
for Malignant Pleural Effusions

Intermittent thoracentesis
Radiation therapy
Chemotherapy
Pleuroperitoneal shunt
Chest tube drainage
Drainage catheter
Pleurodesis
    Talc slurry
    Bleomycin
    Tetracycline
    Thoracoscopic talc insufflation
    Surgical
Pleurectomy

---

sion. Malignant effusions are usually moderate to large in size and associated with dyspnea in half of the cases and with dull, aching chest pain in 25%. Approximately 10% of these effusions will be transudates; an additional 20% will have a low ratio of fluid to serum protein. Most effusions that meet LDH criteria but fail protein criteria for exudates are due to malignancy. The fluid shows a lymphocyte predominance in over half the cases. Eosinophilia is rare. Half of patients will have RBC counts exceeding 100,000/mm^3. Low pH ($<$7.3) and glucose ($<$60 mg/dL) are found in one-fifth of cases and are associated with a large tumor burden, shortened survival time, and failed pleurodesis.

The diagnostic strategy employed in evaluating an effusion with a high index of suspicion for malignancy, as with lymphocytic exudates, is based on the yield and availability of the procedures involved. Typically, pleural fluid cytology is the first step in the evaluation process. Cytology is positive in 66% of cases, but the yield depends largely on the skill and experience of the cytopathologist. The optimal volume of fluid needed for cytological analysis is no greater than 100 mL. Blind pleural biopsy is positive in 45% of cases; when performed in combination with pleural fluid cytology, the diagnostic yield for the two procedures is increased to 73%. Further repeated biopsies increase the overall yield by only 2–4%. Flow cytometry for aneuploidy and immunohistochemical staining for tumor markers may define tumor origin or assist in the diagnosis of indistinct cells. In the remaining undiagnosed patients, medical thoracoscopy is diagnostic in 96% of cases. The negative predictive value of thoracoscopy for malignant pleural disease is 93%.

The majority of malignant effusions carry an ominous prognosis with limited survival. Treatment (Table 4) after an adequate diagnostic evaluation and staging is aimed at palliation. In formulating palliative therapy, the clinician should consider the patient's wishes, underlying performance status, potential for relief of symptoms, and overall prognosis. The best option for severely debilitated patients may be serial outpatient thoracentesis. When the effusion is though to be secondary to hilar lymphatic obstruction, postobstructive pneumonia, or responsive disease—such as small cell carcinoma or lymphoma—radiation or chemotherapy may be of value. Pleuroperitoneal shunting is rarely utilized because it requires daily activation by the patient and placement under general anesthesia; moreover, it is prone to complications, including site infection and shunt obstruction

(25%). Chest tube drainage is successful in as many as 50% of patients; however, it necessitates an inpatient stay.

Pleurodesis is the process by which the pleural space is obliterated by adherence of the parietal and visceral pleural surfaces. Mediastinal shift toward the side of the effusion implies trapped lung, and such patients are often unlikely to benefit from pleurodesis. A variety of agents have been utilized, including tetracycline, bleomycin, and talc. Historically, tetracycline was successful in 70–80% of cases, but it is no longer available in the parenteral form. Bleomycin is successful in 54–84% of cases, but it is expensive and has associated systemic side effects. Asbestos-free talc, a trilayered magnesium sheet silicate, has a 91% success rate. It can be administered as a slurry (81% success) or by direct thoracoscopic insufflation (greater than 90% success). The procedure necessitates chest tube placement and inpatient observation until the output of pleural fluid diminishes. There is currently no definitive standard for the dose utilized (usually 2–6 g), method of sterilization, or method of optimal application. Potential complications associated with talc pleurodesis include fever, pain, bleeding, minor wound infection, pneumothorax following chest tube removal, empyema, cardiac failure, myocardial infarction, and acute respiratory distress syndrome (ARDS). The increased incidence of cancer in talc miners, although thought to be related to asbestos, may limit its utility for nonmalignant conditions. Surgical pleurodesis and pleurectomy necessitate general anesthesia and are associated with greater morbidity and mortality.

Lymphoma.   Lymphomatous pleural effusions are usually present at the time of diagnosis of the malignancy and serve as a poor prognostic sign. As noted, they are common in non-Hodgkin's lymphoma and rare in Hodgkin's disease. Effusions are usually associated with other indicative radiographic manifestations. The postulated mechanisms for fluid accumulation include pleural infiltration by lymphoma cells and obstruction of the lymphatics or the thoracic duct. The effusion is usually unilateral and most commonly exudative, but bilateral, bloody, chylous, and even transudative effusions are seen. The WBC differential reveals a lymphocytic predominance. Symptoms include dyspnea (63%), orthopnea (14%), cough (23%), and chest pain (15%). Some 20% of patients will be asymptomatic.

Malignant Mesothelioma.   Asbestos exposure, especially to the crocidolite fiber, is the major risk factor for development of malignant mesothelioma. Most patients present with pleural effusions. Symptoms at the time of presentation include nonpleuritic chest pain, shortness of breath, weight loss, and a dry, hacking cough. Most effusions are large in size and exudates. The hyaluronic acid level is usually elevated, but this is a nonspecific finding. Some 70% of effusions secondary to malignant mesothelioma have a low fluid pH. Diagnosis is typically challenging. Fluid cytology is positive in 25% of cases, but the cells are difficult to distinguish from adenocarcinoma. Pleural biopsy is diagnostic in one-fifth of cases. Thoracoscopy and thoracotomy are diagnostic in 67–90% of cases. Immunohistochemistry and electron microscopy aid in differentiation of the disease from adenocarcinoma. Overall, the disease carries a poor prognosis, with a median survival of 18 months. Treatment options are usually unsuccessful.

Benign Fibrous Mesothelioma.   Pleural effusions are seen in 10% of cases of benign fibrous mesothelioma. The disease is not associated with asbestos exposure and carries a good prognosis. Symptoms typically include cough (50%), chest pain, dyspnea (40%), and fever (25%). The effusion may be asymptomatic. Systemic hypoglycemia (4%) and hypertrophic pulmonary osteoarthropathy (20%) are associated findings.

Collagen Vascular Disease

Pleural effusions are seen in association with a variety of rheumatologic and autoimmune disease. Most commonly, they are seen in association with rheumatoid arthritis and systemic lupus erythematosus.

Rheumatoid Effusions.   Pleural effusion is the most common intrathoracic manifestation of rheumatoid arthritis and is seen in 5% of patients. Characteristically, the patient with rheumatoid effusion is a male, above 35 years of age, with a history of long-standing articular disease. The effusion can present asymptomatically or with varied symptoms such as intermittent chest pain and symptoms mimicking pneumonia. Likewise, the time course of symptoms may be transient, chronic, or relapsing. Pulmonary rheumatoid nodules and interstitial lung disease are seen in 30% of these patients, and cutaneous rheumatoid nodules are seen in 80%. The fluid characteristically has a yellow-green color and is a neutrophil- or monocyte-predominant exudate. Some 80% of patients have a low pH (<7.0) and glucose (<30 mg/dL). An elevated LDH (>1000 U/L), elevated cholesterol, and low complement levels are seen. The fluid rheumatoid factor is usually greater than 1:320 or greater than the serum value. Cytological analysis reveals multinucleated or elongated macrophages superimposed on a background of necrotic debris. Rheumatoid pleuritis can be accompanied by empyema, pneumothorax (6% of cases), and bronchopleural fistula. The usual course is resolution of the effusion over 1 or more months. Some patients will have a protracted course, with the development of pleural thickening and trapped lung. Rheumatoid effusions will typically respond to corticosteroids and other immunosuppressive agents.

Lupus Pleuritis.   Some 15–45% of patients with systemic lupus erythematosus (SLE) will have pleural effusions. In as many as 5%, it will be the isolated initial manifestation of the disease. Patients are more commonly women and are usually symptomatic, with cough, fever, pleuritic chest pain, and dyspnea. The characteristic radiographic appearance is of small to moderately sized bilateral effusions usually associated with parenchymal infiltrates. The fluid is characteristically an exudate with a neutrophil or monocyte predominance, depending upon the acuity of disease. Usually, the fluid chemistries reveal an LDH < 500 IU/L, pH > 7.30, glucose > 60 mg/dL, and low complement studies. The presence of LE cells is diagnostic, and a fluid ANA titer > 1:160 or greater than the serum value are suggestive but not pathognomonic for disease. Some 5% of patients are seronegative for ANA. Drug-induced lupus has been described with a number of agents (Table 5). Typically, following cessation of the offending agent, the effusion resolves within days to months, but the ANA may persist. Characteristically, chemical analysis is similar to that seen with primary lupus except that complement levels are usually normal. Patients with lupus are at risk for other disorders that can result in pleural effusion formation, including nephrotic syndrome, pulmonary embolism, parapneumonic effusion, and uremia. Lupus pleuritis usually responds to the administration of systemic oral or intrapleural corticosteroids. In resistant cases, there may be a role for pleurodesis, intravenous immunoglobulin (IVIG), azathioprine, or pleurectomy.

Other Causes.   Effusions are seen in a variety of other rheumatologic, collagen vascular, and autoimmune diseases, such as Wegener's granulomatosis (5–55%), mixed connective tissue disorder (6%), Sjögren's syndrome (5%), progressive systemic sclerosis, ankylosing spondylitis (<1%), polymyositis/dermatomyositis (in association with interstitial lung disease), Churg-Strauss vasculitis (30%), eosinophilic myalgia syndrome, and familial Mediterranean fever. In these cases the effusions are usually not clinically problematic. Effusions have been described with Behçet's syndrome in 3% of cases only when

Table 5 Drugs Implicated in Drug-Induced Lupus

Definite Association	Possible Association
Chlorpromazine	Carbamazepine
Hydralazine	D-Penicillamine
Isoniazid	Ethosuximide
Phenytoin	Griseofulvin
Procainamide	Methyldopa
Quinidine	Methysergide
	Oral contraceptives
	Paraaminosalicylic acid
	Penicillin
	Phenylbutazone
	Propylthiouracil
	Primidone
	Reserpine
	Streptomycin
	Sulfonamides
	Tetracycline

there is associated pulmonary involvement or superior vena cava thrombosis. Some 12% of patients with immunoblastic lymphadenopathy, a non-neoplastic proliferation of B cells, will also have pleural effusions.

Pulmonary Embolism

Pleural effusions occur in 50% of patients with pulmonary embolism. The effusion is usually small to moderate in size and unilateral (95%). Presenting symptoms include chest pain (80–98%), dyspnea (80%) that is usually disproportionate to the size of the effusion, cough (50%), apprehension (50%), fever (50%), and hemoptysis (30%). Half of patients with effusion and embolism have a concomitant infiltrate on chest x-ray. Analysis of the fluid finds highly variable results. Some 80% of effusions are exudates. Any cell type can predominate. Gross blood is found in 20–35% of cases; with pulmonary infarction, it is found in as many as 80% of patients. The presence of blood on thoracentesis is not a contraindication to thrombolysis or anticoagulation. In fact, the finding of blood at thoracentesis in the absence of trauma, cardiac injury, or malignancy implies pulmonary embolism. Effusions that progress despite adequate therapy should undergo evaluation for recurrent emboli, hemothorax, infection, and infarction.

Gastrointestinal Diseases

A variety of gastrointestinal illnesses and procedures are associated with pleural effusion formation. These include acute and chronic pancreatitis, esophageal rupture, subdiaphragmatic abscess, abdominal surgery, and improper placement of an enteral feeding tube.

Pancreatitis. Acute pancreatitis results in pleural effusion in 10–20% of cases. Interestingly, alcoholic pancreatitis is much more frequently associated with pleural effusions than is pancreatitis due to biliary tract disease. The effusion is most commonly left-sided (60%; versus 30% right-sided and 10% bilateral) because the left hemidiaphragm reflects lower than the right and reaches under the pancreas. Fluid formation is likely due to either diaphragmatic irritation or transdiaphragmatic transfer of the exudative fluid from the site of inflammation. It is usually small to moderate in size and is associated with dyspnea, chest pain, and cough. A neutrophil-predominant exudate with an elevated amylase is typically found. Recent studies indicate that pleural effusions due to acute pancreatitis predict a more complicated hospital course irrespective of Ranson's criteria. Treatment should focus upon medical therapy for acute pancreatitis.

Pleural effusions associated with chronic pancreatitis are more commonly seen in males with alcoholism. Interestingly, chest symptoms dominate the presentation, with cough, shortness of breath, and chest pain seen in 68% of cases compared with abdominal symptoms, seen in 24%. This is likely due to decompression of a pancreatic pseudocyst via sinus tract formation through the aortic or esophageal diaphragmatic hiatus to permit flow of fluid to the mediastinum and eventually into the pleural space. Characteristically, the fluid amylase is markedly elevated. Serum amylase may be normal or minimally elevated. Treatment options focus on medical or surgical therapy of the underlying disease.

Esophageal Rupture. Esophageal rupture usually presents as a severe illness due to an acute mediastinitis with excruciating chest pain often unrelieved by narcotics. Pleural effusions occur in 60% of cases and are accompanied by pneumothorax in 25%. Time to diagnosis is critical because mortality with delay in therapy greater than 24 h exceeds 50% and rapidly approaches 100%. The effusion is more commonly left-sided and is characterized by an elevated amylase, low pH, and normal glucose. The presence of food particles or squamous epithelial cells in the fluid is diagnostically significant. Most commonly, esophageal rupture is a complication of esophagoscopy (67%). It may also occur with Blakemore tube placement, Boerhaave's syndrome, esophageal carcinoma, gastric intubation, trauma, or esophageal surgery. Treatment usually involves exploration and repair of the perforation with drainage of the pleural space and mediastinum.

Other Causes. A variety of other abdominal processes are associated with exudative effusions. Subdiaphragmatic abscesses—most commonly subphrenic but also pancreatic, splenic, and hepatic abscesses—usually result in a neutrophil-predominant sympathetic effusion. Rarely, the pleural fluid may become infected. Treatment with drainage of the underlying abscess and intravenous antibiotic administration should be sufficient. After intraabdominal surgery, half of patients will have pleural effusions in the first 4 postoperative days, especially when associated with free abdominal fluid, postoperative atelectasis, or upper abdominal surgery. Effusions are seen in as many as 50% of patients who undergo sclerotherapy for esophageal varices. Such effusions will typically resolve spontaneously without intervention. Malpositioning of an enteral feeding tube can lead to perforation of the esophagus or right mainstem bronchus with an associated exudative pleural effusion, empyema, or hemothorax.

Special Considerations

Chylothorax

Chylothorax is the presence of chylomicrons in the pleural space and is characterized by a milky white pleural fluid with an elevated triglyceride level. Chyle accumulates as a result of disruption of the thoracic duct. The most common cause of chylothorax is lymphoma, responsible for 37% of cases. Chylothorax has been described with a variety of other conditions, including metastatic cancer from virtually any primary source, surgical or nonsurgical trauma, lymphangiomyomatosis, protein-losing enteropathy, cirrhosis, re-

Table 6 Causes of Spontaneous
Hemothorax

Arteriovenous malformations
Ascites (bloody)
Cancer
Primary lung
Metastatic
Coagulopathy
Dissecting aortic aneurysm
Endometriosis
Idiopathic
Neurofibromatosis
Pleural infection
Pneumothorax
Retroperitoneal hemorrhage
Sequestration
Vascular anomalies

ticular hyperplasia, and thoracic aortic aneurysm. Conservative therapy includes bowel rest, parenteral nutrition, chest tube drainage, and treatment of the underlying disorder. Pleurodesis, pleurectomy, and pleuroperitoneal shunting may prevent recurrence. Definitive therapy involves thoracotomy and repair of the thoracic duct.

Hemothorax

Hemothorax is defined as a pleural fluid hematocrit exceeding 50% of the serum value. Blunt or penetrating trauma and iatrogenic vascular injury are the two most common causes of hemothorax. Iatrogenic vascular injuries are most commonly a complication of central venous catheter placement. Hemothorax rarely occurs spontaneously and is seen with a variety of disorders (Table 6). The majority of hemothoraces are managed with large-bore chest tube thoracostomy, and thoracotomy is utilized in cases of persistent hemorrhage.

Massive Pleural Effusion

Massive pleural effusions may occupy the entire hemithorax, even resulting in shift of mediastinal structures. It is most commonly associated with malignant effusions (67%) but may also occur with transudative effusions (13%), empyema (9%), hemothorax (7%), or tuberculous effusions (4%).

Effusions in the Intensive Care Unit

Two-thirds of patients admitted to a medical intensive care unit (ICU) will have pleural effusions; 40% have effusions upon admission and 20% develop them during the course of their intensive care stay. Typically, patients with effusions are elderly and more seriously ill as measured by lower serum albumin, higher APACHE (Acute Physiologic Assessment and Chronic Health Evaluation) II scores upon admission, longer ventilator runs, and longer ICU stays. Usually, the effusions are small in size and 80% are due to a noninfectious etiology. The most common cause is CHF, responsible for 35% of ICU effusions. Such effusions are typically bilateral. The most common cause of unilateral effusions is atelectasis, seen in 23% of patients and attributed to patient weakness, sedation, airway

Table 7 Etiology of Pleural Effusions
in AIDS

Kaposi's sarcoma	52%
Parapneumonic effusions	18%
Tuberculosis	15%
Opportunistic infections	10%
Other malignancies	5%

obstruction, and immobility. The portable bedside chest radiograph has been shown to be sensitive in detecting effusions in the ICU. Observation of afebrile patients with bilateral effusions can be safely undertaken. However, the presence of fever, increasing effusion, or consideration of infection should prompt diagnostic thoracentesis and surveillance for the development of a complicated parapneumonic effusion.

Effusions in HIV

Pleural effusions are common among AIDS patients, occurring in 2% of all cases. The most common cause of effusion in AIDS patients is Kaposi's sarcoma (Table 7). Among HIV patients with bacterial pneumonia, parapneumonic effusions occur more frequently than in normal hosts. The mechanism for this finding remains a mystery. Chest tube drainage is more frequently required. With tuberculous effusions, disseminated disease and constitutional symptoms are common. Other disease processes are involved less frequently, including CHF, hypoalbuminemia, histoplasmosis, cryptococcosis, nocardiosis, atypical mycobacterial disease, and lymphoma. Effusions are rarely seen in association with *Pneumocystis carinii* pneumonia.

PNEUMOTHORAX

Introduction

Historically, pneumothorax was used as a therapeutic and diagnostic modality. In tuberculosis patients, pneumothorax was utilized to collapse the infected lung and hasten closure of infected tuberculous cavities. Prior to the era of CT, it was used to distinguish the location of pulmonary parenchymal from extrapulmonic lesions and to determine invasion of the parietal pleura.

Clinical Presentation

Patients present with the acute onset of dyspnea in all cases of pneumothorax. Many patients have associated ipsilateral chest pain or nonproductive cough. Physical findings include tachypnea, tachycardia, diminished breath sounds, and decreased tactile fremitus. Peripheral cyanosis and hypotension are seen in less than 10% of cases. Occasionally, bronchial breath sounds with a metallic quality are auscultable. A pleural friction rub may be noted. When heard, Hamman's sign—a crunching sound synchronous with the heartbeat—suggests concomitant mediastinal emphysema. The constellation of acute onset of respiratory distress, tachycardia, contralateral tracheal deviation, distant heart tones, and peripheral cyanosis implies a tension pneumothorax.

Pathophysiology

Following rupture of an apical subpleural bleb in primary spontaneous pneumothorax, air enters the pleural space and elevates the pleural pressure, which approaches atmospheric pressure. Subsequently, the transpulmonic pressure gradient approaches zero and the lung collapses, resulting in a pneumothorax.

Radiographic Manifestations

On the chest radiograph, a pneumothorax appears as the outwardly convex visceral pleura is separated from the parietal pleura by air. Pneumothoraces are best visualized with end-expiratory chest x-rays. Expiratory films increase the density of the lung while reducing its volume, accentuating the difference between the density of the lung parenchyma and the pleural gas. Supine patient positioning, as seen in the ICU, may impair visualization as the air floats to the most superior location. Loculations appear in the setting of pleural adhesions. Finally, CT may detect small pneumothoraces not visualized by standard chest radiographs. The size of a pneumothorax is determined from a chest x-ray, based on the principle that the volume of the lung and of the air in the pleural space is related to the cube of the radius visualized. Thus, the formula listed in Table 8 estimates pneumothorax size.

Primary Spontaneous Pneumothorax

Primary spontaneous pneumothorax occurs in an otherwise healthy adult without evidence of underlying lung disease. The annual incidence is 40/100,000. It is thought to arise from the rupture of apical subpleural blebs. Typically, patients are tall, thin, young male smokers. The relative risk of pneumothorax is directly related to the amount of tobacco consumed. Other noteworthy risk factors are rapid changes in atmospheric pressure and a family history of pneumothorax. Seen in as many as 10% of cases, hereditary factors follow a pattern of either an autosomal dominant trait with incomplete penetrance or an X-linked recessive trait. Some 25% of patients will have recurrent pneumothoraces within 5 years, with the greatest risk of recurrence in the first year. Likewise, a recurrent pneumothorax markedly increases the likelihood of further recurrence.

Secondary Spontaneous Pneumothorax

Secondary pneumothoraces occur in patients with underlying lung disease. With an annual overall incidence of 8/100,000, secondary spontaneous pneumothorax is most commonly associated with severe chronic obstructive pulmonary disease (COPD) and cystic fibrosis,

Table 8 Estimation of Pneumothorax Size

$$\text{Percent pneumothorax} = 100 - \frac{(\text{diameter of lung})^3}{(\text{diameter of hemithorax})^3}$$

Table 9   Diseases Associated with Secondary Spontaneous
Pneumothorax

Alveolar proteinosis	Necrotizing bacterial pneumonia
Asthma	Paragonimiasis
Berylliosis	Pertussis
Chronic obstructive pulmonary disease	*Pneumocystis carinii* pneumonia
Cystic fibrosis	Primary biliary cirrhosis
Ehlers-Danlos syndrome	Pulmonary fibrosis
Histiocytosis X	Pulmonary infarction
Human immunodeficiency virus	Radiation
Idiopathic pulmonary hemosiderosis	Rheumatoid lung disease
Lung abscess	Sarcoidosis
Lung cancer	Scleroderma
Lung metastasis	Silicosis
Lymphangiomyomatosis	Tuberculosis
Marfan's syndrome	Tuberous sclerosis

but it has been associated with a wide variety of disorders (Table 9). Patients are more commonly male and present with hypoxemia and hypercarbia in 20% of cases. In contrast with primary pneumothorax, secondary disease is usually more severe in presentation and may precipitate respiratory failure. The mortality approaches 10% and is usually related to the underlying lung disease. Pneumothoraces recur in 45% of these patients within 5 years, and each event increases the risk of subsequent recurrence.

Special Considerations

Traumatic Pneumothorax

Blunt or penetrating traumatic injuries may result in pneumothorax. Direct chest penetration is implicated for obvious reasons. In blunt force injury, the injurious force may cause a bronchial or tracheal tear or rib fracture, resulting in laceration of the visceral pleura and lung with resultant pneumothorax. In addition, the sudden rise in alveolar pressure associated with chest trauma may result in alveolar rupture with release of air into the pleural space. Hemoptysis is a noteworthy clinical clue to the diagnosis.

Barotrauma

Occurring in 3–15% of patients receiving mechanical ventilation, pneumothorax is a medical emergency because of its propensity for progression to tension. Barotrauma is associated with elevated peak airway pressure (above 50 cmH$_2$O), high positive end-expiratory pressure (PEEP), and large tidal volumes. It occurs more commonly with controlled mechanical ventilation (CMV) than with synchronous intermittent mandatory ventilation (SIMV) or pressure support ventilation (PSV). It is more common with certain disease states, including acute respiratory distress syndrome (ARDS), aspiration or necrotizing pneumonia, COPD, asthma, and the fibrotic lung diseases. Clinically, the patient may become acutely dyspneic, tachypneic, and begin to "fight" the ventilator. There is an associated sudden rise in the peak airway pressure. Immediate placement of a large-bore chest tube is the treatment of choice.

Catamenial Pneumothorax

Catamenial pneumothorax is the term used to describe recurrent pneumothorax seen with menstruation. Subpleural and diaphragmatic endometriosis are noted in many but not all cases. Some have postulated that air may enter the peritoneum via the fallopian tubes and reach the pleural space by traversing diaphragmatic fenestrations. Some 90% of these are right-sided and usually occur in women between the ages of 20 and 40. Agents that inhibit ovulation, such as danazol and medroxyprogesterone, have been useful in treatment.

Pneumothorax in HIV

The leading cause of pneumothorax among HIV-infected individuals is *Pneumocystis carinii* pneumonia (PCP), occurring in as many as 10% of PCP patients. Pneumothoraces arise from rupture of thin-walled lung cavities on the surface of the lung. Contralateral pneumothorax develops in as many as 50% of patients. Recurrent disease and aerosolized pentamidine prophylaxis increase the risk of developing pneumothorax 15- to 20-fold. Treatment is difficult. The mean time to seal an air leak with chest tube thoracostomy is 20 days. Half of these patients require some form of sclerotherapy, and 25% require open surgical repair. Overall, there is a 20–40% mortality. Pneumothorax in AIDS may also be due to tuberculosis, atypical mycobacterial disease, cytomegalovirus pneumonia, visceropleural Kaposi's sarcoma, or underlying HIV infection.

Iatrogenic Pneumothorax

Various procedures may be complicated by the development of pneumothorax. These include transthoracic needle biopsy, thoracentesis, subclavian central line placement, transbronchial biopsy, and positive-pressure ventilation.

Treatment

Observation and Supplemental Oxygen

Simple observation of a pneumothorax may be indicated in the first episode of a primary spontaneous event when the patient is asymptomatic and the pneumothorax is small (less than 15%). Once the bronchopleural communication is sealed, the pneumothorax will resolve at the rate of 1.25% per day. Supplemental oxygen therapy will increase the rate of gas resorption by raising the partial pressure of oxygen in the capillary bed, resulting in a 4- to 10-fold elevation in the gradient for gas absorption.

Needle Aspiration

Needle aspiration of gas from the pleural space is recommended as initial therapy for symptomatic primary spontaneous pneumothorax. It is successful in 65% of cases. Unfortunately, its success rate in secondary spontaneous pneumothorax is only 40%, and patients usually require more aggressive measures.

Chest Tube Thoracostomy and Pleurodesis

Placement of a small-bore 8- to 12-Fr chest tube in association with a one-way Heimlich valve is successful therapy in 20% of cases but permits outpatient management of the pneumothorax. Frequently, a large-bore (28-Fr or greater) chest tube thoracostomy is necessary. In primary and secondary spontaneous pneumothorax, it is successful in 96 and 80% of cases, respectively. Further therapy with instillation of a sclerosing agent such as minocycline, bleomycin, or talc reduces the recurrence rate by 50%. Sclerotherapy may be utilized even in cases where there is a persistent air leak, but is not recommended when the lung fails to reexpand fully.

Surgical Repair

Patients who fail to reexpand their lung after 5 to 7 days, those with a persistent bronchopleural fistula, and those with recurrent pneumothorax after chemical pleurodesis are candidates for further intervention. Video-assisted thoracic surgery (VATS) may be utilized for talc insufflation, ligation of bullae, bleb ablation or wedge resection, scarification, and pleurectomy. Some 10% of such cases will suffer recurrence. Thoracotomy is more highly successful (99%) but carries a mortality in patients with secondary spontaneous pneumothorax that approaches 10%.

Complications

Tension Pneumothorax

Some 3–5% of patients with spontaneous pneumothorax and 5–15% of those with barotrauma develop tension pneumothorax. A one-way valve mechanism results in a progressive rise in pleural pressure. Soon, the trachea and mediastinum are displaced to the contralateral side and the diaphragm is depressed. The elevated pressure eventually impairs venous return and the patient becomes distressed. Clinically, this is manifest as extreme dyspnea, tachypnea, tachycardia, diaphoresis, cyanosis, and neck vein distention. As hypoxemia worsens and cardiac output falls, hypotension and cardiorespiratory arrest develop rapidly if the condition remains untreated. Placement of a large-bore needle or angiocatheter will rapidly decompress the tension and allow for chest tube placement. Tension pneumothorax is a potentially fatal illness, and its treatment should not be delayed for radiographic confirmation of the diagnosis. Overall mortality rises from 7–30% in such instances when treatment is delayed.

Reexpansion Pulmonary Edema

Reexpansion pulmonary edema is associated with the rapid evacuation of large volumes of air and fluid. In the most severe form, it can result in severe hypoxemia, hypotension, and respiratory failure with a mortality as high as 20%. Multiple mechanisms have been postulated in its pathogenesis, including reperfusion injury, capillary injury resulting from stress on the pulmonary vasculature by large negative pressures, and surfactant loss.

Other Complications

A variety of other complications from pneumothoraces may develop. In 1% of cases, air tracks into the mediastinum, resulting in pneumomediastinum, and may spread into the fascial planes of the neck, resulting in subcutaneous emphysema. Such findings are usually without negative clinical implications. Persistent bronchopleural fistulae occur in less than 5% of cases and require VATS or thoracotomy for repair. Hemothorax develops in less than 5% of patients and is thought to be secondary to tearing of vascularized pleural adhesions between the pleural layers. Treatment involves chest tube placement for lung reexpansion and drainage of accumulated blood.

SUGGESTED READING

1. Bartter T, Santarelli R, Akers SM, Pratter MR. The evaluation of pleural effusion. Chest 1994; 106:1209–1214.

2. Bryant RE, Salmon CJ. Pleural empyema. Clin Infect Dis 1996; 22:747–764.
3. Heffner JE, Brown LK, Barbieri CA. Diagnostic value of tests that discriminate between exudative and transudative pleural effusions. Chest 1997; 111:970–980.
4. Idell S. Granulomatous diseases of the pleura. Semin Respir Crit Care Med 1995; 16:340–345.
5. Jantz MA, Pierson DJ. Pneumothorax and barotrauma. Clin Chest Med 1994; 15:75–91.
6. Kirby TJ, Ginsberg RJ. Management of the pneumothorax and barotrauma. Clin Chest Med 1992; 13:97–112.
7. Light RW. Pleural Diseases, 3d ed. Baltimore: Williams & Wilkins, 1995.
8. Light RW. Management of spontaneous pneumothorax. Am Rev Respir Dis 1993; 148:245–248.
9. Sahn SA. Management of complicated parapneumonic effusions. Am Rev Respir Dis 1993; 148:813–817.
10. Sahn SA. The pleura. Am Rev Respir Dis 1988; 138:184–234.
11. Wyser C, Walzl G, Smedema JP, Swart F, Van Schalkwyk EM, Van de Wal BW. Corticosteroids in the treatment of tuberculous pleurisy: A double-blind, placebo-controlled, randomized study. Chest 1996; 110:333–338.

18

Acute Lower Respiratory Tract Infection

Shawn J. Skerrett
University of Washington
Seattle, Washington

EPIDEMIOLOGY OF ACUTE LOWER RESPIRATORY TRACT INFECTION

Acute lower respiratory tract infections include tracheobronchitis and pneumonia. More than 10 million office visits for bronchitis are made annually in the United States. Two-thirds of these cases are treated with antibiotics, accounting for at least 10% of all out-patient antibiotic prescriptions. There are approximately 4 million cases of community-acquired pneumonia in the United States each year, leading to more than 500,000 hospital admissions. Pneumonia is the sixth leading cause of death in the United States and results in more fatalities than any other infection. The estimated economic burden of pneumonia exceeds $20 billion per year in direct treatment costs and loss of wages.

Risk factors for acute lower respiratory tract infection include chronic airway diseases, aspiration diatheses, recent or concurrent upper respiratory tract infection, advanced age, and immunodeficiency. Chronic airway diseases such as chronic obstructive pulmonary disease (COPD), bronchiectasis, and bronchogenic carcinoma are associated with bacterial colonization of the normally sterile lower respiratory tract as well as defective mechanical clearance of the airways. An increased risk of aspiration is found in conditions associated with impaired consciousness, reduced gag reflex, or impaired glutition, such as alcoholism, seizure disorders, stroke, head and neck cancers, and esophageal disorders. Respiratory viruses such as influenza damage the tracheobronchial epithelium, thereby predisposing to bacterial superinfection. Immunodeficiency states associated with an impaired inflammatory response, diminished antibody production, or defective cell-mediated immunity predispose to opportunistic respiratory tract infections (see Chap. 5).

MICROBIOLOGY OF ACUTE LOWER RESPIRATORY TRACT INFECTION

In considering the microbial causes of acute tracheobronchitis, it is important to distinguish acute infection occurring in the absence of underlying lung disease from acute exacerbations of chronic bronchitis and bronchiectasis (Table 1). Acute bronchitis developing in otherwise healthy persons is usually caused by respiratory viruses such as influenza, parainfluenza, adenovirus, respiratory syncytial virus, and agents of the common cold such as rhinovirus and coronavirus. Measles and herpes simplex virus are rare considerations. Among nonviral pathogens, *Mycoplasma pneumoniae* and *Chlamydia pneumoniae* are relatively common causes of bronchitis, particularly in young adults. *Bordetella pertussis* is increasingly recognized as a cause of tracheobronchitis in the adult population, as a result of waning immunity from childhood vaccination. Pyogenic bacterial infections of the conducting airways are unusual in the absence of underlying disease.

In contrast, patients with chronic airway inflammation often have acute exacerbations associated with the organisms that colonize their lower respiratory tracts. Most patients with chronic bronchitis are colonized below the larynx with nontypeable *Haemophilus influenzae*, *Streptococcus pneumoniae*, and/or *Moraxella catarrhalis*. Patients with bronchiectasis and those with chronic bronchitis who have frequent exacerbations for which they take antibiotics regularly have an increased risk of colonization with antibiotic-resistant gram-negative bacilli, particularly *Pseudomonas aeruginosa*. Adults with cystic fibrosis are nearly all colonized with *Pseudomonas aeruginosa*, but some will harbor other resistant organisms, such as *Burkholderia cepacia* and *Stenotrophomonas maltophilia* (see Chap. 34).

The common microbial causes of pneumonia in patients admitted to hospitals are shown in Table 2. In up to 50% of cases, no specific microbial etiology can be identified despite an intensive diagnostic effort. The organisms that cause less severe infections treated in the outpatient setting are less well defined. It is likely that the spectrum of pathogens is similar but with greater representation by nonpyogenic organisms such as *Mycoplasma pneumoniae*, *Chlamydia pneumoniae*, and the respiratory viruses.

Table 1 Common Causes of Acute Tracheobronchitis

Setting	Pathogens
No underlying disease	Respiratory viruses
	Mycoplasma pneumoniae
	Chlamydia pneumoniae
	Bordetella pertussis
Chronic bronchitis	*Haemophilus influenzae*
	Streptococcus pneumoniae
	Moraxella catarrhalis
Bronchiectasis (long-standing)	*Pseudomonas aeruginosa*

Table 2 Etiologic Agents of Community-Acquired Pneumonia in Hospitalized Adults

Organism	% of Cases
Streptococcus pneumoniae	10–40
Viruses	5–20
Haemophilus influenzae	5–15
Mixed oral flora	3–15
Mycoplasma pneumoniae	2–18
Legionella spp.	2–14
Pneumocystis carinii	2–13
Chlamydia pneumoniae	2–10
Gram-negative bacilli	1–9
Staphylococcus aureus	1–8
Unknown	30–50

CLINICAL PRESENTATION OF ACUTE LOWER RESPIRATORY TRACT INFECTION

Cough is usually the presenting symptom of acute tracheobronchitis. The cough is often productive, and purulent sputum is not a reliable indicator of bacterial infection. In adults with pertussis, the cough is paroxysmal but lacks the whooping quality characteristic of childhood pertussis. Most patients with tracheobronchitis also have active or recent symptoms of upper respiratory infection, such as rhinorrhea, sore throat, hoarseness, and sinus congestion. Chest pain is common and typically related to severe coughing. The vital signs and chest exam are usually normal. Wheezes, rhonchi, and (rarely) crackles can be heard in some patients, but signs of consolidation are absent.

The cardinal symptoms of pneumonia are fever, chills, productive cough, dyspnea, and pleuritic chest pain (Table 3). Upper respiratory symptoms are present in a minority of patients. Occasionally the clinical picture is dominated by other complaints such as headache, myalgias, malaise, gastrointestinal disorders, or neurological symptoms. The presentation of pneumonia in the elderly can be subtle, such as an isolated alteration in mental status. On physical examination, most patients with pneumonia are febrile, and tachypnea and tachycardia are common. The chest exam is focally abnormal in the major-

Table 3 Common Symptoms of Pneumonia

Symptom	%
Cough	86
Fever	72
Shortness of breath	70
Chills	65
Sputum production	65
Pleuritic chest pain	45
Sore throat	31

ity of cases, revealing (in declining order of frequency) crackles, diminished breath sounds, rhonchi, and signs of consolidation, such as bronchial breath sounds, egophony, whisper pectoriloquy, dullness to percussion, and increased tactile fremitus (see Chap. 7). Although most patients with pneumonia will have abnormal vital signs and an abnormal chest examination, the absence of these findings does not exclude pneumonia. No constellation of symptoms and signs can be relied upon to firmly diagnose or exclude pneumonia.

EVALUATION OF PATIENTS WITH SUSPECTED ACUTE LOWER RESPIRATORY TRACT INFECTION

The evaluation of suspected acute lower respiratory infection should be directed toward a determination of whether pneumonia is present, an assessment of the severity of illness, and consideration of the microbial cause of infection. With this information, decisions can be made regarding the need for hospital admission, antibiotic treatment, and follow-up.

When pneumonia is suspected based on symptoms, vital sign abnormalities, and/ or focal findings on chest examination, further evaluation should include posteroanterior and lateral chest radiographs, oximetry, a complete blood count, serum electrolytes and renal function tests, and, when available, expectorated sputum for Gram stain and culture.

The Chest Radiograph

The radiographic demonstration of a parenchymal infiltrate is the reference standard for the diagnosis of pneumonia in a patient with a compatible clinical presentation. False-negative films resulting from severe dehydration, neutropenia, and very early infection are rare. The film should be scrutinized for additional useful information, such as the presence of a pleural effusion, adenopathy, mass lesions, or volume loss suggestive of endobronchial obstruction. Prognostic value can be found in features associated with a complicated course, such as multilobar infiltrates or cavitation. The radiographic pattern of parenchymal infiltration also can offer clues to the infecting pathogen (Fig. 1). Lobar or segmental consolidation usually indicates a pyogenic bacterial infection, whereas bilateral diffuse alveolar and interstitial infiltrates are suggestive of viral, *Pneumocystis*, or (occasionally) *Mycoplasma* infection. Nodular shadows are commonly associated with fungi, mycobacteria, *Nocardia*, and *Legionella*. Cavitation suggests a necrotizing infection caused by anaerobes, *S. aureus*, gram-negative bacilli, hemolytic streptococci, *Rhodococcus equi*, mycobacteria, *Nocardia*, or fungi. *Legionella* pneumonia commonly causes cavities in immunocompromised individuals. Hilar adenopathy suggests an associated malignant or inflammatory condition or an atypical infection. *Mycoplasma* and *Chlamydia* infections often are associated with adenopathy, as are primary tuberculosis, histoplasmosis, coccidiomycosis, tularemia, pertussis, plague, measles, and toxoplasmosis. Pleural effusions are most common with bacterial infections and are evidence against a viral, *Mycoplasma*, or *Chlamydia* etiology.

Microbiological Diagnosis of Pneumonia

Clinical Clues to the Microbiology of Pneumonia

Clues to the microbial etiology of pneumonia may be found by considering host factors and environmental exposures that increase the risk of particular infections. Aspiration

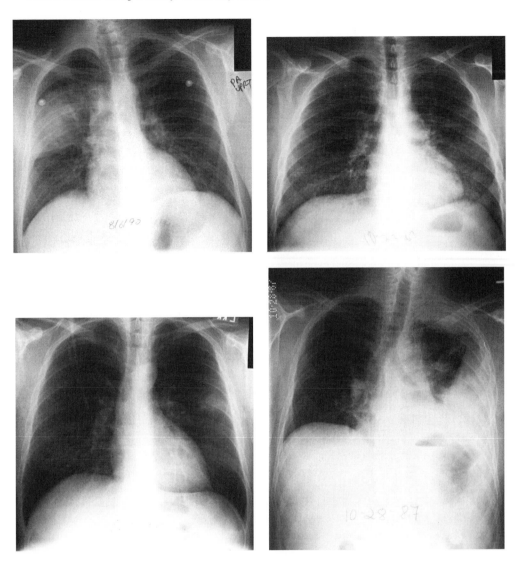

Figure 1 Radiographic patterns helpful in the etiological diagnosis of pneumonia. Top left, segmental consolidation, suggestive of pyogenic bacterial infection. Top right, diffuse alveolar and interstitial infiltrates, suggestive or nonbacterial infection. Bottom left, cavitation of a focal nodular infiltrate with a crescent sign, suggestive of a fungal infection. Bottom right, prominent pleural involvement, suggestive of pyogenic bacterial infection.

diatheses and extensive periodontal disease predispose to infection with mixed aerobic and anaerobic oral flora. Alcoholism, diabetes mellitus, chronic renal failure, and residence in a nursing home are associated with colonization of the upper respiratory tract with gram-negative bacilli and *Staphylococcus aureus*, with an attendant increased risk of pneumonia due to these organisms. The lower respiratory tracts of patients with COPD and bronchiectasis are often colonized with *S. pneumoniae*, *H. influenzae*, or *M. catarrhalis*, predisposing to infection with these agents. *P. aeruginosa* and other resistant gram-nega-

tive bacilli are major concerns in patients with cystic fibrosis and long-standing bronchiectasis.

Specific defects in systemic host defenses also predispose to particular infectious
agents (see Chap. 5). A deficiency in number or function of neutrophils increases the risk
of infection with gram-negative bacilli, *Staph. aureus*, and fungi such as *Aspergillus, Mu-
cor*, and *Candida*. Impairments in humoral immunity, as may be found in multiple myeloma or chronic lymphocytic leukemia, lead to repeated infection with heavily encapsulated organisms such as the pneumococcus and *H. influenzae*. Defective cell-mediated
immunity may result from T-cell malignancies or immunosuppressive drugs and predisposes to infection with a wide variety of opportunistic pathogens, including mycobacteria,
Legionella Nocardia, fungi such as *Coccidioides, Histoplasma, Cryptococcus*, and *Blastomyces*, herpesviruses, and protozoa. The acquired immunodeficiency syndrome is associated with a very broad range of respiratory pathogens because of the associated defects
in both humoral and cellular immunity. Some of the medications used in this disorder can
also cause a drug-induced neutropenia.

An inquiry into potential exposures to infectious agents may be fruitful. Acute respiratory illnesses in the home or community suggest a contagious pathogen, such as a respiratory virus, *Mycoplasma*, or *Chlamydia*. Group housing situations are hazardous for epidemic infections. Nursing home residents are at high risk for outbreaks of influenza,
respiratory syncytial virus, and tuberculosis. Adolescents and young adults housed under
crowded conditions in dormitories and barracks are vulnerable to epidemics caused by
meningococci, *Mycoplasma, Chlamydia*, and viruses. Residents of jails and shelters are
at risk for epidemic pneumococcal disease and tuberculosis. A travel history may suggest
exposure to geographically restricted airborne fungi such as *Histoplasma capsulatum*
(Ohio, Mississippi, and Missouri River valleys), *Blastomyces dermatitidis* (central and
southeastern United States), and *Coccidioides immitis* (southwestern United States), or
regionally distributed bacteria such as the agents of melioidosis (Southeast Asia), lep-
tospirosis (the tropics), and plague (developing world, southwestern United States). Visits
to old hotels, whirlpool spas, or cruise ships are risk factors for legionellosis. Exposure
to animals can be an important clue. Domestic livestock are reservoirs of *Coxiella burnetti*
(Q fever) and brucellosis. Parturient cats also can spread Q fever. Animal hides and wool
can transmit inhalation anthrax. Wild rodents may spread tularemia, plague, and hantavirus. A variety of birds can transmit psittacosis. Tick bites are another source of tularemia.
Elicitation of the patient's occupation and hobbies is important, as this may identify exposure to animals or aerosols containing soil- and water-borne pathogens, such as fungi,
Pseudomonas, Aeromonas, Acinetobacter, and *Legionella*.

Clinical features of the presenting illness may offer some clues to the microbial
etiology of pneumonia. The typical acute pneumonia syndrome—characterized by an
abrupt onset, productive cough, pleuritic chest pain, and leukocytosis—is most often associated with pyogenic bacteria. In contrast, the atypical pneumonia syndrome—characterized by an insidious onset, nonproductive cough, and prominent nonrespiratory symptoms
such as headache, myalgias, and diarrhea—is usually associated with viruses, *Mycoplasma, Chlamydia*, and *C. burnetti*. Unfortunately, many patients do not fit neatly into
one syndrome or another, and the syndromes themselves are poor predictors of microbial
etiology. Abnormalities on the physical examination are occasionally useful in suggesting
particular infections. Periodontal disease and foul-smelling sputum are helpful clues to a
mixed anaerobic infection. The rare case of bullous myringitis should suggest *M. pneumoniae*. Evidence of consolidation on chest exam is suggestive of bacterial infection.

Neurological abnormalities such as confusion, obtundation, and ataxia may be more common with *Legionella* and *Mycoplasma* infections than with other pathogens. Finally, fulminant community-acquired pneumonia presenting with shock or rapidly progressive respiratory failure should prompt particular concern for *S. pneumoniae*, *Legionella*, or gram-negative bacilli such as *Klebsiella*, *Acinetobacter*, and *Pseudomonas*.

Abnormalities in routine laboratory tests such as leukocytosis, hyponatremia, azotemia, and mild increases in liver enzymes are nonspecific. However, evidence of severe hemolysis should prompt consideration of *Mycoplasma pneumoniae* infection. The triad of hemoconcentration, thrombocytopenia, and circulating immunoblasts is characteristic for hantavirus. Acute renal failure in the absence of shock should raise concern for legionellosis and psittacosis.

Tests for the Specific Microbiological Diagnosis of Pneumonia

The single most useful test for the etiological diagnosis of bacterial pneumonia is the Gram stain of expectorated sputum. The sputum Gram stain accurately predicts the etiology of pneumonia when a good specimen is obtained and interpreted according to strict criteria by an experienced observer. A valid Gram stain can be defined by the presence of >25 neutrophils and <10 epithelial cells per low-power field and a clearly predominant pathogen under high power. Such a specimen is an accurate guide to therapy but is obtained in only 30–50% of hospitalized patients with pneumonia. Other helpful patterns include a purulent specimen with a great variety of microorganisms, suggesting oropharyngeal aspiration, and a moderately purulent specimen without visible bacteria, suggestive of an atypical infection. Physicians are more likely to collect adequate specimens than other personnel. Common errors in Gram-stain interpretation include reading a poor specimen, misinterpreting oral flora as pneumococci, and missing *H. influenzae*.

An acid-fast smear is occasionally helpful in the evaluation of pneumonia. A modified Kinyoun stain will detect not only mycobacteria but also weakly acid-fast organisms such as *Nocardia*, *Legionella micdadei*, and *Rhodococcus equi*. Immunological methods for the identification of pneumococcal polysaccharide antigen, such as the Quellung reaction and counter-immunoelectrophoresis, are 70–90% sensitive for the detection of pneumococci in sputum, and their specificity for pneumococcal pneumonia is probably >80%. These tests are popular in Europe but rarely used in North America.

Sputum culture is a sensitive means for detecting potential bacterial pathogens when the specimen is carefully collected and microscopically screened for salivary contamination. However, the sputum culture lacks specificity because it does not distinguish colonization from infection. Thus, the sputum culture should not be interpreted independently of the Gram stain unless a pathogen is recovered that does not colonize the respiratory tract, such as *M. tuberculosis*, *Legionella*, or one of the endemic fungi. Cultures of blood or pleural fluid are very helpful when positive (5–15% of cases).

Legionellosis can be diagnosed by several methods, and the preferred tests will vary with local availability and expertise. Legionellae stain poorly with the Gram stain, but visualization in respiratory specimens can be improved if basic fuchsin is used as the counterstain instead of safranin. The Gimenez stain is a useful albeit nonspecific means of detecting legionellae in bronchoalveolar lavage specimens, and *L. micdadei* is weakly acid-fast. The direct fluorescent antibody (DFA) test of sputum is helpful when positive: it has a specificity greater than 90% in experienced hands, but the reported sensitivity has ranged from 25–75%. The most widely used preparation detects only *L. pneumophila*, which is the most common cause of legionnaires' disease. Sputum culture on specialized media can isolate any of the more than 40 species of *Legionella* and is positive in 50–80% of cases in skilled laboratories. Urinary antigen testing with a commercial kit detects more than 80% of infections caused by *L. pneumophila* serogroup 1 with high specificity, but it misses other serotypes and species. Serologies (a fourfold change in titer or a single titer ≥1:256) are 80% sensitive for *L. pneumophila* infections but have not been standardized for the identification of other species. The detection of legionellae by DNA amplification is now being offered by some reference laboratories. This is a very promising approach but has not yet been fully evaluated.

The diagnosis of *Mycoplasma* and *Chlamydia* infections can be made serologically or by isolation of the organisms from the respiratory tract. *M. pneumoniae* infection can be confirmed with a fourfold change in complement fixation titer or a single titer ≥1:64. Cold agglutinins, IgM autoantibodies that agglutinate red cells at 4°C, are strongly suggestive of *M. pneumoniae* infection when the titer is 1:64 or greater. High titers can be detected at the bedside by collecting blood in a "blue top" tube containing sodium citrate, immersing the tube in ice water for 3–4 min, and then observing macroscopic agglutination of the red cells that disappears with rewarming. *Mycoplasma pneumoniae* can be isolated from respiratory secretions, but cultures require 1–3 weeks of incubation and are not widely available. Similarly, *C. pneumoniae* and *C. psittaci* infections can be diagnosed by isolating the organisms from respiratory secretions or by demonstrating specific serological responses: a fourfold rise, a single IgG titer of ≥1:512, or a single IgM titer of ≥1:16. Unfortunately, methods for culturing chlamydiae and reliable serological tests are not widely available. Nucleic acid detection methods for the diagnosis of respiratory tract infection with *Chlamydia* or *Mycoplasma* are under development.

Fungal pneumonias can be diagnosed using stains, cultures, immunological techniques, and histology. Potassium hydroxide and Calcofluor preparations of sputum are insensitive but specific means of detecting fungi. Cultures of sputum and bronchoalveolar lavage specimens are diagnostic for coccidiomycosis, histoplasmosis, and blastomycosis when positive, as these organisms do not colonize the respiratory tract. Positive cultures for *Cryptococcus neoformans* usually indicate infection, but this organism is a rare saprophyte in patients with chronic airway disease. A positive sputum culture for *Aspergillus* is suggestive of infection in an immunosuppressed patient, but the isolation of *Candida* species from respiratory specimens has no predictive value. Serologies can be helpful in the diagnosis of acute coccidiomycosis and histoplasmosis. Detection of fungal antigens in serum or urine is helpful in the diagnosis of cryptococcosis and histoplasmosis in patients with HIV infection. The demonstration of characteristic fungal forms in lung tissue is definitive and is the only reliable means of diagnosing invasive *Candida* and *Aspergillus* infections.

Pneumocystis carinii pneumonia complicating HIV infection can be diagnosed from induced sputum in 50–80% of cases using silver, Giemsa, toluidine blue, and Papanicoulou stains. A fluorescent antibody test for *P. carinii* improves the yield of induced sputum in less experienced laboratories. Bronchoalveolar lavage is nearly always diagnostic for *P. carinii* pneumonia if bilateral lavages including at least one upper lobe are collected. The diagnosis of respiratory viral infection is made by immunofluorescent staining or culture of nasopharyngeal swabs or bronchoalveolar lavage specimens.

Invasive methods have very limited applications for the diagnosis of community-acquired pneumonia. Transtracheal aspiration will yield a potential pathogen in 75–95% of patients with pneumonia with a specificity of 70–90%. The sensitivity is reduced by prior antibiotic therapy, and specificity suffers in patients with airway diseases associated with chronic colonization. This procedure has largely been abandoned because of potential complications, including subcutaneous emphysema, bleeding, aspiration, infection, and death. Transthoracic needle aspiration will yield a microbial pathogen in 70–90% of cases with presumably high specificity, but it carries a significant risk of pneumothorax and bleeding. This technique is most helpful when the differential diagnosis includes a fungal infection, as in the situation of a nodular infiltrate in a compromised host. Fiberoptic bronchoscopy with quantitative culture of bronchoalveolar lavage fluid or a protected specimen brush can be used to diagnose bacterial pneumonia with a sensitivity >70% and specificity >85% when the cultures yield $\geq 10^3$–10^4 colony forming units per milliliter. Bronchoalveolar lavage is particularly helpful when there is suspicion of *P. carinii*, viral, or fungal infection.

Arguments for and Against Diagnostic Testing

The most compelling argument in favor of diagnostic testing is that the identification of a specific pathogen permits the initiation of narrow-spectrum antibiotic treatment that may be more effective, less toxic, and less costly than empirical treatment. Knowledge of the infecting agent also helps determine prognosis, as some organisms (particularly *Staph aureus* and gram-negative bacilli) are associated with greater morbidity and mortality than other pathogens. Routine diagnostic testing provides information about the local microbial epidemiology of pneumonia, including the prevalence of antibiotic resistance, that can influence empiric treatment strategies. Using narrow-spectrum treatment whenever possible is less likely to exacerbate the growing problem of antibiotic resistance than the routine use of broad-spectrum combinations. Arguments against routine diagnostic testing include the cost of the tests, the fact that no specific pathogen can be identified in up to 50% of cases of pneumonia despite an extensive effort; concerns about the accuracy of commonly used tests, particularly sputum Gram stains and cultures; and the well-established efficacy of empirical treatment in most cases.

Summary: A Reasonable Approach to Microbiological Diagnosis

A reasonable approach to the microbiological diagnosis of pneumonia is to obtain a sputum Gram stain and culture whenever possible and two sets of blood cultures on all patients admitted to the hospital. Pleural fluid should be cultured when present. Other diagnostic studies can be limited to patients with exposure histories or clinical features that suggest particular pathogens, to patients who are immunocompromised, and to those who follow an unexpected clinical course after initial treatment.

Differential Diagnosis of Acute Lower Respiratory Tract Infection

Cough is the dominant symptom of acute lower respiratory tract infection and is among the most frequent reasons for consulting a physician. The differential diagnosis of acute tracheobronchitis includes other causes of recent-onset cough, particularly upper respiratory tract infection. Sinusitis is an important consideration, as sinus infection usually warrants treatment with antibiotics (see Chap. 16). Other entities that can mimic acute tracheobronchitis include asthma, hypersensitivity reactions, gastric or foreign-body aspiration, and toxic inhalations. Pneumonia is the most common cause of an acute febrile

Table 4 Noninfectious Entities That Can Mimic Pneumonia

Atelectasis	Hypersensitivity pneumonitis
Pulmonary edema	Pulmonary hemorrhage
Gastric aspiration	Vasculitis
Foreign-body aspiration	Collagen vascular disease
Malignancy	Sarcoidosis
Pulmonary embolism	Bronchiolitis obliterans organizing pneumonia
Drug toxicity	Eosinophilic pneumonia
Radiation pneumonitis	Idiopathic pulmonary fibrosis

illness associated with radiographic infiltrates, but noninfectious entities occasionally warrant consideration because of suggestive clinical features or an unexpected clinical course. Some of the noninfectious processes that can mimic pneumonia are listed in Table 4.

MANAGEMENT OF ACUTE LOWER RESPIRATORY TRACT INFECTION

Tracheobronchitis

Patients with acute tracheobronchitis in the absence of underlying disease usually require no specific therapy. Analgesics, antipyretics, expectorants, and cough suppressants may provide symptomatic relief, but antibiotics have offered no demonstrable benefit in clinical trials, even when the cough is productive of purulent sputum. Antibiotics may be helpful in reducing symptoms and/or transmission of infection in the subset of patients with tracheobronchitis caused by *B. pertussis M. pneumoniae*, or *C. pneumoniae*, but currently there are no widely available means of rapidly and reliably identifying these infections. However, treatment of the patient with severe symptoms with a macrolide may be reasonable in the setting of a known community outbreak of pertussis or when the patient's history suggests contagion with an incubation period longer than 1 week. A persistent postviral cough can be treated with inhaled ipratropium, albuterol, or corticosteroids.

   In patients with acute exacerbations of chronic bronchitis, treatment of airflow obstruction with bronchodilators and corticosteroids is the major concern. Antibiotics may be helpful in patients with newly purulent sputum and should be directed at the pneumococcus, *H. influenzae*, and *M. catarrhalis*. Trimethoprim/sulfamethoxazole, doxycycline, and amoxicillin are usually effective. The newer cephalosporins, macrolides, fluoroquinolones, and amoxicillin/clavulanic acid all have excellent activity against the expected pathogens but are much more expensive. Sputum cultures are not necessary to guide therapy unless the patient is suspected of harboring a resistant organism or has repeatedly failed empirical treatment.

Pneumonia

Inpatient vs. Outpatient Management

Most patients with pneumonia can be treated as outpatients. The indications for hospital admission include clinical features of a severe illness, risk factors for a complicated course, and suspicion of an opportunistic or unusual infection that warrants further evaluation under observation (Table 5). Hospital admission also should be considered in patients over the age of 65 years, those with underlying chronic diseases that may impair host defenses or pulmonary reserve (such as chronic renal insufficiency, diabetes mellitus, congestive heart failure, and COPD), and patients whose socioeconomic circumstances interfere with reliable treatment and follow-up.

Antibiotics

The antibiotic treatment of pneumonia should be based on the sputum Gram stain and culture whenever possible. Empirical therapy can be directed at the likely etiological agents according to risk factors and clinical presentation (Table 6). Many reasonable options are available.

For most people treated as outpatients, a macrolide such as erythromycin, clarithromycin, or azithromycin is the drug of choice when sputum is unavailable or nondiagnostic. Clarithromycin and azithromycin are more expensive than erythromycin but are better tolerated and more effective against *H. influenzae*. Azithromycin has a very long tissue half-life and is usually given for only 5 days. Fluoroquinolones are also active against most lower respiratory tract pathogens and are reasonable alternatives to macrolides. Only fluoroquinolones with acceptable activity against pneumococci (such as levofloxacin, sparfloxacin, grepafloxacin, and trovafloxacin) should be used in the empirical treatment of

Table 5 Indications for Hospital Admission for Pneumonia

Clinical features of severe illness
  Systolic BP $<$ 100 mmHg or diastolic BP $<$ 60 mmHg
  Heart rate $\geq$125 beats/min
  Respiratory rate $\geq$30/min or labored breathing
  Temperature $<$ 36°C or $>$ 40°C
  Altered mental status
  Hypoxemia: arterial P_{O2} $<$ 60 torr or O_2 saturation $<$ 90%
  Multilobar involvement or cavitation on chest radiograph
  Suppurative complication (e.g., empyema, pericarditis,
    meningitis)
  Severe hematologic abnormality (e.g., marked anemia,
    neutropenia, thrombocytopenia)
  Severe metabolic derangement (e.g., marked hyperglycemia or
    hyponatremia; new azotemia)
High risk for a complicated course
  Immunodeficiency
  Postobstructive pneumonia
  Suspected infection with *S. aureus* or gram-negative bacillus
Suspicion of opportunistic or unusual infection
  Requires further diagnostic evaluation under observation
Admission should be considered for
  Advanced age
  Significant comorbidity: chronic obstructive pulmonary disease,
    renal failure, diabetes, heart failure, neurological disease,
    cancer
  Socioeconomic factors that interfere with reliable treatment and
    follow-up

Table 6 Antibiotics for Empiric Treatment of Community-Acquired Pneumonia

Situation	Preferred Agents	Alternatives
Outpatient	Macrolide[a]	Fluoroquinolone,[b] doxycycline, Amoxicillin-clavulanate, cephalosporin,[c] trimethoprim/sulfamethoxazole
Inpatient	Ceftriaxone, cefotaxime, or cefuroxime ± macrolide or fluoroquinolone	Ampicillin/sulbactam, clindamycin + aztreonam
Fulminant	Antipseudomonal beta-lactam[d] + macrolide or fluoroquinolone ± aminoglycoside	Fluoroquinolone + clindamycin ± aztreonam or aminoglycoside

[a] Macrolides: erythromycin, clarithromycin, and azithromycin.
[b] Fluoroquinolones active against *S. pneumoniae*: levofloxacin, sparfloxacin, grepafloxacin, trovafloxacin.
[c] Oral cephalosporins: cefpodoxime, cefuroxime, cefixime, cefprozil.
[d] Cefipime, imipenem, piperacillin/tazobactam
See text for additional details.

pneumonia. Doxycycline is an inexpensive option in the young adult with mild pneumonia in whom *Mycoplasma* and *Chlamydia* are strong considerations, but the increasing resistance of pneumococci to tetracyclines limits the widespread use of this class. The time-honored use of amoxicillin for the treatment of community-acquired pneumonia is increasingly limited by the growing prevalence of beta-lactamase–producing *H. influenzae* and penicillin-resistant pneumococci. The combination of clavulanate with amoxicillin extends the penicillin spectrum to include all *H. influenzae* and *M. catarrhalis*, most enterics, and most anaerobes.

Amoxicillin/clavulanate is a good choice for patients with a history suggestive of oropharyngeal aspiration. Clindamycin is an alternative in this situation for patients who are allergic to penicillin. Oral cephalosporins with strong activity against *S. pneumoniae* and *H. influenzae* (such as cefpodoxime, cefuroxime, and cefixime) will be effective in most cases, but these agents are ineffective in *Mycoplasma Chlamydia*, and *Legionella* infections and have limited activity against anaerobes. Trimethoprim/sulfamethoxazole is an inexpensive combination that is effective against most strains of *S. pneumoniae* and *H. influenzae* and has some activity against *Legionella*. Its use in pneumonia is limited by meager activity against anaerobes, increasing resistance among pneumococci, and a lack of published experience.

Hospitalized patients requiring empiric therapy should be treated initially with parenteral antibiotics. Monotherapy with a cephalosporin (such as ceftriaxone, cefotaxime, or cefuroxime) or ampicillin/sulbactam will be effective in most cases. The addition of a parenteral macrolide or a fluoroquinolone is advisable when concern for *Legionella*, *Mycoplasma*, or *Chlamydia* is raised on the basis of a potential exposure history or clinical features. It is likely that azithromycin, levofloxacin, or trovafloxacin would be effective as single agents for most patients with community-acquired pneumonia, but experience is greater with beta-lactam–based regimens. Alternatives for penicillin-allergic patients include monotherapy with azithromycin or a fluoroquinolone (levofloxacin or trovafloxacin), a macrolide or fluoroquinolone plus clindamycin when aspiration is a concern, or the combination of clindamycin and aztreonam. Patients with fulminant pneumonia presenting with shock or rapidly progressive respiratory failure should initially be treated very broadly to cover relatively resistant gram-negative bacilli, such as *Acinetobacter* and

Pseudomonas, as well as the pneumococcus, *Legionella*, and *Staph. aureus*. Options in this setting include a broad-spectrum antipseudomonal beta lactam (such as cefipime, piperacillin/tazobactam, or imipenem) plus a macrolide (azithromycin or erythromycin) or a fluoroquinolone. The addition of an aminoglycoside for the first few days of treatment may be wise. Patients who respond well to initial parenteral treatment for pneumonia can be switched to oral antibiotics within 3 days.

The optimal treatment for drug-resistant pneumococcal pneumonia has not been established. However, the available evidence suggests that third-generation cephalosporins, such as cefotaxime and ceftriaxone, or high doses of penicillin G ($\geq$12 million U/day) are effective. These agents achieve blood levels that greatly exceed the minimum inhibitory concentrations for all strains of *S. pneumoniae* that have been isolated to date. Vancomycin and the new fluoroquinolones (levofloxacin, sparfloxacin, grepafloxacin, and trovafloxacin) are the best alternatives, as high-level resistance among pneumococci to these agents has not yet been reported. Whenever possible, the treatment of pneumococcal infection should be guided by in vitro sensitivity testing.

There are limited indications for the use of anti-infectives in treating viral pneumonias. Ganciclovir is clearly effective in reducing the mortality of primary or secondary (reactivation) lung infection with cytomegalovirus. Acyclovir is probably effective in the treatment of lower respiratory tract infection caused by herpes simplex virus. The role of anti-infectives in the treatment of other viral pneumonias is less clear. Amantadine and rimantidine effectively reduce the morbidity associated with influenza A, but their efficacy in treating influenza pneumonia has not been studied. Aerosolized ribavirin reduces the severity of acute respiratory syncytial virus (RSV) infection in infants, and there is anecdotal evidence of its effectiveness in adults with RSV pneumonia. Ribavirin also has activity in vitro against influenza A and B, adenovirus, and parainfluenza, but the role of aerosolized ribavirin in treating pneumonias caused by these agents has not been established. The treatment of fungal pneumonias is discussed elsewhere in this volume (see Chap. 37).

Additional Measures

Supplemental oxygen should be provided as necessary to keep the arterial oxygen saturation greater than 90%. Analgesics are occasionally needed for control of pleuritic pain. Chest physiotherapy and postural drainage can be helpful in patients with lung abscesses and in those who are having difficulty expectorating particularly copious or tenacious sputum.

The use of immunomodulators in the management of acute lower respiratory tract infection is receiving increasing attention, but there are few defined indications. Hyperimmune globulin may be a helpful adjunct to ganciclovir in the treatment of cytomegalovirus pneumonia in transplant recipients. Colony-stimulating factors, such as granulocyte colony-stimulating factor and granulocyte-macrophage colony-stimulating factor are effective in reducing the duration of neutropenia after chemotherapy or marrow transplantation and are indicated in the management of pneumonia in these settings. Whether colony-stimulating factors or other recombinant cytokines have a role in the treatment of respiratory tract infections in less severely immunocompromised individuals has not been clearly established.

Parapneumonic Effusions and Empyema

Parapneumonic effusions should be sampled by thoracentesis whenever possible to help identify a pathogen and guide management. An effusion layering to a thickness of at least

1 cm on a lateral decubitus film can usually be tapped safely. Smaller effusions should be followed radiographically. Loculated effusions should be sampled under ultrasound guidance. Pleural fluid should be sent for Gram stain and culture, LDH, protein, and glucose or pH. Frank pus in the pleural space should be drained. Tube thoracostomy may be sufficient if the empyema is in an early phase of development, and intrapleural fibrinolytics (for example, urokinase) may facilitate drainage of loculated fluid. However, thoracoscopy or thoracotomy is often required for adequate debridement. The management of parapneumonic effusions that are not frankly purulent is controversial. Exudative fluid with a positive Gram stain or culture should probably be drained by thoracentesis or tube thoracostomy; some experts also recommend drainage of uninfected fluid with a pH less than 7.1 (see Chap. 17).

PROGNOSIS AND FOLLOW-UP

Tracheobronchitis resolves over a period of days to weeks. After a respiratory viral infection, cough and postviral airway reactivity can persist for up to 6 weeks. Specific follow-up generally is not required.

Patients with pneumonia should defervesce within 72 h and improve gradually thereafter. Radiographic infiltrates may progress for 24 h after the initiation of effective antibiotic treatment but then should stabilize and slowly clear. Failure to improve is usually a consequence of host factors, such as underlying lung disease that impairs local defenses or immunodeficiency. Other reasons that should be considered include infection with an unusual or resistant pathogen, obstruction to drainage, a suppurative complication, or a noninfectious process masquerading as pneumonia. Further microbiological studies, computed tomography of the chest, and bronchoscopy may be helpful in delineating the cause of a poor response to treatment.

The short-term mortality of community-acquired pneumonia is less than 5% among patients treated in the ambulatory setting, and 10–15% among patients hospitalized for pneumonia. The risk factors for a morbid complication or fatal outcome are listed in Table 5.

All patients with pneumonia who have risk factors for lung cancer should have follow-up chest radiographs after 2–3 months to document resolution. Radiographic clearing is complete by 3 months in 90% of patients.

SUGGESTED READING

1. Bartlett JG, Mundy LM. Community-acquired pneumonia. N Engl J Med 1995; 333:1618–1624.
2. British Thoracic Society Research Committee and Public Health Laboratory Service. Community-acquired pneumonia in adults in British hospitals in 1982–1983: a survey of aetiology, mortality, prognostic factors and outcome. Q J Med 1987; 62:195–220.
3. Fang GD, Fine M, Orloff J, Arisumi D, Yu VL, Kapoor W, Grayston JT, Wang SP, Kohler R, Muder RR, Yee YC, Rihs JD, Vickers RM. New and emerging etiologies for community-acquired pneumonia with implications for therapy: a prospective multicenter study of 359 cases. Medicine (Baltimore) 1990; 69:307–316.
4. Fine MJ, Smith MA, Carson CA, Mutha SS, Sankey SS, Weissfeld LA, Kapoor WN. Prognosis

and outcomes of patients with community-acquired pneumonia: a meta-analysis. JAMA 1996; 275:134–141.

5.   Mackay DN. Treatment of acute bronchitis in adults without underlying disease. J Gen Intern Med 1996; 11:557–562.

6.   Marrie TJ, Durant H, Yates L. Community-acquired pneumonia requiring hospitalization: a five year prospective study. Rev Infect Dis 1989; 11:586–599.

7.   Marrie TJ. Community-acquired pneumonia. Clin Infect Dis 1994; 18:501–515.

8.   Metlay JP, Kapoor WN, Fine MJ. Does this patient have community-acquired pneumonia? JAMA 1997; 278:1440–1445.

9.   Mittl RL Jr, Schwab RJ, Duchin JS, Goin JE, Albelda SM, Miller WT. Radiographic resolution of community-acquired pneumonia. Am J Respir Crit Care Med 1994; 149:630–635.

10. Mundy LM, Auwaerter PG, Oldach D, Warner ML, Burton A, Vance E, Gaydos CA, Joseph JM, Gopalan R, Moore RD, Quinn TC, Charache P, Bartlett JG. Community-acquired pneumonia: impact of immune status. Am J Respir Crit Care Med 1995; 152:1309–1315.

11. Niederman MS, Bass JB Jr, Campbell GD, Fein AM, Grossman RF, Mandell LA, Marrie TJ, Sarosi GA, Torres A, Yu VL. Guidelines for the initial management of adults with community-acquired pneumonia: diagnosis, assessment of severity, and initial antimicrobial therapy. Am Rev Respir Dis 1993; 148:1418–1426.

12. Pallares R, Linares J, Vadillo M, Caballos C, Manresa F, Viladrich PF, Martin R, Gudiol F. Resistance to penicillin and cephalosporin and mortality from severe pneumococcal pneumonia in Barcelona, Spain. N Engl J Med 1995; 333:474–480.

13. Park DR, Skerrett SJ. The usefulness of the sputum Gram stain in the diagnosis of pneumonia. Clin Pulm Med 1995; 2:201–212.

14. Saint S, Bent S, Vittinghoff E, Grady D. Antibiotics in chronic obstructive pulmonary disease exacerbations: a meta-analysis. JAMA 1995; 273:957–960.

15. Skerrett SJ. Diagnostic testing to establish a microbial etiology is helpful in the management of community-acquired pneumonia. Semin Respir Infect 1997; 12:308–321.

19

Acute Respiratory Failure

John J. Marini
University of Minnesota
Regions Hospital
St. Paul, Minnesota

INTRODUCTION

The pulmonary capillary exchanges oxygen for carbon dioxide across a thin, gas-permeable membrane in a process fundamental to sustaining aerobic metabolism and pH homeostasis. Because different physiological processes determine the adequacy of tissue oxygenation and CO_2 elimination, one of these functions usually takes primacy when the system begins to fail, even though dysfunctional elements of both are often present simultaneously. Episodes of respiratory failure, therefore, may be logically subclassified as oxygenation failure or ventilation failure. This discussion examines both primary manifestations of acute respiratory insufficiency with the aim of describing an approach to management that flows from an understanding of the underlying pathophysiology.

OXYGENATION FAILURE

Definitions

Oxygenation failure originates in one or more of the steps necessary to sustain oxygen availability for mitochondrial energy production: (1) ventilation (the transfer of oxygen from the environment to the lungs); (2) pulmonary O_2 exchange; (3) O_2 transport (the delivery of adequate quantities of oxygenated blood to the metabolizing tissue); or (4) tissue gas exchange (the utilization of O_2 and release of CO_2 by the peripheral tissues). Tissue O_2 transport or O_2 delivery ($\dot{D}_{O_2}$), depends not only on lung function, as reflected in the partial pressure of arterial oxygen (Pa_{O_2}), but also on nonpulmonary factors—cardiac output ($\dot{Q}_T$), hemoglobin (Hgb) concentration, and the ability of Hgb to take up and release O_2:

$$\dot{D}_{O_2} = \dot{Q}_t \times Ca_{O_2}$$

In this expression, O_2 content per deciliter of blood (Ca_{O_2}) is determined by the following relationship (Sa_{O_2} is the oxygen saturation of arterial blood expressed as a decimal fraction).

$$Ca_{O_2} = 1.36(Hgb)Sa_{O_2} + 0.003 \, (Pa_{O_2})$$

Cardiogenic shock, profound anemia, and carbon monoxide poisoning provide clinical examples of O_2 transport failure. Laboratory abnormalities characteristic of such conditions are lactic acidosis and an increased arteriovenous O_2 content difference despite adequate arterial oxygen tension.

O_2 uptake failure results from the inability of tissues to extract and utilize O_2. Clinical examples are septic shock—thought to often reflect a problem of microvascular distribution—and cyanide poisoning, a condition in which cytochromes vital to intracellular electron transport are inhibited. Unlike transport insufficiency, these problems of tissue uptake are distinguished by abnormally narrow arteriovenous O_2 content differences and normal or high values for mixed venous oxygen tension, saturation, and content. As with transport insufficiency, lactic acidosis is a helpful laboratory indicator of oxygen deprivation.

Despite the importance of O_2 transport and uptake, respiratory failure is generally understood to imply pulmonary dysfunction. Therefore, the remainder of the present discussion focuses on the performance of the lung in oxygenating the arterial blood.

Mechamisms of Arterial Hypoxemia

The six mechanisms that contribute to arterial oxygen desaturation are outlined in Table 1 and reviewed both below and in Chap. 2, on muscles, nerves, and central control of respiration.

Reduced Inspired Oxygen Concentration

A decrease in the partial pressure of inspired oxygen (PI_{O_2}) occurs in toxic fume inhalation, in fires that consume O_2 in the combustion process, and at high altitude (see Chap. 41).

Hypoventilation

Hypoventilation causes the partial pressure of alveolar oxygen (PA_{O_2}) to fall when alveolar oxygen is not replenished quickly enough in the face of its ongoing removal. Although the alveolar (and arterial) partial pressure of oxygen (PA_{O_2}) may fall much faster than Pa_{CO_2} rises during the initial phase of hypoventilation or apnea, the steady-state PA_{O_2} is estimated by the simplified alveolar gas equation:

$$PA_{O_2} = PI_{O_2} - \frac{Pa_{CO_2}}{R}$$

Table 1 Mechanisms of Hypoxemia

Reduced inspired oxygen concentration
Hypoventilation
Impaired alveolar diffusion of oxygen
Ventilation/perfusion ($\dot{V}/\dot{Q}$) mismatching
Shunting of systemic venous blood to the systemic arterial circuit
Abnormal O_2 desaturation of systemic venous blood

In this equation, PI_{O_2} is the partial pressure of inspired O_2 at the tracheal level (corrected for water vapor pressure at body temperature), and R is the gas-exchange ratio accounting for the difference between CO_2 production and oxygen consumption at steady state (assumed to be a ratio of 0.8). Transiently, however, R can fall to very low values, as alveolar O_2 is taken up faster than CO_2 is delivered.

Impaired Diffusion

Impaired oxygen diffusion implies incomplete equilibration of alveolar gas with pulmonary capillary blood. This potential mechanism has uncertain clinical relevance. However, factors that adversely influence diffusion are commonly encountered in practice: increased distance between alveolus and erythrocyte, decreased O_2 gradient, and shortened capillary transit time of the red cell (e.g., high cardiac output with limited capillary reserve).

Ventilation/Perfusion Mismatching

Ventilation/perfusion ($\dot{V}/\dot{Q}$) mismatching is the most frequent contributor to clinically important O_2 desaturation. Perfused lung units that are poorly ventilated contribute to desaturation, whereas poorly perfused but well-ventilated units contribute to physiological dead space, wasted ventilation, and a high workload, but not to hypoxemia. The relationship of O_2 content to Pa_{O_2}, like that of Pa_{O_2} to hemoglobin saturation, is highly curvilinear (see Chap. 2). Except under hyperbaric conditions, little additional O_2 can be loaded into blood with already well saturated Hgb, no matter how high the O_2 tension in the overventilated alveolus may rise. Blood exiting from different lung units mixes gas contents (not partial pressures); consequently, overventilating some units in an attempt to compensate for others that remain underventilated cannot maintain Pa_{O_2} at a normal level unless inspired oxygen is supplemented. Hence, when equal volumes of blood from well-ventilated and poorly ventilated units mix, the blended sample will have an O_2 content halfway between them but a Pa_{O_2} disproportionately weighted toward that of the lower $\dot{V}/\dot{Q}$ unit.

Supplemental O_2 impressively reverses hypoxemia when $\dot{V}/\dot{Q}$ mismatching, hypoventilation, or diffusion impairment is the cause. At some levels of FI_{O_2}, compensation is complete. In fact, after breathing 100% O_2 for a sufficient time, only perfused units that are totally unventilated (shunt units) contribute to hypoxemia. However, when hypoxemia is caused by alveolar units with very low $\dot{V}/\dot{Q}$ ratios, relatively concentrated O_2 mixtures must be inspired before arterial oxygenation shows a noteworthy improvement.

Shunting

Shunt fraction is the percentage of the total systemic venous blood flow that effectively bypasses aerated alveoli to transfer venous blood unaltered to the systemic arterial system. Alterations of FI_{O_2} fail to influence Pa_{O_2} significantly when shunt is the sole mechanism of hypoxemia and the *true* shunt fraction exceeds 30% (Fig. 1). In contrast, venous admixture resulting from other mechanisms that cause hypoxemia of similar magnitude responds invariably to supplemental oxygen. Shunt can be intracardiac, as in cyanotic right-to-left congenital heart disease, or may result from passage of blood through pulmonary arteriovenous communications. By far the most common cause of shunting, however, is airless lung.

Many indices have been devised to characterize the efficacy of oxygen exchange across the spectrum of FI_{O_2}. Although no index is ideal, the Pa_{O_2}/PA_{O_2} ratio and the alveolar-arterial oxygen tension difference $[P(A-a)_{O_2}]$ are often utilized (see Chap. 2 for examples of the use of $P(A-a)_{O_2}$). In the setting of lung disease, however, both indices are

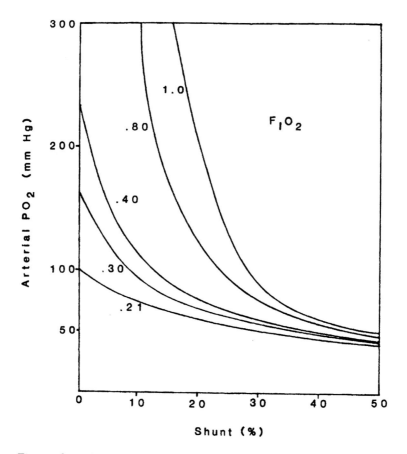

Figure 1   Effect of increasing shunt on arterial PO_2 at different fractions of inspired oxygen (FI_{O_2}). Note that the relative effect of FI_{O_2} depends on the shunt percentage. (From Dantzker DR, Sharf SM. Cardiopulmonary Critical Care, 3d ed. Ed. Philadelphia: Saunders, 1998:45.)

affected by alterations in venous O_2 content, even when the lung itself has not changed its ability to transfer oxygen to the blood. Another imprecise but commonly used indicator of gas exchange is the Pa_{O_2}/FI_{O_2} ratio (the "P/F" ratio). In healthy adults, this ratio normally exceeds 400, whatever the FI_{O_2} may be. Hypoventilation and changes in the inspired O_2 concentration minimally alter these ratios in the absence of FI_{O_2}-related absorption atelectasis or cardiovascular adjustments.

Abnormal Desaturation of Systemic Venous Blood

Admixture of abnormally desaturated venous blood is an important mechanism acting to lower Pa_{O_2} in patients with impaired pulmonary gas exchange and reduced cardiac output. $S\bar{v}_{O_2}$ (the oxygen of mixed venous blood), is influenced by cardiac output ($\dot{Q}$), arterial O_2 saturation (Sa_{O_2}), and O_2 consumption ($\dot{V}_{O_2}$):

$$S\bar{v}_{O_2} \sim Sa_{O_2} - [\dot{V}_{O_2}/(Hgb \times \dot{Q})]$$

This equation illustrates that $S\bar{v}_{O_2}$ is directly influenced by any imbalance between $\dot{V}_{O_2}$ and oxygen delivery. Thus, anemia uncompensated by an increase in cardiac output or a cardiac output too low for metabolic needs can cause both $S\bar{v}_{O_2}$ and Pa_{O_2} to fall unless the lung is normal. In the normal lung, well-ventilated alveoli have adequate oxygenation reserve to compensate for a low $S\bar{v}_{O_2}$. A marked decline in $S\bar{v}_{O_2}$ without arterial hypoxemia occurs routinely during heavy exercise in healthy subjects.

Fluctuations in $S\bar{v}_{O_2}$ tend to exert a more profound influence on Pa_{O_2} when the shunt is fixed, as in regional lung diseases (e.g., atelectasis), than when the shunt varies with changing cardiac output, as it tends to do in diffuse lung injury [acute respiratory distress syndrome (ARDS)]. Furthermore, in normal lungs or lungs in which hypoxemia is due to $\dot{V}/\dot{Q}$ mismatch, such variations in $S\bar{v}_{O_2}$ tend to have greater impact when minute ventilation is fixed than when it is free to increase (Fig. 2). The severity of arterial hypoxemia tends to vary inversely with the effectiveness of hypoxic pulmonary vasoconstriction. Even when $S\bar{v}_{O_2}$ is abnormally low, Pa_{O_2} will remain unaffected if all mixed venous blood gains access to well-oxygenated, well-ventilated alveoli. Abnormal $\dot{V}/\dot{Q}$ matching or shunt is necessary for venous desaturation to contribute to hypoxemia.

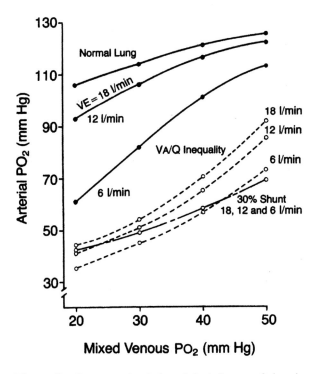

Figure 2 Computer simulation of the influence of changing mixed venous P_{O_2} on arterial P_{O_2} in lungs that are normal or impaired. Effects on arterial P_{O_2} of changes in minute ventilation and mixed venous P_{O_2} is influenced by the mechanism of transpulmonary oxygen transfer—normal, $\dot{V}/\dot{Q}$ inequality, or shunt. (From Dantzker DR, Sharf SM. Cardiopulmonary Critical Care, 3d ed. Philadelphia: Saunders, 1998:42.)

Common Causes of Hypoxemia

Radiographic appearances give important clues to the appropriate management approach to oxygenation failure. Lung collapse (atelectasis), diffuse or patchy parenchymal infiltration, hydrostatic edema, localized or unilateral infiltration, and a clear chest x-ray are common patterns (Fig. 3).

Atelectasis

Atelectasis is classified by morphological type and mechanism. Regional microatelectasis develops spontaneously during shallow breathing when the healthy lung is not periodically stretched beyond its usual tidal range. Plate-like atelectasis may be an exaggeration of this phenomenon due to regional hypodistention (e.g., pleural effusion or impaired diaphragmatic excursion). Micro- and plate-like atelectasis occurs most commonly in dependent regions. Lobar collapse usually results from gas absorption in an airway plugged by retained secretions, a misplaced endotracheal tube, or a central mass. Bronchial compression and regional hypoventilation are important in some patients. Micro- and plate-like atelectasis occurs routinely in patients at prolonged uninterrupted bed rest and in postoperative patients who have recently undergone upper abdominal incisions.

Potential consequences of acute atelectasis are worsened gas exchange, pneumonitis, and increased work of breathing. Pa_{O_2} drops precipitously to its nadir within minutes to hours of a sudden bronchial occlusion, but it then improves steadily over hours to days as hypoxic vasoconstriction and altered regional forces augment pulmonary vascular resistance within the affected region. Whether an individual patient manifests hypoxemia depends heavily on the intensity of the hypoxic vasoconstrictive response, the abruptness of collapse, and the tissue volume involved. If small areas of atelectasis develop slowly, hypoxemia may never surface as a significant clinical problem.

Management of Established Atelectasis.   Mobilization is the best treatment for all types of atelectasis. Periodic sustained deep breaths (yawn equivalents) effectively reverse plate-like and microatelectasis. Relief of chest wall pain helps to reduce splinting and enables more effective coughing. Intercostal or epidural nerve blocks with anesthetic agents such as bupivacaine may be effective. Epidural narcotics may also be effective in

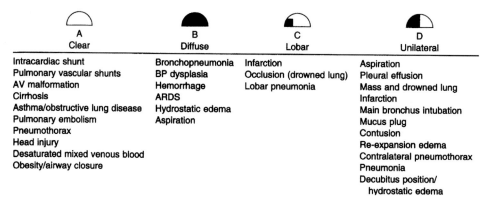

A Clear	B Diffuse	C Lobar	D Unilateral
Intracardiac shunt	Bronchopneumonia	Infarction	Aspiration
Pulmonary vascular shunts	BP dysplasia	Occlusion (drowned lung)	Pleural effusion
AV malformation	Hemorrhage	Lobar pneumonia	Mass and drowned lung
Cirrhosis	ARDS		Infarction
Asthma/obstructive lung disease	Hydrostatic edema		Main bronchus intubation
Pulmonary embolism	Aspiration		Mucus plug
Pneumothorax			Contusion
Head injury			Re-expansion edema
Desaturated mixed venous blood			Contralateral pneumothorax
Obesity/airway closure			Pneumonia
			Decubitus position/ hydrostatic edema

Figure 3   Radiographic patterns associated with hypoxemia. (From Marini JJ, Wheeler AP. Critical Care Medicine—The Essentials, 2d ed. Baltimore: Williams & Wilkins, 1997.)

certain settings. Although rational, the place of positive end-expiratory pressure in treatment of *established* collapse has not been clarified. Retained secretions must be dislodged from the central airways. Vigorous respiratory therapy initiated soon after the onset of lobar collapse can quickly reverse most cases of atelectasis due to airway plugging. Fiberoptic bronchoscopy should be reserved for patients with symptomatic lobar collapse who lack central air bronchograms and who cannot undergo, fail to respond to, or cannot tolerate 48 h of vigorous respiratory therapy. After reexpansion, a respiratory therapy program should be initiated to prevent recurrence.

Diffuse Pulmonary Infiltration

Severe, refractory hypoxemia may result when edema fluid or cellular infiltrates cause alveolar filling. Fluid in the interstitial spaces may cause hypoxemia as a result of compressive peribronchial edema, $\dot{V}/\dot{Q}$ mismatching, and microatelectasis; however, interstitial fluid itself does not interfere with oxygen exchange. Moreover, few clinical problems are confined exclusively to the air spaces or to the interstitium. The major categories of acute disease that produce diffuse pulmonary infiltration and hypoxemia are pneumonitis (infection and aspiration), cardiogenic pulmonary edema, intravascular volume overload, and ARDS. From a radiographic viewpoint, these processes may be difficult to distinguish; however, a few characteristic features are helpful.

A prominent vascular pattern and hilar infiltrates that spare the costophrenic angles suggest volume overload or incipient cardiogenic edema. A gravitational distribution of edema is highly consistent with well-established left ventricular failure or volume overload, especially when accompanied by cardiomegaly and a widened vascular pedicle. Patchy peripheral infiltrates that lack a gravitational predilection and show reluctance to change with position suggest permeability edema (ARDS). Septal (Kerley) lines and distinct peribronchial cuffing are common in congestive heart failure but are seldom seen in ARDS. On the other hand, prominent air bronchograms are quite unusual with hydrostatic etiologies but occur commonly in ARDS and pneumonia.

Hydrostatic edema may occur in multiple settings, with differing implications for prognosis and treatment. Left ventricular failure is the archetype of hydrostatic pulmonary edema (HPE). In this setting, signs of systemic hypoperfusion and inadequate cardiac output often accompany oxygenation failure. However, HPE can develop even with a normally well-compensated ventricle in patients with severe hypoalbuminemia or during transient heart dysfunction (ischemia, hypertensive crisis, arrhythmias). When the myocardium fails to fully relax during diastole (''diastolic dysfunction''), superimposed loading or temporary disturbances of left heart contractility (e.g., ischemia), mitral valve functioning, or heart rate or rhythm may cause rapid, transient alveolar flooding known as ''flash pulmonary edema,'' named for the impressive speed with which extensive radiographic infiltrates develop and resolve.

Acute Lung Injury and Acute Respiratory Distress Syndrome.   ARDS is the most severe form of acute lung injury, and acute lung injury is a general term referring to all degrees of radiographically apparent, diffuse hypoxemic lung injury not attributed purely to hydrostatic forces. The ARDS designation is most useful when restricted to acute noncardiogenic pulmonary edema with certain characteristic features:

1. Brief delay between the precipitating event and the onset of dyspnea
2. Impaired compliance of the respiratory system
3. Markedly reduced aerated lung volume

4. Refractory hypoxemia
5. Delayed resolution

Sepsis, aspiration, pneumonia, and multiple trauma account for the vast majority of cases of ARDS. In general, predisposing illnesses injure the alveolar-capillary membrane from either the gas side (e.g., smoke inhalation, aspiration of gastric acid, pneumonia) or the blood side (e.g., sepsis, fat embolism). Typically, fewer than one-third of all lung units remain aerated. Abnormally increased membrane permeability allows seepage of protein-rich fluids into the interstitial and alveolar spaces, where they directly inhibit or inactivate surfactant, contributing to widespread atelectasis as the inflammatory process degrades the lung's architecture in a three-stage process. The earliest stage of widespread edema and atelectasis (days 1–3) is followed by the proliferative (days 3–7) and resolution (>7 days) stages. Pulmonary artery occlusion pressure usually remains normal, but increased pulmonary vascular resistance and pulmonary hypertension are invariable, especially in the latter stages of severe disease. Extreme pulmonary hypertension is a very poor prognostic sign. Apart from any difference in capillary pressure, permeability edema differs from hydrostatic edema in that it resists clearance by diuretic therapy and initiates the above-mentioned inflammatory response that may require weeks to recede and even longer to heal.

The response of this disease to manipulations of airway pressure (such as PEEP) and drugs (such as corticosteroids) is influenced by the stage of the process and by its etiology. Yet, the core pathophysiology of ARDS and the potential for further injury by misguided ventilation strategies are sufficiently similar to warrant a common treatment approach (see Chap. 25). Excessive fluids must not be given, so as to minimize lung water and improve oxygen exchange. Severe fluid restriction, on the other hand, may compromise perfusion of gut and kidney. Appropriate nutritional support—preferably enteral—and prophylaxis for deep venous thrombosis, skin breakdown and gastric stress ulceration should be considered for all mechanically ventilated or immobile patients.

The routine use of corticosteroids for the early phase of ARDS is not justified because of their adverse effects on immunity, mental status, metabolism, and protein wastage. Corticosteroids are indicated for respiratory distress resulting from vasculitis, fat embolism, or allergic reactions. Corticosteroids may also be lifesaving in certain steroid-responsive diseases that mimic ARDS (e.g., bronchiolitis obliterans organizing pneumonia, pulmonary hemorrhage syndromes, *Pneumocystis carinii* pneumonia). Corticosteroids may help resolve the fibroproliferative stage of ARDS, but there is still no firm consensus on this point.

Because extravascular water accumulates readily in the setting of permeability edema, fluids should be used judiciously, consistent with adequate oxygen delivery. Liberal use of inotropes and other vasoactive drugs can be helpful in certain postoperative or posttrauma settings, but driving the cardiac output to ''supraphysiological'' levels does *not* appear to improve the mortality rate of medical patients with ARDS.

Hypoxemia with a Clear Chest X-Ray

Patients may present with severe hypoxemia without major radiographic evidence of infiltration. In such cases, occult shunting and severe $\dot{V}/\dot{Q}$ mismatching are the most likely mechanisms. Intracardiac or intrapulmonary shunts, asthma, and other forms of airway obstruction, low lung volume superimposed on a high closing capacity (e.g., bronchitis in a supine obese patient), pulmonary embolism, and occult microvascular communications (such as occur in patients with cirrhosis) are potential explanations. Therapeutic vasoactive agents (nitroprusside, calcium-channel blockers, dopamine) can accentuate hypoxia from shunt or $\dot{V}/\dot{Q}$ mismatching.

Unilateral Lung Disease

Marked radiographic asymmetry suggests a confined set of etiological possibilities, which include pneumonia, atelectasis, aspiration, and radiation injury, most of which occur in characteristic clinical settings (Fig. 3).

Techniques to Improve Tissue Oxygenation

Whatever the cause of hypoxemic respiratory failure, important therapeutic aims are to reverse the underlying lung pathology, improve oxygen delivery, relieve an excessive breathing workload, and maintain electrolyte balance while preventing further damage from oxygen toxicity, barotrauma, infection, and other iatrogenic complications. Mechanical ventilation for respiratory failure is reviewed in Chap. 25.

Because oxygen delivery is the product of cardiac output and the O_2 content of each milliliter of arterial blood, O_2 carrying capacity can be improved by increasing hemoglobin (Hgb) concentration. Increasing Hgb tends to elevate mixed venous oxygen saturation as it reduces the need for any rise in cardiac output compensatory to anemia. Lower cardiac output and higher mixed venous O_2 saturation both tend to reduce venous admixture. Reversing alkalemia facilitates O_2 off-loading. As Hgb concentration rises, blood viscosity increases, retarding passage of erythrocytes through the capillary network. O_2 delivery can actually decline as hematocrit (Hct) rises above 50%. Although the optimal Hct in patients with an oxygenation crisis is unknown, it is standard practice to restore the Hct to at least 30%. More extensive supplementation increases the risk of transfusion without proven benefit.

Oxygen Therapy. O_2 toxicity is both concentration- and time-dependent. As a general rule, high inspired concentrations of O_2 can safely be used for brief periods as efforts are made to reverse the underlying process. Sustained elevations in $F_{I_{O_2}} > 0.6$, however, result in inflammatory changes and eventual fibrosis in experimental animals; therefore, it seems prudent to keep $F_{I_{O_2}} < 0.6$ during the support phase of acute lung injury.

Secretion Management and Bronchodilation. Airway edema, bronchospasm, and secretion retention often contribute to hypoxemia. In intubated patients, retained secretions increase endotracheal tube resistance, infection risk, the risk of barotrauma, and maldistribution of ventilation. In some patients with diffuse lung injury, profound bradycardia develops during ventilator disconnections. Although hypoxemia occasionally contributes, this bradycardia is usually reflex in nature and responds to prophylactic (parenteral) atropine or reapplication of positive airway pressure. Circuits that do not interrrupt PEEP during suctioning offer an advantage in this regard.

Reducing Oxygen Requirements. Fever, agitation, overfeeding, vigorous respiratory activity, shivering, sepsis, and anxiety can markedly increase O_2 consumption. Reducing fever may have therapeutic value, but shivering must be prevented in the cooling process. Sedatives and antipyretics rather than cooling blankets make better therapeutic sense.

Although muscle relaxants are a valuable adjunct to reduce O_2 consumption and improve Pa_{O_2} in patients who remain agitated or fight the ventilator even though they are well sedated, lengthy paralysis must be avoided. Paralysis silences the coughing mechanism and creates a monotonous breathing pattern that encourages the retention of secretions in dependent regions. Protracted, unmonitored paralysis may cause weakness or devastating neuromyopathy.

Repositioning. Frequent repositioning of the patient may help to preserve alveolar patency and gas exchange. Use of the prone position should be considered during the early phase of ARDS, as improved oxygen exchange has been confirmed in this setting. Moreover, laboratory work suggests that prone positioning may help protect the lung against ventilation-induced damage or barotrauma.

VENTILATORY FAILURE

Definition

Ventilatory failure is the inability to sustain a sufficient rate of CO_2 elimination to maintain a physiologically appropriate and stable pH without mechanical assistance, muscle fatigue, or intolerable dyspnea. Failure to maintain adequate alveolar ventilation is usually recognized by hypercapnia and acidosis. However, ventilatory failure may be present even in the absence of an elevated Pa_{CO_2} if there is an inadequate respiratory compensation for a metabolic acidosis. For example, a patient with severe COPD may be unable to reduce the Pa_{CO_2} below 40 mmHg in response to urinary sepsis and can, therefore, develop a severe uncompensated metabolic acidosis. Conversely, many patients comfortably maintain a Pa_{CO_2} above 50 mmHg on a chronic basis without satisfying the aforementioned definitions because of an appropriate rise in their serum bicarbonate.

Two categories of disease account for the great majority of episodes of ventilatory failure: obstructive disease of the upper airway or lungs and dysfunction of the ventilatory pump due to neuromuscular disorders, fatigue, or inadequate ventilatory drive. Because airflow obstruction is addressed in Chaps. 3, 26, and 27, attention here is directed toward ventilatory pump failure.

Mechanisms of Ventilatory Failure

In health, quiet tidal breathing is accomplished by active inhalation and passive deflation. The inspiratory muscles comprise the diaphragm (responsible for the major portion of ventilation at all but extreme work rates) and the accessory muscle group, primarily the external and parasternal intercostals, the scalenes, and the strap muscles of the neck. Expiratory muscle activity is required for expulsive efforts (cough, sneeze, defecation), for high levels of ventilation (>20 L/min) and for breathing out against a significant resistive load (as against external PEEP or during an exacerbation of asthma or COPD). Increased ventilatory demand and impaired ventilatory capability often coexist. Maintaining adequate alveolar ventilation requires a pressure gradient sufficient to overcome resistive and elastic forces. Thus, any condition that interferes with the ability to generate negative intrathoracic pressure (e.g., weakness, abnormal thoracic configuration, or muscular incoordination) will stress the system and may lead to ventilatory failure. Alternatively, conditions that increase the force requirement may lead to the same outcome, even without pump impairment.

Ventilatory drive normally adjusts the output of the muscular pump in proportion to metabolic activity so as to maintain pH within narrow limits. To maintain effective ventilation, an appropriate signal must first be sent from the brain to the ventilatory muscles. The muscles must then contract with sufficient force and coordination to generate the fluctuating pleural pressure that drives flow through the airways of the passive lung. The ventilatory work required to sustain this process depends upon the difficulty of gas movement and the minute ventilation requirement. Three major mechanisms cause or contribute to ventilatory failure: deficient central drive to breathe, ineffective muscular contraction, and excessive workload (Table 2). Sustained spontaneous ventilation requires both adequate ventilatory drive and endurance. Impaired ventilatory drive often contributes to CO_2 retention and may be entirely responsible for ventilatory failure in specific settings (e.g., sedative excess). The most common reason, however, is the inability to satisfy ventilatory demand. The total ventilatory workload is determined by the product of expired minute ventilation ($\dot{V}E$) and the energy expended per liter of gas flow.

Ventilatory Demand

Minute Ventilation Requirement.   Three primary factors determine the $\dot{V}E$ requirement: the CO_2 production, efficiency of ventilation, and sensitivity of the central drive mechanism.

CO$_2$ Production. CO_2 production is an obligatory consequence of metabolism; it is determined by body size, nutrient composition, activity level, and other factors. Fever, shivering, pain, agitation, increased work of breathing, sepsis, and overfeeding are common causes of increased CO_2 production. Buffering of hydrogen ion by bicarbonate evolves significant quantities of CO_2 during acidosis. Excess calories may be converted

Table 2 Physiologic Mechanisms of Ventilatory Failure

Increased ventilatory workload	Ineffective musculature
Impedance to thoracic gas movement	Thoracic configuration
Airflow obstruction	Chronic
Parenchymal lung disease	Kyphoscoliosis
Extrapulmonary, intrathoracic restriction	Thoracoplasty
Pleural space	Acute
Chest wall	Pneumothorax
Increased minute ventilation	Pleural effusion
	Flail chest
	Hyperinflation
Muscular weakness	**Inadequate ventilatory drive**
Skeletal muscles	Intrinsic
Weakness	Congenital chronic loading
Neuromuscular impairment	Obesity
Quadriplegia	Severe airflow obstruction
Myopathy	Advanced age
Diaphragm paralysis	Endocrine disturbance
Functional	Extrinsic
Hyperinflation	Drugs and sedatives
Drugs	Sleep deprivation
Electrolytes	Metabolic alkalosis
	Nutritional insufficiency

to fat, generating CO_2 as a metabolic by-product unrelated to energy utilization. Carbohydrate evolves more CO_2 per calorie than fat or protein.

Ventilatory Efficiency.   Alveolar ventilation ($\dot{V}_A$), the component of ventilation that is effective in eliminating CO_2, is the total minute ventilation adjusted for the fraction of wasted ventilation. Breathing efficiency can be characterized by the expression

$$\dot{V}_A = \dot{V}_E (1 - V_D/V_T)$$

where V_D/V_T is the physiological dead-space fraction. Virtually all of the diverse processes that damage the lung or airways of the critically ill patient increase dead space and therefore the minute ventilation required to maintain a stable Pa_{CO_2}. Thromboembolic or vasculitic arterial occlusion or hypovolemia may reduce perfusion to the ventilated lung, thus expanding the alveolar dead space. Small tidal volumes are characterized by a high *anatomic* dead-space percentage. Devices or tubing interposed between the natural airway opening and the source of fresh gas (e.g., between the endotracheal tube and the "Y" of a ventilator circuit) may contribute to ventilatory inefficiency.

Central Drive.   Suppressed ventilatory drive may arise from advanced age, neurological impairment, hypothyroidism, excessive sedation, sleep deprivation, and metabolic alkalosis. Conversely, enhanced central drive due to neurogenic, psychogenic, reflex, or metabolic stimuli augments the ventilatory workload. Drive-stimulating reflexes originating from the lung or chest wall reverse after correction of asthma and acute pulmonary edema. Hypoxemia, hypotension, developing sepsis, and acidosis also accentuate ventilatory demands. Correction of metabolic acidosis reduces central drive. If Pa_{CO_2} is forced below the patient's usual resting value, the ensuing bicarbonate diuresis elevates the $\dot{V}_E$ needed to maintain (cerebral pH) homeostasis. In fact, a somewhat higher than customary Pa_{CO_2} may help to minimize the $\dot{V}_E$ requirement. Supplementation of the inspired O_2 fraction is often an effective way to reduce drive and interrupt hyperpnea accompanied by hypoxemia, especially in a panic disorder or when there are disorganized breathing patterns, as may occur in emphysema.

Work Per Liter of Ventilation.   Ventilatory power is the product of $\dot{V}_E$ and the mechanical work of breathing per liter of ventilation. This mechanical workload in conjunction with neuromuscular efficiency defines how much energy must be expended in breathing. The frictional (resistive) and elastic properties (the reciprocal of compliance) of the respiratory system largely determine the pressure generated per breath of a given depth and speed as well as the external work output per liter of ventilation. For the same level of $\dot{V}_E$, more external work must be done if the compliance of the respiratory system falls or if V_T, auto-PEEP, mean inspiratory flow, or airway resistance increases. Bronchospasm, retained secretions, and mucosal edema are the primary reversible factors that increase resistance. Retained secretions amplify the inspiratory workload in patients with narrowed airways and high minute ventilation. Lung edema and infiltration, high lung volumes, pleural effusions, abdominal distention, and the supine posture reduce respiratory system compliance. Air trapping and dynamic hyperinflation of the respiratory system are more likely if the $\dot{V}_E$ is high, expiratory time is short, and expiratory airway resistance is high.

Ventilatory Capability

The ability to sustain an acceptable effort is determined by respiratory drive and muscle performance. Chronic loading of ventilation (as during a severe bout of asthma) can condition the ventilatory center to tolerate higher Pa_{CO_2}. Minute ventilation occasionally falls markedly during sleep or sedation and accelerates impressively with the return to alertness.

Abnormalities of Muscular Strength, Coordination, and Endurance.   Assuming intact ventilatory drive and normal impedance of the respiratory system, carbon dioxide retention is uncommon if the patient can generate more than 25% of the predicted maximum inspiratory pressure against an occluded airway, or about 30 cmH_2O. The strength of the respiratory muscles is determined by muscle bulk, the intrinsic properties and loading conditions of the contractile fibers, and the chemical environment in which the muscles contract. Poor nutrition causes muscle wasting, and glucocorticoids accelerate protein catabolism. Optimal concentrations of calcium, magnesium, potassium, phosphate, hydrogen ion, chloride, and carbon dioxide are each important in maximizing muscle performance. The resting electrical potential of the skeletal muscle membrane may remain abnormal for several days following sepsis and perhaps in other critical illnesses as well. Moreover, "critical-illness neuropathy" may help to explain the prolonged and impressive muscle weakness observed in many of these patients once the acute phase is past. The extended suppression of neuromuscular excitation by paralytic agents may result in profound weakness for lengthy periods after they are discontinued, especially when corticosteroids have been used concomitantly.

The ability of a muscle to sustain effort is determined by the balance between the supply of and demand for muscular energy. Hypoxemia, anemia, and ischemia are especially important to correct, because working muscles require an adequate flow of well-oxygenated blood for optimal performance. Although the respiratory muscles receive sufficient blood flow under normal circumstances and can recruit a large reserve, even this luxuriant supply may be insufficient under conditions of high stress and a failing cardiac pump. Spontaneous breathing may consume ~25% of total body oxygen consumption in acute respiratory failure and even more during flagrant respiratory distress, as opposed to the normal percentage of ~1%.

Hyperinflation.   The inspiratory muscles normally contract synchronously to either displace volume directly or to stabilize the rib cage or abdomen, so that the inspiratory actions of complementary muscles coordinate and are not offset by simultaneous expiratory activity. Both a stable chest wall and coordinated muscular activity are essential to pump efficiency. However well individual muscle fibers contract, their geometrical alignment determines how effectively the force generated accomplishes ventilation. Inspiratory muscles contract more effectively at *low* lung volumes, at which they are effectively preloaded. On the other hand, a flattened diaphragm develops tension that tends to pull the ribs inward in an expiratory rather than inspiratory action. Partially for this reason, acute hyperinflation represents an important impediment to effective ventilation. Expiratory muscles, on the other hand, contract most effectively at *high* lung volumes.

Common Ventilatory Pump Disorders

Abnormal Chest Wall Configuration

Obesity and Ascites.   Massive obesity and ascites reconfigure the chest wall and afterload the muscles of inspiration (Chap. 43). However, although the elevated diaphragm must contract against the pressurized abdominal contents, impairing diaphragmatic descent, the abdomen also provides a fulcrum around which the diaphragm can flare the rib cage outward. Thus, quiet breathing may be little compromised. Under the stress of increased ventilation requirements, however, higher tidal volumes are needed, and the elastic work of breathing may increase dramatically. The equilibrium position of the chest wall is displaced to a lower volume, so that FRC tends to fall. As compared with normal patients, higher levels of PEEP are needed in those who have chest wall abnormalities in order to produce the physiologically effective changes in lung volume that influence oxygenation. This is especially true in the supine position, where abdominal forces push the underside of the diaphragm cephalad. As FRC falls, airway caliber is compromised, increasing the resistance to breathing. Moreover, the tendencies toward hypoxemia and positional desaturation are increased because the patient often tends to breathe below the "closing volume" of the lung. (This is particularly true in the setting of bronchitis or airway edema.) In managing the obese patient or the patient with ascites, attention must be paid to maintaining a position that minimizes abdominal pressure and to supplementing inspired O_2 when necessary. Large-volume paracentesis may effectively lower abdominal pressure, relieving the work of breathing and allowing expansion of a lung otherwise made atelectatic by excessive abdominal pressure.

Pleural Effusion and Pneumothorax.   Both pleural effusions and pneumothorax may flatten or invert the ipsilateral diaphragm and drive the accessory inspiratory muscles to a "hyperinflated" position. In this configuration, the individual muscle fibers are foreshortened and the resulting geometry does not permit efficient inspiratory motion. Dyspnea may be relieved following thoracentesis or chest tube placement owing to the recovery of an effective mechanical advantage for the diaphragm.

Flail Chest.   A segment of the rib cage that has been separated from the integrated structure by fractures of two or more ribs in two or more places disrupts the structural and often functional integrity of the ventilatory pump. Combined with the pain, contusion, splinting, and atelectasis that usually accompany it, the presence of this flail segment may lead to ventilatory insufficiency as well as impaired oxygenation.

Kyphoscoliosis.   Chronic bony deformity of the chest wall (e.g., kyphoscoliosis and ankylosing spondylitis) may seriously impair the inspiratory capacity, preventing the deep breaths needed for exertion or coughing. Though inspiratory capacity may be limited, functional residual capacity in these specific conditions tends to remain well preserved. Initially, the problem is purely one of distorted and dysfunctional configuration, but the inability to ventilate and to clear secretions effectively from disadvantaged areas can lead to reduced lung compliance and hypoxemia later in the course. Difficulty increases in proportion to the bony deformity. Serious respiratory problems attributable solely to the mechanical disadvantage of scoliosis, for example, are seldom evident until angulation is extreme. Muscles that would ordinarily have an inspiratory action can be placed into a neutral or expiratory alignment by bony distortion. Furthermore, the chest cage becomes difficult to deform with tidal breathing efforts. Severe hypoxemia and cor pulmonale are frequent late complications. In such patients, maintaining the airway free of retained secretions and infection, treatment of hypoxemia, and assuring appropriate electrolyte balance and nutrition are the keystones of effective management.

Impaired Muscular Strength and Coordination

Diaphragmatic paralysis and quadriplegia provide complementary examples of regionalized muscular weakness. As such, both disorders present inherent problems of impaired muscular coordination as well as loss of effective muscle bulk and strength.

Diaphragm Paralysis.   Acute diaphragmatic dysfunction may occur from pneumonia, surgery, radiation, trauma, complications of anesthesia, and idiopathic causes. A paralyzed diaphragm tends to rise rather than fall during the inspiratory phase. As a passive membrane, it moves in proportion to the transmural pressure gradient applied across it. As abdominal pressure rises and intrathoracic pressure falls, the diaphragm tends to ascend into the chest. In the chronic setting, unilateral diaphragmatic paralysis only modestly impairs ventilatory capability, with vital capacity falling approximately 20–30% from its normal value. Quiet tidal breathing is little affected, and many such patients remain relatively asymptomatic throughout life. Symptoms surface only under periods of ventilatory stress or in the presence of a comorbid problem. Although causes of chronic unilateral paralysis can sometimes be identified (e.g., tumor, infection, radiation, trauma, or surgery), the origin of most remains unknown.

By contrast, bilateral diaphragmatic paralysis is a devastating disease that is usually idiopathic. These patients must sustain the entire ventilatory burden using accessory muscles. In the upright position, the expiratory muscles can contract to drive the diaphragm high into the chest at end exhalation. When expiratory tension is released, the falling abdominal pressure sucks the diaphragm caudally, aiding inspiration. This gravity-dependent mechanism cannot function in the supine position, and the abdomen moves paradoxically inward during inspiration. Therefore these patients experience extreme orthopnea and often present with sleep disturbances and headache related to nocturnal CO_2 accumulation. Vital capacity shows significant positional variation, falling by more than 30% in the transition from the upright to supine orientation. Many such patients can sustain ventilation for many hours when upright but need ventilatory support (invasively or noninvasively) for rest periods and in recumbency, especially during sleep. Poor regional ventilation in dependent areas, frequently combined with the need for tracheostomy, causes problems with atelectasis, pneumonitis, and bronchiectasis in basilar regions. Because diaphragmatic function seldom returns, treatment is supportive. Therapy centers on maintaining optimal clearance of secretions, keeping the lungs free of infection, and optimizing nutrition.

Skeletal Muscle Weakness and Paralysis.   The severity of ventilatory problems caused by spinal cord injury relates to the vertebral level of the lesion and, to a lesser degree, to the time elapsed since the injury occurred. Ventilatory effectiveness can improve significantly in the weeks following the injury, as neural function improves, muscle tone alters the compliance of the chest wall, and any functional accessory muscles strengthen. In the usual forms of quadriplegia (levels at or below C5), diaphragmatic function is well preserved. Unfortunately, some accessory inspiratory muscles may be compromised, and a variable fraction of expiratory power is routinely lost. Quadriplegic patients and those with acute myopathy often maintain excellent ventilation during quiet breathing but have little or no reserve. Expulsive activity may be severely impaired. Pneumonitis is potentially life-threatening; secretions cannot be raised, and the ventilatory requirement is increased. Techniques and devices available to assist coughing include manual compression of the upper abdomen, chest vibration, airway oscillation, and cough amplifiers that utilize biphasic (positive-negative) pressure applied at the airway opening.

Some quadriplegic patients breathe more easily when recumbent than when upright. In the former position, enhanced diaphragmatic curvature of the supine position, as well as the larger area of apposition of the diaphragm to the lower rib cage improve mechanical efficiency. Like diaphragmatic paralysis, the focus should center on reducing the ventilatory requirement and on keeping the lungs free of infection. In patients without an effective cough, secretion retention and mucous plugging present a continual risk. Optimal nutrition, prevention of aspiration, optimized bowel motility, prevention of abdominal distention, and prophylactic respiratory therapy—supplemented by assisted coughing (when feasible, indicated, and not contraindicated by abdominal distention, esophageal incompetence, severe thoracic deformity, spinal fracture, etc.)—are essential to health maintenance. When some expiratory force can be generated, abdominal compression may assist the coughing effort by splinting the abdomen and allowing buildup of intrathoracic pressure. Marginal patients often benefit from noninvasive nocturnal ventilatory support. Severely compromised patients who cannot effectively clear their airways with noninvasive assistance or who have other airway, lung, or chest wall diseases will require tracheostomy and conventional ventilation.

PRINCIPLES OF MANAGING RESPIRATORY FAILURE

The discussion of the pathophysiology of respiratory failure has made a deliberate but artificial distinction between hypoxic and ventilatory failure. In fact, many patients with hypercapnic respiratory failure are also hypoxemic, and patients who are primarily hypoxemic often expend so much muscle effort in attempting to compensate that they are at risk of fatiguing their respiratory muscles and developing ventilatory failure as well.

Recognition

The primary physical signs of ventilatory overstress or fatigue are vigorous use of accessory ventilatory muscles, tachypnea, tachycardia, diaphoresis, and paradoxical motion of the chest or abdomen. Patients who exhibit these signs should be placed in a closely monitored care area (emergency department holding area, intensive care unit, or respiratory care unit, depending on the individual hospital's policy). Other patients who must be closely monitored include those who require a high supplemental level of oxygen ($FI_{O_2} > 0.4$) to maintain an oxygen saturation of 89% or who have a significant uncompensated respiratory acidosis (pH ≤ 7.3).

    The respiratory pattern gives important clues to ventilatory compensation. The respiratory frequency (f) is the most sensitive but least specific indicator of developing problems. Early in the course of respiratory muscle fatigue, f increases. As exhaustion sets in, frequency often diminishes—a harbinger of approaching apnea. The respiratory rhythm tends to lose regularity as the fatigue threshold is approached. In late-stage disease, the breathing pattern may become gasping or highly irregular. In responding to an increased ventilatory workload (e.g., increasing exercise), a normal subject will increase both frequency and tidal volume together. When muscular strength is limited, patients tend to meet $\dot{V}E$ requirements by increasing frequency (f) without raising V_T. Although smaller breaths require less effort, the cost of rapid shallow breathing may be increased deadspace ventilation and the need for a higher $\dot{V}E$ to eliminate CO_2. A very high and continuously rising frequency (to rates > 30 breaths per minute) is generally accepted as a sign of ventilatory muscle decompensation and impending fatigue. It should be noted, however, that some patients (especially those with restrictive or neuromuscular diseases) increase f to a stable value > 35 breaths per minute and remain compensated.

    Other features of the respiratory pattern, although harder to quantitate, provide valuable diagnostic clues to impending respiratory failure. At moderate levels of exertion, pressure in the abdomen rises as the diaphragm contracts, displacing the abdominal contents downward and outward. Expiration (which occurs passively at low levels of exertion), often becomes active. Vigorous activity recruits the thoracic musculature, elongating the chest and expanding the rib cage. If diaphragmatic contraction is not forceful enough, the abdomen retracts inward—"paradoxically"—during inspiration. During expiration, the thoracic muscles relax and the abdominal contents return to their original position. When it is observed in the supine position, this phenomenon, known as paradoxical abdominal motion, indicates a high level of exertion relative to capability and suggests a high ventilatory workload that may or may not be tolerable. Much less commonly, overexertion is signaled when the rib cage and abdomen alternate primary responsibility for driving inspiration, a pattern known as respiratory alternans.

Management

Respiratory failure is managed by defining its cause, correcting reversible factors, and providing mechanical support when required. Bedside measurements intended to define the mechanisms of ventilatory failure are especially important. Alertness, agitation, pain or discomfort, body size and temperature, metabolic stress (sepsis, trauma, burns), ventilatory dead-space fraction, nutritional status, and the work of breathing itself help determine the $\dot{V}_E$ requirement. Neuromuscular function is evaluated by observing the ventilatory pattern, tidal volume and breathing frequency, and actions of the respiratory muscles as well as by measuring the maximal inspiratory pressure developed against an occluded airway. The appropriateness of ventilatory drive is often best assessed at the bedside by examining the pH and $PaCO_2$ in relation to breathing effort. (If $PaCO_2$ is high and pH is low, drive may be deficient, muscular reserve inadequate, or both; evidence of patient agitation or dyspnea, suggests primacy of the latter.) The tidal mouth occlusion pressure ($P_{0.1}$), a laboratory research test for more than two decades, is just now coming into clinical use as a quantitative drive index. Ideally, the $P_{0.1}$ should be referenced to the maximal inspiratory pressure, as it is a strength-dependent index.

Correcting Reversible Factors. The search for the cause for ventilatory failure should be guided by a systematic if often qualitative evaluation of ventilatory drive, $\dot{V}_E$, the work of breathing, and neuromuscular performance. Therapy to reverse ventilatory failure should be guided by knowledge of the underlying defect (Table 3). For example, the $\dot{V}_E$, requirement may be lowered by reducing fever, agitation, and dead space. Impedance can be improved by relieving airway obstruction (bronchodilation, secretion clearance, placement of a larger endotracheal tube), increasing parenchymal compliance (reduction of atelectasis, edema, and inflammation), and improving chest wall distensibility (drainage of air or fluid from the pleural space, relief of abdominal distention, muscle relaxation, or analgesia). Neuromuscular efficiency should be optimized by ensuring alertness, maintaining upright posture, relieving pain, reducing dynamic hyperinflation, and correcting electrolyte disturbances, anemia, nutritional deficiencies, and endocrine disorders. Although Addison's disease is rare, adrenal insufficiency is surprisingly common among critically ill and chronically debilitated patients undergoing major physiological stress. Measures that improve cardiac output or arterial oxygenation will also improve neuromuscular performance. Treatable neuromuscular disorders (e.g., myasthenia, myositis, Parkinson's disease) should not be overlooked. Some problems of decreased ventilatory drive are self-limited (e.g., sedative or opiate overdose); others improve with nutritional repletion, hormonal replacement (hypothyroidism), repair of sleep deficit, or recovery or mental status. Few respond to nonspecific ventilatory stimulants such as pro-

Table 3 Reversible Factors in Ventilatory Failure

Excessive ventilation requirement	Impaired muscle strength and endurance
Metabolic acidosis	Nutritional deficiency
Increased CO_2 generation	Electrolyte disturbances PO_4^{-2}, Mg^{2+}, K^+
Fever	Endocrine disorders and corticosteroids
Agitation	Impaired cardiac output
Work of breathing	Neuromuscular disorders
Calories	Hyperinflation
Increased dead space	Drug
Airway apparatus	β Blockers
Hypovolemia	calcium channel blockers
Vascular obstruction	
Increased impedance to ventilation	**Impaired ventilatory drive**
Secretions	Drugs (sedatives and analgesics)
Bronchospasm	Malnutrition
Airway apparatus	Sleep deprivation
Pleural air or fluid	Metabolic alkalosis
Abdominal distention	Hypothyroidism
Auto-PEEP	
Pulmonary edema	

gesterone. Unfortunately, many disorders of ventilatory control are refractory to drug manipulation and must be treated by optimizing ventilatory mechanics with the goal of reducing the work of breathing sufficiently to restore compensation.

Ventilatory Support. Willingness to institute mechanical ventilation should be directly proportional to the risk of deterioration without support and inversely proportional to the anticipated difficulty of eventual weaning. Noninvasive ventilation offers an attractive option for many patients with mild to moderate disease and rapidly reversible etiologies for ventilatory failure (see Chap. 25). To reverse fatigue, a substantial fraction of the imposed workload must be relieved. Support can be assumed adequate if breathing is comfortable. Physiological evidence of subnormal performance can be detected in the laboratory setting for 12–24 h after an acutely fatiguing load has been briefly applied ($<$ 30 mins). Therefore, patients should not be stressed to the point of fatigue, and a rest period of at least 12 h seems appropriate after an episode of acute decompensation.

SUGGESTED READING

1. Curtis J, Hudson L. Emergent assessment and management of acute respiratory failure in COPD. Clin Chest Med 1994; 15:481–500.
2. Derenne J, Fleury B, Pariente R. Acute respiratory failure of chronic obstructive pulmonary disease. Am Rev Respir Dis 1988; 138:1006–1033.
3. Dreyfuss D, Saumon G. Ventilator-induced lung injury: lessons from experimental studies. Am J Respir Crit Care Med 1998; 157:294–323.
4. Feihl F, Perret C. Permissive hypercapnia: how permissive should we be? Am J Respir Crit Care Med 1994; 150:1722–1737.

5. Goldstein R. Hypoventilation: neuromuscular and chest wall disorders. Clin Chest Med 1992; 13:507–521.

6. Kamp D. Physiologic evaluation of asthma. Chest 1992; 101(6 suppl):396S–400S.

7. Leatherman J. Life-threatening asthma. Clin Chest Med 1994; 15:453–480.

8. Leatherman J. Mechanical ventilation in obstructive lung disease. Clin Chest Med 1996; 17: 577–590.

9. Lynn D, Woda R, Mendell J. Respiratory dysfunction in muscular dystrophy and other myopathies. Clin Chest Med 1994; 15:661–674.

10. Marinelli W, Ingbar D. Diagnosis and management of acute lung injury. Clin Chest Med 1994; 15:517–546.

11. Marini J. Evolving concepts in the ventilatory management of acute respiratory distress syndrome. Clin Chest Med 1996; 17:555–575.

12. Marini JJ, Slutsky AS. Physiological Basis of Ventilatory Support. New York: Marcel Dekker, 1998.

13. Marini JJ. Should PEEP be used in airflow obstruction? Am Rev Respir Dis 1989; 140:1–3.

14. Marini JJ, Roussos C, eds. Ventilatory Failure. Berlin: Springer-Verlag, 1991.

15. Marini JJ, Wheeler AP. Critical Care Medicine—The Essentials, 2d ed. Baltimore: Williams & Wilkins, 1997.

16. Nunn JF. Nunn's Applied Respiratory Physiology, 4th ed. London: Butterworth-Heinemann, 1993.

16. Pontoppidan H, Geffin B, Lowenstein E. Acute respiratory failure in the adult. N Engl J Med 1972; 287:690–698, 743–752, 799–806.

17. Rochester D, Esau S. Assessment of ventilatory function in patients with neuromuscular disease. Clin Chest Med 1994; 15:751–764.

18. Tobin MJ. Respiratory muscles in disease. Clin Chest Med 1988. 9:263–286.

20

Evaluation and Management of the Solitary Pulmonary Nodule

T. Glen Bouder
University of Vermont College of Medicine
Fletcher Allen Health Care
Burlington, Vermont

Jay H. Ryu
Mayo Medical School and Mayo Clinic
Rochester, Minnesota

INTRODUCTION

The discovery of a solitary pulmonary nodule (SPN) on a routine chest radiograph is common in clinical practice and raises the important question: Is the nodule malignant? The possibility of a cancerous lesion can make this seemingly simple question an anxiety-provoking problem for patients and a diagnostic dilemma for the practitioner. The often benign causes of solitary pulmonary nodules and the era of cost-efficient medicine emphasize the importance of a logical approach to the evaluation. This chapter reviews the important aspects of the evaluation of a SPN and outlines an approach to the management of this problem.

Definition

A SPN is a discrete, round or oval radiographic opacity that is surrounded by normal lung tissue and not associated with atelectasis or adenopathy. Figure 1 demonstrates a typical chest radiographic appearance of a SPN. The exact size defining a nodule has been reported in the literature in a range from 1–4 cm in diameter. In large case series, lesions larger than 3 cm have demonstrated an increased likelihood of being malignant. On this basis, a nodule is defined as a radiographic abnormality of less than 3 cm in diameter. A lesion greater than 3 cm is considered a mass.

Incidence and Etiology

Solitary pulmonary nodules are seen in 0.1–0.2% of screening chest radiographs. The majority of these are identified on routine radiographic examinations in asymptomatic

329

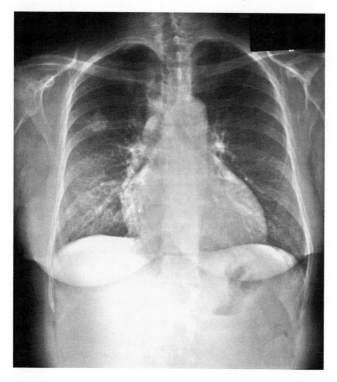

Figure 1 Typical appearance of a solitary pulmonary nodule on chest radiography.

individuals. Prior to the availability of computed tomography (CT), large surgical case series published in the 1970s reported a malignancy rate of approximately 40% among SPNs removed surgically. In more recent reviews, 60–80% have been found to be malignant. This increased malignancy rate is probably due to improved presurgical evaluation resulting in a decreased rate of surgery for benign lesions. The advent of CT scan technology has significantly contributed to improved presurgical evaluation.

Nodules may appear in any location in the lung. Steele, in his report on a multicenter cooperative study of 887 resected and asymptomatic SPNs, found that 73% of the malignant SPNs were located in the upper lobes. Despite the upper lobe predominance, any region of the lungs may have a malignant nodule. Granulomatous disease (except tuberculosis) is found with equal frequency in the upper and lower lung zones.

Bronchogenic carcinoma is the leading cause of malignant SPNs and adenocarcinoma is the most common cell type. The frequency of the cancer cell type of malignant SPNs varies depending on how the authors defined the size of a SPN. Of malignant SPNs, the reported frequency of non-small-cell carcinoma ranges from 41–70%, squamous cell carcinoma from 20–47%, and other types (including small-cell) 6–12%. Approximately 80% of benign nodules are due to granulomatous infections. Histoplasmosis and coccidiomycosis are the most common granulomatous lesions. Table 1 lists benign and malignant causes of SPNs.

Table 1 Causes of Solitary Pulmonary Nodules

Benign	Malignant
Infectious granulomas	Bronchogenic carcinoma
Histoplasmoma	Adenocarcinoma
Coccidioidoma	Large-cell
Tuberculoma	Small-cell
	Squamous-cell
Hamartoma	
	Bronchial carcinoid
Wegener's granulomatosis	
	Solitary metastases
Rheumatoid nodule	Colon cancer
	Renal cell cancer
Arteriovenous malformation	Germ cell tumors
	Breast cancer
Abscess	Head and neck tumors
	Sarcoma
Lipoma	Thyroid cancer
	Others
Localized amyloid	
Bronchogenic cyst	
Ascaris/Echinococcus species	
Lipoid pneumonia	

INITIAL EVALUATION

The evaluation a solitary pulmonary nodule requires a thorough history and physical examination as well as careful consideration of the radiographic features of the nodule. A logical approach is important for everyone in the process.

History and Physical Examination

Most patients are asymptomatic, the nodule having been discovered inadvertently on a routine chest radiograph. Because a history of cigarette smoking is an important risk factor for malignancy, the amount and duration of smoking should be ascertained from the patient. Exposure to other potential carcinogens—for example, asbestos—should be thoroughly sought when recording the history. A previous history of malignancy or the concurrent presence of an extrathoracic neoplasm is a key issue, as approximately 10–30% of malignant nodules are found to be from extrathoracic malignancies. Head and neck cancers and adenocarcinomas of the colon, breast, and kidney are among the more common causes of metastatic nodules. Travel history and a review of geographic areas of past and present residences is important in identifying possible infectious etiologies. For example, coccidiomycosis is endemic in the desert southwest of the United States. Histoplasmosis, however, is commonly found in the Mississippi, Ohio, and St. Lawrence River valleys. *Echinococcus* may be suspected if the patient has lived or traveled to endemic areas.

    Physical signs are absent in most patients with a SPN. No specific chest findings are present in most cases. Digital clubbing may be found occasionally in patients with bronchogenic carcinoma. In patients with pulmonary arteriovenous malformations (AVMs), telangiectasias may sometimes be identified on other areas of the body. Rarely, a pulmonary AVM will be large enough that a bruit may be auscultated, particularly with the aid of a Müller maneuver. This maneuver is accomplished by having the patient make an inspiratory effort with a closed glottis at end expiration. The negative intrathoracic pressure causes engorgement in intrathoracic vascular structures, increasing the intensity of the bruit. Extrathoracic manifestations of underlying systemic diseases may be found in some cases. For example, a rheumatoid nodule might be palpated on the elbow of a patient with rheumatoid arthritis and a rheumatoid lung nodule.

Identifying the Potential for Malignancy

Identification of important factors that increase the likelihood of a SPN being malignant is important. Age is an identified risk factor for malignancy. In case series of patients with SPNs, among patients above 50 years of age, 50–65% of resected SPNs were malignant. Conversely, in patients below 35 years of age with no other risk factors for malignancy, the prevalence of cancer among SPNs was approximately 1%. Thus the age at which the risk of malignancy begins to be a factor is about 35 years, and it increases with aging. Smoking is also an important risk factor for malignancy. The association of tobacco smoke and bronchogenic carcinoma is well established, and the associated risk is increased as the amount and duration of smoking increases. Over time, a reduction in that risk can be gained by cessation of smoking. Secondary exposure to cigarette smoke may also increase the risk of lung cancer, but these data are less certain. Exposure to asbestos or other carcinogens also represents a risk for developing a malignancy. When significant asbestos exposure is combined with cigarette smoking, the risk of lung cancer increases well above that of either alone.

As discussed earlier in this chapter, nodule size is an important feature in considering the malignant potential of a nodule. In retrospective reviews of resected pulmonary nodules, the frequency of malignancy increased as the size of the nodule increased. Nonetheless, in the series reported by Steele, 25% of the 280 carcinomas were 2.0 cm or less in diameter. This finding has been supported in other studies. Thus, large size is a good predictor of malignancy, but small size is a poor predictor of a benign cause.

The relative weight of each of these factors is sometimes difficult to assess. Cummings and coworkers used Bayes theorem to demonstrate that a reasonably accurate estimate of the probability that a SPN is malignant could be calculated using data on the overall prevalence of carcinoma in the population, the size of the nodule, smoking history, and the age of the person. The result, known as P_{ca} (probability of cancer), represents the predicted likelihood that a nodule is malignant. Interestingly, clinical judgment based on a complete evaluation was as good at predicting the probability of malignancy as the actual calculation.

Radiographic Assessment

An important part of the evaluation process is assessing the radiographic features of the nodule. Extrapulmonary structures often create the radiographic appearance of nodular opacities. These include nipple shadows, bone or pleural lesions, and film artifact. These abnormalities should be excluded before further evaluation of a SPN is pursued. Once a true SPN has been identified, the radiographic characteristics of the nodule are evaluated. This information can complement the historical information already obtained. The first step is to observe the general appearance of the nodule. Benign lesions are usually round and well circumscribed. Malignant lesions usually have less well defined, irregular borders and are often spiculated in appearance.

Comparison with old chest roentgenograms is essential in this initial phase of radiographic evaluation. If the nodule is found not to have changed in size over 2 years or more, one may be reassured that it is probably benign. The rationale for this is based on the known growth rates of benign and malignant nodules. Growth rates for nodules are based on doubling time, which is defined as the rate at which the mass of the nodule doubles in volume. With only very rare exceptions, malignancies are known to double in volume at a rate between 20 to 450 days. Nonmalignant nodules either grow at very slow rates or increase in size very rapidly. Therefore a malignant nodule should change in size over a period of 2 years. Volume (V) and radius (r), as measured radiographically, are related by the formula $V = 4/3\pi r^3$. This is important because a 1-cm nodule that doubles in volume increases by only 3 mm in diameter. Any nodule that is growing in size needs further investigation independent of the presence or absence of risk factors for malignancy.

The presence or absence of calcification and its pattern within the nodule are additional radiographic features of SPNs to consider. The nodule in Fig. 2 is a benign hamartoma and demonstrates the classic popcorn pattern of calcification. Benign nodules associated with granulomatous infections often demonstrate dense, central calcification. Overlap in the radiographic features of benign and malignant nodules exists and the calcification pattern should not be used alone in defining the malignant potential of the nodule. Table 2 lists the general patterns of calcification found in SPNs.

When better radiographic definition is desired, a helical CT scan may be obtained. A CT scan demonstrates the nodule characteristics much better than plain chest radiographs (Fig. 2). The same characteristics of nodules evaluated on chest roentogram may also be applied to CT scan images. Thin-section (1 mm) CT scan is a specific radiographic technique used to detect subtle calcification or fat (found in hamartomas). It has significantly improved the ability to evaluate SPNs noninvasively. It is also useful in identifying other nonmalignant causes of SPNs, such as mucous plugs, arteriovenous malformations, round atelectasis, focal scars, and pleural lesions. A CT scan is indicated, and often very helpful, whenever further definition of a suspicious nodule is required.

History, radiographic findings, and risk factors associated with malignancy are the foundation of the initial evaluation of the patient with a SPN. Based on these evaluations and the assessed likelihood of malignancy, the clinician must now decide whether or not further diagnostic testing is appropriate. It is useful to assign the nodule to one of three categories—likely benign, indeterminate, or likely malignant based on the history, physical examination, and radiographic findings. By categorizing SPNs in this way, decisions regarding the need for further diagnostic testing can be made.

DIAGNOSTIC PROCEDURES

Many diagnostic modalities are available for evaluating the SPN. However, prior to any diagnostic procedures, complete pulmonary function testing should be obtained. It is extremely important that this be accomplished in order to (1) assess the risk of the anticipated procedure and (2) to assess postresection morbidity if surgery is indicated. A pneumotho-

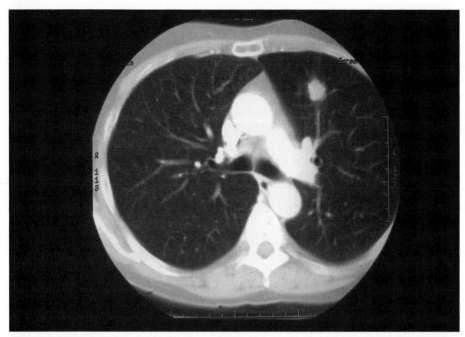

(a)

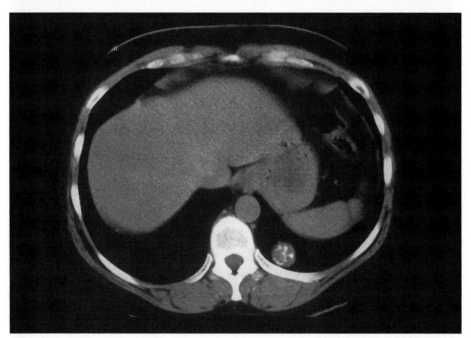

(b)

Figure 2 CT sections demonstrating benign and malignant characteristics. (a) CT section of a malignant nodule—ill-defined, irregular borders of an adenocarcinoma. (b) CT section of a benign nodule—smooth borders and popcorn calcification pattern characteristic of a hamartoma.

Table 2 Calcification Patterns
Found in Solitary Pulmonary Nodules

Likely Benign	Indeterminate
Central	Stippled
Laminated	Eccentric
Diffuse	Absence of calcium
Popcorn	

rax or hemorrhage as a result of a needle biopsy can interfere with optimal pulmonary function testing and thus give the clinician potentially misleading information.

Imaging Techniques

In addition to the chest radiograph and CT scanning, additional methods of noninvasive radiographic testing are being evaluated. Early studies using contrast-enhanced CT scans have been very promising and are now being used routinely in some medical centers. With this technique, malignant nodules exhibit a higher degree of enhancement with the administration of intravenous contrast as compared with benign nodules. Contrast-enhancement studies using magnetic resonance imaging (MRI) and positron emission tomography (PET) technology have also been reported as helpful in improving the accuracy in predicting malignancy. In most hospitals and clinics, cost and availability preclude the routine use of MRI and PET technology.

Bronchoscopy/Sputum Cytology

Bronchoscopy, a useful tool in evaluating patients with a wide range of lung diseases, has limited utility in the evaluation of the patient with a SPN. Using bronchoscopically obtained washes, biopsies, and cytological brushes, the diagnostic yield for lesions smaller than 2 cm is less than 20%. In general, the routine use of bronchoscopy in the evaluation of SPNs is limited.

Evaluation of sputum cytology has been used as an easily obtained and noninvasive technique for diagnosing bronchogenic carcinoma. Unfortunately, in patients with a SPN, studies have shown that the diagnostic yield is less than 20% in patients who are eventually diagnosed with a malignant nodule. Sputum examination is virtually useless in identifying benign disease; therefore, it is not recommended in the evaluation of patients with a SPN.

Transthoracic Needle Aspiration Biopsy

Transthoracic needle aspiration (TTNA) biopsy has become an important tool in the evaluation of the SPN. The ability to directly image the biopsy needle in the nodule by fluoroscopy or CT scan has markedly improved the diagnostic yield of this technique. The skill and experience of the radiographer and the presence of the pathologist at the time of biopsy for rapid cytological evaluation are important factors in obtaining a specific diagnosis. More than one attempt at TTNA is sometimes required to get a satisfactory biopsy. A specimen is considered satisfactory when (1) the operator is reasonably certain that the needle has entered the lesion, (2) the cytologist is confident that the material was obtained from a lesion and not normal lung, or (3) a specific diagnosis is made. In detecting malignancy, TTNA is an excellent tool with diagnostic yields greater than 90% in several large case series. However, the ability of TTNA to definitively determine benign causes of SPNs has not been as high as that for malignancy. This is presumably because the granulomatous infection (the most common cause of benign SPNs) is inactive and the organisms are rare or absent. False-negative rates from 3% to as high as 29% have been reported. TTNA is an excellent test for detecting malignancy, but a negative result does not reliably predict benign disease. Contraindications to TTNA include coagulopathy, platelet count less than 100,000, bullous disease in the immediate vicinity of the lesion, severe pulmonary hypertension, severe respiratory insufficiency, and inability of the patient to cooperate. The most common complications of TTNA biopsy are hemoptysis in 2–14% and pneumothorax in 20–34% of patients. About 5–15% of patients undergoing a TTNA require chest tube placement for the complication of pneumothorax. No deaths have been reported.

Surgery

Surgical removal of SPNs has provided much of the data for our modern approach to this problem. Thoracotomy has been the traditional surgical approach to SPN resection. The advent of less invasive diagnostic techniques has reduced but not eliminated the need for thoracotomy. A mortality risk of 3–7% for resection of malignant nodules via thoracotomy emphasizes the importance of careful preoperative evaluation, particularly in patients with underlying heart and lung disease. The mortality risk for benign lesions is much lower (0.3%), due in part to the smaller surgical resection required. Video-assisted thoracoscopic surgery (VATS) has revolutionized approaches to lung surgery. The reduced complication rate, decreased length of hospitalization, and decreased discomfort make it a very attractive alternative. However, survival rates for the treatment of cancer are better with lobectomy than with less complete resections. In most cases, lobectomy can be accomplished only by converting the VATS procedure to a standard thoracotomy in patients found to have a bronchogenic carcinoma. Thus, VATS becomes a diagnostic procedure like TTNA, not a curative one. From an economic perspective, an overall reduction in the cost of evaluating SPNs exclusively by VATS has not been proven because of this frequent need to convert the procedure to a standard thoracotomy. As a result, the role of VATS in the evaluation and management of the SPN is still being investigated and should not be considered routine.

DECISION MAKING

The many clinical variables associated with each patient can make evaluation of a SPN challenging. A framework for the evaluation process is shown in Fig. 3. The text that follows expands on that framework, providing an approach to the evaluation of patients with SPNs.

The initial step is to review the historical data. Older age and a history of tobacco smoking raise the index of suspicion for malignancy. The radiographic appearance of the abnormality is then reviewed. Concomitantly, a search for previous chest radiographs to be used for comparison should be undertaken. If the nodule was present on prior chest radiographs and is stable in size over a 2-year period, it is likely benign. It is acceptable to observe this patient with chest radiographs on a periodic basis—e.g., once every several

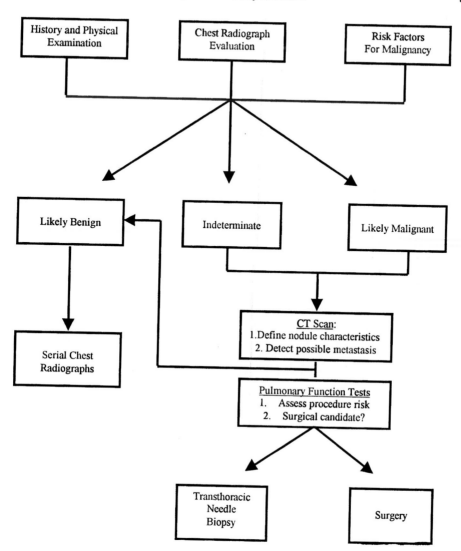

Figure 3 Strategy for evaluating the solitary pulmonary nodule.

years. If the nodule is new but risk factors are absent (age <35 years and no smoking or carcinogen exposure history), a strategy of serial chest radiographs every 3 months for 1 year, every 6 months for 2 years, and yearly thereafter for several more years can be utilized. Similarly, a benign pattern of calcification on chest radiograph in the absence of risk factors is a nodule that is likely benign. This nodule may be followed without biopsy or resection. Often, a CT scan with thin-section cuts through the nodule is obtained to further define the nodule. This may be useful in identifying subtle calcification or fat and may aid in determining which patients may need more diagnostic testing. If a CT scan is performed, subsequent radiographic evaluations of the nodule should utilize this modality. This allows a more accurate measurement of the nodule size. Nodules that enlarge within a 2-year observation period should be considered likely malignant.

Table 3 Estimated Survival in Non-
Small-Cell Lung Carcinoma

Stage	5-Year Survival (%)
I A	67
B	57
II A	34
B	24
III A	25
B	6–8
IV	1

Source: Data from Mountain, CF. Revisions
in the international system for staging lung
cancer. Chest 1997; 111:1710–1717.

Indeterminate and likely malignant nodules require further diagnostic studies. Prior to further diagnostic testing, complete pulmonary function tests and a helical CT scan of the entire chest, liver, and adrenal glands using intravenous contrast should be obtained. Evidence of potential disease elsewhere may indicate a more appropriate biopsy site and significantly influence patient management, particularly with regard to surgical treatment options. In asymptomatic individuals with non-small-cell lung cancer, metastatic lesions to the brain are uncommon and a head CT scan is not routinely performed. After a complete noninvasive evaluation, indeterminate SPNs should be referred for TTNA biopsy. A satisfactory biopsy that is negative for malignancy but without a definite benign diagnosis should be considered for surgical resection. In the absence of a clinical suspicion for malignancy, some authors advocate a watch-and-wait strategy using serial chest radiographs or CT scans. In patients who are elderly or are otherwise poor surgical candidates, this is probably a justifiable approach. For the SPN that is likely to be malignant and in the absence of detectable metastatic disease, direct surgical referral is indicated. Some centers advocate TTNA biopsy for definitive diagnosis prior to surgery. There are no substantive data to support or refute this position.

PROGNOSIS

For patients with a benign SPN the prognosis is obviously excellent. For patients requiring surgery, mortality is related to the extent of resection and comorbid factors. Survival in patients with malignant disease is related to the clinical and pathologic stage. The international TNM classification system is useful in estimating survival for various stage lung cancers. Recent revisions in that system provide improved sensitivity and specificity for identifying patients with similar prognoses and treatment options. Table 3 lists the estimated 5-year survival in non-small-cell lung cancer based on the revised TNM system.

CONCLUSION

The evaluation of the patient with a solitary pulmonary nodule is a common and often challenging problem for the clinician. The excellent 5-year survival of patients with surgically resected stage I non-small-cell lung cancer makes it important to diagnose malignancy in patients with a SPN. Similarly, establishing benign disease prior to thoracotomy reduces the risks associated with that surgery. In evaluating the patient, the guidelines in Fig. 3 serve as a useful framework for the evaluation process. If questions arise, referral to a specialist in this area is recommended. Using the known data on solitary pulmonary nodules and a well-defined diagnostic strategy, a rational approach can be achieved.

SUGGESTED READING

1. Allen MS, Deschamps C, Lee RE, Trastek VF, Daly RC, Pairolero PC. Video-assisted thoracoscopic stapled wedge excision for indeterminate pulmonary nodules. J Thorac Cardiovasc Surg 1993; 106:1048–1052.
2. Calhoun P, Feldman PS, Armstrong P, Black WC, Pope TL, Minor GR, Daniel TM. The clinical outcome of needle aspirations of the lung when cancer is not diagnosed. Ann Thorac Surg 1986; 41:592–596.
3. Cummings SR, Lillington GA, Richard RJ. Estimating the probability of malignancy in solitary pulmonary nodules. Am Rev Respir Dis 1986; 134:449–452.
4. Higgins GA, Shields TW, Keehn RJ. The solitary pulmonary nodule—ten year follow-up of Veteran's Administration—Armed Forces Cooperative Study. Arch Surg 1975; 110:570–575.
5. Khouri NF, Stitik FP, Erozan YS, Gupta PK, Kim WS, Scott WW, Hamper UM, Mann RB, Eggleston JC, Baker RR. Transthoracic needle aspiration biopsy of benign and malignant lung lesions. Am J Roentgenol 1985; 144:281–288.
6. Mitruka S, Landreneau RJ, Mack MJ, Fetterman LS, Gammie J, Bartley S, Sutherland SR, Bowers CM, Keenan RJ, Ferson PF, Weyant RJ. Diagnosing the indeterminate pulmonary nodule: percutaneous biopsy versus thoracoscopy. Surgery 1995; 118:676–684.
7. Siegelman SS, Khouri NF, Leo FP, Fishman EK, Braverman RM, Zerhonni EA. Solitary pulmonary nodules: CT assessment. Radiology 1986; 160:307–312.
8. Steele JD. The solitary pulmonary nodule—report of a cooperative study of resected asymptomatic solitary pulmonary nodules in males. J Thorac Cardiovasc Surg 1963; 46:1:21–39.
9. Toomes H, Delphendahl A, Manke H. The coin lesion of the lung—a review of 955 resected coin lesions. Cancer 1983; 51:534–537.

21
Hemoptysis

David H. Ingbar
University of Minnesota School of Medicine
Fairview University Medical Center
Minneapolis, Minnesota

INTRODUCTION

Hemoptysis is one of the classic symptoms in clinical medicine. Osler and other famous physicians of the past have been interested in it because of its clinical importance; it has served as a sign of tuberculosis and other lung infections. Until recently, it was a common reason for patients to be seen in chest clinics. With the decline in two of the major etiologies of hemoptysis, tuberculosis (TB) and bronchiectasis, hemoptysis is a less common clinical problem. However, it also presents new challenges because the etiological spectrum is now more diverse than in the past, and advances in medicine, such as transplantation and chemotherapy, are changing many of the illnesses with which it is associated.

Hemoptysis is both a sign or symptom of illness and a potentially serious problem in and of itself. As a symptom, it poses difficulty because it may result from life-threatening illness or from less dangerous problems, such as acute bronchitis, especially in individuals with underlying chronic lung disease. Some of the underlying illnesses that lead to presentation with hemoptysis are not readily apparent and can be difficult to diagnose. When bleeding is massive and/or the patient has very little functional lung tissue, hemoptysis may be fatal, owing to asphyxiation. Exsanguination from hemoptysis is extremely rare and usually results when a systemic artery communicates with the bronchial tree—as in some lung or esophageal cancers that erode into great vessels or in tracheoinnominate artery fistulas after tracheostomy.

This chapter examines etiologies of hemoptysis, the diagnostic workup, and management, but it touches only briefly on massive hemoptysis, since this is much less common and is also the subject of recent reviews included in the suggested reading.

ETIOLOGIES

Through the 1940s, the leading causes of hemoptysis were TB, bronchiectasis, and other lung infections. These have become less prevalent, and the etiologies that we now encoun-

341

Table 1   Etiologies of Hemoptysis Reported Since 1980[a]

	UM-KC	Portsmouth	Wadsworth	Tulane	U Rochester
	VA	VA			
Selection Method	Bronch	Bronch Nl/Abnl CXR	Bronch	?ENT	Bronch & Nl CXR
Bronchitis	37%	38%/14%	23%	20%	43%
Cancer	19%	4%/29%	29%	24%	6%
TB	7%	0	7%	2%	1.5%
Idiopathic	4%	2%/10%	22%	20%	32%
Bronchiectasis	1%	4%/20%	1%	4%	3.5%
Upper airway	4%	0 ?	0 ?	10%	2%

Key: Bronch, bronchoscopy; Nl, normal; abnl, abnormal; CXR, chest roentgenogram; ENT, otolaryngologists; ?, uncertain or not specified.
[a] Includes all published series with >100 cases reported.

ter represent a broader spectrum of illnesses. Unfortunately, there are relatively few large, published studies of the etiologies of hemoptysis since 1980 (Table 1). Those published studies likely reflect somewhat skewed populations, such as those treated at Veterans Administration hospitals. In this section, the major etiologies are briefly discussed based on the nature of the disease process; then the relative prevalence of the etiology of hemoptysis is considered.

Specific Etiologies

Congenital

The most common developmental cause of hemoptysis is pulmonary arteriovenous malformations (AVMs). These can be solitary or multiple and may be associated with Osler-Weber-Rendu (OWR, or hereditary hemorrhagic telangiectasia) syndrome. AVMs typically arise from the pulmonary artery and may lead to a high-cardiac-output state. They more typically are in the lower portions of the lung and may lead to an audible chest murmur, especially during inspiration. The chest x-ray and pulmonary arteriogram of a patient with an AVM independent of OWR are shown in Fig. 1.

In patients with OWR syndrome, skin, brain, and other AVMs are also common and pulmonary AVMs occur in 40–50% of patients, with increasing expression with age. The disease is inherited as an autosomal dominant with variable penetrance. Two types of OWR mutations have been defined. Type I has mutations that interfere with production of endoglin, an endothelial protein that binds transforming growth factor (TGF) beta. Type 2 OWR has mutations in the kinase domains of an activin receptor–like kinase that has homology with the TGF-beta$_1$ receptor family. Thus the manifestations of OWR likely arise from abnormalities of transmembrane signaling, possibly related to TGF-beta. Patients with frequent episodes of hemorrhage may also have an iron-deficiency anemia.

Other congenital pulmonary syndromes, such as sequestrations, can rarely result in hemoptysis. This is one instance where the feeding vessel is often systemic in origin. Congenital cardiac disease is also a well-recognized cause of pulmonary hypertension and hemoptysis, although the precise mechanisms are not clearly defined.

Neoplastic

Bronchogenic carcinoma is one of the major etiologies of hemoptysis. Although hemoptysis occurs in only 10–30% of lung cancer cases, it is fear of lung cancer that often leads patients with hemoptysis to seek medical assistance. The typical pattern of hemoptysis from bronchogenic carcinoma is streaking of the sputum with blood for at least 10–14 days or longer. Usually cancers resulting in hemoptysis are endobronchial and fairly centrally located in the airway; thus squamous- and small-cell carcinomas are particularly common. Hemoptysis is the initial presenting manifestation of lung cancer in a relatively small percentage of patients, but because lung cancer now has such a high incidence, it still is relatively common, and excluding it is a very important consideration. Several studies indicate that patients with significant smoking history or age above 35–40 years should be carefully worked up to exclude bronchogenic carcinoma, even in the presence of a normal chest radiograph.

Hemoptysis can occur late in carcinomas of the lung or esophagus and may cause massive hemoptysis if there is central disease eroding through major vascular structures. Hemoptysis is usually felt to be an indication for radiation therapy for inoperable bronchogenic carcinoma.

Other lung tumors may also present with hemoptysis, such as bronchial carcinoid tumors. They typically occur in younger individuals who may have persistent cough, recurrent localized pneumonias, and hemoptysis. On bronchoscopic examination, they may appear as reddish or polypoid lesions of the bronchial wall. On biopsy, they may bleed significantly owing to their vascularity.

Bleeding from tumors metastatic to the lung is relatively uncommon but may be seen with endobronchial metastases, most often from breast carcinoma or melanoma.

Infections

Many different infections can cause hemoptysis. Lung abcess used to be a common cause, but—like TB and bronchiectasis—it has become much less common. However, when bleeding due to lung abcess occurs, it often is massive and may be fatal.

Bacterial infections that cause lung necrosis may also result in bleeding. Typically this occurs in staphylococcal and gram-negative infections, but it may also be seen with mixed anaerobic infections, including aspiration pneumonias. Bleeding is usually not severe but occasionally can be in the setting of thrombocytopenia and/or coagulopathy. Thus this problem is being seen more frequently in patients receiving chemotherapy for cancer.

Fungal and mycobacterial infections of the lung parenchyma commonly cause bleeding. Of the fungi, aspergillosis and mucormycosis are the most dangerous because they are angio-invasive and often produce distal lung infarction. Mycetomas or fungus balls have a high frequency of associated hemoptysis, on the order of 30–50%. As TB has become less common, chronic sarcoidosis has become a common substratum for this problem. In addition, in immunocompromised hosts, localized tracheobronchial ulceration with bleeding can occur with *Aspergillus*.

TB can lead to hemoptysis in multiple ways. First, active cavitary TB can present with small or large amounts of hemoptysis. In general, when this is the etiology, smears for acid-fast bacilli will be positive. In the era of TB sanitariums, small sentinel bleeds sometimes were followed by fatal exsanguinating bleeds, even relatively long after the diagnosis of TB. Previously treated TB also can cause hemoptysis through residual bronchiectasis, reactivation, mycetoma formation in a cavity, or induction of a scar carcinoma. In addition, a sudden, massive, fatal bleed has been attributed to rupture of a Rasmussen's

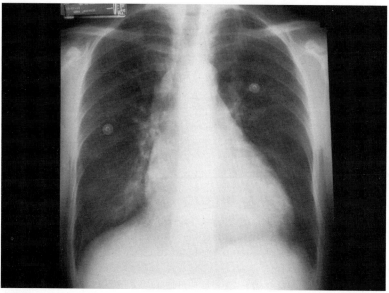

(a)

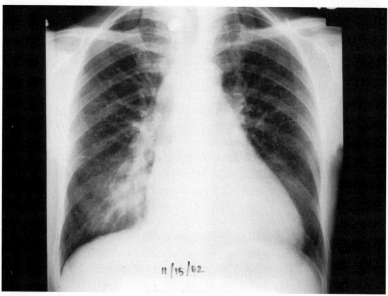

(b)

Figure 1 Pulmonary arteriovenous malformation. (a) Anteroposterior chest radiograph before hemoptysis; (b) after hemoptysis; (c) right pulmonary arteriogram. This 45-year-old woman presented with worsening dyspnea on exertion. Some 24 h after admission she had 150 mL of hemoptysis. Bronchoscopy indicated that bleeding originated from the right middle lobe. Angiographic embolization performed urgently led to cessation of bleeding. The patient was also found to be thyrotoxic; her high-cardiac-output state from this and her pulmonary AVMs were the reason for her dyspnea.

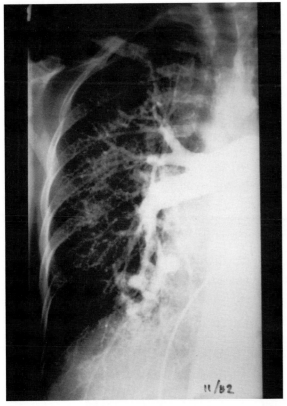

(c)

aneurysm. The belief is that inflammation adjacent to the wall of a vessel permits progressive localized expansion and aneurysm formation with bulging of the aneurysm into an adjacent cavity and eventual rupture. Most pathological studies indicate that the pulmonary artery is most commonly involved, but other publications favor bronchial arterial rupture. How commonly these aneurysms occur in the era of anti-TB chemotherapy is not clear, since almost all studies predate this time period.

Viral infections rarely cause hemoptysis except in the coagulopathic or thrombocytopenic host. An exception is varicella pneumonia, in which hemoptysis is common as vesicles rupture and bleed into airspaces.

Worldwide the most common cause of hemoptysis is paragonamiasis. A variety of other parasitic infections that affect the lung parenchyma are also in the differential diagnosis, especially in immigrants from outside North America. Thus a travel history is of importance in evaluating patients.

Vascular and Cardiac

In addition to AVMs, pulmonary emboli (PE), aortic aneurysms, and pulmonary hypertension can lead to hemoptysis. Hemoptysis due to PE most commonly occurs following smaller, peripheral embolization with infarction syndrome. This is typically accompanied by pleuritic chest pain, a chest radiographic peripheral infiltrate presumably from hemorrhagic and congestive atelectasis, and, sometimes, a small bloody pleural effusion. If the patient has any coagulopathy, the degree of bleeding may be considerable. Rarely, the anticoagulation itself will markedly accelerate the amount of bleeding.

The precise anatomical explanation for the occurrence of hemoptysis in patients with pulmonary hypertension or aortic aneurysm is unknown. In patients at risk for aortic aneurysm from trauma, atherosclerosis, or hypertension and with otherwise unexplained hemoptysis, this diagnosis should be considered.

Another classic etiology for hemoptysis that has become much less prevalent is mitral stenosis (Fig. 2). With the decline in rheumatic fever, it now is relatively rare. When it occurs, the high left atrial and pulmonary venous pressures can lead to diffuse alveolar bleeding. "Cardiac apoplexy" occurs with rupture of the submucosal bronchial varices that are created with reversal of blood flow from pulmonary capillaries into bronchial veins. If this is severe, cardiopulmonary bypass can relieve the bleeding while permitting valve replacement. Shown in Fig. 2 is the chest roentgenogram of a 25-year-old Jamaican male who had a year-long history of exertional dyspnea and had been coughing up small amounts of blood while playing soccer. He presented with severe shortness of breath and hypoxemia at rest.

Tricuspid endocarditis also causes hemoptysis with or without septic emboli and is an etiology of hemoptysis to consider in intravenous drug abusers.

Airway and Lung Parenchyma

Even with the decline of whooping cough and our increased use of outpatient antibiotics, bronchiectasis remains a significant cause of hemoptysis and poses difficult diagnostic and management problems. Bronchiectasis itself has many etiologies. It can occur tran-

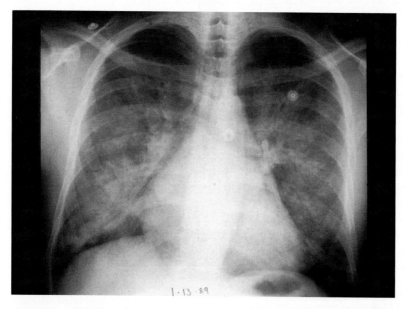

Figure 2 Diffuse alveolar hemorrhage due to mitral stenosis. This 25-year-old male from Jamaica had been having minor episodes of hemoptysis and worsening dyspnea on exertion while playing soccer for 6–8 months. He presented with shortness of breath, this chest radiograph, severe hypoxemia, and small amounts of hemoptysis. Bronchoscopy did not reveal a specific bleeding site; the echocardiogram was diagnostic. The patient remained severely hypoxemic in spite of mechanical ventilation.

siently with lung infection or may become permanent. Proximal bronchiectasis is associated with allergic bronchopulmonary aspergillosis. Distal bronchiectasis occurs in cystic fibrosis, ciliary dysfunction syndromes, and immune-deficiency states, such as IgA, IgG, or IgG subclass deficiencies. Chronic inflammation of the airway causes proliferation and/ or fragility of the bronchial arterial vessels that supply the tracheobronchial tree. Most patients with bronchiectasis have chronic productive cough, but approximately 10% have "dry" bronchiectasis. Establishing the diagnosis of saccular bronchiectasis is usually best done with high-resolution cuts on computed tomography of the chest.

Another frequent cause of small amounts of hemoptysis is bronchitis. A common clinical scenario is the patient with chronic bronchitis, as from chronic obstructive pulmonary disease, who has small amounts of hemoptysis for 1 or 2 days during an acute exacerbation of bronchitis. The hemoptysis can usually be attributed to the bronchitis provided that it lasts less than 1 week and does not recur; otherwise cancer or other important etiologies become a significant concern.

Cystic fibrosis patients commonly have multiple episodes of hemoptysis because of their chronic infections and predisposition to bronchiectasis.

Surprisingly, bullous emphysema can rarely lead to massive hemoptysis. The mechanism of the bleeding is not clear in these patients.

Trauma

Blunt or penetrating chest trauma can lead to alveolar bleeding, reflected in hemoptysis. After deceleration injuries, a ruptured or fractured bronchus may occur and be accompanied by coughing up of blood. This diagnosis is suggested by lobar atelectasis and pneumothorax or pneumomediastinum and may be confirmed bronchoscopically. Aortic aneurysm as a cause of hemoptysis is discussed above. Tracheoinnominate artery fistulae cause sudden massive bleeding and can occur after trauma or tracheostomy.

Systemic and Immune Diseases

Vasculitis, capillaritis, and collagen vascular diseases are often associated with hemoptysis and may cause either focal bleeding or diffuse alveolar hemorrhage.

Diffuse alveolar hemorrhage (DAH) is a manifestation of Goodpasture's syndrome (Fig. 3), idiopathic pulmonary hemosiderosis, systemic lupus erythematosus (SLE), Henoch-Schönlein purpura, capillaritis, and other small vessel vasculitides. Differentiating these causes can be important because of differences in use of cytotoxic drugs and/or plasmapheresis, in addition to glucocorticoid therapy. Renal involvement may be present in many of these illnesses.

In Wegener's granulomatosis (Fig. 4), multiple pulmonary nodules are typically seen on chest roentgenogram, but they may be obscured by retained blood. Microscopically, there often is capillaritis in addition to the granulomatous lesions in medium-sized blood vessels. In approximately 10% of patients, the chest x-ray pattern has linear infiltrates rather than nodules. Diagnosis is now usually made serologically based on the presence of antineutrophil cytoplasmic antibodies.

SLE can involve hemoptysis accompanying either DAH or an acute lupus pneumonitis presentation with localized infiltrate, fever, and hypoxemia. Capillaritis usually underlies the DAH.

Hematological

Disseminated intravascular coagulation (DIC), severe thrombocytopenia, or other severe coagulopathies can lead to diffuse alveolar hemorrhage or bleeding from an underlying localized abnormality.

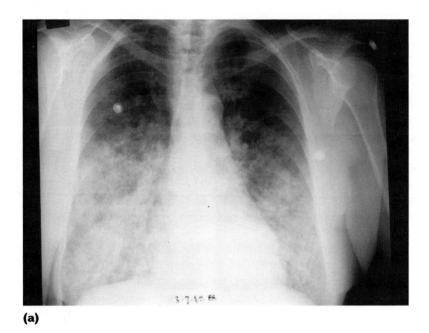

(a)

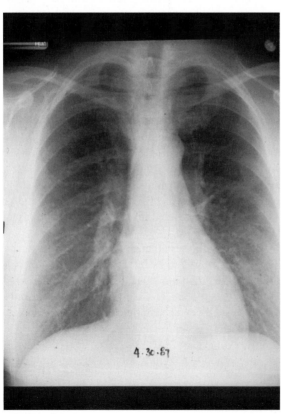

(b)

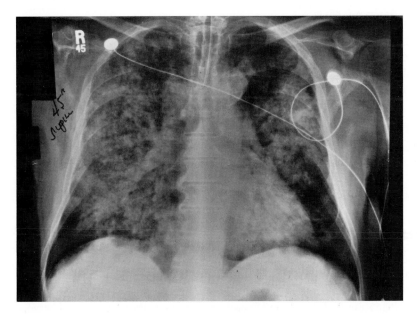

Figure 4 Hemoptysis from Wegener's granulomatosis. This 49-year-old patient had small amounts of hemoptysis for 1 week, followed by increasing hemoptysis and more shortness of breath. The chest radiograph on admission is shown. Renal function was normal. Diagnosis was made by antineutrophil cytoplasmic antibody testing.

Iatrogenic

A number of procedures have the complication of hemoptysis, including bronchoscopy with biopsies, transthoracic needle aspiration, Swan-Ganz catheterization, transtracheal aspiration, and lymphangiography. When pulmonary artery catheters migrate too far distally in the pulmonary artery or are left with the balloon up for too long, they can infarct the parenchyma, usually resulting in small amounts of hemoptysis and a localized infiltrate on the chest roentgenogram. Pulmonary artery rupture occurs more often in patients with underlying pulmonary hypertension. It usually presents as massive, rapid bleeding that can easily cause asphyxiation and has a high mortality.

Figure 3 Hemoptysis due to Goodpasture's syndrome. (a) Admission chest radiograph. (b) Follow-up chest radiograph after 7 weeks of therapy. This 45-year-old female presented with severe dyspnea, ankle edema, scant expectorated blood, and significant renal failure. Bronchoscopy showed fresh blood oozing out of multiple segmental bronchi. Since rapid antiglomerular basement membrane (GBM) antibody testing was not available at that time, diagnosis was made by immunofluorescent studies on a kidney biopsy and subsequently confirmed with a positive anti-GBM antibody test. The patient was treated with glucocorticoids, cytoxan, and plasmapheresis and did very well initially. However, 3 months later, while immunosuppressed, she had vague abdominal symptoms that were due to peritonitis and abdominal sepsis requiring emergent laparotomy.

Miscellaneous

Numerous unusual pulmonary problems can occasionally cause hemoptysis, including amyloidosis of the lung, broncholithiasis, endometriosis of the airway, foreign body, or septic pulmonary emboli. Broncholithiasis may present with the complaint of coughing up gritty, rock-like sputum. A chest roentgenogram or CT scan usually demonstrates calcified mediastinal and/or hilar lymph nodes.

Drugs and Toxins

Hemoptysis has been associated with anticoagulation, especially when greater than therapeutic, and use of thrombolytic drugs or aspirin. Penicillamine and trimetallic anhydride may lead to diffuse alveolar hemorrhage. Solvents and crack cocaine are also known to induce hemoptysis through uncertain mechanisms.

Relative Incidence of Etiologies

With such a multitude of causes of hemoptysis, it is important to place them in perspective. As indicated above, there are few large modern series examining the etiology of either massive or submassive hemoptysis.

Table 1 presents the etiologies found in each series of more than 100 cases of hemoptysis reported since 1980. No series had more than 250 patients and most of them were based on hospitalized patients. The Tulane series was published by otolaryngologists and the selection method was not specified. Several features of this table are important. First, approximately 20% of cases are attributed to bronchitis even with an abnormal chest roentgenogram, compared with 40% of cases with a normal chest roentgenogram. Second, cancer accounted for approximately 20–30% of all cases, and even when the chest roentgenogram was normal, it was a significant cause (4–6%). Third, many cases were designated idiopathic, and bronchiectasis was quite uncommon; I suspect that these surprising values may reflect the lack of high-resolution chest CT scanning in many patients. Finally, these results are heavily influenced by the types of patients studied and the selection criteria used. Thus specific patient groups, such as those with AIDS and other forms of immunocompromise, likely are underrepresented.

Table 2 presents a compiled estimation of the frequency with which different ill-

Table 2 Etiologies of Hemoptysis

Etiology	% Incidence	% Cases with bleeding	% Cases with massive bleeding
Bronchogenic Ca	10–15%	30–50%	10%
Bronchiectasis	20%	25–45%	30%[a]
Pulmonary TB	25–40%	5–20%	20%[a]
Lung abscess	1–6%	10–15%	25%[a]
Bronchial adenoma	1%	40–55%	10%
COPD + exacerbation	10–20%[a]	10%[a]	<5%[a]
Cardiovascular	1–7%[a]	?	?
AVM	10%[a]	40%	25%[a]

Key: AVM, arteriovenous malformation; Ca, carcinoma; TB, tuberculosis; COPD, chronic obstructive pulmonary disease.

[a] Estimated, since little information available in recent literature.

nesses cause hemoptysis, and it indicates the approximate percentage of cases with bleeding for a given etiology; of those with bleeding, the percentage with massive hemoptysis is shown. The frequencies listed in the first column are the approximate mean or core range of many reported series since 1950. Bronchial adenomas and mycetomas have a very high likelihood of associated hemoptysis. When hemoptysis occurs, bronchogenic carcinoma and bronchial adenomas are less likely to have massive amounts. A partial listing of the etiologies associated with massive hemoptysis is given in Table 3.

There is a definite need for comprehensive large series defining the modern etiology of hemoptysis, including a broad range of outpatient presentations, specialized inpatient

Table 3   Common Causes of Massive Hemoptysis

Cardiac	Pulmonary
Mitral stenosis	Bronchiectasis
Tricuspid endocarditis	Pulmonary embolism
Congenital heart disease	Cystic fibrosis
	Bullous emphysema
Hematological	
Coagulopathy	Iatrogenic
DIC	Bronchoscopy
Thrombocytopenia	Swan-Ganz infarction
Platelet dysfunction	Pulmonary artery rupture
	Transtracheal aspiration
Infection	Lymphangiography
Lung abscess	
Mycetoma	Vascular
Necrotizing pneumonia	Pulmonary hypertension
Parasitic	AV malformation
Fungal/TB	Aortic aneurysm
Viral	
	Drugs/Toxins
Neoplastic	Anticoagulants
Bronchial adenoma	Penicillamine
Bronchogenic carcinoma	Trimetallic anhydride
Metastatic cancer	Solvents
	Crack cocaine
Traumatic	Aspirin
Blunt or penetrating chest injury	Thrombolytics
Ruptured bronchus	
Fat embolism	Miscellaneous
Tracheal-innominate artery fistula	Amyloidosis
	Broncholithiasis
Systemic disease	Endometriosis
Goodpasture's syndrome	Foreign body
Wegener's granulomatosis	Cryptogenic
Systemic lupus erythematosus	Septic pulmonary emboli
Vasculitis	
Idiopathic pulmonary hemosiderosis	

Source: Modified from Cahill BC, Ingbar DH. Massive hemoptysis: assessment and management. Clin Chest Med 1994; 15:147.

services, and aggressive diagnostic workup. In a survery of physicians at the American College of Chest Physicians meeting in the late 1980s, chronic bronchitis was felt to be the most common cause of outpatient hemoptysis (72% of respondents); however, lung cancer (11%), TB (5%), bronchiectasis (5%), and idiopathic/uncertain (7%) were each cited by physicians who felt they were the most common etiology observed in their practice. This illustrates the broad range of experience that is not currently reflected in the medical literature.

APPROACH TO DIAGNOSIS AND MANAGEMENT

General Issues

The approach to the individual patient is initially determined by the overall severity of illness, presence of respiratory compromise, and rate of hemoptysis. Management of the individual patient can be difficult because the course of bleeding is hard to predict; sometimes a small sentinel bleed heralds a subsequent massive bleed.

If the patient is unstable, initial efforts need to be directed at ensuring that cardio-respiratory status is stabilized and protected. Oxygenation should be assessed and supported; some patients require intubation to protect the airway or assist in clearance of blood with suctioning. Basic blood work and type- and cross-matching for potential transfusion should be initiated. Pulmonary and, if the bleeding is massive, thoracic surgical consultation should occur without delay.

Assuming that the patient is stable, an important first step is to determine that the bleeding is from the lungs and not of gastrointestinal or upper airway origin. In some patients this may necessitate detailed fiberoptic examinations of these other two areas. Since blood that is coughed up is often swallowed while vomited blood can be aspirated, differentiating the bleeding site is quite difficult in some patients. Upper airway bleeding is a very important diagnostic consideration, especially in smokers.

A second important issue is the amount and rate of bleeding. Quantitation should be attempted through a combination of the patient's or family's history and ongoing collection of any further material brought up. There is no universally accepted definition of massive hemoptysis, with quantities varying from 200–600 mL/24 h. While the prognosis of hemoptysis is much worse with massive hemoptysis, the prognosis likely is determined more by the degree of underlying pulmonary reserve and the amount of blood retained in the lung rather than by the amount expectorated.

A third issue is whether the lung is bleeding at a single site or if the bleeding is mutifocal. The physical examination and chest roentgenogram may be misleading, since aspirated blood may be present at sites that do not have bleeding.

A fourth issue is the specific diagnosis causing hemoptysis. The initial workup should include a careful history and physical examination; blood work specifically looking at hematological, coagulation, and renal function; urinalysis; and a chest roentgenogram. Sputum should be examined for acid-fast bacilli, fungi, and tumor cells. Historical points of particular importance are any prior lung, cardiac, or renal disease; cigarette smoking history; prior hemoptysis or other pulmonary or infectious symptoms; family history of hemoptysis or brain aneurysms (suggesting OWR); travel history; skin rash; drug exposures, including use of aspirin, nonsteroidal anti-inflammatory drugs, cocaine, solvents and trimetallic anhydride; and upper airway or GI symptoms. Occasionally the physical examination is helpful due to skin rashes of vasculitis, SLE, fat embolism, or endocarditis;

splinter hemorrhages; needle tracks; signs of pulmonary hypertension; mitral stenosis or tricuspid regurgitation; an AVM chest bruit; or signs of deep venous thrombosis.

A fifth issue is whether the patient might be a surgical candidate if uncontrollable bleeding were to occur or if a diagnosis were made that would make surgery beneficial. In stable patients, once TB has been ruled out, pulmonary function testing (spirometry at least) should be performed.

Specific Diagnostic Workup

The results of the initial assessment and workup will guide the speed and focus of the diagnostic workup. Another important factor is the likelihood that the patient may have bronchogenic carcinoma. The specific workup includes a combination of bronchoscopy, chest CT scan, and/or arteriography along with other focused diagnostic studies. The order and timing of these tests are individualized.

Bronchoscopy may be useful in several ways. First, it sometimes differentiates bleeding from a single site from multifocal bleeding. This is important, since the presence of bilateral blood does not guarantee diffuse bleeding. Thus the bronchoscopist is looking for sites with active, fresh bleeding that does not clear after some washing. Second, bronchoscopy may localize one specific region that is the site of fresh bleeding. This can be helpful if massive bleeding subsequently occurs, and it can then guide arteriographic studies and embolization or surgery. Third, bronchoscopy may yield a specific diagnosis, such as lung cancer. In prospective studies at multiple institutions, this is one of the most common new significant diagnoses made by bronchoscopy, but obviously many other diagnoses may also result less commonly. The diagnostic yield of bronchoscopy is highest when performed within 24 h of bleeding. For the reasons mentioned above, this is also when it has the greatest chance to help in patient management. Thus, in patients with more than scant bleeding and when the source is uncertain, bronchoscopy usually should be performed within 24 h. The diagnostic yield is greatest for central and mucosal tumors, broncholiths, foreign bodies, and invasive infections. In addition, it may provide a precise histological diagnosis that cannot result from the radiological studies.

An important primary care question is which patients require bronchoscopy to exclude the diagnosis of bronchogenic carcinoma. A normal chest radiograph still has a 4–6% cancer incidence. There is a general consensus that bronchoscopy should be performed in this situation if the patient is above age 40; has bleeding for more than 1 week, has smoked > 40 pack-years of cigarettes, *or*, if smoking, has smoked for > 20 years. Male sex brings a higher risk of cancer and thresholds possibly should be slightly lower for men. The rapid rise in female smoking and lung cancer suggests that this will not be the case for long.

Chest CT scan recently has been used more often for diagnosis in patients with hemoptysis. It is particularly useful in the diagnosis of AVMs, aspergillomas, many lung cancers, and, with high-resolution cuts, bronchiectasis. It detects some bronchogenic carcinomas missed by bronchoscopy and chest radiograph. However, it can be misleading when used during active bleeding, since the blood can obscure findings or lead to the appearance of a pseudotumor, especially in a preexistent cavity. It also can be helpful as a guide to the bronchoscopist or arteriographer in some patients.

Arteriography can be performed on the bronchial, pulmonary, or systemic circulations—all of which are sometimes the bleeding source. Unless the patient is likely to have an AVM, PE, or aortic aneurysm, study of the bronchial circulation first usually produces the highest yield. This requires caution, because of the anatomical variations in the normal bronchial arteries and the fact that they often feed the anterior spinal artery. Thus occlusion or embolization of small materials from a central location can rarely result in paraplegia. Consequently it is important that this procedure be performed by highly qualified angiographers who have had significant experience with the bronchial circulation. In patients with inflammatory diseases, hyperplastic corkscrewed vessels may be seen, but there usually is no frank extravasation of contrast unless bleeding is very rapid. If the bronchial circulation reveals no abnormalities, the pulmonary circulation should be examined. In occasional patients, thorough examination of both circulations shows no abnormality, and potential systemic collaterals may demonstrate the bleeding source. In one study, systemic arteries were involved in 10% of patients, but my experience indicates that it is much less common than this figure.

Less commonly helpful diagnostic tests are done in special circumstances. For example, echocardiography may reveal mitral stenosis, right-sided endocarditis, pulmonary hypertension, or a congenital cardiac lesion. Serological workup for collagen vascular diseases, Goodpasture's syndrome, Wegener's granulomatosis, and other rheumatological disorders is indicated in patients with diffuse alveolar hemorrhage or a renal component, but it is also reasonable when no defined cause for bleeding is found.

In the outpatient setting, it is very important to have a low threshold for diagnostic workup—especially in patients with significant risk of carcinoma. Keeping in mind the broad differential and excluding upper airway and GI sources is also important. In general, it is worth being cautious in attributing hemoptysis to bronchitis. With the changes in etiologies of hemoptysis, modern outpatient studies of the diagnosis and outcome of patients presenting with submassive hemoptysis are needed to develop better diagnostic algorithms. The approach to the management of massive hemoptysis has been discussed in detail in several of the references listed and is not reviewed here.

TREATMENT

While the diagnosis is being pursued, general management includes supplemental oxygen as needed, small amounts of codeine to suppress cough without causing too much sedation, and reversing any coagulopathy.

Specific therapies obviously depend upon the cause. For pulmonary renal syndromes, steroid therapy with possible addition of cytotoxic drugs and/or plasmapheresis may be appropriate. For proximal mucosal lesions of bronchogenic carcinoma, radiation therapy, laser bronchoscopy, or brachytherapy may be indicated.

In addition to these specific treatments, arteriographic embolization and surgery are two other major considerations. Embolization is helpful for massive hemoptysis or for patients with diffuse lung disease and continuing bleeding when lung preservation is desirable. Common examples of the latter situation are cystic fibrosis and multifocal bronchiectasis. Embolization is successful in stopping bleeding 90–95% of the time. However, there are early rebleeds at less than 1–2 months in approximately 10%; these are presumably due to incomplete embolization of the involved vessels. Later rebleeding is typically due to recanalization, newly developed collateral vessels, or a new bleeding site. Thus embolization, when done in good hands, is a very effective short-term procedure; however, it has a small but significant failure rate in the long term. This raises the question of whether elective surgical treatment should be used in addition for selected patients.

Surgery is the most definitive therapy but has significant morbidities. This is particularly true when done emergently for massive hemoptysis, since there is a high frequency of postoperative empyema and air leak. In the elective setting, little recent information is available, but older literature suggests it has much fewer complications. Absolute contraindications are severely compromised lung function, diffuse bleeding, inoperable cancer, and active TB without treatment. Some situations pose major difficulty in decision making about whether surgery is truly beneficial, such as massive bleeding from a unilateral aspergilloma in a patient with chronic sarcoidosis and bilateral lung scarring and cavities. It is clear that if all patients who qualify as surgical candidates are considered, there is no major survival advantage to aggressive surgical therapy. Thus, with increasing use of arteriographic embolization and other relatively conservative treatments, surgery is now used much less often for the management of hemoptysis.

Patients who undergo aggressive diagnostic workup, including bronchoscopy and chest CT, but who do not have a bleeding source determined are labeled as having cryptogenic hemoptysis. When the hemoptysis has been submassive, then the long-term prognosis is very good, with a low incidence of cancer or other serious illnesses accounting for hemoptysis later being discovered. However, this is not established for cryptogenic massive hemoptysis. Thus the diagnostic challenge is particularly important in these patients.

SUGGESTED READING

1. Cahill BC, Ingbar DH. Massive hemoptysis: assessment and management. Clin Chest Med 1994; 15:147.
2. Haponik EF, Chin R. Hemoptysis: clinicans' perspectives. Chest 1990; 97:469.
3. Johnston H, Reisz G. Changing spectrum of hemoptysis: underlying causes in 148 patients undergoing diagnostic flexible fiberoptic bronchoscopy. Arch Intern Med 1989; 149:1666.
4. Knott-Craig CJ, Oostuizen JB, Rossouw G, Jouber JR, Barnard PM. Management and prognosis of massive hemoptysis: recent experience with 120 patients. J Thorac Cardiovasc Surg 1993; 105:394.
5. Leatherman JW, Davies SF, Hoidal JR. Alveolar hemorrhage syndromes: diffuse microvascular lung hemorrhage in immune and idiopathic disorders. Medicine 1984; 63:343.
6. McGuiness G, Beacher JR, Harkin TJ, Garay SM, Rom WN, Naidich DP. Hemoptysis: prospective high-resolution CT/bronchoscopic correlation. Chest 1994; 105:1155.
7. Miller RR, McGregor DH. Hemorrhage from carcinoma of the lung. Cancer 1980; 46:200.
8. Muller NL. Hemoptysis: high-resolution CT vs bronchoscopy. Chest 1994; 105:982.
9. Primack SL, Miller RR, Muller NL. Diffuse pulmonary hemorrhage: clinical, pathologic and imaging features. AJR 1995; 164:295.
10. Rasmussen V. On haemoptysis, especially when fatal, in its anatomical and clinical aspects. Edinburgh Med J 1868; 14:385.
11. Santiago S, Tobias J, Williams AJ. A reappraisal of the causes of hemoptysis. Arch Intern Med 1991; 151:2449.
12. Thompson AB, Tescheler H, Rennard SI. Pathogenesis, evaluation and therapy for massive hemoptysis. Clin Chest Med 1992; 13:69.

22

Oxygen Therapy

Walter J. O'Donohue, Jr.
Creighton University School of Medicine
Omaha, Nebraska

INTRODUCTION

This presentation focuses on the use of oxygen for the long-term management and rehabilitation of patients with chronic lung disease and hypoxemia, recognizing that oxygen is also a critical component of therapy in acute respiratory failure but with different goals and applications. Multicenter studies conducted in North America and the United Kingdom have demonstrated the value of long-term oxygen therapy (LTOT) in patients with chronic obstructive pulmonary disease (COPD) and hypoxemia. In these clinical trials, it has been shown that oxygen not only increases survival but also improves quality of life, measured in both physiological and functional parameters. In patients with COPD and hypoxemia at rest, nearly continuous oxygen was found to be superior to oxygen administered for shorter periods of time during the day or night. Subsequent studies have suggested that "true" continuous oxygen therapy may provide even greater benefits than those found in the Nocturnal Oxygen Therapy Trial (NOTT) conducted in North America, where nearly continuous oxygen for 18 h/day was superior to nocturnal oxygen to improve survival and quality of life.

REGULATIONS AND REQUIREMENTS FOR HOME OXYGEN THERAPY

The Health Care Financing Administration (HCFA) classifies oxygen and oxygen delivery equipment as durable medical equipment (DME); therefore, home oxygen therapy (HOT) is reimbursable at 80% of allowable charge as a Medicare benefit. In order to qualify for this benefit, Medicare patients must have evidence of hypoxemia to the extent, as follows:

1. Either $PaO_2 \leq 55$ mmHg or $SaO_2 \leq 88\%$.
2. Or PaO_2 of 56–59 mmHg or SaO_2 of 89%, with one of the following conditions:
   a. Edema due to congestive heart failure.
   b. Evidence of cor pulmonale.
   c. Erythrocythemia with hematocrit > 56.

Oxygen may also be authorized during sleep or exercise if the following conditions are met:

1. Exercise: $PaO_2 \leq 55$ mmHg or $SaO_2 \leq 88\%$.
2. Sleep: $PaO_2 \leq 55$ mmHg or $SaO_2 \leq 88\%$ during sleep, a fall in PaO_2 of more than 10 mmHg, or a fall in SaO_2 of more than 5% with signs or symptoms of hypoxemia (e.g., cognitive process, restlessness, or insomnia).

Hypoxemia documented only during sleep or exercise does not justify a prescription for continuous oxygen therapy.

In addition to these arterial blood gas or oxyhemoglobin saturation measurements, there are several other requirements mandated by HCFA for authorization of therapy. These include the following:

1. The measurement of arterial PaO_2 or SaO_2 must be made by a Medicare-qualified laboratory and not by the supplier.

NAME _____

ADDRESS _____ DATE _____

℞

1. Oxygen flow:
☐ Continuous: Liters/min _____ . (FiO2 _____ for assisted ventilation) <u>and/or</u>
☐ Noncontinuous: (liters/min) walking _____ , sleeping _____ , exercise _____ .

2. Oxygen equipment (check one):   **3. Delivery System:**
☐ Stationary only (eg nocturnal or bedbound)   ☐ Nasal Cannula
For portable or ambulatory* systems, patient   ☐ Transtracheal catheter
regularly goes beyond the limits of a stationary   ☐ Reservoir cannula
system with 50-ft tubing for times indicated below: ☐ Mask (eg CPAP or BiPAP)
☐ Stationary and portable   ☐ Other: _____
(less than 2 h/day, minimum 2 hr/wk)
☐ Stationary and ambulatory*
(more than 2 hr/day, minimum 6 hr/wk)
☐ Portable only ☐ ambulatory* only
(eg walking or exercise only)

* Ambulatory systems weigh less than 10 lbs,
are designed to be carried and will last at least 4 hrs
at a flow equivalent to 2L/min (eg liquid refillable units
or light-weight cylinders and regulators,
with or without oxygen conserving devices)

_____**M.D.**

Figure 1   Model prescription for initial ordering of home oxygen therapy, indicating the type of oxygen delivery equipment and flow rates desired.

2. The patient must be clinically stable and receiving optimal medical management before LTOT is authorized.
3. The physician must sign a Certificate of Medical Necessity (CMN), which can be completed only by the physician or a member of his or her staff.
4. If the initial PaO_2 is >55 mmHg or the SaO_2 is >88%, retesting of the PaO_2 or SaO_2 is required in 60–90 days.
5. Recertification but not retesting is required at the end of 1 year.
6. Further recertification is necessary only if there is a change in the prescription.

Currently, HCFA is in the process of redesigning the CMN (FORM HCFA-484) so that it contains more billing information and no longer serves as a comprehensive oxygen prescription. This revision is predicated on the requirement that the oxygen supplier will have a written or verbal prescription on file and will specify the type of equipment being supplied on the CMN when it is sent to the physician for completion and signature. The physician is instructed not to sign the form if the oxygen delivery system that was prescribed is not being supplied to the patient by DME provider. The physician will also have the opportunity to indicate different O_2 flow rates at rest, during sleep, and during exercise. The appropriate diagnostic codes (ICD-9-CM) must be provided by the physician or the office staff. Previously there was a checklist of usual diagnoses from which a selection could be made. The home oxygen provider will not be reimbursed by Medicare until the CMN has been completed, the prescription verified, and the form signed by the physician. A major concern relative to these proposed changes is how the written or verbal prescription will be transmitted to the home oxygen supplier in a comprehensive enough format that the supplier will provide the type of oxygen delivery system that is best suited for the patient—e.g., portable or ambulatory, liquid or gaseous system with a nasal cannula, transtracheal catheter, or oxygen-conserving device. Figure 1 demonstrates a model prescription form that could serve well for initiation of HOT.

PHYSICIAN RESPONSIBILITY IN LONG-TERM OXYGEN THERAPY

In addition to the requirements of Medicare and other third-party payers for documentation of need and completion of the CMN, there are other important considerations for appropriate therapy. Measurement of arterial blood gases should be the standard for certifying the need for lifetime continuous oxygen therapy. Even though Medicare allows arterial oxygen saturation measurements to document hypoxemia, this measurement is not appropriate as the ultimate test in patients who require LTOT. Arterial oxygen saturation measurements are practical to assess hypoxemia during sleep or exercise and are commonly used to monitor therapy and to titrate the oxygen flow rates required to correct hypoxemia at rest and during other activities of rehabilitation and daily living. Since the oxygen requirements will differ during rest and exercise in most patients with hypoxemia, titration of the dose (flow) during rest and walking is recommended. When oxygen-conserving devices are being used, titration is even more important, because higher flow-rate settings that are greater than those for continuous flow rates may be necessary during exercise. Despite these higher settings, there are still substantial savings in oxygen utilization by using oxygen-conserving devices.

Patients who are clinically unstable when oxygen therapy is begun, such as those who are hospitalized with an acute cardiopulmonary illness, may need short-term oxygen until the acute or subacute problem is resolved. This should not be a prescription for continuous oxygen indefinitely, and retesting should be done in 1–3 months when the patient is clinically stable and receiving optimal medical management. It is also the responsibility of the physician to monitor the therapy being provided by the home oxygen supplier and to periodically reassess the needs of the patient and the adequacy of the prescribed flow rates in correcting hypoxemia. This includes the assurance that patients who are mobile and physically active are provided modern ambulatory devices to encourage full rehabilitation.

The physician also must be prepared to advise patients about travel, including air travel with its many nuances. Many patients who require continuous oxygen therapy are physically active and should be encouraged to travel if they so desire. Air travel does require a prescription for each leg of the flight and prearrangements by the patient with the carrier. Patients can also contract with their oxygen supplier to have oxygen provided in airports and at their final destination. The air carrier must provide the oxygen during flight; patients cannot carry oxygen-filled canisters on their person or as baggage. Some airlines refuse to provide oxygen for patients during flight, but most will accommodate this need with proper medical authorization and prescriptions from the patient's physician.

OXYGEN REIMBURSEMENT ISSUES

Home oxygen is currently reimbursed by HCFA on a prospective payment basis, with all oxygen delivery systems considered to be equal for payment purposes. Initially, the amount of payment was predicated on the historical cost of the mixture of liquid and gaseous systems being supplied. Current Medicare data indicate that about 80% of Medicare recipients are receiving oxygen from an oxygen concentrator. Since oxygen concentrators are the least expensive systems for oxygen delivery, it has been assumed by HCFA that Medicare is paying too much for HOT. Congress, HCFA, and the executive office have all recently proposed a 30% reduction in oxygen reimbursement for medicare patients. A major fallacy in this assumption of overpayment is the fact that Medicare data cannot identify whether a patient may be receiving oxygen by a dual system, such as a concentrator for stationary use and a liquid oxygen system or lightweight compressed gas cylinders for portability or ambulation. Since most patients who qualify for HOT are ambulatory and not bed-bound, it is unreasonable to assume that 80% are using a stationary source (e.g., a concentrator) alone. A reduction in reimbursement of this magnitude (30%) would undoubtedly have a negative impact on patient care by forcing many suppliers to provide the least expensive delivery systems possible without regard for the rehabilitative needs of the patient. Any policy that discourages the use of ambulatory equipment by patients who are willing and able to be active outside of their homes will have a negative impact on health care and individual productivity.

OXYGEN DURING SLEEP AND EXERCISE

As previously stated, Medicare and most third-party payers agree that oxygen is indicated if there is evidence of hypoxemia during sleep or exercise. Unless there is evidence of tissue hypoxia, however, the efficacy of oxygen therapy is unclear, and there is the potential for costly misuse of therapy.

Sleep

There is a spectrum of sleep disorders that may be associated with nocturnal oxyhemoglobin desaturation (NOD). Some are without known clinical consequences and some may be associated with pulmonary hypertension, cor pulmonale, right heart failure, erythrocythemia, and decreased survival. Central or obstructive sleep apnea is usually not correctable by supplemental oxygen therapy alone and requires mechanical aids for treatment.

Studies in both the United States and Europe have indicated that between 25 and 40% of patients with chronic obstructive pulmonary disease (COPD) who have arterial oxygen tensions above 60 mmHg while awake will demonstrate periods of significant NOD during sleep. When pulmonary artery catheters are inserted, many of these patients have been found to have pulmonary hypertension. Although there is evidence suggesting that nocturnal oxygen therapy may be beneficial to these patients, there are no definitive studies to substantiate efficacy. The current cost of HOT in the United States is estimated to be approximately 1.4 billion per year (for 600,000–700,000 patients). Since there are about 14 million patients with COPD living in the United States, if nocturnal oxygen were provided to 25% of these individuals—who would be expected to have evidence of NOD if studied—the cost of therapy would increase by fivefold to more than $7.2 billion each year. At this time, it is recommended that nocturnal oxygen therapy be prescribed only for persons with evidence of hypoxic end-organ dysfunction, such as pulmonary hypertension, cor pulmonale, or erythrocytosis.

Exercise

In patients with hypoxemia at rest, the use of oxygen while walking and performing other activities of daily living is an essential component of therapy. In patients without hypoxemia at rest who desaturate during an exercise test, the value of oxygen with activities of daily living is unproven. Exercise studies using treadmills, ergometers, and 6-min walk tests have shown increased exercise tolerance and endurance in patients with cardiopulmonary disease while receiving supplemental oxygen, even when hypoxemia is not present. To date, there are no long-term studies demonstrating the value of supplemental oxygen during usual activities of daily living in patients who are not hypoxemic at rest but who desaturate during an exercise test or while performing a walk test (the usual way to assess "exercise" desaturation).

Previous studies have indicated that 30–39% of patients with COPD who are not hypoxemic at rest experience oxyhemoglobin desaturation during an exercise test. If 30% of the 14 million patients with COPD in the United States were provided with ambulatory oxygen delivery systems for desaturation during activities of daily living, the cost of HOT, based on the results of a standard exercise test, would increase more than $6\frac{1}{2}$ times and be greater than $9.5 billion per year. It is apparent that we need better methods to demonstrate the need for supplemental oxygen during activities of daily living other than the usual exercise tests. Long-term studies are also required to document the efficacy of this therapy in patients who are not hypoxemic at rest. This has proven to be a costly problem in other nations where oxygen suppliers are allowed to document the need for HOT by exercising patients to demonstrate oxyhemoglobin desaturation.

OXYGEN DELIVERY SYSTEMS

Oxygen Cylinders

Although HOT began with the use of large, high-pressure steel cylinders, these are rarely used today as a source of continuous oxygen therapy. These cylinders are unattractive when placed in the home and have to be refilled frequently, even when multiple cylinders are employed. Small steel cylinders (E or D size) are still utilized for portable oxygen and are often mounted on wheels because they are too heavy to be carried. Lightweight aluminum or fiber-wrapped aluminum cylinders with aluminum regulators have become increasingly popular as sources of ambulatory oxygen. Units that are small enough to be carried in a fanny pack and weigh less than 5 lb. will last up to $7\frac{1}{2}$ h at a flow equivalent to 2 L/min using an oxygen conserving device. Larger units that weigh less than 10 lb can last more than 24 h using the same technology (Fig. 2). It is now possible to refill these cylinders in the home from a stationary oxygen concentrator.

OXYGEN CONCENTRATORS

Oxygen concentrators are molecular sieves that separate nitrogen from oxygen and can usually provide 90–95% oxygen at flows of 4–6 L/min. Initially these units were as large as refrigerators and were noisy, with substantial heat production. Today they are quiet, produce little heat, and usually weigh no more than 40–60 lb. They also require very little

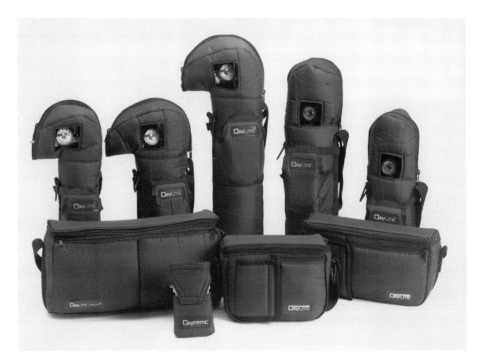

Figure 2   Family of lightweight aluminum and fiber-wrapped aluminum cylinders with aluminum regulators and an external pulse device, weighing from 3.7 to 9.5 lb and lasting from 2.3 to 24 h at a flow equivalent to 2 L/min continuous flow.

maintenance and are equipped with alarms to warn if the oxygen concentration falls below a critical level. Compliance with therapy and maintenance can be monitored using some models (Fig. 3). The cost of electricity to power these units may range from $25–$45 per month and is not reimbursed by any payer.

Portable concentrators that operate from either a 12-V battery or from standard AC current are available for use outside of the home and for travel. A portable concentrator weighing 32 lb is manufactured in the United States and packaged in a suitcase. Flow is limited to 2 L/min, however. A portable concentrator recently introduced from Italy weighs 19 lb and can be mounted on a stroller with wheels. It can deliver a higher equivalent flow rate using a demand oxygen delivery system at settings above 2 L/min (Fig. 4). There is currently no concentrator that weighs 10 lb or less and would qualify as an ambulatory device.

Liquid Oxygen

The advent of liquid oxygen systems heralded the introduction of ambulatory oxygen units that could be transfilled from a stationary oxygen source in the home. The stationary

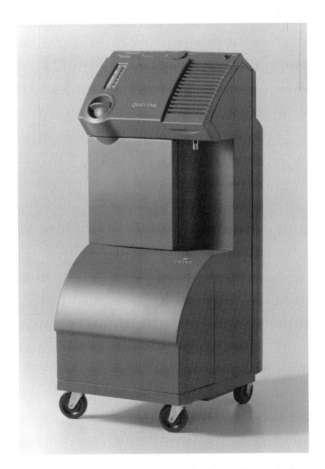

Figure 3   Oxygen concentrator weighing 60 lb with built-in monitor for compliance and maintenance. This unit delivers up to 6 L/min of $> 90\%$ O_2 with a noise level of 45 dB.

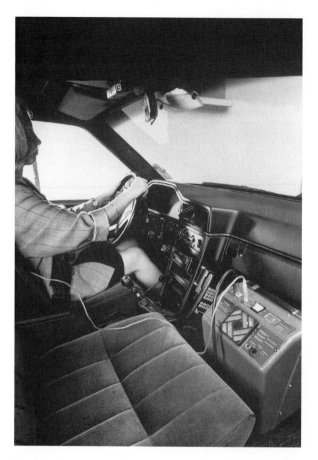

Figure 4 Portable oxygen concentrator weighing 19 lb and operating from a 12-V DC automobile battery.

canisters weigh from 60–120 lb and are refilled by the home oxygen supplier. Since liquid oxygen is cold, these canisters function as insulators, but there is some loss of oxygen through venting as warming occurs if the oxygen is not being used constantly. Small, portable, or ambulatory canisters can be safely transfilled by the patient in the home, since liquid oxygen is a low-pressure system. Ambulatory liquid oxygen systems that weigh less than 6 lb can last up to 8 h at a flow equivalent to 2 L/min using a built-in demand oxygen delivery device (Fig. 5). Although liquid oxygen is inexpensive, supplying it is relatively costly because of the requirements for frequent visits to refill the stationary units and the large investment in the vehicle that is necessary for transporting liquid oxygen and refilling the canisters in the home.

Oxygen-Conserving Devices

Oxygen-conserving devices utilize one of the following two techniques:

1. A mechanical or anatomical reservoir stores a volume of about 20–50 mL of 100% oxygen, which is delivered immediately with initiation of each inspiration.

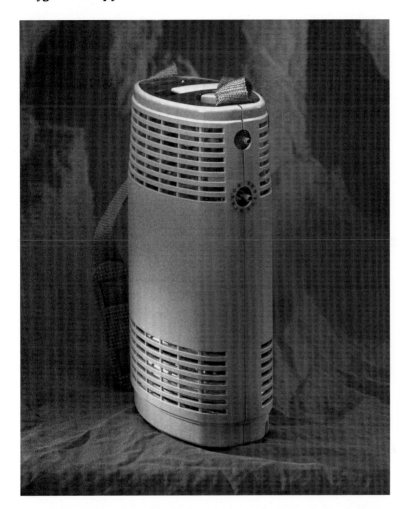

Figure 5 Liquid oxygen ambulatory unit with a built-in demand oxygen delivery device that is flow-activated. This unit weights 5.5 lb when filled and will last for about 8.5 h at a flow equivalent to 2 L/min continuous flow.

2. A pulse of 100% oxygen is delivered during the first 25–50% of inspiration. Both the volume and timing of the pulse of oxygen may vary depending upon the design of the device and the equivalent flow setting.

The mechanical reservoir devices currently in use are the nasal reservoir cannula and the pendant reservoir cannula (Fig. 6). Both are marketed by the same oxygen equipment manufacturer and both utilize a reservoir with a collapsible membrane that allows filling with 100% oxygen during exhalation and emptying during early inhalation. The nasal pendant contains about 20 mL of 100% oxygen when filled, it is soft and comfortable to wear but obtrusive in appearance because of its mustache configuration. The pendant reservoir holds about 40 mL of 100% oxygen when filled, but the effective oxygen delivery during early inspiration is about 20 mL from the conducting tubing between the nasal cannula and the pendant. The pendant can be concealed beneath clothing and is therefore

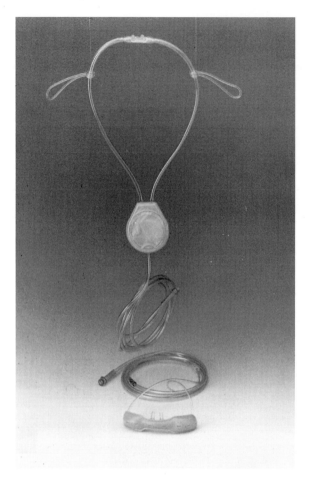

Figure 6   Nasal reservoir (below) and pendant reservoir (above) oxygen-conserving systems with collapsible membranes, capable of oxygen conservation of 50–60% at rest.

less conspicuous; however, the conducting tubing is relatively large and rigid and less comfortable than the nasal reservoir cannula. Transtracheal oxygen therapy utilizes the anatomical reservoir of the trachea and upper airway for filling with 100% oxygen near end-exhalation. All of the reservoir systems can provide oxygen savings of 50–60% at rest, but the degree of conservation may be less when higher flows are required and during exercise.

Demand oxygen delivery systems (DODS) are currently the most commonly used technology for oxygen conservation. There are multiple manufacturers in the United States, and each unit is somewhat different in design. Most are powered by a rechargeable or replaceable battery with considerable variability in the operational time before recharge or replacement. One unit is flow-activated and requires no power source. The timing of the oxygen delivery also varies from early in inspiration to throughout the first half of inspiration. Most DODS increase the pulse volume as the flow rate is increased, while one unit utilizes a fixed volume and varies the frequency of pulse activations from one in every fourth breath to one with nearly every breath, corresponding to flow settings of

1–4 L/min, respectively. Obviously, some of these units are more efficient than others, but all that are currently marketed appear to be effective and capable of long-term operational reliability. The arterial oxygen tension or saturation correlation with continuous oxygen is usually good at rest but may not be as good during exercise and at higher flow rates. Any patient using an oxygen-conserving device should have the flow rates titrated for rest and usual exercise with the specific device being utilized.

Transtracheal Oxygen Therapy

In addition to being an oxygen conserving technique, transtracheal oxygen (TTO) is a program for LTOT that has both clinical and physiological benefits. Once installed, the transtracheal catheter is more comfortable and almost universally preferable to the nasal cannula (Fig. 7). One therapeutic advantage that appears to have far-reaching physiological implications is that TTO assures continuous (24 h/day) oxygen therapy in most patients. The transition to TTO in patients who have been using nasal oxygen for months or years has been shown to be associated with further reductions in pulmonary artery pressure, reduced hematocrits in subjects with persistent secondary erythrocytosis, reduced alveolar-arterial oxygen gradients, and increased exercise tolerance. A previous study in patients with COPD using nasal cannulae showed that removal of supplemental oxygen for only 2–3 h each day is associated with increased pulmonary artery pressures and impaired cardiac function. In the NOTT study, patients who were prescribed continuous oxygen therapy used the oxygen for only 18 h each day (by diary) and therefore continued to experience approximately 6 h of hypoxemia daily.

Transtracheal oxygen is more invasive and does require more patient and physician

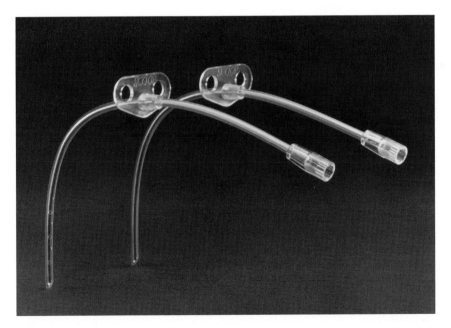

Figure 7 SCOOP transtracheal oxygen catheters. SCOOP I catheter (rear) has a single distal outlet and SCOOP II catheter (foreground) has multiple side ports.

responsibility for management. The major complications have been related to long-term therapy and the formation of mucous balls at the end of the catheter that can result in mucous plugging of the airways. Regular removal and cleaning of the catheter can usually prevent this complication. With the technique of needle-guidewire insertion of the catheter used in the past, many patients have difficulty reinserting the catheter and are reluctant or unable to remove it for cleaning. A new technique of catheter insertion using a "minitracheostomy" can eliminate this problem. Studies are now in progress to evaluate the benefits of transtracheal augmented ventilation (similar to insufflation ventilation) using high flows of a humidified oxygen-air mixture delivered through a transtracheal catheter during sleep in patients with COPD and hypoventilation. Preliminary studies suggest that high flows of 10 L/min may reduce inspiratory work of breathing and dead-space ventilation.

CONCLUSION

Although oxygen therapy is authorized in any patient with hypoxemia of the degree previously stated, it should be recognized that most of the studies that have demonstrated increased survival and long-term benefit have been in patients with COPD. Correction of hypoxemia may be one factor in reducing dyspnea; however, hypoxemia alone is rarely a cause for severe incapacitating shortness of breath. Even though quality of life may be improved in patients with interstitial lung disease, chronic cardiac failure, or malignancy of the lung by the use of oxygen therapy when hypoxemia is present, life expectancy is unlikely to be significantly changed. The use of oxygen for palliative therapy or to correct dyspnea when hypoxemia is not present cannot be medically justified.

Finally, the goal of therapy is to correct hypoxemia in a manner that will provide maximum therapeutic benefit. In most disease states, there is an attempt to normalize all abnormal laboratory tests. In patients with hypoxemia, the "ideal" therapeutic arterial oxygen tension is often unclear. In most studies, the goal of therapy has been to maintain the arterial Pa_{O2} at levels between 60 and 80 mmHg; in patients with COPD, this has been associated with both increased survival and improved quality of life. Currently, there is no definitive answer to the question of what is an "ideal" target for correction of hypoxemia. Although there are many other questions regarding LTOT that remain unanswered, the benefits in patients with chronic hypoxemia are substantial and the use of HOT is increasing in most nations throughout the world. A very useful patient information booklet describing home oxygen therapy and the oxygen delivery systems available has been developed by the National Association for Medical Direction of Respiratory Care (NAMDRC), at 5454 Wisconsin Avenue, Suite 1270, Chevy Chase, MD 20815.

SUGGESTED READING

1. Barker AF, Burgher LW, Plummer AL. Oxygen conserving methods for adults. Chest 1994; 105:248–252.
2. Christopher KL, Spofford BT, Betrun MD, McCarty DC, Goodman JR, Petty TL. A program for transtracheal oxygen delivery: assessment of safety and efficacy. Ann Intern Med 1987; 107:802–808.
3. Conference Report. Further recommendations for prescribing and supplying long-term oxygen therapy. Am Rev Respir Dis 1988; 138:745–747.

4. Conference Report. New problems in supply, reimbursement and certification of medical necessity for long-term oxygen therapy. Am Rev Respir Dis 1990; 142:721–724.

5. Conference Report. Problems in prescribing and supplying oxygen for Medicare patients. Am Rev Respir Dis 1986; 134:340–341.

6. Fletcher EC, Luckett RA, Goodnight-White S, Miller CC, Qian W, Costorangos-Galarza. A double-blind trial of nocturnal supplemental oxygen for sleep desaturation in patients with chronic obstructive pulmonary disease and daytime PaO$_2$ above 60 mmHg. Am Rev Respir Dis 1992; 145:1070–1076.

7. Levi-Valensi P, Weitzenblum E, Rida Z, Aubry P, Braghiroli A, Domer C, Aprill M, Zielinski J, Wurtenberger G. Sleep related oxygen desaturation and daytime pulmonary hemodynamics in COPD patients. Eur Respir J 1992; 5:301–307.

8. Lipkin A, Christopher K, Yaeger E, Diehl S, Jorgenson S. Otolaryngologist's role in transtracheal oxygen therapy. Otol Head Neck Surg 1996; 115:447–453.

9. Nocturnal Oxygen Therapy Trial Group. Continuous or nocturnal oxygen therapy in hypoxemic chronic obstructive lung disease: a clinical trial. Ann Intern Med 1980; 93:391–398.

10. O'Donohue, WJ Jr, Plummer AL. Magnitude of usage and cost of home oxygen therapy in the United States. Chest 1995; 107:301–302.

11. O'Donohue WJ Jr. Home oxygen therapy. Med Clin North Am 1996; 80:611–621.

12. Report of the Medical Research Council Working Party. Long term domiciliary oxygen therapy in chronic hypoxic cor pulmonale complicating chronic bronchitis and emphysema. Lancet 1981; 1:681–685.

13. Selinger SR, Kennedy TP, Buescher P, Terry P, Parham W, Godfried D, Melinger A, Spagnolo SV, Michael JR. Effect of removing oxygen from patients with chronic obstructive pulmonary disease. Am Rev Respir Dis 1987; 136:85–91.

14. Tarpy SP, Celli BR. Long-term oxygen therapy. N Engl J Med 1995; 333:710–714.

23

Smoking Prevention and Smoking Cessation

Roger H. Secker-Walker
University of Vermont College of Medicine
Burlington, Vermont

SCOPE OF THE PROBLEM

Burden of Ill Health

The harmful effects of cigarette smoking on health have been extensively documented since the report of the Royal College of Physicians from the United Kingdom in 1963 and the Surgeon General's Report from the United States in 1964. Harmful effects of tobacco use, particularly in relation to cancers of the mouth and lung, had been suspected for many years before these reports. Cigarette smoking is firmly established as the major cause of lung cancer and chronic obstructive pulmonary disease, a major risk factor for coronary artery disease, and for other cancers, such as those of the pharynx, larynx, esophagus, kidney, pancreas, and bladder. Cigarette smokers are also at higher risk for cervical and anal cancer. Chewing smokeless tobacco is a major cause of oral cancer.

Among women who smoke during pregnancy, miscarriage, antepartum hemorrhage, placenta previa, and premature rupture of the membranes are all more common. On average, infants born to women who smoke are 200–300 g lighter than the infants of nonsmokers, or of women who quit early in pregnancy. Exposure to their partners' cigarette smoke among nonsmoking pregnant women is also associated with lower birth weight in their offspring. Women who smoke during pregnancy are also more likely to have low-birth-weight infants ($\leq$2,500 g) than nonsmokers.

Infants raised by parents who smoke are more likely to suffer from bronchitis, pneumonia, and ear infections in their first year of life than infants in nonsmoking families. Exposure to tobacco smoke during childhood may cause asthma in some children and certainly exacerbates childhood asthma. Adult nonsmokers exposed to environmental tobacco smoke—that is, the smoke wafting from a lit cigarette and to a lesser extent the smoke exhaled by smokers—are clearly at greater risk for lung cancer and heart disease. The lung function of nonsmokers working with smokers is also adversely affected, as is the lung function of children growing up in families where one or both parents smoke.

The number of deaths attributable to smoking is well over 450,000 per year in the United States and approaches 4–5 million worldwide. The number of productive years of life lost before age 65 attributable to smoking is greater than that resulting from any other human behavior, although alcohol consumption is a close second. The World Health Organization predicts that tobacco use will be the leading cause of lost disability-adjusted life years worldwide before the year 2005.

The prevalence of adult smoking in the United States is now about 20–25%, and has been falling steadily since the 1964 Surgeon General's report. Current adult smokers tend to be less well educated, have lower incomes, are heavier smokers, and are more likely to suffer from depression than smokers of 10–20 years ago.

In the last 3–5 years, there has been a disturbing increase in the prevalence of cigarette smoking among teenagers and young adults after several years of declining prevalence among both boys and girls. This increase began shortly after the introduction of generic cigarettes, which were substantially cheaper than named brands, and also at a time of increased promotional efforts by the tobacco industry. Use of smokeless tobacco, which has also been heavily promoted, is also on the increase, particularly among boys.

Nicotine Addiction

Most children experiment with cigarette smoking, often first trying a smoke at ages 11 or 12 but occasionally much younger. Important influences are the smoking behavior of their parents or siblings and their attitudes to smoking. Of even more importance is the smoking behavior of their friends and peers. These social influences, together with adolescent's misperception that most kids smoke, play key roles in shaping their attitudes toward and norms concerning cigarette smoking. Addiction to nicotine builds up slowly after smoking initiation, usually taking several years to become fully established. This addiction is strongly reinforced by the repetitive sequence of puffing on the cigarette, each inhalation being followed almost at once by activation of nicotine receptors in the brain and feelings of both relaxation and alertness.

Most smokers experience well-recognized withdrawal symptoms when they attempt to quit smoking. These symptoms—which include craving for nicotine, irritability, frustration or anger, anxiety, difficulty concentrating, restlessness, and an increased appetite—usually taper over the course of 3 or 4 weeks after stopping smoking and are as severe in adolescents as they are in adults. The craving for nicotine is often lifelong. The strength of addiction is not reliably measured, but the Fagerstrom scale, a short eight-item questionnaire, is widely used in research. In practice, time to first cigarette after waking and number of cigarettes smoked per day are useful clinical guides: the sooner the first smoke and the more cigarettes smoked per day, the more highly addicted the smoker is and the more difficulty that smoker will have stopping smoking.

Benefits of Quitting Smoking

The health benefits of quitting smoking are well recognized. The symptoms of chronic bronchitis—cough and phlegm—diminish rapidly, often after an initial increase in the symptoms for a few days after the last cigarette. The bronchial epithelium slowly recovers, becoming almost normal within about 5 years. Lung function, as measured by forced vital capacity or forced expiratory volume in 1 s, increases a little, on average about 100 mL, during the first year after stopping smoking. Within about 3 years, the rate of loss of lung function returns to the normal rate of 25–30 mL/year. The risk of heart attack diminishes rapidly, by 50%, a year after quitting. By 5 years, the risk approaches that of never smokers. Compared to never smokers, the risk of lung cancer diminishes slowly over 15–20 years. Stuffy noses clear, the sense of smell returns, and appetite increases. For pregnant women who quit smoking before 20 weeks gestation, pregnancy and birth outcome and average infant birth weight are the same as for nonsmokers. On average there is weight gain of 5–10 lb within the first year after quitting, although in about 10% of quitters, gains of up to 30 lb may be seen. At today's price of about $2 a pack, a successful quitter would save about $730 in the first year.

SMOKING PREVENTION

School Programs

Early school-based smoking prevention curricula focused on imparting knowledge of the health effects of cigarette smoking. These were generally unsuccessful in preventing the onset of smoking among teenagers. In the last two decades, curricula incorporating social influence theory and modeling refusal skills have been introduced. The effectiveness of these curricula has been well established by numerous trials, especially in the United States. Most delay the onset of smoking but do not prevent it. An exception is the Life Skills Training curriculum, which addresses smoking, alcohol use, and other substance use. It was designed to be taught in 30 classes in grades 7–9 and has been shown to have lasting effects in preventing the onset of cigarette smoking into young adulthood.

Community Programs and Mass Media

Several other smoking prevention programs have had favorable effects that lasted at least through high school. One of these, the Minnesota school smoking prevention curriculum, was combined with communitywide antismoking activities and was shown to reduce the onset of smoking into young adulthood. Another multicomponent intervention—which addressed smoking, alcohol use, and other substance use and involved school, community, and mass media components—reduced the onset of smoking through high school. A third program, the University of Vermont's Smoking Prevention Through Mass Media and School Programs project, compared a 4-year mass media and school program with a school program only. It was shown to reduce the onset of smoking by more than 30% among students, initially in grades 4–6, who were followed into grades 10–12 in high school.

The role that physicians can play in preventing the onset of smoking has not been well defined. Pediatricians, family physicians, and internists who treat adolescents all have opportunities to address smoking, particularly at examinations for student participation in sports. Pediatricians also have the opportunity to discuss smoking issues with parents, especially in relation to passive smoking issues.

Key concepts that have guided the successful smoking prevention programs described above can be used as a framework in which to discuss smoking and other substance use: these stress the immediate health consequences of smoking rather than the distant ones, point out that young people who do not smoke can have a good time and are socially acceptable, make it clear that most young people do not smoke, and have them think of and rehearse ways of refusing cigarettes.

Legislation

Another important approach to reducing the onset of smoking is through legislation. Raising cigarette excise taxes is an effective way of reducing adolescent consumption of tobacco. Studies from several countries have shown that increasing the cost of cigarettes by 10% is accompanied by a 14% reduction in tobacco use by youth, with 12% of young people not starting to smoke and 2% cutting down or quitting. Clean air policies in schools, substance use curricula, and laws restricting under-age access may all help reduce teenage smoking, but the evidence supporting these efforts is not strong at this time. Recently, it was shown in Massachusetts that successful efforts to reduce the purchase of cigarettes by underage youth to less than 20% were not accompanied by a reduction in the prevalence of smoking among young people in communities where these efforts were in progress. All communities will need to be involved in these efforts to restrict access, because without uniform enforcement, young people will purchase tobacco products in nearby communities with lax enforcement of laws banning the sale of these products to youth.

SMOKING CESSATION

Human Behavior Change

Several theories related to human behavior change have been used to guide approaches to smoking cessation. Underpinning much of this work are the theory of reasoned action and social learning theory. In the theory of reasoned action as applied to smoking cessation, a smoker's intention to quit is seen as based on level of motivation to quit, which, in turn, is based on perceived positive and negative consequences of quitting and also the level of confidence that the smoker would succeed if an attempt were made. Increasing a smoker's awareness of the health risks of continued smoking and of the benefits of quitting has been shown to increase motivation to quit, which, in turn, increases intention to quit. Social learning theory emphasizes the importance of self-efficacy—that is a person's confidence in his or her ability to undertake a planned behavior change as a key to success in making a change. Self-efficacy can be measured by a smoker's responses to a series of questions about the level of confidence in being able to resist smoking in a variety of different circumstances. Self-efficacy can be increased, especially by seeing other people such as friends or peers, model the behavior, by practicing the behavior, and also by being rewarded for successfully accomplishing the behavior.

The transtheoretical model of stages of behavior change provides a practical approach to delivering smoking cessation advice. This model takes into account the smoker's level of readiness to change his or her smoking behavior and allows the advice to be tailored to the smoker's readiness to quit. The model, which draws on a broad theoretical base, including the theory of reasoned action and social learning theory, was developed through detailed observations of the cognitive, emotional, and behavioral processes that occur as smokers quit spontaneously. Several levels of readiness—or stages of change, as they are called in this model—are recognized: precontemplation, in which the smoker enjoys smoking and has no thought of quitting; contemplation, in which the smoker is actively thinking about stopping in the next 6 months and in which the perceived benefits of smoking no longer outweigh the perceived advantages of quitting; preparation, in which the smoker intends to quit in the next month and has begun to take steps to do so; action, arbitrarily defined as the first 6 months after a serious quit attempt and the stage during which most attempts will fail; maintenance, or successful abstinence from smoking for more than 6 months; and relapse, much of which occurs in the first week or two after a quit attempt. Most smokers who have relapsed after a quit attempt return to the contemplation stage.

Although developed from observations of smoking behavior change, these same stages have now been recognized for many other health-related behaviors, including quitting cocaine, taking up regular exercise, sunscreen use, safer sex, consistent condom use, weight control, reduction of dietary fat, modifying delinquent behavior, screening mammography, and physicians intervening with smokers.

For physicians and other providers engaged in helping smokers quit, recognizing a smoker's stage of change will indicate what approach is most appropriate and most likely to help. For example, discussion of the pros and cons of quitting, especially the benefits of quitting, and reductions in consumption would be appropriate for precontemplators; discussion of quitting methods for contemplators; modeling quitting techniques and rehearsing skills to resist urges to smoke for those in preparation; and rehearsal of strategies to resist relapse for those in action.

Cessation Methods

The vast majority, more than 85%, of smokers who succeed in quitting smoking do so by setting a date and quitting "cold turkey." Smokers who reduce their cigarette consumption without setting a quit date tend to revert to their previous levels of smoking. Once a decision has been made to quit, several important steps are associated with success. These include setting a quit date, preparing for that date by reducing the number of cigarettes smoked, getting rid of all smoking materials, letting friends know of the plan and asking for their support, and preparing for situations in which the smoker anticipates that he or she will be at high risk for relapse. Most smokers make several quit attempts before succeeding.

As aids to these efforts, there are tip sheets, self-help booklets, manuals, books, and videotapes modeling smoking cessation. Each of these may help. In trials of their success, quit rates of 5–20% at 1 year have been achieved.

More intensive methods, such as smoking cessation classes, have greater success, with quit rates in the range of 15–25% at 1 year. Sometimes members of these classes continue to meet as their own stay-quit support groups to help prevent relapse after the classes are over. Cessation classes are usually attended by smokers who are highly motivated to quit; but among smokers in general, only a small proportion are interested in taking part in such classes, and that proportion is lower among male (5–10%) than among female smokers (10–15%).

There are other strategies that have been shown to increase the likelihood that a quit attempt will succeed. Arranging for follow-up visits to discuss progress and provide support for the quit attempt has had varied success, but making several supportive telephone calls during the first few weeks has been more consistently successful in achieving long-term abstinence from smoking.

The most successful aid to smoking cessation has been nicotine replacement therapy. Use of either the transdermal nicotine patch or nicotine gum clearly increases long-term quit rates, usually by a factor of about 2. The severity of withdrawal symptoms is reduced. Cognitive behavioral support increases the likelihood of success with the gum and may also do so with the patch. Both types of nicotine replacement are available over the counter, but their cost—about $56 for 2 weeks' supply of the patch and $38 for 48 pieces of the gum, which might last only a week—may seem excessive to many smokers. A pack-a-day smoker spends about $14 per week on cigarettes. Other devices to deliver nicotine as replacement therapy are available, including a nasal spray and an inhaler. Use of these devices is accompanied by quit rates similar to those seen with transdermal nicotine or nicotine gum.

Recently, several studies have reported success with the antidepressant drug bupropion (Wellbutrin). A sustained-release preparation of bupropion (Zyban), which was approved by the Food and Drug Administration for use in smoking cessation in 1997, has been shown to approximately double the quit rate at 1 year compared to placebo in nondepressed moderate to heavy smokers, who also received brief counseling. There was no effect on withdrawal symptoms. In another study, direct comparison with a transdermal nicotine patch showed that sustained-release bupropion was more effective than the patch but that the combination of the patch and sustained-release bupropion was only slightly but not significantly more effective than sustained release bupropion alone. In these trials, the use of sustained-release bupropion was associated with about half the weight gain seen in the placebo control group while on the medication, but there was a smaller difference at 6 months. This limitation of weight gain could prove a useful feature of the use of bupropion as an aid to smoking cessation, as there is no consistent evidence that the use of nicotine replacement therapy limits the extent of the usual long-term weight gain that follows smoking cessation.

Numerous other methods have been tried to help smokers quit. The clonidine patch enjoyed brief success but is rarely used now. In general, the other methods—such as hypnosis, acupuncture, meditation, and other drugs such as lobeline—have not been well evaluated in randomized controlled trials, and their efficacy is not clearly established.

Environmental Factors

As with adolescents, there are environmental factors that influence cigarette consumption and smoking cessation among adults. These include tobacco excise taxes and the price of cigarettes and smoking policies in public places and worksites. Because adults tend to have more disposable income than adolescents, the effect of a price increase on adult cigarette consumption is substantially less: an increase of 10% in the cost of cigarettes reduces adult smoking by about 4%. There is also evidence that strict worksite smoking policies also reduce adult smoking. Banning smoking in public places changes the norms for those who live in such communities or states and may also help reduce adult smoking. It certainly makes the environment safer and more pleasant for nonsmokers and especially for asthmatics.

Guideline and Systems for Physicians

In 1996, the Agency for Health Policy and Research produced a consensus statement called the *Smoking Cessation Clinical Practice Guideline*. This statement was based on careful review and some further analyses of scientific articles on smoking cessation published between 1975 and 1994. Guideline recommendations were made for three groups of health professionals: primary care clinicians, tobacco cessation specialists and programs, and health care administrators, insurers, and purchasers.

The guideline for primary care clinicians is based on four key activities, the four A's: *ask* about tobacco use, *advise* users to quit, *assist* those who are interested, and *arrange* follow-up.

The first A, *ask*, means asking all patients about tobacco use status at each visit. An important aspect of this recommendation is setting up an office system ensuring that tobacco use is checked and documented at each visit. Such a system could, for example, be an expanded vital signs record in the chart, to include tobacco use, for example as current, former, or never. Stickers on each patient's chart have also been used, as have computerized medical record systems. An important part of implementing such a system is to have a member of the office health care team responsible for updating tobacco use status at each visit, especially among continuing smokers and recent quitters.

Although categorizing a patient's smoking status as current, former, or never (the latter usually defined as having smoked fewer than 100 cigarettes ever) is essential for tracking progress, other details of current smoker's history of tobacco use can provide useful information in discussions of quitting. Age at onset of smoking, years smoked, current number of cigarettes per day, time after waking to first cigarette, number of quit attempts and length of longest time quit, provide indications of the strength of the addiction and the smoker's experience with quit attempts.

The second A, *advise*, means strongly urging all smokers to quit. The advice should be personalized and unambiguous. For example: ''I am concerned about your smoking, because smoking is harmful to your health. Therefore, I strongly recommend that you quit smoking.'' It is helpful to follow such a direct statement with a question, such as ''How do you feel about quitting?'' This allows the smoker to let the provider know how he or she feels about quitting, and these comments give a good indication of the smoker's readiness to quit. All that is needed from the provider is an acknowledgement of the situation. A more certain method of assessing readiness to change can be obtained by asking the smoker about his or her level of intention to stop smoking in the near future, for example: ''Do you intend to quit smoking in the next month?'' Smokers who say no are clearly in the precontemplation stage, while those who say yes or maybe are in the contemplation or preparation stages.

The next step depends on the level of intention. If the patient is not interested in stopping smoking, a few words about the benefits of quitting, both short and long-term, rather than the harm from continued smoking, may help move them along the path toward contemplation. Having patients weigh up the pros and cons of smoking, by asking what they get out smoking, what worries them about smoking, and then asking they would like to do about it, may help some smokers become more motivated to quit.

The third A, *assist,* comes into play for smokers who intend to quit in the next month. Here the provider helps to develop a quit plan. A key part of this plan is to elicit a quit date. The following words are an efficient way of doing this: ''Most smokers who succeed in quitting smoking do so by setting themselves a quit date. Would you be willing to set a quit date?'' The response can be yes or no. If yes—and about 50% of smokers who say they intend to quit in the next month will say yes—a date in the next week or two is sought and the date recorded in the chart. Brief advice on ways to prepare for the quit date should be given—such as getting rid of all smoking materials; telling family, friends, and coworkers of the impending attempt and seeking their support; and planning what to do in circumstances that may have led to relapse in the past or which the smoker recognizes as posing a high risk for smoking, such as drinking or being with other smokers.

If the response to setting a quit date is no, there are two courses of action. The simplest is to let the matter rest there, with some comment about the benefits of quitting and encouragement to consider a quit date in the future. A second approach, perhaps more appropriate for patients who are being seen frequently, is to ask if the smoker is willing to cut down, say to half the present level, and if so, to set a date for that. Such action requires follow-up, either by phone or during the next office visit, when further progress toward quitting may be accomplished. For smokers like this, who are unable or unwilling to quit, a harm-reduction strategy aimed at long-term reduction in the daily number of cigarettes smoked may be pursued.

For smokers who set a quit date, the guideline strongly supports the use of nicotine replacement therapy, either the patch or the gum, and providers are recommended to encourage the use of such therapy for smoking cessation except in special circumstances. The special circumstances are pregnancy, within 4 weeks of a previous myocardial infarction, in the presence of serious arrhythmias, and in patients with serious or worsening angina. In pregnancy, although there have been no randomized controlled trials of its effectiveness, nicotine replacement therapy is recommended only after cognitive/behavioral methods have failed and the risks of using the patch or gum are felt to outweigh the continued risk of smoking.

The transdermal nicotine patch has the advantage of ease of use, being applied each morning to a different hairless part of the upper torso and taken off either at night or the following morning. Insomnia and bad dreams may occur with nicotine excess. Apart from skin irritation, there are few side effects. Most skin reactions are mild and self-limiting, but some progress and may need treatment with a topical steroid ointment. Those with allergies to nicotine transdermal patches should avoid them in the future. Great care should be taken when disposing of used patches, as they contain substantial amounts of unabsorbed nicotine and, if swallowed, can poison children and pets.

For most smokers, the usual course would be a month or two with a high dose patch (15–22 mg), followed by 2–4 weeks at the intermediate strength (10–14 mg) and another 2–4 weeks at the lowest dose (5–7 mg). One brand has two strengths, a higher one (22 mg) and a lower one (11 mg), each used for 4 weeks. Light smokers—that is, patients smoking less than 10 cigarettes per day—or patients weighing less than 100 lb should start with an intermediate-strength patch. There is some evidence that treatment with transdermal nicotine patches for 8 weeks is as effective as treatment longer time periods. However, a few smokers who have succeeded in quitting with the patch may benefit by continuing their use beyond the recommended 8-week period.

Nicotine gum comes with either 2 or 4 mg per piece. The 4-mg gum is best for highly addicted smokers and those who have failed the 2-mg gum but are still interested in quitting. Up to 20 pieces of the 4-mg gum and 30 pieces of the 2-mg gum may be chewed daily. The gum should be chewed slowly and intermittently and kept between cheek and gum between chews to aid nicotine absorption. Regular use every hour or two may be more beneficial than ad lib use. Mouth soreness, hiccups, dyspepsia, and jaw ache are common adverse effects but are usually transient and tend to resolve with proper chewing technique.

Duration of use should be tailored to the patient's needs, but 3 or more months are often needed, and a small proportion of users continue to use the gum for an extended period of time beyond this. Relapse to smoking is more likely to occur when too few pieces are chewed over too short a time period.

Sustained-release bupropion's place as an aid to smoking cessation has yet to be firmly established, but it has the advantages of being in pill form, not containing any nicotine, and possibly reducing postcessation weight gain. Sustained-release Bupropion is started a week before the quit date, at a dose of 150 mg daily for the first 3 days and then 150 mg twice daily. It is continued for 6–12 weeks after the quit date. Brief supportive counseling—for example, by telephone or at an office visit—should be an integral part of this treatment.

Common side effects include nausea and insomnia. Seizures are very rare, but bupropion is contraindicated in patients with seizure disorder, bulimia, or anorexia nervosa, those on monoamine oxidase inhibitors, and those with allergies to this medication.

For success in quitting smoking, total abstinence is essential. Even a single puff can lead to relapse. But relapse should be seen as a learning experience and used to help plan what skills need to be acquired or what situations avoided during the next quit attempt. The situations in which relapse is likely to occur are well recognized: being around other smokers, experiencing negative emotions, having cravings for cigarettes, withdrawal symptoms, and having concerns about weight gain. Planning how to deal with each of these ahead of time will reduce the likelihood of relapse. Several techniques may be helpful to smokers who are trying to quit. When they are around other smokers, they should try not to smoke, to leave the situation, or to use distraction strategies by doing something else with their hands, mouth, or mind.

When a smoker is experiencing negative emotions—such as stress, anxiety, anger, frustration, sadness, loneliness, boredom, or depression—he or she must have coping strategies available other than the passive strategy of smoking. Undertaking some physical activity, employing relaxation strategies, or just venting ones feelings may help. Other coping strategies include seeking social support, cognitive strategies such as deliberately thinking about positive events and achievements, and actively seeking a solution, if possible, to the problem or problems associated with the negative emotion. Distraction techniques may be tried, but these tend to be least successful.

For cravings, the best strategy is to change the routines associated with smoking. For heavy smokers, this can be a major undertaking and perhaps better directed at the most important cigarettes first. It is best to do something when one is experiencing a craving rather than trying to wait for it to pass. Making it hard to get a cigarette helps.

For withdrawal symptoms—which are certainly ameliorated by nicotine replacement therapy but not by bupropion—asking friends and family to be especially tolerant of one's irritability, inability to concentrate, restlessness, and sleeplessness for the next 3 or 4 weeks may help.

Weight gain after smoking cessation, which tends to be more of a concern for women than men and often leads to relapse, needs to be anticipated. Attempts to prevent weight gain by simultaneous dieting may undermine the attempt. A prudent approach is to advise potential quitters to accept some weight gain and adopt a healthy lifestyle that includes regular exercise, eating plenty of fruits and vegetables, and limiting alcohol consumption. A serious attempt at weight loss should, if necessary, be postponed for 6 or more months, by which time the new ex-smoker should have gained sufficient confidence and experience to maintain a nonsmoking status.

Self-help materials—which can be obtained from several sources, such as the American Cancer Society, the American Lung Association, the American Heart Association, and the National Cancer Institute—may be offered to those smokers interested in using them. To facilitate and encourage their use, such materials should be readily available in the provider's office.

A few primary care clinicians do their own smoking cessation counseling; others have a nurse or health educator in their practice who has this responsibility. However, most practices must rely on whatever is available in the local community. Smoking cessation classes tend to occur sporadically. Having regularly scheduled cessation classes, individual support, and ''stay quit'' support groups available locally would go a long way to providing the help that many primary care clinicians perceive as necessary to support their efforts.

The fourth A, *arrange*, refers to arranging to follow the progress of the quit attempt

and to continue to offer encouragement and help in problem solving and addressing anticipated relapse situations. Many quit attempts fail within the first 2 weeks. Thus, the first
follow-up contact, which can be done by phone, should occur soon after the quit date and
further contacts made after that. The guideline recommends a second contact within the
first month, but consideration should be given to varying the frequency of contacts to
match the needs of the person undertaking the attempt. For patients being seen for other
reasons, office visits may be used for follow-up, but scheduled office visits specifically
to discuss progress with quitting smoking tend to be skipped.

The preceding discussion has focused on cigarette smoking, for it is among cigarette
smokers that almost all the research has been done. Pipe and cigar smokers who have
switched from cigarettes inhale almost as much nicotine, carbon monoxide, tars, and other
noxious products of tobacco combustion as cigarette smokers, but lifelong pipe or cigar
smokers inhale substantially less. The office-based techniques used for smokers can be
applied to pipe and cigar smokers and are likely to be more efficacious for lifelong pipe
and cigar smokers as they tend to be less addicted. Similar office-based techniques have
been tried with users of smokeless tobacco, with similar modest levels of success.

Cost Savings

There is good evidence that health care costs are reduced following smoking cessation.
Reductions are seen in both the direct medical costs and in the indirect costs related to
disability. However, because smokers who quit live longer than those who continue to
smoke, they incur both greater Social Security and pension costs and substantial medical
costs in their old age. In a recent analysis from the Netherlands, the cost benefits associated
with men quitting smoking became equal to the cost associated with their longer lives 26
years after quitting, with no discounting, 31 years at a 3% discount rate, 37 years at a 5%
discount rate, and more than 50 years, if ever, at a discount rate of 10%.

From a health policy perspective, a cost-effectiveness analysis is a more appropriate
way to look at smoking cessation interventions. In such analyses, the cost per life-year
gained, or the cost per quality-adjusted life-year gained, can be used to compare different
preventive and therapeutic strategies. Thus policy decision makers, working within a bud-
get, can implement those interventions that yield the best returns in terms of quality-
adjusted life-years gained. The use of mass media to prevent smoking has been shown to
be economically attractive; that is, the cost per life-year gained is relatively low. Similarly,
the use of mass media to promote smoking cessation has also been shown to be economically attractive. Several studies have examined the cost-effectiveness of smoking cessation
interventions provided by physicians, the use of nicotine gum, and also the use of the
transdermal nicotine patch. Each was shown to be more cost-effective than other medical
interventions such as treatment for hypertension, hyperlipidemia, coronary artery bypass
surgery, breast cancer screening, and markedly more cost-effective than renal dialysis or
liver transplantation.

A metanalysis of studies of physicians' advice to quit smoking showed that face-
to-face contact, advice from physicians and other health professionals, and repeated contact are key factors associated with smoking cessation. In this analysis, quit rates averaged
about 8.4% higher than in control groups at 6 months and about 5.8% higher at 1 year.
Such low success rates lead many clinicians to think that their efforts are not worthwhile.
However, two observations suggest otherwise: first, an increase of 5–6 percentage points
approximately doubles the population of smokers' spontaneous quit rate; second, in the

study of the cost-effectiveness of physicians' smoking cessation advice, quit rates at 1 year of 1 and 4.4% were both shown to be economically attractive.

SUGGESTED READING

1. Ajzen I, Fishbein M. Understanding Attitudes and Predicting Social Behavior. Englewood Cliffs, NJ: Prentice-Hall, 1980.
2. Bandura A. Social Learning Theory. Englewood Cliffs, NJ: Prentice Hall, 1977.
3. Bandura A. Self-Efficacy: The Exercise of Control. New York: Freeman, 1997.
4. Barendregt JJ, Bonneux L, van der Maas PJ. The health care costs of smoking. N Engl J Med 1997; 337:1052–1057.
5. Cummings SR, Rubin SM, Oster G. The cost-effectiveness of counseling smokers to quit. JAMA 1989; 261:75–79.
6. Fiscella K, Franks P. Cost-effectiveness of the transdermal nicotine patch as an adjunct to physicians' smoking cessation counseling. JAMA 1996; 275:1247–1251.
7. Hughes JR. The future of smoking cessation therapy in the United States. Addiction 1996; 91:1797–1802.
8. Kottke TE, Battista RN, DeFreise GH, Brekke ML. Attributes of successful smoking cessation interventions in medical practice. JAMA. 1988; 259:2883–2889.
9. Murray JL, Lopez AD, eds. The Global Burden of Disease: A Comprehensive Assessment of Mortality and Disability from Diseases, Injuries, and Risk Factors in 1990 and Projected to 2020. Vol. 1. Cambridge, MA: Harvard University Press, 1996:295–324.
10. Prochaska JO, DiClemente CC. Stages and process of self-change of smoking: toward and integrative model. J Consult Clin Psychol 1983; 51:390–395.
11. Prochaska JO, DiClemente CC, Norcross JC. In search of how people change. Am Psychol 1992; 47:1102–1114.
12. The Smoking Cessation Clinical Practice Guideline Panel and Staff. The Agency for Health Policy and Research Smoking Cessation Clinical Practice Guideline. JAMA 1996; 275:1270–1280.
13. Tobacco and the Clinician: Interventions for Medical and Dental Practice. Smoking and Tobacco Control Monograph Number 5. NIH Publication No. 94-3693. Rockville, MD: U.S. Department of Health and Human Services, Public Health Service, National Institutes of Health, 1994.
14. U.S. Department of Health and Human Services. Preventing Tobacco Use Among Young People: A Report of the Surgeon General. Washington, DC: U.S. Department of Health and Human Services, Public Health Service, Centers for Disease Control and Prevention, National Center for Chronic Disease Prevention and Health Promotion, Office of Smoking and Health, 1994.
15. U.S. Department of Health and Human Services. The Health Benefits of Smoking Cessation: A Report of the Surgeon General. DHHS Publication No. (CDC) 90-8416. Rockville, MD: U.S. Department of Health and Human Services, Public Health Service, Centers for Disease Control, Center for Chronic Disease Prevention and Health Promotion, Office of Smoking and Health, 1990.
16. U.S. Department of Health and Human Services. The Health Consequences of Using Smokeless Tobacco: A Report of the Advisory Committee to the Surgeon General. NIH Publication No. 86-2874. Bethesda, MD: U.S. Department of Health and Human Services, Public Health Service, 1986.
17. Warner KE, Slade J, Sweanor LLB. The emerging market for long-term nicotine maintenance. JAMA 1997; 278:1087–1092.

24
Lung Transplantation

James H. Dauber
University of Pittsburgh
Pittsburgh Veterans Administration Medical Center
Pittsburgh, Pennsylvania

INTRODUCTION

Inclusion of a chapter on pulmonary transplantation in a textbook devoted to the management of pulmonary disease is appropriate, since this form of therapy for end-stage cardiopulmonary disease is now widely accepted by health care providers and third-party payers. Such acceptance is a relatively recent development. The field of pulmonary transplantation did not achieve such a status until the beginning of the last decade of the twentieth century, years after the acceptance of renal, hepatic, and cardiac transplantation. The clinical challenges leading to the late blossoming of pulmonary transplantation will become apparent to the reader as the chapter unfolds. Advances in recipient selection, organ preservation, operative technique, and immunosuppression have markedly improved the early survival of lung recipients. Approximately 75% of lung recipients worldwide will survive at least 1 year; 5-year survival, however, is just reaching 50% and lags well behind that for other solid organs, which approaches 75%. The principal cause for late mortality following lung transplantation is the bronchiolitis obliterans syndrome, which is believed to be a manifestation of chronic rejection of the lung allograft. Much effort is being devoted to understanding the pathogenesis of chronic rejection and to developing strategies for its prevention and management. As these efforts begin to bear fruit, it is likely that survival following lung transplantation will equal that of other major solid organs, firmly establishing this technique as a treatment for patients who have failed conventional medical therapy.

DEFINITIONS AND SURGICAL CONSIDERATIONS

Currently there are several procedures that fall under the heading of pulmonary transplantation. The simplest is a single-lung transplant in which the new lung is implanted through a standard thoracotomy. There are two vascular and one airway anastomoses. In some patients it is not possible to do just a single lung transplant, in which case two lungs must be implanted. Most often this is accomplished by doing sequential bilateral single-lung transplants. In instances where there is irreversible dysfunction of the left ventricle, a combined heart and lung transplant must be performed. In this instance the airway anastomosis is at the level of the distal trachea and the vascular anastomoses include the vena cava and aorta. In contrast, airway anastomoses in lone pulmonary transplantation are at the distal mainstem bronchi and the vascular anastomoses at the pulmonary artery and left atrium. The justification for doing a tracheal anastomosis in the combined heart-lung transplant is that some of the bronchial arteries are derived from the coronary arteries, which provide better circulation to the donor airways than might be the case if the proximal airways of the donor along with their bronchial arteries were excluded by doing bibronchial anastomoses. In the latter instance, proximal donor airways are supplied by retrograde flow derived from bronchopulmonary anastomoses at the level of the small airways. Cardiopulmonary bypass is required for heart-lung transplantation and in lone pulmonary transplantation when the native lung and newly transplanted allograft cannot provide sufficient gas exchange. This type of circulatory support should be avoided whenever possible, however, due to the risk of bleeding from anticoagulation. Explanting of the native lungs is both tedious and dangerous in an anticoagulated subject with dense pleural adhesions and hypertrophic bronchial arteries. There are several other aspects of the surgical technique and early postoperative care that are important to outcome, such as approaches to preservation of the donor lung and induction of immune suppression, but these are not developed here as they are less relevant to the goals of this chapter. The interested reader is directed to several excellent reviews.

DISEASES AMENABLE TO TRANSPLANTATION

There are four broad categories of lung disease that have the potential to benefit from pulmonary transplantation (Table 1).

Chronic Obstructive Pulmonary Disease

This is the category for which the majority of lung transplants are performed today. Disease in the vast majority of this group of recipients is related principally to tobacco abuse even when alpha$_1$-antitrypsin deficiency is present. The majority of these patients do well with a single-lung transplant, but some centers advocate double-lung transplantation for young recipients in order to maximize life expectancy and long-term functional status.

Interstitial Lung Disease

This category is also well suited to single-lung transplantation except when moderate to severe pulmonary hypertension is present. In the latter instance, the increased vascular reserve of a double-lung allograft lessens morbidity and mortality in the early postoperative period in the event of primary graft failure, which occurs as a consequence of severe acute lung injury. This situation is further aggravated if there is persistent pulmonary hypertension following a single-lung transplant. Transplantation has been performed for a wide variety of interstitial lung diseases, but the leading condition is idiopathic pulmonary fibrosis because of its poor response to conventional medical therapy. Recurrence of the underlying disease in the lung allograft has been reported in recipients transplanted for sarcoidosis, hard metal pneumoconiosis, and lymphangiolyomyomatosis. To date there

Table 1 Categories of Lung Disease Amenable to Transplantation

Disease Type	Procedure
Chronic obstructive lung disease	
Cigarette-induced	Single > double
Alpha₁ antitrypsin deficiency	Single or double
Bronchiolitis obliterans	
Idiopathic[a]	Single
Graft-versus-host disease from bone marrow transplantation	Single
Post–lung transplantation[a]	Single
Interstitial lung disease	
Idiopathic pulmonary fibrosis	Single
Sarcoidosis[a]	Single
Scleroderma/CREST/rheumatoid Arthritis/mixed CTD	Single
Eosinophilic granuloma	Single
Pneumoconioses	Single
Silicosis	
Asbestosis	
Heavy metal disease[a]	
Lymphangiolyomyomatosis[a]	Single
Pulmonary vascular diseases	
Primary pulmonary hypertension	Single or double
Eisenmenger's syndrome *with* correctable cardiac effect	Single or double
Eisenmenger's syndrome *without* correctable cardiac defect	Heart-lung
Chronic LV faillure with reactive pulmonary hypertension	Heart-lung
Septic lung disease	All require double lung transplant
Cystic fibrosis	
Idiopathic bronchiectasis	
Post lung transplantation	
Immune deficiency	?

Key: CTD, connective tissue disease.
[a] Denotes diseases that have recurred in lung allograft.

are no reports of recurrence of idiopathic pulmonary fibrosis or pulmonary fibrosis associated with collagen vascular disease. In fact, the native lung in such recipients may show gradual radiographic improvement in the posttransplant period.

Pulmonary Vascular Disease

This condition may be either primary or secondary to congenital heart disorders or collagen vascular disease. Some centers advocate a double-lung allograft, but the majority of recipients receiving a single lung for this indication have also done well. As with interstitial lung disease that is complicated by pulmonary hypertension, the risk of primary graft failure due to acute ischemia-reperfusion injury is heightened when the majority of the cardiac output flows through the newly transplanted lung. Severe decompensation in lung function later in the postoperative course due to infection and/or rejection is also more likely in single-lung recipients transplanted for pulmonary hypertension than in recipients who receive a double allograft for this indication. Nonetheless, transplantation of a single lung for patients with pulmonary hypertension remains an accepted approach because there does not seem to be a major difference in outcome, and single-lung allografting is a more efficient utilization of a scarce resource. When the congenital heart defect that caused the pulmonary hypertension is not correctable, combined heart and lung transplantation is necessary.

Septic Lung Disease

This final category is characterized by chronic infection, typically with *Pseudomonas* species, in the lower respiratory tract. All diseases in this category require double-lung and occasionally heart-lung transplantation in order to eliminate the reservoir of infection that would quickly soil a single lung allograft. Once thought to be an absolute contraindication to lung transplantation, cystic fibrosis (CF) is now the leading indication for double-lung transplantation and the second most common indication for lung transplantation overall. Although the other manifestations of this disease persist following a transplant, adult recipients with CF enjoy a survival rate and quality of life that are equivalent to those of other recipient groups. Patients with idopathic bronchiectasis also benefit from double-lung transplantation, but the jury is still out for patients whose bronchiectasis is related to underlying immune deficiencies such as hypogammaglobulinemia.

Diseases Not Suited for Transplantation

Not all conditions producing chronic respiratory insufficiency are amenable to transplantation. The most notable examples are neuromuscular diseases and kyphoscoliosis. In these conditions, injury to the lungs is secondary to the primary abnormality, which will not be corrected by replacing the lungs. Transplantation is also not indicated for cure of lung cancer with the possible exception of bronchioloalveolar cell carcinoma. The are a handful of anecdotal reports of long-term survival following double-lung transplantation for this form of lung cancer. Distinguishing between metastatic adenocarcinoma with pulmonary involvement and multicentric bronchioloalveolar carcinoma is critical. When this is done successfully, however, cancer-free survival following transplantation for the latter disorder has exceeded 5 years. There seems to be no role for lung transplantation presently in the treatment of other forms of bronchogenic carcinoma. The immunosuppression required to prevent rejection of the allograft will likely diminish tumor surveillance and promote the growth of any metastases that occurred prior to resection of the primary tumor.

SELECTION OF RECIPIENTS

Severe end-stage pulmonary or cardiopulmonary disease causing marked functional impairment and shortened life expectancy in subjects who have the potential to regain a normal lifestyle are the principal criteria for lung transplantation. To avoid becoming bogged down in the intricacies of the selection process for a wide range of end-stage lung diseases, it is convenient to define who is *not* an ideal candidate by considering the absolute and relative contraindications for lung transplantation (Table 2).

Contraindications

Infection with the human immunodeficiency virus (HIV) or the presence of an active malignancy are absolute contraindications that are universally accepted at the present time. The exception to the latter condition is bronchioloalveolar cell carcinoma, which may not recur after a double-lung transplant, but this area remains controversial. Ongoing substance abuse will also disqualify a candidate. Most programs demand a period of abstinence of at least 6 months from tobacco and of 12 months for alcohol. Prior to the introduction of combined multiple organ transplants, the presence of end-stage liver or renal disease was usually an absolute contraindication as well. In the few centers capable of performing combined lung-liver or lung-kidney transplants, hepatic and renal insufficiency may no longer stand in the way; realistically, however, such insufficiency remains an absolute contraindication in the vast majority of programs. Poorly controlled psychiatric disease is also a strong contraindication.

Recipients must have the potential to become fully ambulatory after a successful transplant. Thus, most centers require that candidates be ambulatory prior to the transplant. Walking at least 600 ft in 6 min is the minimum acceptable in many programs. However, candidates with severe limitation of cardiac output from end-stage primary pulmonary hypertension are not consistently held to this standard, since this amount of exertion might produce syncope and accelerate heart failure.

Individuals with active coronary artery disease amenable to angioplasty should un-

Table 2 Contraindications to Pulmonary Transplantation

Absolute
Infection with human immunodeficiency virus
Active malignancy
Ongoing substance abuse
Uncontrolled psychiatric disease
Multiple organ failure
Relative
Nonambulatory state
Poorly controlled coronary artery disease
Inadequate family and/or social support
History of poor medical compliance
Inadequate financial support
"Panresistant" bacteria in the respiratory tract
Severe diabetes mellitus with end-organ insufficiency
Pharmacological doses of corticosteroids
Gross obesity
Severe malnutrition
Severe osteoporosis with compression fractures

dergo this procedure prior to evaluation. Those with uncontrolled coronary artery disease will need a heart-lung transplant. Even when events in the posttransplant period are favorable, recipients still require much family and social support to maintain the regimen required for successful function of the new organs over the long term. Without such support and demonstrated compliance with previous medical regimens, recipients are at risk for losing their new organs and potentially their lives in the event of a major complication. Adequate financial resources are also mandatory in today's climate. The cost of the procedure is what most recipients focus on, but expenses after a successful transplant are not trivial and often produce severe financial strain for recipients with inadequate medical benefits.

Chronic infection of the lower respiratory tract with *Pseudomonas* and related species deserves special mention. Resistance of such bacteria in vitro to all currently available antibiotics will usually exclude transplantation. Multiple resistance has become a relative contraindication, but less so if synergy between different classes of antibiotics can be demonstrated in special testing. Infection with the organism *Cepacia burkholderia* (formerly *Pseudomonas cepacia*) is also a very strong contraindication. Although this bacterium is not as virulent as many strains of *Pseudomonas aeruginosa*, it is typically resistant to all antibiotics in vivo. It has the potential to cause fatal postoperative infection in recipients who harbored this agent preoperatively, but this is not a universal outcome. For this reason, candidates with *Cepacia burkholderia* in their sputum must be considered individually, and those with few other relative contraindications have the potential for doing well after a double-lung transplant.

Insulin-dependent diabetes mellitus was at one time a rather strong contraindication, but it is much less so now. It remains an issue if there are significant complications such as renal insufficiency, vascular disease, and severe neuropathy. Regimens of high-dose corticosteroids were at one time absolute contraindications for lung transplantation because of the fear of poor wound healing, particularly at the airway anastomosis. As surgical technique has improved, however, concern about the doses of corticosteroids has diminished. Nonetheless it is desirable to minimize exposure to steroids as much as possible prior to transplant because of the increased risk for infection and complications such as perforation of colonic diverticuli in the early postoperative period.

The nutritional status of individuals referred for transplantation is an important consideration. Under optimal circumstances, candidates should be within 80–120% of their ideal body weight. When they fall outside of this range, the rate of postoperative complications increases, but this is not a ground for exclusion at the present time. Overweight individuals should be given the opportunity to lose weight, which is an indication that they are able to comply with demanding medical regimens. Underweight individuals often find it necessary to rely on tube feeding, most often through the gastric or jejeunal route. Problems with nutritional status often persist in the posttransplant period. Severe osteoporosis with a history of compression fractures should serve as a warning. The high doses of steroids used in the early postoperative period to prevent and treat acute rejection will only aggravate this situation, and there is evidence that drugs such as cyclosporine will accelerate bone loss.

Timing of Listing for Transplant

Striking a balance between the candidate who becomes too debilitated to survive the rigors of a transplant and one whose life expectancy could potentially be shortened rather than extended by the procedure is not always a straightforward exercise. The United Network for Organ Sharing (UNOS) presently controls the distribution of organs nationwide. It is the policy of the network that priority for receiving a lung allograft is based principally on time spent on the national waiting list. In addition, organs are distributed preferentially to the region where they were donated. In the last 5–7 years the number of transplant programs has increased much more rapidly than the size of the donor pool. Consequently, the number of candidates on waiting lists (around 2500) has grown disproportionately to the number of procedures done each year (around 1500). This has greatly increased the time that most candidates wait before receiving an allograft. For large, established transplant centers located in regions with medium to low population densities, the waiting time for a single lung ranges from 12–18 months and that for a double lung from 18–24 months. Candidates for a heart-lung block may need to wait for 3 or more years. But even for newer programs with shorter waiting lists located in regions with high population densities, the waiting time for a single lung may be as long as 8–12 months.

The long wait for an organ forces the transplant team to predict when a candidate will need to receive a new lung and usually leads to the early listing of candidates who are ''too healthy'' for a transplant at the time they are first evaluated. It also places a responsibility on candidates and transplant teams to maintain the functional status of candidates at the highest level possible until the appropriate organs become available. This goal can be achieved only through a combined effort on the part of the primary care providers, transplant teams, and candidates, which involves meticulous attention to the details of management of the underlying disease and close communication between all three parties. Periodic reevaluation of candidates at the transplant center after they have been listed will help to identify intercurrent problems that might compromise the outcome after transplantation. Some centers require that candidates move to the area as their names begin to come to the top of the list. This requirement assures rapid access to the candidate when an organ becomes available and allows the transplant team to monitor the status of the candidate more carefully just prior to transplant. The disadvantage of this approach is that it often totally disrupts the lifestyle of the candidate and takes him or her away from their local family and social support systems.

There are published criteria for when to refer patients with a variety of diseases for lung transplantation. The best course of action for primary physicians, however, is to refer individuals ''earlier rather than later.'' It is far superior to evaluate individuals in a systematic and unhurried manner and to deactivate individuals on the waiting list because they are too healthy to accept the risks of the procedure than it is to watch them die before they can receive an organ.

SELECTION OF A DONOR

The criteria for selecting donor organs are relatively straightforward but require that some consideration be given to the widening disparity between the numbers of candidates and donors. In the early days of pulmonary transplantation, when the numbers of candidates were few and donors relatively abundant, transplant surgeons were highly discriminating in the selection of the donor in order to optimize outcome from this standpoint. The pressure to increase the donor pool has led to relaxation of some of the early criteria used to identify an adequate donor. The criteria presently used by the majority of centers are listed in Table 3.

Table 3 Criteria for Donor Selection

Function of donor lung
  Clear chest radiograph
  Adequate oxygenation ($Pa_{O_2} > 350$ torr on
    Fi_{O_2} of 1.0 or $Pa_{O_2}/Fi_{O_2} > 250$ torr)
  Static lung compliance between 15 and 30
    cmH_2O
  No abnormal findings at bronchoscopy
  Normal gross appearance of the lungs at time
    of harvest
Demographics of suitable donors
  Age < 65 years
  No history of clinically significant lung
    disease
  Cigarette exposure of < 30 pack-years

Function of the Donor Lung

The major determinants are a clear chest radiograph and an adequate $(A-a)_{O_2}$ gradient while the potential donor is breathing 100% oxygen. Ideally the latter should be less than 200 mmHg ($Pa_{O_2} \geq 450$ torr), but at times organs will be used when gas exchange is slightly poorer ($Pa_{O_2} > 350$ torr) if the ischemic time will be short. The chest radiograph must be free of localized or diffuse infiltrates. Bronchoscopy is performed routinely as part of the donor evaluation to exclude the presence of foreign bodies, aspirated oral and gastric contents, and purulent secretions in the large airways. It is particularly important to look for blood in the major bronchi, since its presence is usually a sign of aspiration from the upper airway. Bronchial washing should also be prepared for a Gram stain. The presence of mixed flora consisting of both gram-positive and gram-negative organisms is a good indication of aspiration of oral secretions. Aspiration of gastric contents and upper airway secretions is a risk factor for poor allograft function in the immediate postoperative period due to previous chemical injury to the donor lung that was not evident at the time of harvest.

Donor Characteristics

Ideally the donor should be a nonsmoker with no evidence of chronic obstructive airways disease. This is not always the situation, as the prevalence of smoking in donors tends to be higher than that in the general population. A history of mild asthma should not exclude donation, as new onset of asthma in a recipient without a previous history is rare. There is presently no absolute age limit for donation, but most centers draw the line at 65 years. Matching the age of the recipient and donor is an attractive concept but a goal that is often difficult to achieve in practice. At the present time, the donor and recipient are matched for size and major blood group. The principal determinant for size is the height of the recipient, but some adjustment for the relative size of the thoracic chambers must be taken into account. Recipients with preexisting obstructive airways disease who have severe hyperinflation will do better with a larger donor, whereas recipients with preexisting restrictive lung disease who have a small, "frozen" thorax do better with a smaller donor. In the former instance, a lung from a donor matched exactly for height will often fail to expand completely in the early postoperative period, creating a persistent pneumothorax that may take 1–3 weeks to resolve. In the latter case, the donor lung may not fit into a disproportionately small hemithorax. Attempting to force the oversized lung into place is usually associated with atelectasis, hypoxemia, pulmonary hypertension, and systemic hypotension from inadequate cardiac output. Finally donors must be free of active systemic and pulmonary infections and neoplastic disease.

Discrepancy Between Numbers of Donors for Lungs and for Other Organs

Injury to the lung during the event leading to an individual becoming a donor results in the majority of these individuals being disqualified for donating lungs despite their being suitable donors for hearts, livers, and kidneys. Only one in five donors of a heart will also yield a lung. The disparity is greater for liver and the greatest for kidney, where less than one of ten donors will also be suitable for lung donation. This limitation to lung donation is not easily overcome and will likely perpetuate the discrepancy between the numbers of lung transplants performed compared with transplants of other solid organs for some time to come.

PRINCIPLES OF IMMUNOSUPPRESSION

The human lung is highly immunogenic. Presently there are no effective ways to induce adequate specific tolerance to the human lung allograft without pharmacological intervention, and living donation from an identical twin is not practical. For this reason, drug-induced suppression of the recipient's immune system is essential to prevent rapid destruction of the newly transplanted lung. There are three phases of immune suppression following lung transplantation, as with other solid organs: induction, maintenance, and augmentation for treatment of intercurrent rejection. Each is discussed separately below.

Induction

The response to donor antigens is potentially most intense and injurious in the early post-transplant period, when the lung allograft is highly vulnerable owing to the trauma of transplantation. Consequently, virtually all centers use more intense immunosuppression in the perioperative period than later for maintenance. Almost all programs employ high doses of intravenous methylprednisolone, combined with cyclosporine or tacrolimus, and azathioprine given either parenterally or orally. In addition, some centers use antilymphocyte globulins in the form of either horse antihuman thymocyte globulin (ATGAM) or mouse antihuman CD3 monoclonal antibodies (OKT3). The addition of cytolytic antisera at this stage may reduce the prevalence of acute rejection and delay the onset of chronic rejection, but it also seems to increase the rate of infection in the early postoperative period. Consequently there is no consensus for the use of such therapy at present.

Maintenance

The cornerstone of maintenance immunosuppression is either cyclosporin A (Sandimmune or Sandimmune Neoral) or tacrolimus (Prograf, also frequently referred to by its early designation of FK-506). Both of these drugs are potent suppressors of T-cell activation. They inhibit a calcium-dependent phosphatase, which is critical in the induction of the interleukin-2 (IL-2) gene. Tacrolimus is more potent than cyclosporin A on a weight basis and seems to be more effective in the prevention of rejection of both liver and lung transplants. The frequency and severity of toxicity for the two agents seems to be similar when blood levels are kept within the therapeutic range. The major manifestations of toxicity for both are renal insufficiency and neurological symptoms, of which tremor and headache are the most common. Since renal failure ensues in 1–2% of all lung transplant recipients as a direct consequence of these and other drugs, careful monitoring of renal function and adjustment in the dose of cyclosporine or tacrolimus is essential. It is also important to realize that the toxicity of these drugs is related to the amount of free (unbound) drug in the blood. Conditions that reduce the degree of protein binding of these drugs have the potential to increase toxicity despite whole blood levels being in the therapeutic range. Anemia, hypoalbuminemia, and uremia all increase the amount of free drug. When these conditions prevail, keeping the blood level at the lower therapeutic range will help to reduce toxicity. An even more critical issue with the use of these agents is the potential for drug interactions. Many drugs used to treat complications in organ recipients interfere with the metabolism of tacrolimus and cyclosporine A. Table 4 lists the agents known to affect blood levels in recipients on stable doses of either drug. It is *vitally important* for any physician treating organ recipients to be aware of these interactions when a new medication is being prescribed, since an unexpected increase in blood levels will cause toxicity, whereas a marked decline may promote a rejection episode.

Although cyclosporine A and tacrolimus are very potent immunosuppressive agents,

Table 4   Drugs That Alter the Concentration of Cyclosporine or Tacrolimus in Blood

Raise Blood Levels	Decrease Blood Levels
Calcium-channel blockers	Anticonvulsants
Diltiazem	Phenytoin
Verapamil	Carbamazepine
Nicardipine	Phenobarbital
Methylprednisolone (Medrol)	Antibiotics
Antifungal agents	Rifampin
Ketoconazole (Nizoral)	Nafcillin
Itraconazole (Sporanox)	Other drugs
Fluconazole (Diflucan)	Ticlopidine (Ticlid)
Macrolide antibiotics	Octreotide (Sandostatin)
Erythromycin	
Clarithromycin (Biaxin)	
Whole grapefruit and grapefruit juice	
Other drugs	
Allopurinol	
Bromocriptine	
Danazol	
Metoclopramide (Reglan)	

they are usually ineffective when administered alone, particularly in the early posttransplant period. Adjunctive agents are usually required for adequate control of rejection at this time. Corticosteroids and azathioprine are drugs of choice at present. A new agent, mycophenolate mofetil (Cellcept), which interferes with DNA synthesis in lymphocytes, has recently been shown to be as effective as azathioprine in the prevention of rejection after renal and cardiac transplantation when given with cyclosporine A. Its exact role in lung transplantation remains to be established. Adjunctive agents also produce toxicity, which is usually dose-dependent. The principal toxicity of azathioprine is bone marrow suppression, manifest primarily by leukopenia. For mycophenolate mofetil, it is diarrhea and leukopenia. Corticosteroids are associated with a variety of problems, many of which the recipients have already experienced prior to transplantation. One steroid complication that is assuming greater importance is osteoporosis. Inactivity in the preoperative period along with chronic steroid use often produces a significant degree of bone demineralization prior to transplant. High doses of corticosteroids and treatment with cyclosporine A in the early postoperative period greatly aggravates bone loss, leading to an unacceptable rate of pathological fractures; these severely impair rehabilitation.

Most transplant recipients require a combination of three different agents initially. As time progresses, the tendency to reject diminishes in the majority of recipients, which allows reduction in the doses of these agents and at times even discontinuation of corticosteroids and azathioprine. In rare instances it may be necessary to discontinue cyclosporine or tacrolimus because of unacceptable toxicity. This may be done without rejection occurring immediately if the doses of azathioprine and corticosteroids are increased, but whether the recipient can be maintained for an extended period off these drugs remains to be demonstrated. At present there are no good clinical laboratory markers indicating adequate levels of maintenance immunosuppression. The emergence of rejection usually indicates that the doses are too low, the appearance of toxicity suggests that the doses are too high. Finding clinically applicable methods to quantitate the degree of immunosuppression is one of the most important challenges facing the field of solid-organ transplantation today.

Augmentation of Immunosuppression

Maintenance immunosuppression frequently does not prevent rejection of the human lung allograft, particularly within the first 6 months after transplantation. When clinically evident rejection supervenes in a previously quiescent allograft, augmentation of immunosuppression is needed to restore a more tolerant state. Most commonly this is in the form of intravenous methyl-prednisolone at a dose of 500–1000 mg/day for 3 consecutive days. Oral steroids starting at a dose of 1.5 mg/kg of prednisone and tapering down to the previous maintenance dose in 10 days is used when the rejection episode is less severe. Rejection episodes that seem to be resistant to corticosteroid therapy or those that recur within a few months after treatment of the original episode are usually treated with anti-lymphocyte globulins such as ATGAM or OKT3, but other regimens such as oral methotrexate, total lymph node irradiation, colchicine, plasmapheresis and photopheresis have been employed. Regional immunosuppression with an aerosol of cyclosporine A has also proven successful in treating persistent rejection, but its widespread application awaits development of a more efficient delivery system. Multicenter trials are needed to compare the efficacy of current immunosuppressive regimens and to develop more effective methods to prevent rejection.

OUTCOMES OF LUNG TRANSPLANTATION

Survival

The rates of survival after lung transplantation based on pretransplant diagnosis are shown in Table 5. Recipients transplanted for obstructive airways disease enjoy the best rates, whereas those transplanted for diseases such as pulmonary hypertension (both primary and secondary), idiopathic pulmonary fibrosis, or cystic fibrosis experience a higher mortality. Much of the excessive mortality for the latter group occurs in the first 3 postoperative months where the death rate is relatively steep for all recipients. Thereafter, the mortality rate slows, but a steady rate of attrition continues, leading to a 5-year survival rate of only 50%. This rate is substantially poorer than that for other solid organs such as heart and liver, where 5 year survival exceeds 70%. Other preoperative factors that have a negative impact on mortality are mechanical ventilation at the time of transplant, age greater than 40 years, and retransplantation. Survival at 1 year in recipients who were not ambulatory when transplanted is only one-third that of ambulatory patients. In those who were retransplanted, survival is less than one half that of first-time transplants.

Causes of Death

These are listed in Table 6. In this analysis two time periods are considered. The first covers days 0–90 and the second is that after the ninetieth postoperative day. In the first period, infection is the leading cause of death. In the second, rejection assumes this posi-

Table 5 Survival Based on Pretransplant Diagnosis

Indication for Transplant	1 Year %	3 Years %	5 Years %
Emphysema/COPD	80	62	42
Alpha$_1$ antitrypsin deficiency	72	59	48
Cystic fibrosis	73	58	54
Idiopathic pulmonary fibrosis	68	52	NA
Primary pulmonary hypertension	69	53	NA
Congenital lung disease	62	53	NA
Repeat lung transplant	42	32	NA
Other	72	57	46
Overall survival	73	57	46

Source: Data from the 1996 UNOS Annual Report for the cohort of transplants performed between October 1987 and December 1994. The data and analyses reported in the 1996 Annual Report of the UI S. Scientific Registry of Transplant Recipients and the Organ Procurement and Transplantation Network have been supplied by UNOS. The authors alone are responsible for the reporting and interpretation of these data.

Table 6 Causes of Death After Pulmonary Transplantation

Postoperative Day 0–90		Postoperative Day >90	
Cause	% of Deaths	Cause	% Deaths
Infection (not CMV)[a]	29	Rejection	29
Other	21	Other	26
Cardiac failure	9	Infection (not CMV)	24
Multiorgan failure	6	CMV	5
Hemorrhage	6	Neoplasm	6
Rejection	5	Hemorrhage	4
Airway Complication	5	Multiorgan failure	3
Primary graft Failure	5	Cardiac failure	2
CMV	5	Primary graft failure	0
Neoplasm	0	Airway complication	0

[a] Cytomegalovirus.
Source: Data from the April 1996 report of the St. Louis International Lung Transplant Registry.

tion, but with infection running a close second. These two complications are considered in more detail in the next section because they will be encountered by physicians whose major focus in not transplantation medicine but who treat recipients after they are discharged from the transplant center. Risk factors for death in the two periods are as follows. Early death (<90 days): cytomegalovirus (CMV) serological mismatch, no prophylaxis for CMV infection, and infection other than CMV. Late death (>90 days): CMV mismatch, no prophylaxis against CMV infection, presence of CMV disease, cyclosporine instead of tacrolimus, adult respiratory distress syndrome from acute diffuse alveolar damage in the early posttransplant period, a score of >10% on a reactive antibody panel, and mismatch in the HLA-DR locus. The impact of infection and rejection on death is quite evident from such analysis.

Quality of Life

Results of the relatively few studies to date that examine the impact of pulmonary transplantation on the quality of life suggest a positive effect. More than 90% of recipients indicate that they are satisfied with the result. Perceptions of general and mental health, social functioning, physical functioning, and role activity improve once recipients recuperate from the operation itself. The perception of pain, however, may not improve. The higher quality of life persists if allograft function does not deteriorate. But, as expected, quality declines if complications arise that diminish the function of the allograft, the most important of which is chronic rejection. In the opinion of many recipients, the degree to which quality of life improves after transplantation offsets any potential reduction in the quantity of life as a consequence of the procedure. The vast majority of recipients will recommend transplantation to other patients with similar end-stage lung disease.

Impact of Transplantation on Respiratory Physiology

Static Pulmonary Function Tests

In the vast majority of instances there is clear improvement in lung volumes, flow rates, and gas transfer following transplantation. The degree of improvement after a successful double-lung or heart-lung transplant is greater than that for a single lung transplant, with values for the FVC and FEV_1 exceeding 80% of predicted in recipients without significant complications. Improvements after single-lung transplantation are not as great but still are often substantial and lead to a marked improvement in overall functional status. One exception to this generalization concerns recipients transplanted for pulmonary vascular disease. Not infrequently, they have nearly normal lung volumes and flow rates prior to surgery. Transplantation of a single- or double-lung allograft in these cases usually does not lead to marked improvement in spirometric values, but it does reduce the pulmonary artery pressure to a normal or near-normal levels.

Following single-lung transplantation for restrictive disease, the FVC may achieve a level of nearly 70% of predicted. The final value in the absence of major complications seems to be related to the predicted value of the donor. Following single-lung transplantation for obstructive lung disease, the FEV_1 eventually increases to a value of 45–60% of predicted. In both instances the allograft receives the majority of ventilation and perfusion, leading to good ventilation perfusion matching in both the allograft and the native lung. The same is not true following single-lung transplantation for pulmonary hypertension. Here, more than 80% of the cardiac output usually goes to the allograft, but ventilation between the native lung and allograft is more evenly balanced. Although this creates a major ventilation/perfusion mismatch with wasted ventilation in the native lung, the effects on gas exchange are usually minimal. However, when there is a complication in the allograft that interferes with ventilation, hypoxemia may become quite profound. This is particularly important when transbronchial biopsies are being contemplated in single-lung recipients transplanted for pulmonary hypertension.

Exercise Capacity

Despite the fact that transplantation greatly reduces (or even abolishes) the ventilatory limitation to exercise that existed prior to surgery, lung recipients rarely if ever achieve a normal peak oxygen consumption even after a course of intense rehabilitation. Instead they reach a level that is 45–60% of predicted. This limitation is not related to abnormal gas exchange or inadequate cardiac response. It may be explained in part by mild anemia, which is quite common even in healthy recipients, but the deficit occurs even in the face of a normal hemoglobin. The leading explanation for this finding is that oxygen uptake in the periphery is limited by a reduction in the capillary bed of the muscles. A similar limitation in peak oxygen consumption is seen in subjects with chronic obstructive pulmonary disease (COPD), where the mechanism is thought also to be a defect in muscle capillaries. Other factors that have the potential to limit oxygen consumption by muscles in transplant recipients include steroid-induced myopathy (an all too common complication), a direct effect of cyclosporine on metabolism of muscle mitochondria or muscle blood flow, and mild uremia secondary to drug-induced nephrotoxicity. This is an important area that demands further study to determine whether limitation of oxygen uptake is irreversible.

COMPLICATIONS

This discussion emphasizes those complications that are common and have a high likelihood of being encountered by physicians who provide primary care to recipients after they are discharged from their initial and subsequent hospital stays at the transplant center. It is important for the primary physicians to understand the major complications and the principles of the diagnosis and management of these challenging patients. This will allow them to participate in a more meaningful way and optimize their care. The complications with the greatest impact on mortality are infection and rejection. For this reason, they are given the greatest attention in this discussion. Although other complications that occur after transplant also have the potential to affect the survival of recipients negatively, either by their frequency or timing, they are not encountered nearly as often by primary care physicians as infection and rejection. For this reason they are dealt with in a less detailed manner.

Acute Rejection

Description

The term *acute rejection* has different connotations for different audiences. For clinicians, it stands for a clinical syndrome that is most frequently encountered in the first 6 months after transplantation; for the pathologist, it describes a type of inflammatory reaction in the lung allograft that can be seen even years after a transplant. Acute rejection is almost the rule after lung transplantation. Only 5% of recipients transplanted at the University of Pittsburgh Medical Center since 1990 did not experience an episode in the first 2 postoperative years. The majority of episodes occur within the first 6 months, with the first as early as the fifth postoperative day. Hyperacute rejection, manifesting as graft failure in the first 12–24 h, is exceedingly rare, possibly because of proper matching of major blood groups, avoidance of transplanting candidates with high titers of preformed antibodies, and the fact that severe injury may be attributed to inadequate preservation. The time of onset of acute rejection may be later if cytolytic therapy is given as induction immunosuppression, but there is no convincing evidence that the overall rate of acute rejection and the eventual development of chronic rejection is lessened when antilymphocyte globulins are administered in the early postoperative period.

Clinical Findings

Early episodes of acute rejection typically manifest as cough, chest tightness, and worsening dyspnea on exertion. Laboratory findings include leukocytosis and new or worsening radiographic infiltrates and pleural effusions. One of the most sensitive abnormalities is widening of the $(A-a)_{O_2}$ gradient, particularly when the radiograph is normal and the recipient does not have a problem with retained secretions. Unfortunately, this finding lacks specificity for rejection. Episodes of acute rejection occurring after the first 3 months are usually associated with less dramatic clinical findings than episodes occurring earlier; in a substantial number of instances, there may be totally asymptomatic. Spirometry may reveal either a plateau or even a decline in the FVC and FEV_1, but—due to improvements in chest wall and pulmonary mechanics—this is not always the case, particularly for double-lung recipients, whose values may continue to increase even in the face of acute rejection. Declines in spirometric values are also not specific for rejection, since a variety of infections can produce the same result.

Diagnosis

Because of the high frequency of both rejection and infection in the first 2 years after a lung transplant and the relative inability to distinguish between the two on the basis of clinical findings alone, clinicians should have a low threshold for performing bronchoscopy whenever the recipient's condition suggests a complication in the allograft. The preferred approach to diagnosis of acute rejection is transbronchial lung biopsy. When six to eight adequate-sized specimens are provided to an experienced pathologist, the sensitivity and specificity of this approach exceed 90%. Bronchoalveolar lavage unfortunately has not yielded any findings specific for acute rejection, but it should be done routinely to establish whether potential pathogens exist in the lower respiratory tract that could be the cause of the new symptoms and complicating the treatment of acute rejection. Occasionally a clinical diagnosis of acute rejection will be made when the picture is strongly suggestive and other complications such as acute lung injury from inadequate preservation and infection are excluded. This most frequently occurs in the early postoperative period, when doing a transbronchial lung biopsy carries more risk.

There is also evidence that surveillance transbronchial lung biopsies, performed according to a predetermined protocol in the absence of symptoms, are justifiable. Most centers practicing this policy will perform a biopsy at 3,6,9, and 12 months postoperatively. This approach has discovered clinically significant positive findings in 25–71% of procedures during this time frame. The most common finding are low grades of acute rejection and CMV pneumonitis. At the University of Pittsburgh, trained transplant physicians frequently made an incorrect diagnosis of ''no infection or rejection'' in asymptomatic recipients based on findings from an extensive clinical evaluation that did not include results of a transbronchial lung biopsy. In nearly half of all recipients evaluated at 1, 3, and 6 months who had no complaints, the transbronchial biopsy performed after the evaluation was completed revealed a clinically significant finding that necessitated a change in management. Thereafter, the rate of unexpected findings in healthy recipients from surveillance transbronchial lung biopsy diminished but was still as high as 15% during the second postoperative year. It dropped to less than 8% in succeeding years. Not all centers practice surveillance biopsies, claiming that this approach does not lead to better overall survival rates. This issue should be addressed in multicenter trials because, on the one hand, the cost associated with surveillance procedures is not trivial. On the other hand, the outcome following lung transplantation is still not optimal by any standard and all avenues to improve outcome should be systematically evaluated.

Treatment

The histological severity of acute rejection is typically graded according to a scheme devised by the Lung Rejection Study Group, which has recently been revised. There are five histological grades (A0 through A4) that are based principally on the severity of perivascular mononuclear inflammatory cell infiltrates (Table 7). Grade A0 indicates absence of infiltrates, whereas grade A4 indicates that the perivascular infiltrates have spread to involve the alveolar space. The severity of the histological inflammatory infiltrates often corresponds well with the clinical manifestations of acute rejection. Histological grades

Table 7 Grading System for Acute Rejection of the Lung Allograft

Grade	Nominal Severity	Extent of Perivascular Infiltrates
A0	No rejection	No significant abnormality.
A1	Minimal	Infrequent perivascular mononuclear cell infiltrates mainly surrounding venules with a thickness of just a few cells.
A2	Mild	More frequent infiltrates involving veins and arteries which are more than several cells thick.
A3	Moderate	More exuberant mononuclear cell infiltrates that extend from the perivascular space into the alveolar interstitium.
A4	Severe	Infiltrates extend into the alveolar space with pneumocyte damage; there may necrosis of vessels and lung parenchyma.

Source: Adapted from the Lung Rejection Study Group Revised Working Formulation.

A3 and A4 are felt to be sufficient to warrant therapy even if the individual is relatively asymptomatic, which is unusual. Grade A2 is more controversial, and asymptomatic individuals commonly will not be treated. Most centers do not treat grade A1.

Therapy of acute rejection episodes involves augmenting immune suppression. The first episode is usually treated with intravenous methylprednisolone, 1 g/day for 3 days. Mild episodes may be treated with oral prednisone, typically starting with 100 mg and decreasing by 10 mg/day until the previous maintenance dose is reached. A follow-up transbronchial biopsy should be performed 2–6 weeks after completion of therapy. This is crucial, since persistent or recurrent rejection was detected in 63% of recipients who were deemed to have responded to previous therapy on the basis of clinical evaluation alone. The second episode is also usually treated with intravenous corticosteroids. Treatment of subsequent episodes varies from center to center and includes polyclonal horse antihuman lymphocyte globulin (ATGAM) or murine OKT3 monoclonal antibody, plasmapheresis, photopheresis, and total lymphoid irradiation. In addition to such augmentation, tacrolimus may be substituted for cyclosporine and methotrexate for azathioprine. Regional immune suppression with an aerosol of cyclosporine has also proved effective. Refractory rejection occurs in only 10–15% of recipients, but successful management is crucial, since afflicted recipients appear to be at the highest risk for contracting chronic rejection or losing the allograft to persistent rejection, which is not uncommonly fatal. Prophylaxis for CMV should be given during treatment of subsequent episodes of acute rejection, particularly for recipients who receive cytolytic therapy and are at risk for a primary infection or those who have already manifested CMV disease. Antibacterial prophylaxis should also be considered for those recipients being treated for recurrent rejection who have had bacterial pneumonia in the allograft and are colonized with potential pathogens such as *P. aeruginosa* and *Staphylococcus aureus*.

Before moving on to a discussion of chronic rejection, the reader is invited to compare the features of the two complications in Table 8.

Chronic Rejection

Definition

Late-graft dysfunction that is characterized by airflow obstruction secondary to inflammation and scarring of small airways is frequently given the name of *chronic rejection*. The

Table 8 Comparison of Acute and Chronic Rejection Syndromes

Feature	Acute Rejection	Chronic Rejection
Clinical findings		
Onset	Tends to be abrupt early; tightness	Usually subtle; dyspnea on exer-
Symptoms	in chest, cough, dyspnea	tion; cough (often productive)
Hematological	Leukocytosis	Normal
Physiological	Oxygen desaturation	Normoxia until late
	Primarily restrictive disease	Primarily obstructive disease
Radiological	Diffuse infiltrates, effusions	No abnormality until late
Histological	Perivascular mononuclear cell infil-	Obliterative bronchiolitis; venous
	trates ± airway inflammation	and arterial sclerosis ± perivas-
		cular mononuclear cell infiltrates
Response to therapy	Usually responds briskly to pulsed	Progressive decline in lung func-
	doses of steroids but often re-	tion over months to years is the
	curs (most recipients have more	rule
	than one episode)	

primary histological abnormality is obliterative bronchiolitis (OB), but there is also damage to blood vessels, particularly veins, which undergo sclerosis. At many centers, transbronchial lung biopsy is not sensitive in detecting OB. In addition, there are other causes for this histological finding that are not due to an immunological response to donor antigen, such as infection, chronic aspiration of gastric contents, and drug reactions. For this reason there has been strong movement toward defining late graft dysfunction due to airflow obstruction as the bronchiolitis obliterans syndrome (BOS) when no other cause for the decline in lung function can be demonstrated. This diagnosis does not require confirmation of histological OB, but it does depend on the exclusion of other conditions in the allograft, such as acute rejection and infection, which usually requires bronchoscopy with bronchoalveolar lavage and transbronchial lung biopsy.

The severity of BOS is based on the degree of decline in the FEV_1 compared to its best posttransplant baseline, which is usually determined by calculating the average of two best readings taken 3–6 weeks apart. Four stages are recognized based on the percentage change from the best FEV_1 (Table 9). Each stage contains two subcategories, a and b, which respectively signify that OB was not or was histologically confirmed. This grading scheme is useful in comparing the prevalence and severity of BOS from center to center and in characterizing the course of an individual recipient. One limitation of this system is that it tends to deemphasize the importance of early OB that is not associated with a significant decline in the FEV_1. In the minds of many clinicians, Stage O BOS, subcategory b (presence of OB) does not imply much of threat, yet failure to treat OB at a stage when function is still well preserved may well be missing the best opportunity to control this complication.

Clinical Characteristics

As the name implies, the appearance of chronic rejection is delayed. The mean time of onset is around 18 months, but it has been detected as early as the third postoperative month, with the risk extending to years after the transplant. Typically the onset is subtle, with the recipient experiencing more shortness of breath than expected for the degree of exertion. In some instances a productive cough is the presenting symptom, often with no

Table 9 Staging of
Bronchiolitis Obliterans
Syndrome

Stage	% Decline in FEV$_1$[a]
0	<20%
1	20% to 35%
2	35% to 50%
3	>50%

[a] Change in FEV$_1$ is calculated by following formula:
[(Current baseline FEV$_1$ − best baseline FEV$_1$)/best baseline FEV$_1$] × 100%.
The best baseline FEV$_1$ represents the average of the two highest levels of FEV$_1$ measured at least 3–6 weeks apart.

pathogen identified in the sputum. Less commonly the onset is abrupt, presenting with a rapid and substantial decline in allograft function. The biopsy may reveal histological changes of both acute and chronic rejection. The acute rejection usually responds histologically to treatment, but often this response is not associated with improvement in spirometry and the findings of chronic rejection persist. The prevalence of BOS varies from center to center, but in most it approaches 50% of recipients who survive for more than 3 months.

In the early stages, the physical examination is usually normal. As the disease progresses, inspiratory rales appear at the lung bases, often being more noticeable anteriorly than posteriorly. Wheezing is distinctly uncommon but occurs in a small fraction of recipients later in the course. Reactive airways disease is not a usual feature of chronic rejection, but there is a subset of recipients with this disorder who develop severe wheezing at bronchoscopy. The chest radiograph is often unchanged at the onset of disease. With progression of chronic rejections, linear parenchymal infiltrates and chronic effusions may appear, particularly in recipients who have developed intercurrent infection as a consequence of treatment with augmented immunosuppression. Computed tomography of the chest may reveal bronchiectasis, attenuation of peripheral vascular markings, and air trapping. Such findings help to confirm the diagnosis, which is based on the results of bronchoscopy and pulmonary function tests.

Diagnosis

Transbronchial lung biopsy is often insensitive in detecting OB. This is related to the fact that the distribution of OB is patchy and that even optimal transbronchial biopsy specimens often contain only a few small airways for examination. Increasing the number of biopsy specimens will help to improve sensitivity, but even under the best of circumstance, the sensitivity is still under 90%. Nonetheless, bronchoscopy with transbronchial biopsy is the cornerstone of diagnosis, since the results will permit exclusion of other conditions, such as infection and acute rejection, that are also capable of causing a decline in spirometric values. A transthoracic lung biopsy is seldom called for, but in complicated situations, it may be justifiable.

Treatment

Chronic rejection is treated in much the same fashion as acute rejection. The first time chronic rejection is suspected or confirmed, treatment usually consists of intravenous methylprednisolone and maximization of maintenance immunosuppression. This approach reverses airflow obstruction in only a small minority of recipients. More typically, it only stabilizes lung function for a matter of weeks before the decline sets in again. Some recipients are totally refractory to corticosteroids and continue to experience a decline in flow rates. In the last two instances, other forms of therapy are tried next. Most often this consists of cytolytic therapy, but other modalities—such as methotrexate, total lymphoid irradiation, and aerosolized cyclosporine—may be used. These treatments stabilize function for a period of time in the majority of recipients, but the tendency for relapse with a further decline taking place months to years later is notable. Any treatment given after multiple relapses, by which time there is obliteration of many small airways and dropout of associated distal lung units, has little chance at improving allograft function. A small proportion of afflicted recipients appear to be resistant to all forms of conventional therapy and develop end-stage obstructive and restrictive lung disease within 6 months after the onset of chronic rejection. Chronic rejection is the single greatest cause of mortality in the late postoperative period, with rates varying from 25–30%. It also decreases the quality of life and adds to the cost of care. Accordingly it has become the major barrier to long-term success of lung transplantation.

Prevention and Control of Risk Factors

Efforts to control chronic rejection must of necessity turn to prevention and interruption of the fibrotic response, since conventional treatment with augmented immunosuppression is relatively ineffective. Much has been written about the risks factors for chronic rejection. There is universal agreement that recurrent early acute rejection is the most important. This suggests that reducing the rate and severity of acute rejection should lessen the risk of chronic rejection. Prevention of acute rejection will require more effective immunosuppression and/or the induction of greater tolerance to the lung allograft. Improved tolerance may be achieved by creating a "microchimeric" state within the donor owing to the persistence of donor-derived cells that have migrated from the allograft. Persistence of donor-derived cells in the recipient may be enhanced by infusing donor bone marrow at the time of lung transplantation. Although this approach has not appreciably reduced the frequency of *acute rejection* after lung transplantation, recent evidence from studies at the University of Pittsburgh suggests that the frequency of *chronic rejection* is lower in recipients who received donor marrow versus contemporaneous controls who did not (A. Zeevi, personal communication). More subjects and a longer observation time are needed to confirm such an advantage for microchimerism. Maintenance immunosuppression based on tacrolimus also seems to lessen the risk of chronic rejection as compared with a cyclosporine-based regimen, despite the fact that the rate of acute rejection was not decreased in the tacrolimus group. Promising new immunosuppressive drugs such as mycophenolate mofetil have recently been released and others such as rapamicin are coming to clinical trials. Hopefully, salvage and maintenance regimens employing these agents will prove to be effective in reversing or preventing acute and chronic rejection of the lung allograft.

Other factors that may predispose to chronic rejection include CMV pneumonia, severe early acute lung injury, and bacterial pneumonia in the late transplant period. The latter is strongly linked with chronic rejection, possibly because treatment of chronic rejection with augmented immunosuppression predisposes the damaged allograft to bacterial infection. It is also tempting to speculate that bacterial infection promotes chronic rejection through cytokine release and upregulation of donor MHC antigens in the airway.

The challenge of gaining a better understanding of the pathogenesis of chronic rejection is not trivial, since there are no good animal models for this condition. Nonetheless, work with rodent models of tracheal allografts may yield insight and point the way to the use of antagonists to cytokines and growth factors that promote fibrosis in the rejecting lung (e.g., platelet-derived growth factor, basic fibroblast growth factor, and transforming growth factor beta). The ideal outcome would be to prevent this complication entirely rather than treating it once it is established.

Infection

Bacterial Pneumonia

Even though the prevalence is greatest in the early postoperative period, where it is the leading cause of death, bacterial pneumonia occurs all too frequently throughout the entire postoperative course. In the perioperative period, gram-negative rods and *P. aeruginosa* in particular are the leading cause. When *S. aureus* is found in cultures from the donor trachea, however, there is a risk of pneumonia in the allograft from this organism. Prophylaxis with broad-spectrum antibiotics has greatly reduced the incidence of infection at this time. Prophylaxis typically includes ceftazidime and clindamycin as a minimum and other agents as suggested by the flora in the lower respiratory tract of both the recipient and donor. Bacterial pneumonia may also occur later, after the recipient returns to a more normal lifestyle. *Pseudomonas* remains the leading cause of late pneumonias and is frequently associated with allograft injury related to chronic rejection and augmentation of immunosuppression. Even in the absence of documented chronic rejection, the lower airways of recipients may become colonized with this organism, and this type of colonization occurs earlier in recipients transplanted for CF versus those transplanted for all other diseases. Although much less common than the organisms mentioned above, *Streptococcus pneumoniae* is identified as the cause of lobar pneumonia in ambulatory recipients. In this case it is important to determine antibiotic sensitivities because of the increasing prevalence of penicillin resistance. Prophylaxis with inhaled tobramycin or colistin should be considered in recipients with recurrent pneumonia from *Pseudomonas* and other gram-negative rods.

Viral Infections

With better control of bacterial pneumonia, viral infection is assuming greater importance as a cause of morbidity and mortality. The types of clinically significant viral infections following lung transplantation are summarized in Table 10. The major cause of viral pneumonia following lung transplantation is cytomegalovirus (CMV), but herpes simplex, adenovirus, influenza, parainfluenza, and respiratory syncytial virus have also been implicated. The primary impact of infection with Epstein-Barr virus (EBV) is on the development of posttransplant lymphoproliferative disease. The present discussion centers on CMV and EBV infection.

Cytomegalovirus Infection.   As in other forms of solid-organ transplantation, CMV is the major viral pathogen. The risk of developing infection depends on whether the recipient or the donor had been infected before transplant. Recipients who were not in-

Table 10 Viruses Causing Clinically Significant Infections in Lung Transplant Recipients

Virus	Time of Risk	Syndrome
Herpes simplex virus (HSV)	POD 1–7	Stomatitis, pneumonia
Cytomegalovirus (CMV)	POD 30–180	Pneumonia, gastroenteritis
Epstein-Barr virus (EBV)	POD 45–90	Mononucleosis, PTLD
Respiratory syncytial virus	Sporadic	Pneumonia
Adenovirus	Sporadic	Pneumonia
Parainfluenza virus	Sporadic	Sinusitis, bronchitis, and asthma
Influenza A and B	Influenza season	Bronchitis

Key: POD, postoperative day; PTLD, posttransplant lymphoproliferative disease.

fected prior to transplant and who receive an organ from an uninfected donor (R_{neg}/D_{neg}) have the lowest risk, but even when CMV-negative blood products are employed in this population, the rate of infection in this group of recipients is 15%. The risk is much higher for other combinations: R_{neg}/D_{pos}(71%), R_{pos}/D_{pos}(69%), and R_{pos}/D_{neg}(58%).

Infection with CMV usually indicates that viral replication is taking place at a sufficient rate for virus to be detectable in body fluids by usual culture techniques. When viral replication is rapid and widespread enough to be detected by viral inclusion bodies in tissue, the resulting inflammatory response is usually sufficient to produce symptoms and organ dysfunction. This type of infection is referred to as CMV disease and produces considerable morbidity and mortality in lung transplant recipients despite prompt treatment with potent antiviral agents. Disease occurs in about 80–85% of recipients with primary infection (R_{neg}/D_{neg} and R_{neg}/D_{pos}) and in 33 and 25% of recipients with secondary infection (R_{pos}/D_{pos} and R_{pos}/D_{neg}), respectively. Pneumonitis is the most common form of CMV disease in lung recipients, but gastritis and colitis also occur. In the era prior to CMV prophylaxis, CMV pneumonitis commonly occurred when recipients were still recovering from surgery, heavily immunosuppressed, and at the highest risk for acute rejection. In this setting, CVM pneumonitis produced a clinical syndrome that mimicked rejection. With effective prophylaxis, pneumonitis tends to occur later but still can be confused with rejection because it often follows treatment of rejection, particularly when a previous episode of rejection was treated with antilymphocyte globulins. Diagnosis of CMV disease is usually confirmed by detecting viral inclusions in affected tissue. For the lung allograft, this may be achieved with either cytological analysis of secretions from the lower respiratory tract or transbronchial biopsy. The former technique is highly specific but relatively insensitive. For this reason transbronchial lung biopsy is the technique of choice, providing excellent sensitivity with acceptable risk.

Treatment of CMV disease is based on intravenous ganciclovir, which has proven to be effective in the vast majority of cases when given for 21 days. Some centers will add hyperimmune CMV globulin, particularly if organ function is badly compromised or if the disease has relapsed after initial therapy. For severe disease, consideration should be given to reducing maintenance immunosuppression, but this may increase the likelihood of rejection at a later time. Nonetheless, if the recipient appears near death from CMV disease, a drastic reduction in immunosuppression is justifiable. Relapse of disease after initial therapy is certainly not the rule, but it occurs often enough that it must be watched for carefully. Repeat transbronchial biopsy is indicated 1–2 weeks after completion of therapy. This biopsy will also help to clarify whether rejection is present, since the inflammatory response to CMV may mask acute and chronic rejection. Persistence of inclusion bodies in the tissue at this time warrants another course of ganciclovir and testing for ganciclovir resistance in the CMV isolate. If resistance is documented or clinically suspected, foscarnet should be given in place of ganciclovir. CMV disease may relapse weeks to months after the first episode, particularly if the recipient has received augmented immunosuppression in the form of antilymphocyte globulin. Relapsing disease is associated with loss of memory cells specific for CMV antigens in peripheral blood. When memory cells are present in peripheral blood, the risk of relapse is negligible.

Despite the marked reduction in mortality achieved with ganciclovir, morbidity continues to be a major problem. This has led to a variety of methods directed at prevention. The most widely employed rely on intravenous ganciclovir given before there are any findings suggesting infection. Typically, uninfected recipients receive the same regimen in the early postoperative period that recipients being treated for established CMV disease receive later on. The goal is to totally prevent or at least delay the onset of disease until a time when the recipient is better able to tolerate it. Recipients at risk for a primary infection (R_{neg}/D_{pos}) often receive ganciclovir prophylaxis for more than 3 weeks and in some instances for up to 180 days. Whether oral ganciclovir will suffice for long-term prophylaxis remains to be established. The role of passive immunization with CMV-specific immunoglobulin in prophylaxis is still under investigation, but this regimen has proven effective in liver and kidney transplantation. An alternative approach is to treat only those recipients who develop CMV infection as early as it can be detected and presumably before it causes disease. Centers employing this approach rely on frequent monitoring of peripheral blood for evidence of viremia. Once viremia is detected, the recipient immediately receives standard therapy with intravenous ganciclovir. This approach has the potential for decreasing the amount of ganciclovir used in prophylaxis but requires frequent testing of peripheral blood for a minimum of several months. Although short-term results appear promising, long-term efficacy remains to be established.

Epstein-Barr Virus. The principal reason for discussing this virus is its association with lymphoma after solid-organ transplantation, which is termed posttransplant lymphoproliferative disease (PTLD). The vast majority of such cases can be traced to a primary infection or reactivation of latent EBV infection. The prevalence of primary infection depends on the serological status of the donor and recipient pools. Because most adult recipients have been infected before they come to transplant, primary infection is relatively uncommon. It occurs when a seronegative recipient receives an organ from a seropositive infected donor. In this setting, the recipient will almost invariably become infected within 6 weeks, but usually the infection is asymptomatic, when symptoms occur, they are not specific. On the other hand, the vast majority (75%) of primary infections will lead to clinically significant PTLD. Reactivation of latent infection as a consequence of treatment of rejection with intensified immunosuppression also carries a risk for PTLD, but this situation accounts for only a small minority of cases of PTLD. The clinical manifestations and management of PTLD are discussed below.

The diagnosis of primary infection has traditionally been made serologically. Periodic monitoring of seronegative recipients for the appearance of specific antibodies to early antigens in the first several postoperative months is necessary to determine the onset of infection. Techniques to measure the amount of EBV-specific RNA in peripheral blood mononuclear cells have recently been introduced. The extent of viral replication correlates with the burden of EBV RNA in peripheral blood. The risk of developing PTLD seems to be greater in the face of active viral replication. Therefore, monitoring of the burden of EBV RNA in peripheral blood may identify those recipients at high risk for contracting PTLD. Unfortunately, at this time there are no antiviral drugs that are effective in controlling EBV infection.

Other Viruses. Most recipients are seropositive for the herpes simplex virus (HSV) at the time of surgery, and this usually precludes life-threatening infection. However, reactivation of oral disease is not uncommon in the immediate postoperative period (days 1–7) due to the stress of surgery and intensity of immunosuppression. Prophylaxis with low-dose acyclovir (600 mg tid) will frequently prevent this annoying complication, which may interfere with eating at a time when the recipient's appetite is already limited for other reasons. Seronegative individuals are at risk for HSV pneumonitis, which may be fatal. Prophylaxis should be continued for 60 days unless ganciclovir is given for CMV.

Respiratory syncytial virus and adenovirus are relatively uncommon pathogens but have been reported to cause life-threatening pneumonia in adult recipients. These two viral infections should be suspected in recipients with pneumonia from whom no bacterial pathogens or other viral pathogens are isolated. Parainfluenza virus is a relatively rare cause of severe bronchitis that is frequently associated with symptoms of acute sinusitis and asthma. High doses of corticosteroids may reduce the level of airway inflammation and relieve bronchospasm. There may be a role for inhaled ribavirin in the treatment of these viral infections.

Influenza virus occasionally produces a febrile respiratory tract infection in lung recipients, but it is not considered a major pathogen. The diagnosis is often missed, since appropriate cultures are usually not done. Most centers advocate yearly vaccination for influenza, but there is little information to support the idea that vaccinated recipients develop adequate immunity.

Fungi

Aspergillus. By far the most important fungal pathogen in lung recipients is *Aspergillus fumigatus*. This organism causes life-threatening infection in both the early and late postoperative periods. The ischemic bronchial anastomosis is the primary target early after transplant. Later the donor bronchial mucosa and lung parenchyma are prone to infection, particularly after intense immunosuppression for control of acute and chronic rejection. Less commonly, infection involves the native lung; this possibility must always be kept in mind when new infiltrates appear in a symptomatic recipient. Infection may also be disseminated, involving the central nervous system, abdominal organs, and even bones. Invasive disease ideally should be confirmed whenever possible by isolation of the organism from the involved area and demonstration of tissue invasion. The latter is often difficult to establish, particularly for parenchymal lung infection. Treatment should be initiated with systemic amphotericin B or one of the new lipisomal complexes of this drug, which are more expensive but less toxic to the kidneys. Once control is established, itraconazole may be relied on for long-term therapy and suppression. Inhaled amphotericin may also be used to treat bronchial invasion, but usually in conjunction with itraconazole.

A. fumigatus is isolated from bronchoalveolar lavage (BAL) fluid in up to one-third of long-term survivors who have no evidence of tissue invasion. This condition is referred to as *colonization*. The relationship between colonization and invasive infection is somewhat controversial. Most centers believe that organisms found in the lower airways of the allograft are capable of causing invasive infection under the proper circumstances. Consequently, these recipients are often treated with itraconazole for 6–12 months. This approach is very effective at suppressing colonization; since it has been practiced at the University of Pittsburgh, the death rate from aspergillosis has declined. Centers that do not treat colonized recipients claim that morbidity and mortality from aspergillosis is no greater than at centers that do treat colonized recipients. The relationship between colonization prior to transplant and development of invasive disease is also controversial. Not infrequently, patients with septic lung disease have *Aspergillus* isolated from their sputum preoperatively. These recipients seem to be at high risk for invasion of the bronchial anastomosis in the early postoperative period. Therefore, it is not unreasonable to treat colonized candidates with itraconazole 3–6 months before the anticipated date of transplant. Such a policy is not practiced at all centers, however. There is still much to learn about this organism, which is a common cause of serious infection in all forms of organ transplant.

Candida. These organisms may colonize the airway of both the donor and recipient, particularly if either has been on high-dose corticosteroids just prior to transplant. Before the advent of aggressive prophylaxis, or preemptive therapy, this organism frequently caused life-threatening infection involving the airway anastomosis, surgical wounds, mediastinum, and aortic anastomoses in heart-lung transplant recipients. The donor and recipient airway should always be carefully examined for the presence of *Candida* and the identification of this organism at either site is grounds for beginning fluconazole or a short course of intravenous low-dose amphotericin B. Even with such prophylaxis, however, invasive disease of the airway anastomosis may still occur. *Candida* pneumonitis is very rare. Invasive disease should be treated until evidence of infection can no longer be found. With involvement of the airway anastomosis, repeated bronchoscopic examination with endobronchial biopsy is indicated.

Pneumocystis carinii

Prior to the introduction of aggressive prophylaxis, this organism was a common cause of pneumonitis that frequently was subclinical and detected only with bronchoscopy and BAL. It also caused fatal pneumonitis when treatment was not instituted early in symptomatic infection. Since the advent of prophylaxis, this infection has become a rarity. It still produces clinically significant pneumonitis sporadically, but these cases usually occur in recipients who are not practicing adequate prophylaxis. The most effective form of prophylaxis is a single-strength tablet of trimethoprim sulfamethoxazole (TMP/SMX) given daily or every other day. For recipients who are intolerant of these doses, it may be given every third day, usually with adequate prevention. Other prophylactic agents include inhaled pentamidine and oral dapsone, but neither appears to be as effective as TMP/SMX.

Severe Early Graft Injury

Despite many efforts to improve preservation of the lung after it is harvested, severe acute graft dysfunction attributed to ischemia-reperfusion injury remains all too common, afflicting 10–15% of recipients, prolonging time on the ventilator, and occasionally leading to multisystem organ failure. The differential diagnosis includes pulmonary venous occlusion, acute rejection, and infection. Detection of each of these possibilities is relatively straightforward. Transesophageal echocardiography reliably shows obstruction of the venous anastomosis. Fiberoptic bronchoscopy with transbronchial lung biopsy is very helpful in excluding the last two possibilities and is also useful for assessing the degree of injury to the donor airway and the integrity of the bronchial anastomosis. With good supportive care (which may include a short period of extracorporeal membrane oxygenation, inhalation of nitric oxide, and prompt treatment of intercurrent infection or rejection), the majority of afflicted recipients survive and eventually achieve an acceptable level of allograft function, albeit at a slower rate than in recipients who did not suffer this complication. Reported mortality rates range from 13–16%. Recipients who survive severe early graft dysfunction may be more likely to develop chronic rejection than recipients who do not experience early dysfunction.

Phrenic Nerve Injury

With careful dissection of the native lung and avoidance of cold-induced injury, phrenic nerve damage is a relatively rare complication and occurs in less than 5% of patients. It is of little consequence in a double-lung recipient but can be a major problem in single-lung recipients transplanted for restrictive diseases. Poor diaphragmatic function in this setting will produce respiratory insufficiency and inadequate clearance of secretions. This combination leads to prolonged mechanical ventilation and slowed recovery. Nonetheless, the recipient with diaphragmatic dysfunction seems ultimately to adapt with no serious long-term consequences.

Airway Complications

Although the frequency of life-threatening complications with airway anastomoses has decreased dramatically as compared with the early days of lung transplantation, up to 20% of all recipients still experience a clinically significant problem at this site. Stenosis at the anastomosis is the most common abnormality, which results from granulation tissue growing into the lumen, loose sutures to which mucus has attached, scarring with anatomical narrowing, or bronchomalacia. In the former three instances, obstruction to airflow occurs throughout the respiratory cycle and tends to cause a plateau in the inspiratory and expiratory arms of the flow-volume loop. With bronchomalacia, obstruction is a problem principally during forced expiration. When the degree of dynamic obstruction is severe, expiratory flow rates at middle to low lung volumes are disproportionately low, mimicking the abnormality seen in chronic rejection. Fiberoptic bronchoscopy is the most efficient method for detecting an airway complication, but it is important to observe the airway when the recipient is breathing spontaneously in order to assess the degree of obstruction during expiration.

Granulation tissue and fibrous webs are quite amenable to laser therapy. Balloon dilatation provides temporary relief from narrowing due to diffuse scarring, but patency usually persist for only a few weeks. Bronchial stents offer a longer-term solution. Initially solid stents were employed, but they have recently been largely replaced by expandable wire stents, which have the advantage of permitting more normal mucociliary transport and a larger airway lumen. They may also be modified once inserted to assure optimal distribution of airflow and clearance of secretions. Long segments of malacia affecting the entire bronchus intermedius and lower lobe bronchi are difficult to manage with stents, but shorter segments of malacia in these regions have the potential to be stabilized with a wire stent of appropriate size.

Dehiscence of the airway anastomosis is very rare and is usually treated with supportive therapy. Reoperation or retransplantation for acute airway complications is not widely employed owing to poor outcomes. Once the recipient has stabilized, it is possible to repair an area of stenosis by sleeve resection if the anatomy of the region permits.

Neoplastic Disease

Posttransplant Lymphoproliferative Disease

Lymphoma is the most common malignant neoplasm in lung transplant recipients. There are a variety of types, including Hodgkin's disease and non-Hodgkin's lymphomas. As mentioned earlier, these lymphomas are often referred to as posttransplant lymphoproliferative disease (PTLD) and are frequently related to an active infection with Epstein-Barr virus. Polyclonal or oligoclonal B lymphocytes make up the vast majority of PTLD. The cells usually demonstrate the phenotype of the recipient. The prevalence is about 6% in adult recipients and higher in the pediatric population due to the greater rate of primary EBV infection in this group. The process usually presents within the first 3–6 months, most commonly in the lung allograft as either a solitary deposit or multiple nodules. In this case, the recipient is asymptomatic unless the burden of tumor is large. Other sites include the gastrointestinal tract and peripheral lymph nodes. An all too common presentation is abdominal pain from partial bowel obstruction. The risk of perforation in this setting is high, necessitating resection of involved portions of the gut. Treatment at most centers begins with a dramatic reduction in the level of maintenance immunosuppression. This produces a beneficial response in the majority of cases but is frequently associated with acute rejection. Other approaches include surgical resection, particularly in the bowel; and/or treatment with ganciclovir, alpha interferon, anti-B-cell monoclonal antibodies, and host natural killer cells that have been activated with IL-2 in vitro. Conventional chemotherapy is usually ineffective and toxic. Death from progression of the tumor is less common with the approaches listed above, but mortality from chronic rejection and complications of therapy remains unacceptably high. One- and two-year survival rates of the first 20 cases of PTLD at our institution were only 50% and 19% respectively. The strong association between primary infection with EBV and PTLD has led some centers to avoid transplanting candidates who are EBV-seronegative due to the difficulty in matching a seronegative recipient with a seronegative donor and the high rate of mortality when there is a mismatch.

Other Neoplasms

Cancers that are common in the nontransplant population do not seem to occur more frequently than expected in solid-organ recipients. Given the large number of lung recipients transplanted for emphysema caused by heavy cigarette consumption, careful monitoring of the native lung for bronchogenic carcinoma is warranted. At the University of Pittsburgh, there have been five cases of bronchogenic carcinoma among approximately 300 recipients who have survived for at least a year. In all but one case the disease progressed very quickly once it became clinically evident, with death occurring from 2–6 months after diagnosis. Only one case was resectable at the time of diagnosis, owing to metastases in the other cases. Cancers that are more common in organ transplant recipients than in the nontransplant population include carcinoma of the skin, lip, vulva and perineal area, and cervix as well as Kaposi's sarcoma.

SUMMARY

The intent of this chapter is to summarize the current practice of pulmonary transplantation. It is not meant to be exhaustive in scope, because excellent detailed and extensive reviews are available. Instead, the focus is on selected features that are particularly relevant to pulmonary medicine specialists who manage patients with end-stage lung and pulmonary vascular disease and who refer them for transplantation. Advances in survival and related outcomes have been sufficient to ensure that lung transplantation will be widely practiced in the future. Consequently, pulmonary medicine specialists and pulmonary care providers will be taking a greater role in the postoperative management of the patients they refer for this procedure. There still is much room for improvement. The major factors limiting the widespread application and success of this technique are chronic rejection and donor-organ shortage. Solutions to the problem of chronic rejection are largely the responsibility of transplant physicians, surgeons, immunologists, and pharmacologists. Dealing with the shortage of donor organs is the responsibility of everyone interested in this technique. It would be an oversight to end this chapter without an appeal to the reader to consider ways to increase organ donation at his or her institution.

SUGGESTED READING

1. Aris RM, Neuringer IP, Weiner MA, Egan TM, Ontjes D. Severe osteoporosis before and after lung transplantation. Chest 1996; 109:1176–1183.
2. Armitage JM, Kormos RL, Stuart RS, Fricker FJ, Griffith BP, Nalesnik M, Hardesty RL, Dummer JS. Posttransplant lymphoproliferative disease in thoracic organ transplant patients: ten years of cyclosporine-based immunosuppression. J Heart Lung Transplant 1991; 10:877–887.
3. Bando K, Armitage JM, Paradis IL, Keenan RJ, Hardesty RL, Konishi H, Komatsu K, Stein KL, Shah KN, Bahnson HT, Griffith BP. Indications for and results of single, bilateral and heart-lung transplantation for pulmonary hypertension. J Thorac Cardiovasc Surg 1994; 108:1056–1065.
4. Gibbons WJ, Levine SM, Bryan CL, Segarra J, Calhoon JH, Trinkle JK, Jenkinson SG. Cardiopulmonary exercise responses after single lung transplantation for severe obstructive lung disease. J Thorac Cardiovasc Surg 1991; 100:106–111.
5. Gross CR, Savik SK, Bolman RM, Hertz MI. Long-term health status and quality of life outcomes of lung allograft recipients. Chest 1995; 108:1587–1593.
6. Guilinger RA, Paradis IL, Dauber JH, Yousem SA, Williams PA, Keenan RJ, Griffith BP. The importance of bronchoscopy with transbronchial biopsy in the management of lung transplant recipients. Am J Respir Crit Care Med 1995; 152:2037–2043.
7. Iacono AT, Smaldone GC, Keenan RJ, Diot P, Dauber JH, Zeevi A, Burckart GJ, Griffith BP. Dose-related reversal of acute lung rejection by aerosolized cyclosporine. Am J Respir Crit Care Med 1997; 155:1690–1698.
8. Keenan RJ, Konishi H, Kawai A, Paradis IL, Nunley DR, Iacono AT, Hardesty RJ, Weyant RJ, Griffith BP. Clinical trial of tacrolimus versus cyclosporine in lung transplantation. Ann Thorac Surg 1995; 60:580–85.
9. Lynch JP, Trulock EP. Recipient selection. Semin Respir Crit Care Med 1996; 17:109–117.
10. Paradis IL, Williams PA. Infection after lung transplantation. Semin Respir Infect 1993; 8:207–215.
11. Penn I. Neoplastic complications of transplantation. Semin Respir Infect 1993; 8:233–239.
12. Sharples LD, Tamm M, McNeil K, Higgenbottam T, Stewart S, Wallwork J. Development

of bronchiolitis obliterans syndrome in recipients of heart-lung transplantation—early risk factors. Transplantation 1996; 61:560–566.

13. Snell GI, Esmore DS, Williams TJ. Cytolitic therapy for the bronchiolitis obliterans syndrome complicating lung transplantation. Chest 1996; 109:874–878.

14. Tamm M, Higenbottam TW, Dennis CM, Sharples LD, Wallwork J. Donor and recipient predicted lung volume and lung size after heart-lung transplantation. Am J Respir Crit Care Med 1994; 150:403–407.

15. Trulock EP. State of the art: lung transplantation. Am J Respir Crit Care Med 1997; 155:789–818.

25

Principles of Mechanical Ventilation

Theodore W. Marcy
University of Vermont College of Medicine
Fletcher Allen Health Care
Burlington, Vermont

GOALS OF MECHANICAL VENTILATION

Mechanical ventilation is a supportive therapy for patients who are unable to maintain adequate gas exchange because of neuromuscular impairment, cardiovascular failure, diffuse lung disease, or disordered central respiratory drive. The primary goals of mechanical ventilation are to improve arterial oxygenation, decrease energy consumption by the ventilatory muscles, facilitate carbon dioxide (CO_2) elimination, and preserve acid-base homeostasis. Ventilatory support is continued until the condition responsible for respiratory failure improves and the patient can successfully resume spontaneous respiratory efforts.

A secondary goal is to prevent or minimize the adverse effects and complications that can occur with this intervention. For example, the risk of barotrauma or hemodynamic compromise is greater in patients with airflow obstruction or acute respiratory distress syndrome (ARDS) and often necessitates specific ventilatory strategies. In other patients, their condition allows a trial of noninvasive ventilatory techniques that avoid the hazards of artificial airways. Thus, the appropriate method of mechanical ventilation depends on the clinical problem for which ventilatory support is required. Examples of this type of clinical decision making follow a review of the physiological principles and terminology of mechanical ventilation.

CLASSIFICATION OF VENTILATOR MODES

Ventilator Control Variables

To move a volume of gas into the lungs, a pressure difference (P_{tot}) must be applied across the respiratory system to overcome both the elastic recoil of the lung and chest wall (P_{el}), and the resistance of the anatomical and artificial airways (P_{res}). This relationship can be approximated by a simplified form of a linear differential equation called the *equation of motion* for the respiratory system:

413

$$P_{tot} = P_{el} + P_{res} \tag{1}$$

or

$$\text{Pressure} = \frac{\text{volume}}{\text{compliance}} + \text{flow} \times \text{resistance} \tag{2}$$

While this equation is only an approximation, its value is that it illustrates the relationship of applied pressure to flow and volume and allows us to better understand the intimidating terminology of modern mechanical vantilators.

One classification system for describing forms of ventilation is based on this *equation of motion*. The classification system first states which side of the equation the ventilator directly regulates or controls (pressure, or flow and volume). It then describes whether pressure, flow, or volume is limited to a preset value or limit, and which variables determine the phase of the respiratory cycle—i.e., how inspiration is triggered and when inspiration ends or cycles.

For example, a ventilator can be set to *control* the magnitude and pattern of flow applied during inspiration. The inspired gas volume is *limited* in that the inspiratory flow ends after delivery of the tidal volume set by the respiratory clinician ("clinician-set"). The pressure applied by the ventilator to generate this flow and volume is a dependent variable determined not by the clinician but by the elastic recoil and resistance properties of the respiratory system. As flow and volume are so closely related (flow is the derivative of volume and volume is the integral of flow), flow/volume ventilation is conventionally called *volume-control ventilation*, even though most modern ventilators in this mode actually regulate flow (Fig. 1).

Alternatively, the ventilator can be set to regulate the pressure applied at the airway opening; flow and volume then become dependent variables determined by respiratory system compliance and resistance and the duration of time over which the pressure is applied (*pressure-control ventilation*). The flow required to generate the clinician-set pressure is initially high, reflecting the pressure difference between the airway opening and the alveoli, but it then decreases as the pressure at the alveolar level rises with increasing lung volume. Pressure is *limited* in that the pressure never exceeds the clinician-set value during inspiration (Fig. 2).

During either pressure- or flow/volume-controlled ventilation, each breath can be *triggered* at a set time after the last breath (*time- or machine-triggered*) or in response to the patient's respiratory efforts as detected by changes in airway pressure or flow (*pressure- or flow-triggered*). During flow/volume-controlled-ventilation, inspiration ends, or *cycles*, when the clinician-set volume is delivered (*volume-cycled*). During pressure-controlled ventilation, the ventilator cycles off after a clinician-set inspiratory time (*time-cycled*). The time interval can be expressed as an absolute time (for example, 1s), as a ratio of inspiratory to expiratory time (for example, an I:E ratio of 1:2), or as percentage of the total breath length (for example, an inspiratory time of 33%).

The most common form of ventilation used in adult patients requiring full ventilatory support and who are making no spontaneous efforts would be most accurately called *flow-controlled, time-triggered, volume-cycled ventilation*. If pressure-controlled ventilation is utilized, it would be termed *pressure-controlled, time-triggered, time-cycled ventilation*. The advantage of flow-controlled volume-cycled ventilation is that the tidal volume and minute ventilation are generally assured. The disadvantage is that the ventilator may apply dangerously high levels of pressure to the lung to deliver the set tidal volume. Pressure-

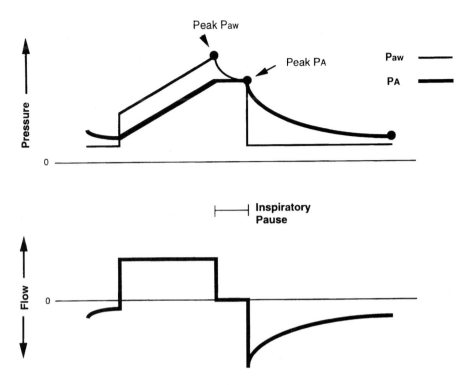

Figure 1 Schematic of pressure and flow during volume- or flow-controlled volume-cycled ventilation. The thin line indicates the ramped airway pressure (Paw) applied during the inspiratory phase to overcome resistance and elastic forces; the thick line indicates the change in alveolar pressure (PA) with increasing lung volume. An inspiratory pause is included to illustrate a method to estimate the pressure required to overcome elastic forces.

controlled ventilation limits the amount of pressure applied and can be a more comfortable mode for patients making respiratory efforts, as this mode better matches the inspiratory flow demands of the patient. However, tidal volume and minute ventilation will vary with the changing resistance and elastic properties of the respiratory system when, for example, secretions accumulate or pulmonary edema either resolves or worsens. In addition, minute ventilation is not a linear function of the respiratory rate and instead will plateau above a certain rate that depends on the characteristics of the lung. Alveolar ventilation may actually fall and Pa_{CO_2} rise with increases in the respiratory rate as the delivered tidal volume decreases to approach the volume of the anatomical dead space. This can be confusing for clinicians not familar with this mode of ventilation.

Interacting with Patient Efforts

Mechanical ventilators must sense the patient's respiratory efforts and then interact with these efforts with an appropriate response as selected by the clinician. *Modes of ventilation* refer to these different patterns of response to the patient's efforts. Microprocessor-equipped ventilators provide a bewildering variety of modes of ventilation, some of which

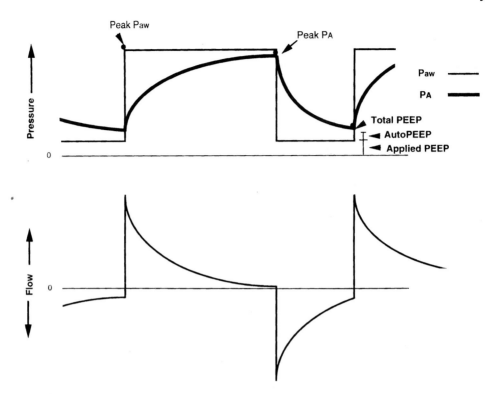

Figure 2 Schematic of pressure and flow during pressure-controlled, time-cycled ventilation (PCV). The thin line indicates the idealized square wave of airway pressure (Paw) applied during the inspiratory phase; the thick line shows the change in alveolar pressure (PA). The I:E ratio is inverted in this schematic to demonstrate the development of auto-PEEP from a short expiratory time. Total PEEP is the measured end-expiratory pressure and represents the sum of both applied PEEP and auto-PEEP.

have never been clinically tested. The following section reviews the principal modes of ventilation that are in common use in clinical medicine.

When a patient makes no respiratory efforts because of the effects of the underlying disease, sedation, or paralysis, he or she contributes nothing to the work of breathing. All breaths are time-triggered and the characteristics of the breath are set by the clinician within the limits of the ventilator in use. *Controlled mechanical ventilation* (CMV) is the simplest and mechanically most reliable method of ventilation. In this mode, the clinician must set the respiratory rate and tidal volume appropriately to deliver a minute ventilation that maintains an adequate Pa_{CO_2} and an appropriate acid-base balance.

The patient's minute ventilation requirement is a function of two factors: (1) the patient's metabolic rate, reflected in the CO_2 production rate; and (2) the efficiency of CO_2 elimination by the lung, reflected by the degree of dead space or wasted ventilation. Patients with high metabolic rates from fever or sepsis, or patients with lung disease and high dead space to tidal volume ratios require a higher minute ventilation. As the patient's clinical condition changes there must be a reassessment of the patient's pH and Pa_{CO_2} so that the minute ventilation is appropriately adjusted.

Many patients on full ventilatory support continue to make respiratory efforts either in response to their physiologic requirements or because of pain and agitation. While the clinician can suppress these efforts with additional sedatives or neuromuscular blocking agents, these medications have many hazards. Instead, the ventilator can trigger a full machine breath (either flow/volume controlled or pressure controlled) in response to the patient's effort—a mode called *assist-control ventilation* (ACV). This is probably the safest initial mode of ventilation as it allows the patient to compensate for higher minute ventilation requirements with the least effort.

Alternatively, the clinician can set a minimum (backup) number of machine breaths triggered by the ventilator or the patient, and allow the patient to have additional unsupported breaths above this backup rate without machine support—a mode called *intermittent mandatory ventilation* (IMV). The acronym becomes SIMV if the supported breaths are *synchronized* with patient efforts as shown in Fig. 3. SIMV has been used most widely as a method of gradually removing the patient from ventilatory support.

Yet another option is *pressure-support ventilation* (PSV), commonly used to gradually withdraw ventilatory support, or to assess a patient's ability to ventilate spontaneously while compensating for the additional resistance of the endotracheal tube. During this mode, the patient triggers every breath and the ventilator provides only enough additional flow to maintain a clinician-set pressure at the airway. When the flow required to maintain this pressure falls—as it will when the patient completes inspiration—the ventilator cycles off. PSV can be combined with SIMV to provide support for patient initiated breaths above the backup rate. However, as in any pressure-controlled mode of ventilation, the delivered tidal volume will vary with the changing resistance and elastic properties of the respiratory system. If secretions, bronchospasm, or edema develop, the ventilator may fail to provide an adequate minute ventilation. In addition, there is no backup ventilator rate if the patient's central respiratory drive fails.

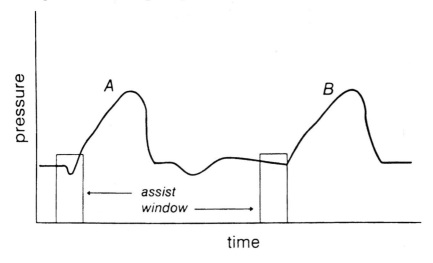

Figure 3 Schematic diagram of airway pressure during sychronized intermittent mandatory ventilation (SIMV). Assist windows occur at a frequency determined by the clinician-set SIMV respiratory rate. An assisted machine breath is triggered either by the patient's inspiratory effort during this window (A) or by the ventilator if the patient makes no effort (B). Between these windows, the patient's inspiratory efforts are unsupported. (From Kacmarck RM, Mess D. Basic principles of ventilatory machinery. In Tobin M, ed. *Principles and Practice of Mechanical Ventilation.* New York: McGraw-Hill, 1994, with permission.)

It is important to realize that patients who are triggering breaths while on full-support modes such as assist/control may continue to make significant respiratory muscle efforts. In a *passively* ventilated patient, the pressure that generates changes in flow and volume (P_{tot} in the equation of motion) is equal to the change in airway pressure. During *assisted* ventilation, P_{tot} is the sum of the change in airway pressure applied by the ventilator and the absolute change in pleural pressure that reflects the patient's own efforts. When a patient triggers a mechanically assisted breath, the inspiratory muscles continue to contract, though the load on these muscles should be decreased by the "push" generated by the ventilator. However, if the flow rate to the patient does not match the patient's flow demand or if the tidal volume is set inappropriately low, the patient "pulls" against both the elastic and resistive forces of the respiratory system and that of the machine circuitry. The patient may expend as much energy during an assisted breath as during unsupported breathing. This "flow dyssynchrony" will contribute to patient agitation and respiratory muscle fatigue.

The Interface Between the Patient and the Ventilator

Positive-pressure ventilation must be applied either with an artificial airway (endotracheal tube or tracheostomy) or with a nasal or full face mask. Placing an endotracheal tube or a tracheostomy can be hazardous and should be performed only by individuals experienced in these techniques. Hemorrhage, mucosal injury and edema, or aspiration of gastric contents are risks with repeated attempts at oral or nasal translaryngeal intubation. Prolonged attempts or unrecognized esophageal intubation may result in seizures or cardiac arrest. Once in place, the endotracheal tube can become dislodged from the airway, migrate into a main bronchus, or be occluded by inspissated secretions. A tracheostomy tube, particularly within the first several days following surgery, can be malpositioned into the pretracheal fascia and occlude the trachea. Even a perfectly placed and maintained artificial airway violates anatomical barriers to bacterial contamination of the lower respiratory tract and, along with repeated suctioning, may alter the mucosal surfaces in ways that promote bacterial adherence and colonization. The risk of nosocomial pneumonia—a serious and life-threatening complication—increases linearly with the duration of intubation.

Because of the risks associated with artificial airways, there has been expanded use of noninvasive forms of ventilatory support for patients with acute respiratory failure and those who require chronic but part-time (4–12 h/day) ventilatory support for chornic respiratory insufficiency. Tight-fitting nasal masks or face masks are the interface between the patient and either a conventional ventilator using any of the modes described above. Alternatively, a Bilevel Positive Airway Pressure (BiPAP) machine may be utilized. This device is a modification of the standard nasal continuous positive airway pressure (CPAP) machine used to treat patients with obstructive sleep apnea. It can augment the patient's respiratory efforts by cycling to a higher applied inspiratory pressure (IPAP) from a set baseline expiratory pressure (EPAP) in response to the patient's efforts or, in some machines, at a set backup rate. The difference between the inspiratory and expiratory applied pressures represents a "pressure boost" analogous to that during PSV. Noninvasive ventilation requires skilled clinicians who can achieve a mask fit that causes neither skin injury nor excessive leaks. The ventilator must be carefully adjusted to patient tolerance yet achieve adequate ventilation. Monitoring of the patient is more difficult, as the BiPAP machine does not have alarms and tidal volumes and minute ventilation cannot be measured.

Initial Ventilator Settings and Monitoring for Complications

Using the above terminology, the clinician can systematically approach ventilator orders. The sequence of decisions with suggested initial settings are listed in Table 1. Volume/flow-controlled ventilation is used in most adult patients. An exception may be patients with severe ARDS in whom pressure-controlled ventilation may be both safer and better tolerated. When initiating mechanical ventilation, one usually selects the ACV mode to provide nearly full support. The tidal volume and machine respiratory rate establish the minimum minute ventilation. Standard settings for tidal volume are in the range of 8–12 mL/kg but may need to be set lower and, in any case, do not exceed one liter so that applied pressures are not excessive. The respiratory rate depends on the patient's minute ventilation requirement. Once the patient has stabilized, the backup rate should be set to provide 80% of the patient's observed minute ventilation in the event that the patient's central respiratory drive or ventilatory muscles fail. As the patient's condition changes, this backup rate will need to be adjusted.

The positive end-expiratory pressure (PEEP) represents the minimum airway pressure applied throughout the respiratory cycle. Levels of 5 cmH_2O are usually set to limit the development of atelectasis, particularly in patients receiving small tidal volumes (less than 10 mL/kg). In patients with pulmonary edema, higher levels of PEEP are used to recruit alveoli, prevent alveolar collapse, and improve oxygenation. PEEP and the fraction of inspired oxygen (FI_{O_2}) are the two settings that have the most effect on oxygenation.

Table 1 Typical Ventilator Settings for Full Support

From of ventilation	Flow/volume controlled
	(Pressure control in some patients with ARDS)
Mode of ventilation	
Initial	Assist control (ACV)
Evaluation for extubation	Intermittent mandatory ventilation (IMV)
("weaning")	Pressure-support ventilation (PSV)
	Intermittent T-piece, or low-level PSV
Tidal volume	8–12 mL/kg
	(May be smaller in patients with ARDS or severe airflow obstruction)
Respiratory rate	
Initial	12–20 breaths per minute
Maintenance	Backup rate to provide 80% of minute ventilation
Fraction of inspired oxygen (FI_{O_2})	
Initial	0.60 to 1.0
Maintenance	Adjusted to lowest FI_{O_2} that maintains oxygen saturation > 92–95% (lower in special circumstances)
Positive end-expiratory pressure (PEEP)	
Initial	5 cmH_2O
Maintenance	Increased in steps up to 18–20 cmH_2O to improve oxygenation if FI_{O_2} requirement greater than 0.60
Flow rate and pattern	Flow rate adjusted to patient comfort.
	Decelerating flow is often the best match to the patient and may improve gas exchange

In those patients making inspiratory efforts, the pattern of flow and the inspiratory flow rate are adjusted to match the patient's own inspiratory flow demand so as to limit the risk of flow dyssynchrony described above.

Once the patient is on ventilatory support, the clinician must monitor airway pressures, corresponding volume and minute ventilation changes, and indices of gas exchange. The current ventilator settings, total respiratory rate, airway pressures, delivered tidal volume, and minute ventilation are displayed on most ventilators and should be reviewed in sequence. Common measurements of gas exchange include intermittent arterial blood gases and continuous oximetry. Some intensive care units are equipped to monitor exhaled CO_2 concentration (capnography) as an index of changes in Pa_{CO_2} and to identify specific abnormalities in ventilation. Newer ventilatory strategies use these measurements of pressure, volume, and gas exchange as targets or limits in an attempt to minimize the risk of mechanical ventilation while providing adequate oxygenation and ventilation to support organ function.

Peak airway pressure (PAP) is the maximal pressure measured at the airway opening during inspiration. During flow/volume-controlled ventilation, the profile of applied airway pressure is a function of the impedance of the respiratory system and the inspiratory flow rate and pattern selected (Fig. 1). For a set tidal volume and flow pattern, peak airway pressures will rise with an increase in airway resistance, a decrease in respiratory system compliance, or with the development of dynamic hyperinflation (air trapping). The incidence of barotrauma is reported to be 40% when peak airway pressure exceeds 70 cmH_2O, though it is uncertain whether increases in peak airway pressure directly contribute to barotrauma or indirectly reflect the presence of alveolar overdistention. In patients with severe airflow obstruction, for example, much of the applied airway pressure is dissipated across the airways before reaching the alveoli. High peak airway pressure appears to be better tolerated by these patients than by others.

An estimate of the average *peak alveolar pressure*—called the *plateau pressure*— is obtained by measuring airway pressure after an end-inspiratory hold or pause of at least 0.5 s. This pressure reflects the degree of lung inflation at the end of inspiration—a quantity that is difficult to estimate by other means (Fig. 1). Alveolar overinflation is considered an important factor in the development of lung injury. High plateau pressures indicate alveolar overinflation unless there is an increase in pleural pressure from increased chest wall stiffness, large pleural effusions, or abdominal distention. There is an emerging consensus that peak alveolar pressures exceeding 30–35 cmH_2O may increase the risk of lung injury. Newer ventilator strategies in ARDS patients maintain plateau pressures below these levels, even though this may result in hypercapnia (discussed below).

Dynamic hyperinflation occurs primarily in patients with airflow limitation when there is insufficient time for the lung to deflate to its resting equilibrium volume. In the passively ventilated patient, the magnitude of auto-PEEP—defined as the difference between the alveolar pressure and the airway pressure at end-expiration—estimates the degree of dynamic hyperinflation (Fig. 2). The most common method of measuring auto-PEEP is to perform an end-expiratory port occlusion that allows the ventilator manometer to estimate auto-PEEP once pressures within the circuit and the respiratory system equilibrate (Fig. 4). In the passively ventilated patient, dynamic hyperinflation and auto-PEEP increase pulmonary vascular resistance and right ventricular afterload and decrease venous return (preload). These effects can cause significant hypotension that clinicians may misinterpret as evidence of cardiogenic shock or tension pneumothoraces unless the presence

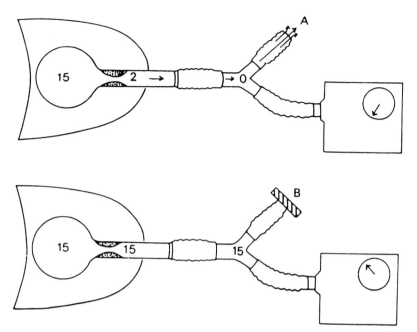

Figure 4 Schematic diagram illustrating auto-PEEP and one method—end-expiratory port occlusion—of its measurement. Because there is inadequate time to allow the lung to deflate to its resting equilibrium volume, alveolar pressure remains positive at the end of expiration (15 cmH$_2$O) and flow continues. The ventilator manometer approximates auto-PEEP only when pressures equilibrate following occlusion of the expiratory port at end-exhalation (lower panel). (From Pepe PE, Marini JJ. Occult positive end-expiratory pressure in mechanically ventilated patients with airflow obstruction: the auto-PEEP effect. Am Rev Respir Dis 1982; 126:166–170, with permission.)

of auto-PEEP is identified. In this situation, the clinician must reduce the respiratory rate or tidal volume in addition to treating bronchospasm and improving secretion clearance.

VENTILATOR SETTINGS IN SPECIFIC CLINICAL SETTINGS

Central Nervous System and Neuromuscular Disorders

There are a variety of acute and chronic disorders that impair the function of the "ventilatory pump"—that part of the respiratory system responsible for gas movement into the lungs. Respiratory failure can occur if there is impairment of the thoracic cage, the muscles that act as pressure generators and the nerves that innervate them, or the centers in the central nervous system (CNS) that coordinate respiration. In addition, the lung parenchyma may be secondarily injured by aspiration of gastric contents or by atelectasis and pneumonia from ineffective cough and secretion clearance.

Patients with respiratory failure or unconsciousness from acute reversible disorders of the CNS (e.g., drug overdosage) are usually supported with assist/control ventilation and intubation so that control of the airway is attained, secretions can be suctioned, and minute ventilation is assured. Exacerbations of certain neuromuscular disorders (e.g., myasthenia gravis), or prolonged support of patients with chronic respiratory muscle impairment (e.g., muscular dystrophy) can often be managed with noninvasive ventilatory support using BiPAP or conventional ventilators with nasal or face masks. Exceptions to this are patients with Guillain-Barré syndrome who require ventilatory support. These patients often have autonomic instability and are at risk for arrhythmias or hypotension during manipulation of the airway. They should be electively intubated by a skilled operator when indices of muscle strength suggest impending respiratory failure.

The ventilator settings in patients with CNS or neuromuscular disorders are straightforward as long as there is no significant atelectasis, aspiration, or other parenchymal lung disease. The usual mode is ACV with flow/volume-control ventilation using standard tidal volumes. The flow rate is then adjusted to patient comfort. The backup respiratory rate is set to maintain an adequate minute ventilation as assessed by periodic arterial blood-gas measurements. PEEP is applied at a level of 3–5 cmH$_2$O to combat progressive atelectasis. The most challenging aspect in ventilator management is establishing when these patients can resume spontaneous, unsupported respiration (discussed below).

Cardiogenic Pulmonary Edema

There are physiological benefits of prompt ventilatory support for patients with cardiogenic edema who fail initial medical therapy. First, up to 60% of total oxygen requirement of patients with acute cardiorespiratory failure may be consumed by the respiratory muscles. Mechanical ventilation can reduce diaphragmatic activity to as little as 10% of that during spontaneous respiration, allowing diversion of the limited cardiac output in patients with ventricular dysfunction to other organs. Second, positive-pressure ventilation and the subsequent increase in intrathoracic pressure can improve hemodynamics by decreasing systemic venous return (preload) and by effectively decreasing left ventricular afterload. Afterload falls because the positive intrathoracic pressure is transmitted to the outside wall of the myocardium, decreasing the transmural pressure difference and thereby reducing the myocardial muscle tension required to maintain a constant stroke volume. CPAP alone benefits patients with cardiac failure by these hemodynamic mechanisms, even though CPAP does not provide any ventilatory support.

Initial ventilator settings are usually an assist/control mode with flow/volume-controlled ventilation that performs much or all of the work necessary to maintain an adequate minute ventilation. PEEP should be set at a minimum of 5 cmH$_2$O and can be gradually increased if the F$_{IO_2}$ requirement is greater than 0.60. While many of these patients rapidly improve with diuresis, treatment of ischemia, and afterload reduction, one needs to remember the beneficial hemodynamic effects of ventilatory support when the patient is evaluated for extubation. Though seemingly comfortable while on mechanical ventilation, these patients can decompensate when challenged again with a trial of spontaneous ventilation. Careful appraisal of the patient's fluid status, evaluation for ischemia, and review of the patient's cardiac medications should precede any attempt to discontinue mechanical ventilation.

Noncardiogenic Pulmonary Edema

Patients with ARDS secondary to sepsis, aspiration, pneumonia, or other medical conditions often have a much different course than those with cardiogenic pulmonary edema.

The underlying pathophysiology—disruption of the alveolar capillary membrane—will progress until the primary medical problem is identified and controlled. Even then, severe gas-exchange abnormalities persist unless the lung is able to repair itself, requiring a prolonged period of ventilatory support.

Patients early in the course of ARDS have a relatively small aerated lung volume—only one-third to one-half of the lung tissue participates in gas exchange; the rest of the alveoli are collapsed, filled with fluid, or severely damaged. If one attempts to deliver a standard tidal volume based on the patient's size into these "small" lungs, the remaining normal alveoli will be overdistended and disrupted, extending the initial injury. For this reason, plateau pressures—an indication of peak alveolar distention—should be maintained below 30–35 cmH$_2$O. On the other hand, PEEP levels of 5–20 cmH$_2$O must often be applied to recruit alveoli, improve oxygenation, and prevent the collapse of unstable alveoli at end-expiration. To stay within these pressure limits, small tidal volumes (5–8 mL/kg) or pressure-controlled ventilation with peak pressures less than 30 cmH$_2$O are used even if the Pa$_{CO_2}$ gradually rises and respiratory acidosis develops—a strategy termed *permissive hypercapnia*. Patients in some studies had pH levels of 7.2 and some had Pa$_{CO_2}$ levels above 100 mmHg. Initial reports suggest that this lung-protective approach is associated with improved outcome, though the safe limits of acidosis and hypercapnia have not been established.

Chronic Obstructive Pulmonary Disease and Asthma

Respiratory failure in patients with airflow obstruction occurs because the respiratory muscles are unable to maintain an adequate minute ventilation against the increased resistive load. The indications for initiating ventilatory support include respiratory arrest, altered mental status, or a pH less than 7.15. However, several published reports suggest that many patients with severe asthma and respiratory acidosis respond to aggressive medical management and close observation without mechanical ventilation. Patients with exacerbations of chronic obstructive pulmonary disease (COPD) and impending respiratory failure may improve with noninvasive ventilatory support, avoiding the need for intubation.

In those patients who are intubated, expiratory flow rates may be too low to allow the lung to deflate to its resting equilibrium volume before the next ventilator cycle (dynamic hyperinflation or auto-PEEP as outlined above). Since high levels of minute ventiation will increase the risk of dynamic hyperinflation, it may be hazardous to completely correct the respiratory acidosis of many patients with COPD or asthma. Instead, it may be necessary to tolerate some degree of hypercapnia and respiratory acidosis in patients with severe airflow obstruction, similar to the strategy used in patients with ARDS.

Recent ventilator strategies that reduce minute ventilation to avoid dynamic hyperinflation have had a much lower incidence of complications. Initial ventilator settings use relatively small tidal volumes (6–10 mL/kg), with low respiratory rates depending on both the measured auto-PEEP and plateau pressures. Controlling the respiratory rate and minute ventilation may require significant sedation, particularly in patients with asthma. Brief infusions of neuromuscular blocking agents are sometimes necessary but should be limited as these drugs in combination with steroids have been associated with an acute myopathy. Pressure-control ventilation is avoided, as rapid changes in airway resistance will lead to large changes in delivered tidal volume.

EVALUATING FOR DISCONTINUATION
OF VENTILATORY SUPPORT

Assessment of Medical Stability and Appropriateness

The vast majority of patients on ventilatory support can resume spontaneous ventilation once their underlying illness resolves or improves. In these patients, the precise method of withdrawing ventilator support is not critical and does not determine success or failure. Instead, the clinician's primary task is to assess whether the timing of extubation is appropriate.

A checklist reviewed on a daily basis can help identify problems that require further evaluation (Table 2). Is the patient medically stable both from the inciting illness and from any intervening complications—infections, electrolyte imbalance, arrhythmias, or other problems? Is the patient alert enough to protect his or her airway and participate in pulmonary toilet? Does the patient have a cough effective enough to clear secretions, and are the secretions neither copious nor tenacious? The latter assessment requires input from the nursing and respiratory care staff who actually do the suctioning. Is the patient able to be oxygenated on an FI_{O_2} that can be delivered by face mask (conservatively, an FI_{O_2} less than or equal to 0.40)? Finally, does the patient have the central drive and muscle endurance to sustain an adequate minute ventilation against the load on the respiratory muscles? The patient should meet all of these criteria before being extubated. Some patients intubated for acute CNS disorders (seizures, drug overdosages) may be extubated rapidly following review of this checklist and a brief bedside trial of spontaneous ventilation.

Evaluating the patient's ventilatory ability is often the most difficult part of the

Table 2 Evaluating for Discontinuation of Ventilatory Support

Is the patient medically stable?	Initial illness improving
	Acute infections resolved or improving
	Electrolytes normal; acid-base balance stable
	No serious arrhthymias or other complications
Is the patient's level of consciousness adequate?	Can protect airway
	Able to participate in pulmonary toilet
Can the patient clear secretions?	Patient has an effective cough
	Secretion neither copious or tenacious
Can the patient be oxygenated once extubated?	Adequate Pa_{O_2} on an FI_{O_2} equal to or less than 0.40
Can the patient sustain an adequate spontaneous minute ventilation?	Minute ventilation requirement not high–Less than 10–15L
	Respiratory system load (elastic and resistive forces) not excessive
	Respiratory muscle strength adequate Vital capacity greater than 10 mL/kg Negative inspiratory force (NIF) greater than 20 cmH$_2$O
	Respiratory muscle endurance adequate f/Vt ratio less than 100 Tolerates trial of spontaneous ventiltation for 1 h

assessment. Several of the "weaning parameters"—negative inspiratory force, vital capacity, spontaneous tidal volume—measure respiratory muscle strength, not endurance. Based on the observation that patients with impending respiratory failure often have rapid shallow breathing, an index reflecting this pattern of breathing—the ratio of respiratory frequency in breaths per minute to tidal volume in liters (f/Vt ratio)—has been evaluated as a predictor of weaning success. In some studies, a f/Vt ratio of less than 100 proved to be quite accurate in predicting successful extubation provided that the patients were otherwise stable, and an f/Vt ratio greater than 100 predicted failure. For example, a patient observed during a brief trial of spontaneous ventilation to have a respiratory rate of 30 breaths per minute with tidal volumes less than 300 mL would not be expected to tolerate extubation. In most patients, however, a 1- to 2-h trial of spontaneous ventilation accompanied by clinical assessment and a satisfactory arterial blood-gas analysis remains the best indication of ventilatory capability in patients with cardiorespiratory or neuromuscular disorders.

Prolonged Ventilator Dependence

Approximately 10% of patients placed on mechanical ventilation require prolonged ventilatory assistance. A number of factors contribute to ventilator dependence, including hemodynamic instability, persistent lung disease, psychological dependency, malnutrition, and unresolved medical problems. Many times there is an imbalance between the patient's ventilatory capability and the demand imposed by both the minute ventilation requirement and the elastic and resistive load on the respiratory muscles. Malnutrition, corticosteroids, and metabolic abnormalities contribute to muscle weakness and limited endurance. Minute ventilation requirements will be higher if there is elevated CO_2 production secondary to fever, metabolic acidosis, excessive caloric intake, or increased dead-space ventilation from lung disease. Lung diseases also decrease lung compliance and increase airway resistance. All of these potential factors must be sought for and corrected, if present, before any mode of ventilatory withdrawal is likely to be successful.

If patients have been on ventilatory support for an extended period of time, they may not tolerate an abrupt conversion to spontaneous ventilation. Instead, ventilatory support may need to be withdrawn gradually. The clinician can use SIMV with a gradual decrease in the backup rate, PSV with decreasing pressure-support levels, or low-level PSV ventilation (nearly equivalent to T-piece trials) for increasing time intervals. Controlled trials comparing different weaning techniques have been inconclusive, and individual patients may do better with one mode than with another. Gradual withdrawal of support should be done in the daytime, with rest on full-support modes at night. Once the patient is tolerating spontaneous ventilation throughout the day, withdrawal of nocturnal ventilation often proceeds relatively quickly.

LONG-TERM VENTILATION

Despite all efforts, there will be patients who remain dependent on ventilatory support either continuously or for portions of the day and yet are otherwise able to leave the hospital. Increasingly, these ventilator-assisted individuals (VAIs) are discharged either to home or to an extended-care facility with long-term ventilatory support. It is estimated that the number of VAIs in the United States currently exceeds 10,000 patients. Both the number of VAIs and the conditions treated with prolonged ventilatory support are increasing. The availability of resources required for long-term ventilatory support has gone hand in hand with increased physician utilization. It is likely that many primary care physicians will assist in the care of these patients.

The underlying diseases can be classified into four diagnostic groups: (1) ventilatory muscle disorders, (2) central hypoventilation syndromes, (3) restrictive lung disease, and (4) obstructive lung diseases. The most prevalent underlying diseases are poliomyelitis, cervical trauma, amyotrophic lateral sclerosis, COPD, and muscular dystrophy. Some of these patients, usually with a history of poliomyelitis, have been on ventilatory support for over 20 years.

For those patients with ventilatory muscle disorders, adequate ventilation is relatively easy to attain. Some patients may tolerate periods of spontaneous ventilation and then rest for a portion of the day (up to 12 h) on noninvasive ventilatory support such as BiPAP. Ventilator settings are more challenging in patients with significant parenchymal lung disease, but home ventilators are increasing in their sophistication. Ventilator settings and airway management should be reviewed periodically by the pulmonary consultant. The clinician should be aware of the complications related to the patient's tracheostomy, and have access to an ear, nose, and throat physician. Plastic-cuffed tracheostomy tubes should be changed by a trained nurse or respiratory care practitioner every 2 to 3 weeks, and the stoma inspected for tissue erosions or cellulitis. Metal tracheostomies need to be cleaned regularly. Significant air leaks may herald the development of tracheal injury and dilatation, and increasing secretions or abdominal distention may signal the development of a tracheal esophageal fistula. These patients are at an increased risk of lower respiratory tract infections, which may precipitate worsening of their respiratory status and require urgent hospitalization.

There are both personal and financial advantages for most VAIs to return home, if possible. However, they require a great deal of time and support from family, friends, the home equipment provider, and available social services. Prior to discharge, there must be careful training and coordination of care. The care providers in the home, whether family or a trained personal care attendant, should be observed performing care tasks in the hospital or long-term-care facility before discharge. With good care, we have seen some of these patients at home or in long-term-care facilities gradually improve to the point that they no longer require ventilatory assistance.

SUGGESTED READING

1. ACCP Consensus Conference on Mechanical Ventilation. Chest 1993; 104:1833–1859.
2. Amato M, Barbas C, Medeiros D, Schettino G, Filho G, Kairalla R, Deheinzelin D, Morais C, Fernandes E, Takagaki T, DeCarvalho C. Beneficial effects of the ''open lung approach'' with low distending pressures in acute respiratory distress syndrome. Am J Respir Crit Care Med 1995; 152:1835–1846.
3. Chatburn R. A new system for understanding mechanical ventilators. Respir Care 1991; 36: 1123–1155.
4. Corbridge T, Hall J. The assessment and management of adults with status asthmaticus. Am J Respir Crit Care Med 1995; 151:1296–1316.
5. Leatherman JW. Mechanical ventilation in obstructive lung disease. Clin Chest Med 1996; 17: 577–590.

6. Make B, Gilmartin M. Care of ventilator-assisted individuals in the home and alternative sites. In: Burton G, Hodgkin J, Ward J, eds. Respiratory Care. Philadelphia: Lippincott, 1991:669–690.
7. Marcy T, Marini J. Respiratory distress in the ventilated patient. Clin Chest Med 1994; 15(1): 55–73.
8. Meduri GU. Noninvasive positive pressure ventilation in patients with acute respiratory failure. Clin Chest Med 1996; 17:513–554.
9. Rasanen J, Nikki P, Heikkila J. Acute myocardial infarction complicated by respiratory failure: the effects of mechanical ventilation. Chest 1984; 85:21–28.

26
Asthma

William J. Calhoun
University of Pittsburgh
Pittsburgh, Pennsylvania

INTRODUCTION

Asthma is associated with increasing prevalence, costs, and mortality. However, it is a disease that largely can and should be cared for in the primary care setting. Because most asthmatic patients can be very well controlled with current therapy, it is gratifying for both the treating physician and the patient to witness the improvements in symptom frequency, pulmonary function, and quality of life that can be achieved with proper asthma management. The objective of this chapter is to convey concepts and information to facilitate optimal care of asthmatic patients in the primary care setting.

The understanding of asthma has fundamentally changed in the past two decades. Asthma had previously been considered to be a disorder of airway hyperresponsiveness (''twitchy airways'') and variable airway obstruction. With this (mis)understanding of pathogenesis, treatment strategies were logically focused on bronchodilator agents that both treated the airway obstruction and, via functional antagonism, served to reduce airway hyperresponsiveness. Current definitions and understandings of asthma now include airway inflammation as a *central* characteristic, which implies that anti-inflammatory therapies should have a *central* role in treatment. Thus, airway hyperresponsiveness and airflow obstruction are consequences of the primary abnormality, airway inflammation, and it is the primary abnormality that is the target of therapy. Detailed review of the pathogenesis of asthma is not an aim of this chapter. Additional information about this point can be obtained through the list of suggested readings.

GOALS OF ASTHMA MANAGEMENT

The goals of asthma management outlined in Table 1 are condensed and consolidated from the National Heart, Lung, and Blood Institute (NHLBI) Expert Panel Report II (EPR II). Patients see physicians because of symptoms, and it is symptoms that most adversely affect quality of life. Achieving and maintaining control of asthma symptoms must therefore be a primary goal. Another important goal is to normalize measures of pulmonary

429

Table 1 Goals of Asthma Management

Prevent chronic symptoms of asthma
Maintain normal or nearly normal pulmonary function
  and prevent progressive loss of function over time
Maintain normal levels of activity and exercise
Prevent exacerbations, hospitalization, and emergency
  department visits
Minimize adverse effects of pharmacotherapy
Meet expectations of patients and their families

Source: Adapted from National Heart, Lung, and Blood Institute Expert Panel Report II.

function. Patients with asthma may perceive their existing airflow limitation poorly and thus underestimate the severity of their asthma. In asthmatic patients, symptoms and "objective" measures of pulmonary function do not always correlate well. The lack of correlation does not necessarily imply that symptoms and physiology are unrelated to asthma control. Rather, it is likely that symptoms and pulmonary function measures provide complementary information, all of which is important to the clinician—and to the patient—in assessing the level of asthma control. To rely on symptoms alone, an insensitive index of airway obstruction, could lead to undertreatment of asthma.

Minimizing morbidity and mortality depends on reducing or eliminating asthma exacerbations, because virtually all mortality and most morbidity are related to exacerbation. As amplified below, there are concrete steps that can provide early identification and treatment of asthma exacerbations. Minimizing the costs of asthma care should always be subjugated to optimal management, even in managed care settings. Clearly, the majority of asthma costs are associated with exacerbations requiring emergency department visits or inpatient hospitalizations. Costs of maintenance medications, even with complex controller regimens, are always small in comparison with those of even a single inpatient hospitalization. Thus, regardless of the payer situation, the focus should remain on optimizing the care of asthmatic patients.

Finally, it is important to minimize progressive loss of pulmonary function. Clearly, some patients with long-standing asthma, despite no significant history of tobacco abuse, develop fixed airway obstruction. Whether or not this loss of lung function can be prevented with current anti-inflammatory therapy has not been shown unequivocally. One report demonstrates that early institution of inhaled steroid therapy prevents the loss of pulmonary function that occurs in untreated patients. Whether or not this beneficial effect is present in the long term (years to decades) is not known. Nonetheless, it is reasonable to presume, by analogy with inflammatory interstitial lung disease, that control of airway inflammation would at best control and ameliorate peribronchial fibrosis and at worst have no effect.

APPROACH TO ASTHMA DIAGNOSIS

The diagnosis of asthma is made in the setting of a compatible clinical history and physical findings, with confirming physiological testing. Thus, asthma diagnosis is conceptually a two-step process: (1) establish a presumptive diagnosis of asthma by careful history and physical examination and (2) confirm the diagnosis by demonstrating excessive bronchial responsiveness to either bronchodilator or bronchoconstrictor agents.

Common Presenting Symptoms and Signs

Symptoms and Complaints

A characteristic feature of most asthma is the episodic nature of symptoms. Patients may complain of shortness of breath, wheezing, cough, chest tightness, or a variety of other descriptive terms to convey the concept of difficult breathing. Dyspnea at rest, or dyspnea that is consistently provoked by activity and quickly relieved by rest, is atypical for asthma. Much can be learned by careful history taking as to the frequency, duration, and clock time of episodes. Nocturnal symptoms of wheezing, dyspnea, or cough are of particular concern because of the association between frequent nocturnal symptoms and asthma mortality. The timing of clusters of attacks can offer important insights in seasonal asthma (see "Allergic Asthma," below), from which, in connection with skin testing or other assessment of allergic sensitivities, helpful advice on allergen avoidance can be offered. Factors consistently associated with asthma exacerbation should be sought (e.g., workplace, pets, drugs, viral infections), as should situations in which asthma attacks are unusual (e.g., vacation, travel). The duration of symptoms, and response to any previous therapy (such as inhaled beta$_2$-agonists) are also important historical facets. (For a more detailed discussion about obtaining a pulmonary history, see Chap. 7).

Cough productive of sputum is atypical for uncomplicated asthma but may occur intermittently in the context of viral infections or allergen exposure, chronically with "postnasal drip," or in that overlap syndrome sometimes called *asthmatic bronchitis*. Dry or nonproductive cough, in contrast, is a common presenting symptom in asthma (see also Chap. 15).

Physical Findings

The physical examination should focus on the entire respiratory tract and on manifestations of allergic disease. Wheezing, if present, can be helpful but is neither specific for asthma nor particularly sensitive. That is, wheezing may be present in many disorders other than asthma, and asthma of mild or moderate severity can present with entirely normal chest findings. Forced expiratory maneuvers can be used to evoke wheezing, but it is important to distinguish adventitious sounds originating from the small airways (true wheezing) from those produced in the larynx. Examination of the nose to determine the presence of pale blue nasal mucosal discoloration (suggesting allergic disease), mucopurulent discharge (suggesting sinusitis), or polyps is an important aspect of the evaluation. In addition, signs of conjunctivitis can, in the appropriate clinical setting, be helpful in assessing the presence of allergic sensitivity.

Confirming Physiological Tests

Measures of Expiratory Flow

The best objective test of pulmonary function used to confirm the diagnosis of asthma is simple spirometry. Equipment used to assess pulmonary function should meet accepted standards of the American Thoracic Society (ATS) for accuracy and precision. If airway obstruction is present, follow-up testing 10–20 min after inhalation of two puffs of a beta$_2$ agonist is generally indicated. Criteria for a significant bronchodilator response vary somewhat by organization and authority. However, those of the ATS are typical and broadly employed. A significant bronchodilator response is seen if the FEV$_1$ improves by at least 12% (using the screening FEV$_1$ as the denominator, not the "percent predicted"), and the absolute change in FEV$_1$ is at least 200 mL.

Peak expiratory flow rate (PEFR) is a measure of pulmonary function used primarily for monitoring, not for initial diagnosis. From the PEFR record, the absolute values (in liters per minute), the percent of personal best, and the diurnal variation (percent of baseline) can be obtained.

Methacholine Bronchoprovocation

It is not uncommon for screening spirometry to be within the limits of normal, particularly with asthma of intermittent or mild persistent severity (see Table 2). In these cases, bronchoprovocation with methacholine can be helpful. Each pulmonary function laboratory will have its own standard protocol and normative data. The interpretation of the test is generally performed by a pulmonary specialist. A methacholine challenge test indicating bronchial hyperresponsiveness in the context of an appropriate history of episodic chest tightness, wheezing, or cough can be used as a confirming test for asthma.

Useful Supplementary Tests

Pulmonary Function Tests

Complete pulmonary function testing, including lung volumes, diffusion capacity for carbon monoxide, and arterial blood-gas analysis can help to characterize the physiological abnormalities in asthma. However, none of these tests would likely be of critical importance in intermittent or mild persistent asthma. Measurement of lung volumes (FRC, TLC, RV) may be useful in assessing air trapping in asthma. Measurements of diffusion capacity are most useful in differentiating emphysema (associated with low diffusion capacity) from chronic bronchitis and asthma (in which diffusion capacity is generally normal). Likewise, arterial blood-gas (ABG) analysis can provide useful differentiating information in chronic, stable obstructive diseases. Retention of carbon dioxide is distinctly unusual in uncomplicated asthma but may be evident in chronic bronchitis and in more severe emphysema. Analysis of ABGs can be helpful in the assessment of acute asthma presenting to the emergency department or other urgent care setting.

Assessments of Atopy

Allergies are a risk factor for developing asthma, and allergen exposure is a common trigger of asthma attacks. Allergen avoidance is an important part of the more general concept of trigger avoidance. In order to recommend rational allergen avoidance, it is necessary to understand which aeroallergens are important for the individual patient. This information can be obtained most simply and cost-effectively by prick-puncture skin testing. Intradermal skin testing is an alternative thought to be more sensitive, but it is more costly, minimally more risky, and somewhat less predictive. In those patients in whom skin testing cannot be performed because of pregnancy, concomitant medications, or other reasons, radioallergosorbent (RAST) testing can be conducted. RAST tests are minimally invasive (venipuncture), and confer no risk on the patient. However, RAST testing is often considerably more expensive than skin testing.

Measurement of total circulating IgE can be helpful in some circumstances. A nor-

Table 2 Classification of Asthma

	Intermittent, Mild Step 1	Persistent		
		Mild, Step 2	Moderate, Step 3	Severe, Step 4
Number of attacks and symptoms	≤2/week, brief exacerbations	>2/week; <once daily	Daily symptoms	Multiple daily or continual symptoms
Nocturnal symptoms	≤2/month	>2/month	>1/week	Several per week to nightly
Lung function	Normal PEFR between exacerbations, FEV_1 ≥ 80% predicted	FEV_1 ≥ 80% predicted	FEV_1 between 60% and 80% predicted	FEV_1 ≤ 60% predicted

Source: Consolidated and abstracted from the Expert Panel Report II.

mal level does not exclude significant atopy (at least as assessed by skin testing), but an elevated level might prompt a more vigorous search for allergic triggers, including specific allergy testing. Marked elevations of IgE are associated with allergic bronchopulmonary aspergillosis (ABPA), and serial measurements of IgE can be used to monitor response of ABPA to therapy.

Chest Radiography

A chest radiograph is most commonly normal in chronic stable asthma. Hyperlucency, suggesting hyperinflation, may be seen in patients with air trapping from peripheral airway obstruction. Most patients with intermittent or mild persistent asthma can probably be appropriately managed without routine chest radiography. Patients who present with asthma of more severe degree may benefit from a chest film to exclude structural lesions, infiltrates (suggesting infection, vasculitis, ABPA, or other disorders), or cardiac disease. A chest radiograph is not mandatory in the assessment of uncomplicated asthma exacerbations unless other clinical information (such as fever, purulent sputum production, leukocytosis, physical findings on lung ascultation), dictates a search for pneumonia, vasculitis, or other disorder associated with pulmonary infiltrates.

Differential Diagnosis

The differential diagnosis of asthma is fairly broad, including chronic bronchitis, emphysema, other obstructive airway diseases (see appropriate chapters in this text), laryngeal dysfunction, congestive heart failure, tracheal abnormality (congenital or acquired), tracheobronchial foreign body, and a variety of other conditions. Generally, a careful history, cardiopulmonary physical examination, and spirometry will serve to clarify the diagnosis, but complete pulmonary function testing, chest radiography, and occasionally direct fiberoptic visualization of the airway may be necessary. When the differential diagnosis is difficult or complex, consultation with an asthma specialist can be helpful.

Classifying Asthma Severity

Asthma can be classified as intermittent or persistent. Intermittent asthma is always mild, and persistent asthma can be further subdivided into mild, moderate, and severe varieties. The NHLBI Expert Panel Report II offers a framework for understanding asthma severity and its classification (Table 2). A number of clinical parameters may aid the clinician with this assessment; however, there may be some initial ambiguity in making the determination of severity. Although many patients will present with symptoms and pulmonary function testing which are consistent with a single level of severity, others may have daytime or nighttime symptoms suggesting one level of severity, and pulmonary functions consistent with another. When these discrepancies occur, it is generally best to treat at the higher severity level, and later reduce therapy as possible (see discussion of medications below). Figure 1 depicts an algorithm for defining asthma severity at an initial visit. Spirometry information should be integrated into the overall assessment of asthma severity.

Symptom Frequency and Duration

Intermittent and persistent asthma are primarily differentiated by symptom frequency: asthma symptoms that occur more than twice weekly indicate persistent asthma and conse-

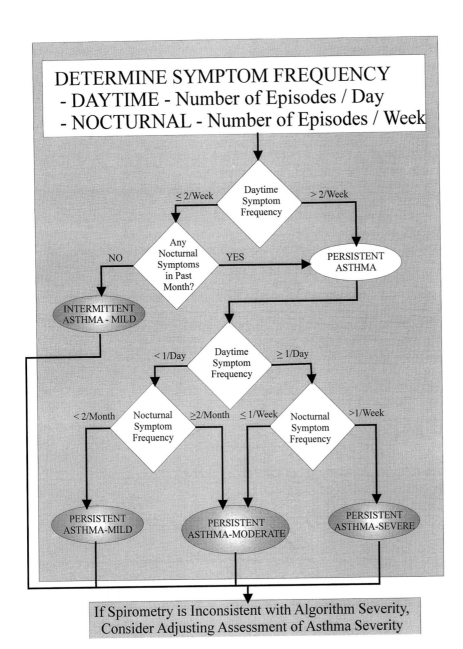

Figure 1 Asthma severity algorithm.

quent need for daily controller therapy. Symptom frequency twice weekly or less is consistent with intermittent asthma. Within persistent asthma, mild, moderate, and severe levels can be differentiated, to a first approximation, by symptom frequency of less than once daily (mild), daily (moderate), and more than once daily (severe). Symptom duration also parallels asthma severity. In intermittent asthma, exacerbation duration is typically short (2–24 h), whereas in moderate and severe asthma, exacerbations may last for days.

Presence or Absence of Nocturnal Symptoms

Nocturnal symptoms may occur as a consequence of well-described diurnal variation in pulmonary function. This variation is such that airway obstruction is maximal at 4 A.M. and minimal at 4 P.M. in patients acclimated to a typical daytime schedule. Some controversy exists regarding the precise mechanisms by which the diurnal variation occurs, but it is clear that the degree of variation in pulmonary function, nighttime to daytime, bears a direct relationship to asthma severity and is a marker for suboptimally controlled asthma. Nocturnal symptoms can occur nightly in patients with severe asthma and quite infrequently in patients with mild intermittent disease. A large study in England suggests that the frequency of nocturnal symptoms may be considerably greater than recognized, with weekly nocturnal asthma symptoms present in the majority of patients. Moderate asthma is generally associated with nocturnal symptoms at least once weekly. If nocturnal asthma symptoms are more frequent than expected on the basis of daytime symptom frequency, one may consider initiating anti-inflammatory therapy at a higher level (see Table 2).

Pulmonary Function

Pulmonary function testing via spirometry is another important index of asthma severity and should be obtained in every asthmatic patient. The Expert Panel Report II (EPR II) guidelines offer representative examples of pulmonary function in asthma of varying severity (see Table 2). If pulmonary function suggests asthma severity greater than that indicated by symptoms, one may consider treating for the more severe classification.

APPROACH TO ASTHMA MANAGEMENT

Understanding Asthma as Inflammatory Disease of the Airway

The 1997 NIH Expert Panel Report II states that "asthma, *whatever the severity*, is an inflammatory disease of the airways." Although it is not clear that airway inflammation causes airway hyperresponsiveness (AHR) (or if causal how inflammation might produce AHR), it is clear that these two central features of asthma are quite closely related. In fact, histological measures of inflammation do significantly correlate with methacholine AHR. Treatments that reduce inflammation, such as inhaled corticosteroids, also reduce AHR, although the magnitude of the change in AHR can be somewhat modest. The understanding of inflammation as central to asthma pathogenesis implies that appropriate asthma management will include therapies that mitigate airway inflammation.

Patient Education Issues

Proper Use of Devices

Virtually all asthmatic patients should use three devices for management and monitoring: (1) metered-dose inhaler(s) (MDIs), (2) a chamber or spacer for drug delivery, and (3) a peak flowmeter to monitor function. The first two are important for ensuring that medications are delivered with maximal efficacy and minimal adverse effects and the third is essential for monitoring efficacy of therapy, daily asthma control, and to provide objective warning of the onset of exacerbations. It is clear that without both initial and *ongoing* patient education efforts to develop and maintain skills in the use of MDIs, proper technique is rare.

Medications and Their Uses

Patients should understand the reasons why each of their medications were prescribed and should have reasonable expectations about their effects. For example, patients should understand that their short-acting beta$_2$ agonist will provide relief of symptoms but does not control the underlying process of inflammation in asthma. They should understand that their controller medications will not provide acute relief of symptoms and must be used daily. Thus, patients should have general expectations of their medications consistent with their pharmacological actions.

Recognizing and Responding to Exacerbations

Patients must have clear guidelines for determining whether an asthma exacerbation is developing. Increasing daytime symptom frequency, need for rescue beta$_2$ agonists, increasing or newly developing nocturnal symptoms, or a fall in PEFR of more than 20% from baseline are some signals that asthma control is failing. Peak flow measurements consistently less than 50% of personal best suggest a severe exacerbation that will require urgent medical intervention. It is helpful to determine, when possible, what factors might have been responsible for the exacerbation. For example, viral infections, bacterial sinusitis, exposure to allergens or irritants, and exercise are common triggers of asthma exacerbations. A plan of action for responding to asthma exacerbation should be provided to each patient. Depending on the severity of exacerbation, patients might be advised to call the physician, make an unscheduled office visit, or present to the emergency department.

Controller (Maintenance) and Reliever (Rescue) Therapies

Controller Therapies

Common controller therapies are listed in Table 3. A variety of controller agents are useful in achieving and maintaining relief of asthma symptoms and improving pulmonary function.

Table 3 Controller Therapies in Asthma

Inhaled corticosteroids
Oral corticosteroids
Salmeterol aerosol
Theophylline
Leukotriene blockers (zileuton, zafirlukast, montelukast)
Cromones (cromolyn, nedocromil)

Clearly the most effective single class of therapy in adult asthmatic patients is inhaled corticosteroids. These agents vary by potency and mass delivery. A comprehensive direct comparison of the available inhaled steroids using a panel of important outcomes (improvement in pulmonary function, reduction in exacerbation rate, control of asthma symptoms, pharmacological parameters, etc.) has not been made. However, several more limited comparisons have led to a consensus statement published in the EPR II. This information is summarized in Table 4. Inhaled corticosteroids have limitations, however, which include physical difficulty in coordinating use of an inhaler device, local side effects (such as dysphonia, oral candidiasis, and hoarseness), and, in pediatric populations, evidence of a quantitatively small reduction in the growth rate of the long bones. This observation must be balanced against the reduction in growth rate that may occur with poorly controlled asthma. At higher doses, inhaled steroids may be associated with measurable effects on the hypothalamic-pituitary-adrenal axis (of uncertain clinical significance) and on bone metabolism. Use of concomitant calcium and vitamin D supplementation, with or without replacement estrogen, may reduce or prevent the development of osteopenia. These effects on bone metabolism are most prominently observed at the high doses used to reduce dependence on oral steroids, and the magnitude of systemic effects from inhaled steroids is very small compared with the effects of chronic oral corticosteroids.

Chronic oral corticosteroids should be reserved for patients with severe persistent asthma. Many patients who appear to require oral steroids have one or more complicating factors. These patients should almost always be managed in conjunction with an asthma specialist. Conversely, short courses of oral corticosteroids have a critical role in managing acute exacerbations of asthma. The oral steroids may be given in a short burst of 7–10 days in doses of up to 1 mg/kg/day (either as a single dose or in two divided doses).

Leukotriene (LT) blocking agents (zafirlukast, montelukast, pranlukast, and zileuton) interfere with the generation or activity of a class of compounds, cysteinyl LTs, with demonstrable relevance to asthma and other allergic diseases. Each of these compounds has demonstrated efficacy in the management of mild persistent asthma. These data support the positioning suggested by the NHLBI Expert Panel and present LT blockers as an alternative to low-dose inhaled steroids. In addition, preliminary and published data suggest that leukotriene blockers can be used to achieve an added measure of symptom and physiological control in patients whose asthma is not completely controlled by the use

Table 4 Approximate Dose Equivalence of Inhaled Corticosteroids in Adults

Agent			Dose (puffs per day)		
Generic Name	Trade Name	Dose (µg/puff)	Low	Medium	High
Beclomethasone dipropionate	Beclovent	42	4–12	12–20	>20
	Vanceril	42	4–12	12–20	>20
	Vanceril DS	84	2–6	6–10	>10
Triamcinolone acetonide	Azmacort	100	4–10	10–20	>20
Flunisolide	Aerobid	250	2–4	4–8	>8
	Aerobid M	250			
Budesonide	Pulmicort	200	1–2	2–3	>3
Fluticasone propionate	Flovent 44	44	2–6	—	—
	Flovent 110	110	2	2–6	>6
	Flovent 220	220	—	1–2	>3

of inhaled corticosteroids. Both zileuton and zafirlukast block eosinophilic inflammation in human models of airway inflammation, but it has not yet been demonstrated in long-term studies that LT blockers suppress airway inflammation in asthma. Head-to-head comparisons of the LT blockers are not available; however, to a first approximation, the efficacy in asthma of these four agents appears to be equivalent. The lukasts (LT receptor antagonists) are generally free of significant adverse events. Zileuton (5-lipoxygenase inhibitor) has been linked to a quantitatively small ($\approx 5\%$) but statistically significant incidence of liver transaminase elevations; these do require monitoring. Additional clinical trials and clinical experience will be necessary to refine the proper positioning of LT blockers, both with respect to other members of the class and with respect to other asthma controller therapies.

The cromones (sodium cromoglygate, nedocromil) can be useful as mild anti-inflammatory agents, particularly in pediatric and adolescent patients. These compounds have an enviable record of safety. They may act by stabilizing mast cells and preventing mediator release or by an effect on chloride channels. Whatever the specific mechanism, they block both immediate and late-phase responses to allergen challenge. Clinical trials have shown efficacy in adult asthma patients, and there is laboratory evidence of an anti-inflammatory effect on allergic responses. These agents may be used as prophylaxis prior to exercise. However, not all patients respond well to cromones, and aside from the generally favorable response in pediatric patients, demographic and clinical predictors of response are unreliable.

Theophylline can be used to control asthma symptoms and has been used for decades for this purpose. Enthusiasm for theophylline has waned in recent years due to gastrointestinal, cardiovascular, and central nervous system adverse effects, and because the bronchodilation is modest compared with that achievable with inhaled beta$_2$ agonists. Further, there was little evidence of a disease-modifying or anti-inflammatory effect. However, there is now some evidence that theophylline may reduce infiltration of eosinophils and other inflammatory cells and that it reduces markers of inflammatory cell activation. Additional study will be required to answer definitively the question of whether or not theophylline has significant anti-inflammatory activity in asthma. A recent study demonstrated that addition of low-dose theophylline to inhaled steroids, sufficient to produce a serum theophylline concentration of about 9 µg/mL, produced better improvement in pulmonary function and nocturnal symptoms than did doubling the dose of inhaled steroids. Adverse effects can be minimized with acceptable efficacy by maintaining serum theophylline concentration between 5 and 10 µg/mL. Regardless of the mechanism of action, theophylline can be especially useful in the management of nocturnal asthma. Interactions with asthma medications and other agents used in asthmatic patients (e.g., macrolide antibiotics) can occur, and serum theophylline concentrations require monitoring. In particular, zileuton can increase serum theophylline levels by up to 100%.

Finally, long-acting bronchodilators have an important role in achieving and maintaining control of asthma symptoms and lung physiology in some patients. Although beta$_2$ agonist bronchodilation can be achieved with either a compound that has an intrinsically long half-life (salmeterol) or by sustained-release oral preparations (oral albuterol, sustained release), the tolerability of oral beta$_2$ agonist preparations is much less than that of inhaled salmeterol. Thus, inhaled salmeterol is the agent of choice for sustained beta agonist–dependent bronchodilation. Salmeterol can be added to an inhaled steroid or other anti-inflammatory regimen to improve pulmonary function and reduce asthma symptoms. Two well-controlled clinical trials have now confirmed that the addition of salmeterol to low-dose inhaled steroids provides better control of pulmonary function and symptoms than doubling the dose of inhaled steroids. With few exceptions, long-acting bronchodilators should be used in asthma only in conjunction with an effective anti-inflammatory agent and not as monotherapy. One such exception to this general rule may be the patient who requires consistent long-term (>8 h) exercise prophylaxis. Salmeterol can be useful in such situations.

An emerging theme in asthma therapy is that combination therapy may provide better control of asthma symptoms and physiology than high-dose monotherapy and do so with less adverse effects. Thus, addition of either theophylline or salmeterol to moderate doses of inhaled steroids appears to improve asthma symptoms and pulmonary physiology to a greater degree than doubling the dose of inhaled steroids. LT modifiers also appear to provide added asthma control beyond that achieved with inhaled steroids. However, the question of comparative efficacy of LT modifiers, theophylline, or salmeterol in the context of inhaled steroid therapy has not been definitively answered.

Reliever Therapies

There are two situations in which reliever (or "rescue") therapy may be needed: (1) relief of acute symptoms in patients with chronic stable asthma and (2) urgent or emergent care of asthma attacks. Short acting beta$_2$ agonists, delivered by the inhaled route, are drugs of choice in either situation. In the urgent or emergent setting, there are additional options. Table 5 summarizes useful rescue medications.

Beta$_2$-selective agonists should be delivered by the inhaled route to minimize systemic effects and maximize pulmonary delivery. The specific device used to achieve aerosol delivery is a choice ultimately best left to the physician. Some general guidelines can, however, be given. Delivery of drug by metered-dose inhalers (MDIs) or powder delivery systems is equivalent to that achieved by air-powered nebulizers *if the patient is able to use the MDI appropriately*. Thus, for most patients with chronic stable asthma, the MDI with a spacer or chamber device is most appropriate, as it is more convenient, portable, and considerably less costly. Patients who cannot appropriately use a standard MDI, owing to inability to coordinate inspiration with activation of the device, may be helped by a inspiration-activated delivery system. Some patients, however, are better treated with traditional jet (wet) nebulizers. Such patients may include those who have difficulty with breath-holding or coordination of inspiration and device activation. In emergency situations—in which dyspnea is severe, tachypnea is present, and breath-holding may be im-

---

Table 5 Reliever Therapies for Asthma

Short acting inhaled beta$_2$ agonists (quick onset)
  Albuterol, MDI, HFA MDI, rotahaler, or
    solution for nebulization
  Pibuterol autohaler
  Metaproterenol
  Bitolterol
  Terbutaline
Ipratropium bromide (longer onset)
  MDI or solution for nebulization
Systemic corticosteroids (delayed onset)

Key: MDI, metered-dose inhaler; HFA, hydrofluoroalkane propellant.

possible—delivery of a beta$_2$ agonist by jet nebulizer is probably preferable to dosing with an MDI.

The frequency of use of beta$_2$ agonists is an important index of asthma control. Rescue inhaler use greater than eight puffs (four doses) per day is a sign of suboptimal asthma control. In fact, a case can be made for intensifying anti-inflammatory therapy if rescue beta$_2$-agonist use is as much as four puffs (two doses) per day (see discussion of initial therapy, below).

Ipratropium bromide, delivered by MDI or aerosol, can be used to relieve bronchospasm mediated by excessive cholinergic activity. There are no studies that convincingly demonstrate the efficacy of ipratropium bromide in the long-term management of chronic asthma. However, it is the agent of choice for patients with asthma attacks precipitated by beta blockers, because beta blockers substantially diminish or entirely abrogate the bronchodilator response to inhaled beta$_2$ agonists. There is theoretical support for the use of ipratropium bromide in asthma exacerbated by viral infections, but convincing clinical trials are lacking.

In urgent or emergency settings, a systemic corticosteroid may be used as a reliever agent provided that aggressive inhaled bronchodilator therapy is also undertaken.

Selecting Initial Asthma Therapy

Determining Asthma Severity

On the basis of information gathered in the initial assessment, a judgment of presenting asthma severity can be made. Comparison of daytime and nighttime symptom frequency, symptom duration, and spirometric measures with EPR II guidelines for asthma severity (Table 2) will usually lead to an internally consistent assessment of asthma severity. An algorithm is illustrated in Fig. 1. From this initial determination of asthma severity, an appropriate management program and follow-up schedule can be developed.

Establishing Initial Therapy

The EPR II guidelines offer therapeutic flexibility to the prescribing physician. As noted above, patients with persistent asthma should receive controller therapy that mitigates airway inflammation. All patients with asthma should be provided with a short-acting inhaled beta$_2$ agonist for relief of symptoms. This approach is reflected in Table 6.

It is important to offer advice about avoiding asthma triggers at the initial visit or as soon thereafter as information on allergic sensitivity is available. Environmental tobacco smoke, indoor and outdoor pollutants, avocational and vocational irritants, and sensitizers are a few of the areas for counseling.

Monitoring Response to Therapy

Historical Information

The frequency of daytime and nocturnal asthma symptoms is an important measure of response to therapy. Most patients can be encouraged to record symptoms daily, for review by the physician. Alternatively, the patient's recall of symptom frequency may be used. Rescue beta$_2$ agonist use should be recorded, in addition to daytime and nighttime symptoms. This information should be compared with the frequency of symptoms and rescue inhaler use recorded during initial assessment.

In optimally controlled asthma, symptoms should not appear every day and noctur-

Table 6 Recommendations for the Management of Asthma in Adult Patients Based on Severity of Disease

Severity stage	Intermittent	Persistent		
	Mild	Mild	Moderate	Mild
	Controller Medications:			
1	None	Low-dose ICS or LT blocker or Cromone	Moderate-dose ICS	High-dose ICS
2	None	Add salmeterol or theophylline SR 400 mg qhs	Add salmeterol or theophylline SR 400 mg qhs	Add salmeterol or theophylline SR 400 mg qhs
3	None	N/A	Add LT blocker or Double ICS dose	Add LT blocker or Double ICS dose
4	None	N/A	Double ICS dose or Add LT blocker	Double ICS dose or Add LT blocker
5	None	N/A	N/A	Oral corticosteroids (e.g., prednisone 10–40 mg qd or qod)
	Reliever Medicines:			
	Selective β_2 agonist up to qid prm	Selective β_2 agonist up to qid prm	Selective β_2 agonist up to qid prm	Selective β_2 agonist up to qid prm

Key: ICS, inhaled corticosteroid; SR, sustained release; N/A, not applicable; LT, leukotriene; qid prm, 4 times daily, as needed.

[a] In pregnancy, the judgment of the physician with regard to the risk: benefit ratio of any specific therapy is a critical factor.

nal symptoms should be rare. Use of rescue beta₂ agonists should generally be less than twice daily. Certainly use of rescue medication of more than eight puffs per day, and perhaps more than four puffs per day, suggests incomplete control of airway inflammation.

Measures of Pulmonary Function

Due to differences among peak flowmeters of different design and manufacture, patients should use a single device for their serial measurements. Patients should measure and record their morning peak expiratory flow rate daily, shortly after arising. Implementation of effective anti-inflammatory therapy is usually associated with improvement in morning PEFR. Several pieces of information can be gleaned from the peak flow record. First, the absolute change in PEFR (attributable to therapy) can be determined by comparing the peak flow in the first day or so of therapy with that recorded at the follow up visit. Second, the variability in peak flow for a given week can be computed. Finally, the PEFR can be normalized to the patient's individual personal best PEFR as a percentage. According to the EPR II, good control is indicated by PEFR in the ''green zone'' of 80% of personal best PEFR or better. ''Yellow zone'' values from 50–80% of personal best suggest need for additional therapy. As noted elsewhere (in the discussion of patient education, above, and that of responding to exacerbations, below), PEFR measures consistently less than 50% of personal best indicate a severe exacerbation requiring prompt medical intervention.

At the second or third visit, repeat spirometry should be performed to assess the change in FEV_1 attributable to therapy. Similarly, spirometry should be repeated to assess physiological changes after any substantive changes in therapy (Fig. 2). Finally, as part of ongoing monitoring to detect progressive loss of lung function, it is reasonable to assess spirometry at 6- to 12-month intervals.

What if Initial Therapy Does Not Control All Symptoms? (''Step Up'')

Initial assessment will suggest a therapeutic regimen likely to improve asthma symptoms and airway physiology. Some patients will have incomplete resolution or suboptimal relief of symptoms and incomplete resolution of airway obstruction despite implementation of appropriate therapy. If aggravating factors and poor compliance can be excluded (see below, under ''Confounding Factors''), additional therapy may be considered. Many possibilities may be appropriate, but one strategy that can be used is the stage approach, shown in Fig. 2 and Table 6, which offers a rational sequence for added therapy. In general, therapy that combines inhaled corticosteroids with a long-acting bronchodilator may offer better control of symptoms and physiology than increased corticosteroid doses. LT blockers combined with inhaled steroids may provide added control over inhaled steroids alone, but the clinical trial evidence is less well developed than for salmeterol or theophylline (see discussion of controller and reliever therapies, above).

Does My Patient Need All These Medications? (''Step Down'')

In patients with acceptable control, it is reasonable to attempt to reduce therapy so as to use the minimum amount of controller agents. The key questions are defining what is ''acceptable control'' and determining the rate at which controller therapies can be withdrawn and in what order. No clinical trials have been conducted to answer these questions,

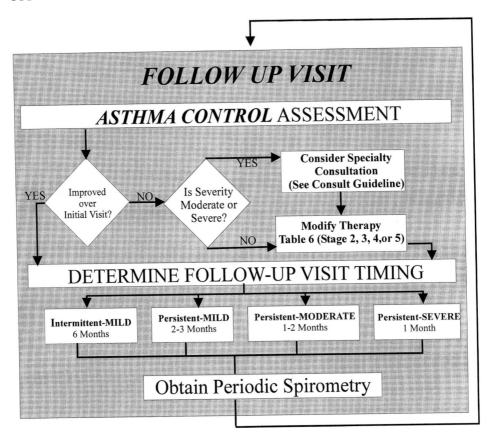

Figure 2   Asthma management algorithm.

so they remain a matter of clinical judgment. Most concepts of acceptable control would include the absence of interval exacerbations, the stability of peak flow measurements, infrequent nocturnal symptoms, and minimal daytime symptoms. Asthma is a variable disease; sufficient time should elapse between adjustments in therapy that it is clear that the asthma is actually stable and that there is not merely temporary downturn in activity. In general, "step-down" adjustments should be made no more frequently than every 2–4 months.

Recognition and Management of Asthma Exacerbations

Early recognition of asthma exacerbations is key to effective management. Exacerbations may be recognized by increasing frequency of daytime or nighttime symptoms, increasing need for rescue beta$_2$-agonists, declining PEFR, or a fall in FEV$_1$ by formal spirometry. The EPR II guidelines suggest that the severity of exacerbation can be assessed partly by comparing the measured PEFR during exacerbation to personal best PEFR. Mild exacerbations are associated with a PEFR of 80%, moderate exacerbations with a PEFR of 50–80%, and severe exacerbations with a PEFR below 50% of personal best. Management of exacerbations requires clinical judgement. The EPR II recommends increased frequency of beta$_2$-agonist use, and double-dose inhaled steroids for mild exacerbations in patients already on inhaled steroids. Patients with moderate or severe exacerbations will likely require oral corticosteroids as well as medical evaluation. Whatever treatments are instituted for the exacerbation should be continued until symptom frequency and PEFR return to baseline.

Confounding Factors in Asthma Management and Their Mitigation

If patients fail to respond to management, the possibility of confounding factors should be considered. Such factors would include triggers of asthma that were not recognized in the initial assessment, difficulty with adherence to the regimen, or unrecognized aggravating factors.

Unrecognized Trigger Factors

Careful historical information should be sought on the factors associated with asthma exacerbations, including triggers contacted in the occupational, avocational, or recreational setting. Environmental tobacco smoke, animal danders, house dust mite allergy, and chemical irritants and sensitizers encountered in the home, shop, or workplace should be sought.

Suboptimal Adherence to Regimen

The questions ''How are you taking your medications?'' and ''Are you having any problems with your medications?'' should be part of each visit. Active recall of medical regimen during history taking accomplishes several goals. First, the information may be more accurate than if the patient is simply asked to nod assent to a list of medications from the physician or nurse. Second, it reinforces the concept that the patient must be an active participant in the management of his or her own asthma. Finally, it opens lines of communication with the patient by acknowledging that all medications may have some side effects and that the physician is specifically interested in minimizing those adverse effects.

Aggravating Factors

When response to therapy is less than optimal, the presence of aggravating factors should be considered. Such factors include subclinical sinusitis, gastroesophageal reflux, aspirin sensitivity syndrome (rhinosinusitis, nasal polyposis, and asthma), uncontrolled rhinitis and postnasal drip, and unrecognized drug adverse effects (beta blockers, angiotensin-converting enzyme inhibitors, etc.), and recurrent viral infections. When such effects are present, aggressive therapy should be directed at the aggravating factor with the expectation that a beneficial effect on asthma control will be observed.

Indications for Specialty Consultation

Most asthmatic patients can be appropriately managed in the primary care setting. Many of those who will benefit from specialty consultation can continue to receive the bulk of their asthma care from a primary care provider, with periodic consultative visits with the asthma care specialist. Indications for subspecialty consultations are summarized in Table 7.

Table 7   Indications for Specialty Consultation in Asthma

Life-threatening asthma, including patients with one or
   more episodes of intubation and mechanical
   ventilation
Difficult differential diagnosis
Asthma complicated by significant chronic sinusitis,
   allergic bronchopulmonary aspergillosis,
   eosinophilic vasculitis, gastroesophageal reflux
Apparent requirement for oral steroid therapy
Severe persistent asthma
Need for specialty testing or procedure (allergy skin
   tests, allergy immunotherapy, methacholine
   challenge test, rhinoscopy or bronchoscopy, etc.)
Inadequate response to therapy after three office visits

Patients whose asthma is not well controlled (see discussions above of asthma therapy and monitoring) after two or three visits with the general internist, family physician, pediatrician, or other primary care provider may benefit from subspecialty expertise. Consultation may be sought from pulmonary specialists, allergists, or other physicians with special training and expertise in the management of asthma. Certainly patients with life-threatening asthma manifesting as the need for mechanical ventilation or intensive care unit management should be cared for in collaboration with an asthma specialist. Asthma patients whose disease is complicated by eosinophilic vasculitis, allergic bronchopulmonary aspergillosis, chronic sinusitis, unremitting rhinitis, or severe gastroesophageal reflux exemplify patients who may benefit from subspecialty comanagement.

SPECIFIC ASTHMA SYNDROMES

Allergic Asthma

The majority of asthmatic patients have a component of allergy. Mitigation of allergic exposure should be an integral part of the overall asthma management program. Allergic asthma is exacerbated by exposure to allergens. Thus, both seasonal and perennial patterns of symptoms may be encountered. If consistent seasonality is present, then avoidance of allergens present during those times is warranted. For example, a history of yearly asthma exacerbations in May–June could suggest that grass pollens might be a factor. Perennial symptoms do not exclude an allergic basis for asthma, because perennial allergens, such as pet danders or house dust mite antigen, can be associated with this pattern. Because of the prevalence of atopy among asthmatic patients, assessment of allergic sensitization by skin prick-puncture or RAST testing is indicated in patients with persistent asthma. Allergen exposure may produce two phases of bronchial obstruction. The immediate phase lasts up to an hour and is characterized by release of histamine, cysteinyl LTs, and mediator-induced bronchial obstruction. In more than half of all allergic asthmatics, a late-phase bronchial response may occur 4–8 h after exposure. This airway obstruction may be greater in magnitude than the immediate response. Late-phase responses are characterized by cellular infiltration and activation, production of larger quantities of cysteinyl LTs, and a reduced bronchodilator response to inhaled beta$_2$-agonists. Understanding the dual nature of allergic asthma has therapeutic implication: if the exacerbation is clearly related to allergen exposure, both the patient and physician should be aware that a late wave of airway obstruction requiring additional therapy may occur. Allergic asthma should be managed with allergen avoidance, control of trigger factors, and, in persistent disease, appropriate controller medications.

Nocturnal Asthma

The majority of patients with uncontrolled asthma will report nighttime symptoms. Pulmonary function is minimal about 4 A.M. in both asthmatic and normal individuals, but the magnitude of the variation is much greater in asthma. Lung inflammation also appears to vary in the same circadian cycle, with increased inflammation seen at 4 A.M. versus 4 P.M. Control of these nocturnal asthma episodes, and the underlying variable airway obstruction, is a principal goal of asthma management. Nocturnal asthma symptoms are a marker of uncontrolled disease and are associated with asthma morbidity and mortality. There remains controversy about whether nocturnal asthma is fundamentally a different disorder or a more severe end of the spectrum of asthma. Literature exists on both sides of that question. Nonetheless, nocturnal asthma symptoms are of sufficient clinical import that their presence and frequency should be sought at each visit. Management of nocturnal asthma generally requires anti-inflammatory controller therapies. Some patients may report excellent control of daytime symptoms but persistent flares at night. In these individuals, inhaled salmeterol or oral sustained-release theophylline may control the nocturnal breakthrough.

Virally Induced Asthma

Viral infections are associated with exacerbations of asthma. In adults, the rhinoviruses are most commonly implicated. In children, respiratory syncytial virus (RSV) is associated with exacerbations. RSV may alter the host's immune response so as to favor allergic sensitization. The mechanisms by which rhinoviruses produce asthma exacerbations is not fully understood. However, it appears that these viruses amplify allergic responses by increasing the quantity of mediators released during allergic reactions. In addition, other viruses may increase cholinergic neurotransmission through vagal ganglia, which may result in increased bronchial obstruction and secretion of mucus. For this reason, the use of anticholinergics such as ipratropium bromide during exacerbations due to viral infection makes theoretical sense; however, there are no convincing clinical trial data to support this use. Because specific therapy for these viral infections is not available and prevention is difficult, early recognition of viral infections should lead to more frequent PEFR monitoring and early implementation of increased anti-inflammatory therapy.

Exercise Asthma

Exercise is a frequent trigger of asthma exacerbations. Occasionally, the history is of exacerbation solely with exercise or cold air exposure, but more typically, exercise is only one of several clinically important triggers. Exacerbations due to exercise add to the weekly symptom count in determining asthma severity. Thus, exercise-induced asthma occurring three or more times weekly suggests that the patient has persistent asthma requiring controller therapy. With appropriate controller therapy, exercise may become a less potent trigger of bronchial obstruction.

Prophylaxis of exercise-induced asthma can be achieved with an beta$_2$ agonist or cromolyn delivered 15–30 min prior to exercise. If exercise prophylaxis is required for more than 4–5 h, inhaled salmeterol can provide protection for up to 12 h.

Cough Variant Asthma

Patients may present with symptoms of cough without wheezing, shortness of breath, or sputum production. The differential diagnosis for such cough is truly wide (see Chap. 15) but includes asthma, or bronchial hyperresponsiveness, as a frequent cause. Evaluation often includes methacholine challenge testing. This diagnosis is best made in collaboration with an asthma specialist.

Aspirin-Intolerant Asthma

Aspirin-intolerant asthma (AIA) is an unusual type of asthma from which a great deal has been learned about the pathogenesis of asthma. Patients with AIA historically present with rhinitis, sinusitis, nasal polyposis, and, finally, asthma, often moderate or severe. Ingestion of aspirin may result in life-threatening asthma, gastrointestinal symptoms, and frank anaphylaxis. These patients have excessive baseline production of cysteinyl leukotrienes, which is dramatically augmented following aspirin challenge. Leukotriene pathway inhibitors, such as zileuton or the lukasts (cysteinyl leukotriene receptor antagonists), block the development of both systemic symptoms and bronchial obstruction. Although it is reasonable to use leukotriene blockers in this clinical setting, it should be emphasized that patients with AIA should assiduously avoid aspirin and other nonsteroidal anti-inflammatory drugs, whether or not they are treated with a leukotriene blocker.

SUMMARY

Asthma is characterized by airway inflammation, airway hyperresponsiveness, and variable airflow obstruction. Airway hyperresponsiveness is closely associated with inflammation and is a key factor underlying variable airway obstruction. Diagnosis is based on history and compatible measurements of airway function. Spirometry should be used in medical diagnosis in preference to a peak flowmeter. Peak flowmeters, in contrast, are ideal for ongoing, long-term monitoring of airway function by the patient. For all but the mildest asthma, management plans should include medications that control the underlying inflammation. When an initial dose of anti-inflammatory medication fails to control symptoms adequately, combination therapy with several effective controllers may be better than increased doses of inhaled steroids. Long-acting bronchodilators (salmeterol and theophylline) and leukotriene antagonists can be effective controller agents in combination with inhaled steroids; for mild persistent asthma, a leukotriene blocker may suffice as monotherapy. Patient education should include careful and repeated instruction on the use of devices (peak flowmeter, metered-dose inhalers, and spacer/chambers), recognition and management of exacerbations and trigger factor avoidance. If acceptable asthma control is not established within two to three visits or if the patient has evidence of severe persistent asthma, consultation with an asthma specialist is advised.

SUGGESTED READING

General Asthma References

1. ATS Official Statement: Standards for the diagnosis and care of patients with chronic obstructive pulmonary disease and asthma. Am Rev Respir Dis 1987; 136:225–244.
2. Expert Panel Report 2: Guidelines for the Diagnosis and Management of Asthma. NIH Publication 97-4051. National Institutes of Health, Bethesda, Maryland, April 1997.
3. Goldstein RA, Paul WE, Metcalfe DD, Busse WW, Beece ER. NIH Conference: Asthma. Ann Intern Med 1994; 121:698–708.
4. Martin RJ, ed. Clinics in chest medicine. Asthma 1995; 16:557–744.
5. Weiss KB, Gergen PJ, Hodgson TA. An economic evaluation of asthma in the United States. N Engl J Med 1992; 326:862–866.

Inhaled Corticosteroids

1. Barnes PJ. Drug Therapy: inhaled glucocorticoids for asthma. N Engl J Med 1995; 332:868–875.
2. Johnson M. Pharmacodynamics and pharmacokinetics of inhaled glucocorticoids. J Allergy Clin Immunol 1996; 97:69–176.

Leukotriene Antagonists

1. Henderson WR. The role of leukotrienes in inflammation. Ann Intern Med 1994; 121:684–697.
2. Holgate ST, Bradding P, Sampson AP. Leukotriene antagonists and synthesis inhibitors: new directions in asthma therapy. J Allergy Clin Immunol 1996: 98:1–13.

Specific Asthma Syndromes

1. Calhoun WJ. Asthma: what next when your patient does not respond to therapy? Consultant 196; 36:1853–1858.
2. Corne JM, Holgate ST. Mechanisms of virus induced exacerbations of asthma. Thorax 1997; 52:380–389.
3. Israel E, Fischer R, Rosenberg MA, Lilly CM, Callery JC, Shapiro J, Cohn J, Rubin P, Drazen JM. The pivotal role of 5-lipoxygenase products in the reaction of aspirin-sensitive asthmatics to aspirin. Am Rev Respir Dis 1993; 148:1447–1451.
4. Martin RJ. Nocturnal asthma. Clin Chest Med 1992; 13:533–550.

27

Chronic Obstructive Pulmonary Disease and Emphysema

John W. Kreit and Robert M. Rogers

University of Pittsburgh
Pittsburgh, Pennsylvania

INTRODUCTION

Chronic obstructive pulmonary disease (COPD) is an extremely common disorder and a major cause of morbidity and mortality throughout the world. In the United States, COPD afflicts an estimated 14 million people and is the fourth most common cause of death. In 1994, the last year for which statistics are available, 101,628 Americans died from COPD. It is essential, then, that physicians have a clear understanding of how to both diagnose and treat this disease.

The relationship between chronic bronchitis, emphysema, COPD, and other forms of obstructive lung disease is illustrated in Fig. 1. According to the American Thoracic Society, COPD is characterized by the presence of chronic bronchitis or emphysema combined with airflow obstruction that is, at most, partially reversible. Chronic bronchitis is defined clinically by the presence of a productive cough for at least 3 months in each of 2 successive years, whereas emphysema is defined in anatomical terms as permanent airspace enlargement due to the destruction of alveolar walls. These diseases coexist in the majority of patients. Other disorders leading to airflow obstruction such as asthma, bronchiectasis, and obliterative bronchiolitis are excluded from the definition of COPD.

PATHOPHYSIOLOGY

In patients with COPD, airflow obstruction, defined as a reduction in the rate of expiratory flow, initiates a pathophysiological cascade that results in dyspnea, exercise limitation, and abnormal gas exchange.

Lung Mechanics

Airflow obstruction results from several different mechanisms. In emphysema, destruction of alveolar walls leads both to a reduction in lung elastic recoil and loss of the normal

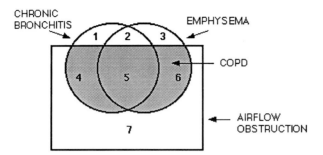

Figure 1 Classification of obstructive lung disease. This nonproportional Venn diagram shows that COPD is defined by the combination of airflow obstruction and chronic bronchitis (subset 4), emphysema (subset 6), or both (subset 5). In the absence of airflow obstruction, patients with either disease (subsets 1, 2, and 3) are not considered to have COPD. Other forms of obstructive lung disease (subset 7) are also excluded from the definition of COPD. (Modified from Ref. 2, with permission).

"tethering" effect by the pulmonary parenchyma on the small, noncartilaginous airways. These factors, in turn, produce expiratory slowing by decreasing alveolar driving pressure and allowing small airway collapse. In chronic bronchitis, airflow obstruction results primarily from intrinsic airway narrowing due to inflammation, edema, and excessive production of mucus. Regardless of its mechanism, airflow obstruction may lead to incomplete exhalation, which, coupled with loss of elastic recoil, produces an increase in lung volume, a process referred to as hyperinflation.

Respiratory Muscle Function

Hyperinflation causes the normally dome-shaped diaphragm to flatten, thereby reducing the zone of apposition with the lower ribs and interfering with its ability to expand the lungs and chest wall. In addition, in the setting of marked expiratory slowing, inspiratory effort may begin before the respiratory system returns to its equilibrium or resting volume. The respiratory muscles must, therefore, generate sufficient pressure to balance inward elastic recoil before inspiration can begin. The presence of this inspiratory "threshold load" coupled with decreased diaphragm efficiency may lead to chronic respiratory muscle fatigue.

Pulmonary Hemodynamics

Pulmonary hypertension is common and results from both local hypoxia and emphysema-induced destruction of the alveolar capillary bed. With time, increasing afterload may lead to right ventricular failure.

Gas Exchange

Airway narrowing and loss of alveolar capillaries lead to altered ventilation/perfusion ($\dot{V}/\dot{Q}$) relationships and abnormal gas exchange in patients with COPD. Lung regions with impaired ventilation relative to perfusion (low $\dot{V}/\dot{Q}$) contribute to arterial hypoxemia, whereas decreased perfusion to well-ventilated regions (high $\dot{V}/\dot{Q}$) increases physiological ''dead space'' and the minute ventilation required to maintain a normal arterial P_{CO_2}. Hypercapnia occurs when severe airflow obstruction prevents this compensatory rise in minute ventilation. Exercise-induced desaturation is common in patients with emphysema and results primarily from obliteration of the alveolar capillary bed.

Dyspnea and Exercise Limitation

In patients with COPD, dyspnea with activity, and ultimately at rest, results from alterations in lung mechanics, respiratory muscle function, pulmonary hemodynamics, and gas exchange. Airflow obstruction prevents a sufficient increase in expiratory flow (and minute ventilation) to accommodate increased ventilatory demands. In addition, increases in the respiratory rate and/or tidal volume place added strain on the respiratory muscles and may even result in worsening function by reducing expiratory time and increasing hyperinflation. Pulmonary hypertension and arterial hypoxemia may also contribute to dyspnea, and both may worsen significantly during exercise.

CLINICAL FEATURES

History

Patients with COPD typically have a long history of cigarette smoking. Although other factors such as passive smoke inhalation, occupational exposures, and alpha$_1$-antitrypsin deficiency may give rise to COPD, absence of a smoking history makes the diagnosis unlikely. Patients usually present after the age of 50 and complain of gradually progressive dyspnea, although a much more abrupt onset is occasionally described. The dyspnea has little variability and is usually worsened or precipitated only by exertion. Complaints of wheezing and chest tightness are usually not prominent. If previously treated, patients typically report little or no subjective improvement with inhaled bronchodilators or systemic corticosteroids. Cough is common, chronic, and usually productive of mucoid sputum. Cough and sputum production are most prominent in the morning but may occur throughout the day. Patients often report intermittent, acute exacerbations characterized by increased dyspnea, cough, and purulent sputum production.

Physical Examination

Airflow obstruction is demonstrated by the presence of a prolonged expiratory phase. Early in the course of COPD, this may be detected only with forced expiration but becomes evident even during tidal breathing in the advanced stages of the disease. Expiratory wheezes may be present but are usually not prominent. Coarse rales and rhonchi are common in patients with chronic bronchitis, especially during an acute exacerbation, and reflect the presence of secretions in the large airways. In patients with hyperinflation, hyperresonance to percussion and distant breath and heart sounds are common, and the anteroposterior (AP) diameter of the chest may be noticeably increased. Patients with severe disease may have cyanosis as well as signs of pulmonary hypertension and right ventricular failure, including a prominent pulmonic component of the second heart sound, jugular venous distention, hepatojugular reflux, and edema.

Chest Radiography and Computed Tomography

The chest radiograph is often normal in patients with mild COPD. With the development of hyperinflation, frontal and lateral views demonstrate an increased AP diameter, flattening of the hemidiaphragms, and increased size of the retrosternal space. In patients with complicating pulmonary hypertension and right ventricular failure, enlargement of the main pulmonary arteries and encroachment of the right ventricle on the retrosternal space is seen. The radiographic hallmarks of emphysema are hyperlucency of the lungs and the presence of bullae, radiolucent areas bordered by thin rims of lung parenchyma. Although usually evident in patients with severe emphysema, these findings are often absent in the setting of mild to moderate disease.

Computed tomography (CT), especially with high-resolution scanning, is a very sensitive technique for detecting a variety of disorders affecting the pulmonary parenchyma and small airways. In patients with emphysema, centrilobular or panlobular airspace enlargement is usually evident even in the presence of mild disease and a normal chest radiograph. Figure 2 illustrates the radiographic and CT findings in a patient with severe emphysema.

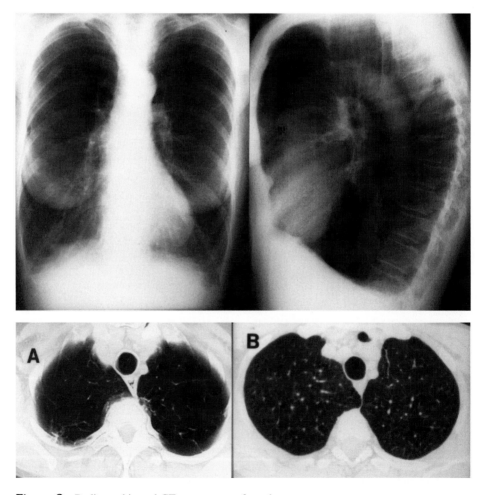

Figure 2   Radiographic and CT appearance of emphysema.

Pulmonary Function Measurements

By definition, spirometry demonstrates the presence of airflow obstruction. The forced expiratory volume at 1 s (FEV_1) is decreased out of proportion to any reduction in the forced vital capacity (FVC), producing a decrease in the ratio of these two volumes (FEV_1/ FVC). Although complete reversibility excludes the diagnosis, up to 20% of patients with COPD have at least a 15% improvement in FEV_1 or FVC following bronchodilator administration. Lung volume measurements are usually normal in patients with mild COPD. As the disease worsens, hyperinflation is demonstrated by an increase in the functional residual capacity (FRC), residual volume (RV), and total lung capacity (TLC). In patients with emphysema, destruction of the alveolar capillary bed reduces the diffusing capacity for carbon monoxide (DL_{CO}) in proportion to disease severity.

Arterial Blood Gas Measurements

Although unusual in patients with mild disease, resting arterial hypoxemia and hypercapnia become increasingly common once the FEV_1 falls below 50% of the predicted value. Exercise-induced hypoxemia occurs almost exclusively in patients with emphysema and a DL_{CO} less than 55% of predicted.

DIAGNOSIS

Differential Diagnosis

Several disorders must be considered in patients who present with airflow obstruction accompanied by dyspnea and/or cough. These are listed in Table 1, and most are discussed

Table 1 Differential Diagnosis of Airflow Obstruction

Chronic obstructive pulmonary disease
    Emphysema
    Chronic bronchitis
Asthma
Cystic fibrosis
Bronchiectasis
    Postinfectious
    Allergic bronchopulmonary aspergillosis
    Immunodeficiency states
    Primary ciliary dyskinesia
Obliterative bronchiolitis
    Idiopathic
    Inhalational injury
    Postinfectious
    Drug-induced
    Associated with other diseases
        Organ transplantation
        Connective tissue disease
Pneumoconiosis
    Silicosis
    Coal workers pneumoconiosis
Lymphangioleiomyomatosis

in detail in other chapters of this text. In most cases, COPD can be distinguished from other forms of obstructive lung disease by the history, physical examination, chest radiograph and spirometry. On occasion, however, additional information is needed. For example, CT is helpful in the diagnosis or exclusion of bronchiectasis, bronchiolitis, and disorders affecting the pulmonary interstitium and often demonstrates the presence of emphysema in patients with a nondiagnostic chest radiograph.

The most common diagnostic challenge is to distinguish between COPD and asthma, since these diseases may have a considerable degree of overlap. For example, patients with asthma may have a history of cigarette smoking and present late in life, having constant dyspnea, a productive cough, and evidence of hyperinflation by physical examination and chest radiograph. On the other hand, patients with COPD may have a relatively brief smoking history, present in the fourth or fifth decade, and have a nonproductive cough, intermittent dyspnea and wheezing, and a normal chest radiograph. These diseases may also be indistinguishable by spirometry, since asthmatics may demonstrate only partial reversibility, even with long-term therapy. Further blurring the distinction between COPD and asthma is the fact that a large percentage of patients (85% of women and 59% of men) with clinically diagnosed COPD have airway hyperresponsiveness as demonstrated by methacholine inhalation.

In difficult cases, these two diseases can usually be distinguished by the response to a trial of systemic corticosteroids. Spirometry should be performed before and at the end of a 14-day course of prednisone. Complete resolution of airflow obstruction is diagnostic of asthma, whereas lack of significant improvement is strongly suggestive of COPD. Patients who have a large but incomplete response may have COPD with a significant reversible component or asthma with fixed airflow obstruction. Since both of these disorders should be treated with an aggressive anti-inflammatory and bronchodilator regimen, further attempts to separate them are unnecessary.

Additional Evaluation

Once a diagnosis of COPD has been made, additional testing is indicated in selected patients.

Gas Exchange

Arterial blood gas measurements should be performed in patients with an FEV_1 less than 50% of predicted to screen for resting hypoxemia and hypercapnia. Patients with resting hypoxemia, severe emphysema, marked exercise limitation, or a DL_{CO} less than 55% of predicted should be assessed for exercise-induced desaturation using pulse oximetry (see below).

Alpha₁-Antitrypsin Deficiency

Although it accounts for less than 1% of all cases of COPD, alpha₁-antitrypsin deficiency is an important disorder, since it is the only known genetic cause of emphysema and requires specific therapy. Alpha₁-antitrypsin (AAT) is a serine protease inhibitor that is synthesized and secreted by the liver and whose major function is to neutralize neutrophil elastase in the lung. Four major alleles of the AAT gene have been identified and, in order of decreasing enzyme production, are referred to as M, S, Z, and null. The protease inhibitor (Pi) phenotype is determined by the two inherited parental alleles. The normal AAT phenotype, Pi MM, is associated with enzyme levels ranging between 150 and 350 mg/dL. Patients with severe AAT deficiency (defined as less than 80 mg/dL) have a significantly increased risk of emphysema and almost always have the Pi ZZ, Pi Z-null, or Pi null-null phenotype. These patients develop rapidly progressive dyspnea that typically begins between 30 and 50 years of age. Characteristically, the chest radiograph demonstrates emphysema that predominates at the lung bases. Rarely, patients with severe AAT deficiency develop chronic hepatitis that progresses to cirrhosis and hepatic failure. AAT deficiency should be suspected in patients with (1) onset of emphysema at a young age, especially in the setting of minimal or no smoking history; (2) a chest radiograph showing emphysema predominately at the lung bases; (3) a family history of AAT deficiency or early-onset emphysema; and (4) emphysema accompanied by cirrhosis of unknown etiology. AAT deficiency is diagnosed by measuring serum enzyme concentrations. Patients with abnormally low levels should have phenotyping performed to confirm the diagnosis. In addition to standard therapy, patients with emphysema and severe AAT deficiency should receive augmentation therapy with human AAT.

MANAGEMENT OF STABLE COPD

Smoking Cessation

Cigarette smoking is perpetuated by both psychological and pharmacological factors, making smoking cessation extremely difficult. The techniques used to address these factors as well as the many health benefits of smoking cessation are described in detail in Chap. 23. In this section, only the benefits of smoking cessation that relate directly to COPD are discussed.

Lung Function

Subjects who have never smoked experience a yearly decrease in FEV_1 of 25 to 30 mL per year beginning at about age 35. Susceptible smokers have a more rapid rate of decline that varies directly with both the duration of smoking and the number of cigarettes smoked each day (commonly quantified in ''pack-years''). As shown in Fig. 3, smoking cessation

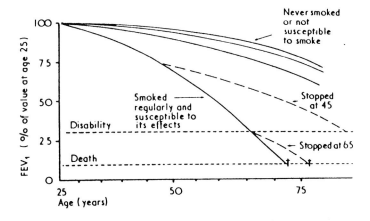

Figure 3 Effect of smoking and smoking cessation on lung function. Never-smokers and nonsusceptible smokers have a gradual decline in FEV_1 with increasing age. Susceptible smokers experience a much more rapid deterioration. Smoking cessation returns the rate of decline to that of never-smokers. (Reproduced from Br Med J 1997; 1:1646. With permission.)

rapidly decreases the rate of decline in FEV_1 to that of age-matched never-smokers. Although smoking cessation is beneficial in all patients, it is evident that its impact decreases with advancing age and worsening pulmonary function. For example, Fig. 3 demonstrates that a hypothetical patient who stops smoking at age 45 may never develop significant dyspnea, whereas discontinuing cigarettes at the age of 65 does little to alter the course of the disease.

Morbidity and Mortality

Smoking cessation is accompanied by a rapid and often dramatic decrease in the frequency of cough and sputum production. Improvement in dyspnea is much more variable and, when it occurs, is typically modest. Smoking cessation has also been shown to reduce mortality in patients with COPD. Interestingly, the death rate of former smokers actually exceeds that of continued smokers for as long as 10 years, probably because of the high prevalence of severe lung disease in patients who stop smoking. Following this initial increase, COPD-related mortality progressively falls with increasing duration of abstinence.

Pharmacological Therapy

Bronchodilators

Although COPD is often considered a disease of fixed airflow obstruction, a subset of patients have a significant response to one or more of the three classes of bronchodilators—beta$_2$-adrenergic agonists, anticholinergic agents, and theophylline. Since improvement in pulmonary function may occur only with chronic therapy or with a single class of drug, bronchodilator therapy should not be withheld based on the lack of an immediate response to an inhaled beta agonist.

Beta$_2$-Adrenergic Agonists.   Beta agonists produce smooth muscle relaxation and bronchodilation by activating adenylate cyclase, which, in turn, catalyzes the conversion of ATP to cyclic AMP. Beta agonists may be administered orally or by inhalation, but the oral route is associated with a high incidence of tremor and tachycardia and has no role in the management of COPD. Inhaled beta agonists may be divided into those with an intermediate (3- to 6-h) and a long (>12-h) duration of action. The intermediate-acting drugs are metaproterenol (Alupent, Metaprel), albuterol (Ventolin, Proventil), bitolterol (Tornalate), pirbuterol (Maxaire), and terbutaline (Brethaire). These drugs are interchangeable with the possible exception of metaproterenol, which is less beta$_2$-selective. Initial therapy should consist of one to two puffs from a metered dose inhaler (MDI) every 4 h as needed. In some patients, higher doses are associated with further symptomatic improvement, although dose is typically limited by sympathomimetic-induced side effects. Patients must be given detailed instructions regarding the use of MDIs and shown the proper technique. Spacer devices and reservoirs enhance the delivery of respirable particles and may both increase bronchodilation and reduce systemic absorption and side effects. Although several beta agonists are available for delivery via a jet nebulizer, no advantage has been demonstrated in patients who are able to use a MDI properly with a spacer device. Use of a jet nebulizer should, therefore, be restricted to a small minority of patients with stable COPD. Salmeterol (Serevent) is the only long-acting beta agonist available in the United States and is administered in a dose of two puffs twice a day. Its role in the management of COPD has not been well defined, although it may be useful in patients with moderate to severe chronic dyspnea and in those with prominent nocturnal symptoms.

Anticholinergic Agents.   Several synthetic atropine derivatives, referred to as quarternary ammonium compounds, produce bronchodilation by inhibiting the effect of acetylcholine on bronchial smooth muscle. Of these, only ipratropium (Atrovent) is approved for use in the United States. Ipratropium may be administered via either a MDI/spacer combination or a jet nebulizer, but the latter should be used only when patients are unable to master proper inhaler technique. Ipratropium is at least as effective as and often more effective than beta agonists in producing bronchodilation in patients with COPD and is virtually free of side effects. Because of its slower onset and longer duration of action, ipratropium should be used on a regular rather than an as-needed basis and therapy should be initiated at a dose of two puffs four times a day. In some patients, a dose-related increase in bronchodilation occurs, and a dose of four to six puffs every 6 h is required. Given the distinct mechanisms of action of anticholinergic agents and beta agonists, it is not surprising that many (but not all) studies have shown them to have additive effects, and combination therapy is routinely prescribed. Recently, a single MDI containing both albuterol and ipratropium (Combivent) has become available and may be of benefit by improving patient compliance.

Theophylline.   Until relatively recently, theophylline was considered a first-line drug for the treatment of COPD. Because of its potential for toxicity and the advent of specific beta$_2$-adrenergic agonists and anticholinergic agents, however, theophylline has now been relegated to a much less important role. Nevertheless, this drug has several properties that may be of benefit to patients with severe COPD. Theophylline produces an additive bronchodilator effect when combined with a beta agonist or with a beta agonist plus ipratropium. Theophylline also decreases the sensation of dyspnea and improves exercise tolerance in some patients with COPD, even in the absence of an objective improvement in pulmonary function. This is believed to result from a number of actions that are independent of its effect on airway smooth muscle. For example, theophylline has been shown to increase both the strength and endurance of the diaphragm, improve gas exchange, and enhance mucociliary clearance. Theophylline may also decrease pulmonary and systemic vascular resistance and improve both right and left ventricular function, effects that may further enhance the functional capacity of patients with COPD.

Although theophylline has a number of documented beneficial effects, it also has a large potential for toxicity. Headache, nausea, anorexia, and abdominal discomfort are common, even at therapeutic levels, and seizures and life-threatening cardiac dysrhythmias may occur at high serum concentrations. Because of its narrow therapeutic index, theophylline should be used only in patients with an inadequate response to ipratropium and beta agonists and should be discontinued if no objective or subjective improvement occurs within several months. The incidence of adverse effects can be reduced by starting at a low dose and gradually increasing it until a serum concentration between 10 and 15 mg/L is achieved. Periodic monitoring of serum concentration is recommended. It is important to note that a number of commonly used medications interfere with theophylline clearance and may lead to acute toxicity. A complete list of drugs that alter serum theophylline concentration is provided in Table 2.

Corticosteroids

Although corticosteroids are essential in the pharmacological therapy of asthma, their role in patients with COPD appears to be limited. Oral corticosteroids produce a significant improvement in airflow in only 10–20% of patients with stable COPD, and inhaled corticosteroids are beneficial in an even smaller number, typically a subset of those who respond

Table 2 Drugs Affecting Serum
Theophylline Concentration

Increased Concentration	Decreased Concentration
Quinolone antibiotics	Phenytoin
Clarithromycin	Phenobarbitol
Erythromycin	Carbamazepine
Tetracycline	Rifampin
Propranolol	Moricizine
Verapamil	Sulfinpyrazone
Mexilitine	
Cimetidine	
Oral contraceptives	
Fluvoxamine	
Methotrexate	
Pentoxifylline	
Ticlopidine	
Zileuton	

to oral therapy. Because of disabling and even life-threatening side effects—including myopathy, osteoporosis, osteonecrosis, diabetes mellitus, cataracts, and immune suppression—corticosteroids should be considered only in patients who remain severely limited despite optimal therapy and used only in those who are truly steroid-responsive. Since this cannot be predicted by any clinical parameter, including response to inhaled bronchodilators, appropriate patients can be identified only by assessing the objective response to a short trial of corticosteroids. Spirometry should be performed during a period of clinical stability, therapy instituted with prednisone in a dose of 40 mg/day, and spirometry repeated after approximately 2 weeks. Corticosteroids are immediately discontinued in patients with less than a 15% improvement in FEV_1. In patients with a significant objective response, therapy is initiated with high-dose inhaled corticosteroids, and prednisone is tapered to the lowest daily or alternate-day dose that maintains the objective improvement.

For many years, there has been a great deal of interest in whether the long-term use of inhaled corticosteroids can slow the rapid decline in lung function characteristic of COPD. To date, studies have been plagued by a number of methodological problems, and results have been contradictory. Several large multicenter trials are now attempting to answer this question. Based on currently available information, however, the routine use of inhaled corticosteroids in patients with COPD cannot be recommended.

Mucoactive Drugs

In patients with chronic bronchitis, hypertropy of mucous glands and goblet cells leads to excessive production of mucus. This, in turn, contributes to airflow obstruction by occluding the small airways and reducing the clearance of inflammatory cells and mediators. Therapy directed at enhancing the mobilization of mucus from the peripheral airways would, therefore, appear to be beneficial. In the United States, two drugs guaifenasin and potassium iodide, have been approved for use as expectorants, and both are believed to reduce sputum viscosity by increasing the transport of water into the airway lumen. Studies examining these and other mucoactive drugs, however, have reported conflicting results. Although some have noted a decrease in dyspnea as well as cough frequency and severity, others have found no symptomatic improvement. A trial of a mucoactive agent is reasonable in patients who complain of difficulty expectorating sputum, but the drug should be discontinued in the absence of a subjective response.

Approach to Therapy

Based on the concepts discussed above, a step-care approach to the pharmacological therapy of COPD is recommended and is outlined in Table 3.

Long-Term Oxygen Therapy

In patients with COPD, correction of arterial hypoxemia has been shown to reduce pulmonary artery pressure, increase exercise tolerance, and improve neuropsychological function. More importantly, however, two large, prospective, randomized trials conducted in North America and Great Britain have shown that long-term oxygen therapy (LTOT) reduces patient mortality in direct proportion to the number of hours of daily use. That is, continuous oxygen therapy is superior to intermittent or nocturnal use, which, in turn, is more effective than no oxygen at all. Although the mechanism by which oxygen improves patient survival remains unproven, it is widely believed to relate to the observed improvements in pulmonary hemodynamics, which reduce right ventricular work and improve systemic oxygen delivery. Because of these beneficial effects, LTOT is essential in the management of patients with arterial hypoxemia.

Oxygen therapy, including oxygen supply and delivery systems, is described in detail in Chap. 22. Here, discussion is limited to the prescription of LTOT in patients with COPD.

Table 3 Step-Care Approach to Pharmacotherapy of COPD

Step 1: Mild, intermittent symptoms
Intermediate-acting beta agonist, two puffs every 4–6 h as needed
Step 2: Mild to moderate continuous symptoms
Ipratropium, two to six puffs every 6 h *plus*
Intermediate-acting beta agonist, two to four puffs every 4–6 h as needed
Step 3: Response to step 2 is inadequate
Add sustained-release theophylline *and/or* long-acting beta agonist two puffs every 12 h; consider use of a mucoactive drug
Step 4: Response to step 3 is inadequate
Objective trial of oral prednisone, 40 mg/day for 14 days
If no response, discontinue prednisone
If significant response, begin therapy with inhaled steroids and taper prednisone off or to a low daily or alternate day dose

Indications for LTOT

Based largely on published studies, Medicare reimbursement guidelines for LTOT have been established by the Health Care Financing Administration (HCFA) and adopted by private insurance companies throughout the United States. These guidelines, which are now generally accepted by the medical community as indications for LTOT, are listed in Table 4.

Patient Evaluation

All patients with moderate to severe COPD must undergo an orderly evaluation to assess the need for LTOT. First, arterial blood-gas measurements are performed to detect resting hypoxemia. Although pulse oximetry is useful in assessing exercise or sleep-related desaturation (see below), a prescription for continuous, lifelong oxygen therapy should be based on the more accurate, direct measurement of arterial P_{O_2}. If the criteria for continuous LTOT are met, oxygen flow is titrated using pulse oximetry to achieve an arterial hemoglobin saturation (Sa_{O_2}) greater than 90%, and this should be confirmed by repeat arterial blood-gas analysis. Next, oxygen requirements during exercise must be determined. In patients with resting hypoxemia, pulse oximetry is monitored during activity that simulates the patient's maximum level of exertion, and oxygen flow is increased, if necessary, to maintain Sa_{O_2} greater than 90%. Exercise testing can be performed on a treadmill or cycle ergometer, or the patient can simply be monitored during typical strenuous activities, as walking or climbing stairs. Patients who do not qualify for continuous oxygen therapy should be assessed for exercise-induced desaturation in the presence of severe emphysema, a DL_{CO} less than 55% of predicted, or marked exercise limitation. Finally, nocturnal oxygen requirements must be determined. Since nighttime desaturation is common, oxygen flow is routinely increased by 1 L/min during sleep in patients requiring continuous oxygen therapy. Pulmonary hypertension, cor pulmonale, or erythrocythemia in the absence of daytime hypoxemia should raise the possibility of isolated nocturnal desaturation or

Table 4 Indications for Long-Term Oxygen Therapy

Continuous oxygen therapy
1. $Pa_{O_2} < 56$ mmHg or $Sa_{O_2} < 89\%$, or
2. Pa_{O_2} 56–59 mmHg or Sa_{O_2} 89%, with
   a. Edema caused by congestive heart failure, or
   b. Pulmonary hypertension or cor pulmonale,
      determined by measurement of pulmonary artery
      pressure, gated blood pool scan,
      echocardiogram, or "P pulmonale" on ECG, or
   c. Erythrocythemia with a hematocrit $> 56\%$
Nocturnal oxygen therapy
1. $Pa_{O_2} < 56$ mmHg or $Sa_{O_2} < 89\%$ during sleep, or
2. A decrease in $Pa_{O_2} > 10$ mmHg or $Sa_{O_2} > 5\%$
   during sleep when associated with erythrocythemia
   or signs of pulmonary hypertension or cor
   pulmonale
Oxygen with activity only
1. $Pa_{O_2} < 56$ mmHg or $Sa_{O2} < 89\%$ during activity

sleep apnea. In such patients, polysomnography is indicated both for diagnosis and for the accurate titration of oxygen flow and positive airway pressure.

Prescribing LTOT

Once the need for either continuous or intermittent LTOT has been established, the physician must write an oxygen prescription that specifies the indication for therapy, the flow rate(s) required to correct hypoxemia at rest, with activity, and during sleep, the stationary and portable oxygen source, and the type of delivery system. For Medicare patients, this entails completion of a certificate of medical necessity, HCFA Form 484. Similar forms are provided by private insurance companies.

Patients who are found to require LTOT during a period of clinical stability should receive lifelong therapy. Oxygen requirements should be periodically reassessed to ensure the continued correction of hypoxemia. Since oxygen may improve gas exchange as a consequence of its favorable hemodynamic effects, however, improvements in oxygenation do not justify the termination of therapy. On the other hand, patients who are prescribed oxygen during an acute respiratory illness may require only short-term therapy and should be retested after recovery.

Pulmonary Rehabilitation

Despite smoking cessation and optimal medical management, many patients with COPD continue to have significant dyspnea with activity or even at rest. This functional impairment leads to further deconditioning, social isolation, anxiety, and depression. These patients are candidates for pulmonary rehabilitation, a multidisciplinary program whose goal is to improve quality of life by reducing dyspnea, increasing exercise tolerance, and improving functional status. Although the elements of pulmonary rehabilitation have not been strictly defined, most comprehensive programs have four major components: education, breathing retraining, nutritional assessment and therapy, and exercise training. These programs may, therefore, employ the expertise of a variety of health care professionals including pulmonologists, nurses, physical and occupational therapists, dietitians, and exercise physiologists.

Patient Education

Patients are instructed about their disease and its clinical manifestations, the purpose and proper use of prescribed medications including oxygen, and the symptoms and signs that require medical attention. This allows patients to have a greater sense of control and to participate more actively in their own care—a concept referred to as collaborative self-management. Other important educational topics include smoking cessation, proper nutrition, and relaxation and energy-conserving techniques.

Breathing Retraining

Two techniques that alter the breathing pattern, namely pursed-lips and diaphragmatic breathing, are effective in reducing the sensation of breathlessness in many patients with COPD. Although the mechanism(s) by which these techniques relieve dyspnea is not entirely clear, both have been shown to increase tidal volume and decrease respiratory frequency, a ventilatory pattern that reduces respiratory muscle work. Because of their simplicity and effectiveness, these techniques are an important component of a rehabilitation program.

Nutritional Assessment and Therapy

Both malnutrition and obesity have significant adverse consequences for patients with COPD. Obesity reduces exercise capacity by increasing the work required of the respiratory muscles, whereas protein-calorie malnutrition (PCM) leads to functional impairment through the progressive loss of skeletal and respiratory muscle mass. In addition, PCM is a predictor of increased mortality in patients with COPD. Weight loss and PCM result primarily from decreased caloric intake. In many patients with severe disease, eating is associated with a marked increase in dyspnea and may also be accompanied by arterial desaturation. Anorexia and early satiety are also common and may be caused by depression, medications (especially theophylline), and displacement of the stomach by the flattened diaphragm.

Nutritional assessment and therapy are, therefore, important in the management of patients with COPD and can easily be incorporated into a comprehensive pulmonary rehabilitation program. Nutritional screening can be performed by taking a dietary history and comparing the patient's actual weight with an "ideal" body weight (IBW) based on published standards. A more detailed assessment can be performed by calculating the percentages of body fat and lean tissue mass using anthropometric measurements such as triceps skin fold thickness and middle-arm circumference. Underweight patients (less than 90% of IBW) and those with normal weight but a low lean tissue mass should be instructed regarding proper nutrition and techniques for managing anorexia, early satiety, and meal-related dyspnea. Nutritional supplements may also be useful in some patients. Overweight patients (greater than 120% of IBW) should also receive nutritional counseling. In these patients, exercise training is essential not only to improve functional status but also to facilitate weight loss.

Exercise Training

Lower Extremity Exercise.   There is considerable evidence that lower extremity exercise, using a treadmill or cycle ergometer, is effective in reducing dyspnea and increasing the exercise tolerance and capacity of patients with COPD. The basis of these observed benefits is unclear, however, since studies have repeatedly shown no improvement in either pulmonary function or respiratory muscle strength or endurance. It is currently believed that exercise tolerance improves by a number of mechanisms including improved mechanical efficiency, desensitization to dyspnea, and increased confidence and motivation. In addition, several investigators have documented a physiological adaptation to training characterized by a reduction in minute ventilation and lactate concentration at a given work rate and an increase in the oxidative capacity of skeletal muscle.

Significant improvements in exercise capacity have been shown to occur using a wide variety of training protocols; however, the optimum type, intensity, and duration of lower extremity exercise have not been determined. At the University of Pittsburgh, a baseline treadmill exercise test is performed to determine the patient's maximum work rate (Wmax). Patients then perform supervised, symptom-limited treadmill exercise with a target workload of approximately 80% of their baseline Wmax. Between outpatient visits and following completion of the program, patients are encouraged to perform daily exercise that simulates the intensity of their supervised sessions.

Upper Extremity Exercise.   For many patients with COPD, the most dyspnea-provoking activities are those everyday tasks requiring use of the arms, such as lifting and carrying objects, dressing, and grooming. This is believed to result from the inability of the chest musculature to simultaneously stabilize the arms and participate in lung and chest wall expansion. Since exercise training is generally muscle- and task-specific, upper extremity exercise has been incorporated into many pulmonary rehabilitation programs. This may take the form of arm cycle ergometry or unsupported exercise such as repetitive arm abduction and extension. Upper extremity training does, in fact, improve arm exercise capacity and is accompanied by a decrease in metabolic and ventilatory requirements. Since these improvements are largely task-specific, however, it is unknown whether they are translated into improved patient functional status. At our institution, patients perform a variety of unsupported arm exercises during each supervised session and are encouraged to repeat them two or three times each day.

Inspiratory Muscle Training. Patients with COPD are predisposed to chronic respiratory muscle fatigue because of both a high resistive load and reduced muscle strength and efficiency. Chronic fatigue may, in turn, contribute to the disabling dyspnea that is so common in this disease. Inspiratory muscle training (IMT) has been investigated as a means of increasing the strength and endurance of the respiratory muscles, decreasing dyspnea, and improving exercise tolerance. Inspiratory muscle training has been performed using several techniques designed to provide low-intensity, high-frequency exercise. The most common method is threshhold loading, in which a set pressure must be generated by the patient in order to initiate inspiratory flow. Studies have clearly demonstrated that IMT increases respiratory muscle strength and endurance, and most, but not all, have reported an associated improvement in exercise capacity. Recently, several investigators have reported that IMT combined with lower extremity training improves exercise capacity significantly more than lower extremity exercise alone. It appears, therefore, the IMT is a useful adjunct to upper and lower extremity training in patients with COPD.

Most pulmonary rehabilitation programs are conducted in outpatient facilities and require patients to attend between two and four sessions a week for 8–12 weeks. The optimum frequency and duration of these sessions has, however, not been determined, and there is now increasing interest in shifting pulmonary rehabilitation to the home. Regardless of the specific characteristics of the rehabilitation program, it is essential that patients perform upper and lower extremity exercise between sessions and after the completion of the program. Not surprisingly, exercise gains made during a rehabilitation program are quickly lost if patients resume a sedentary lifestyle.

Although pulmonary rehabilitation has become a widely accepted form of therapy for patients with COPD, its utilization has been limited by erratic and often inadequate reimbursement by third-party payers. For example, Medicare payments are not based on a uniform national standard, and this has led to widely differing regional reimbursement policies. In fact, in most states, payment cannot be obtained for the rehabilitation program itself. Instead, reimbursement must be sought for procedures performed during the program, such as pulmonary function testing, cardiopulmonary exercise testing, and exercise oximetry. Similar problems are encountered when dealing with most private insurance companies. Efforts are currently under way to change these policies, and they may ultimately be successful. In the meantime, patients referred to a pulmonary rehabilitation program must be informed about all nonreimbursible costs.

Surgical Approaches to COPD

Lung Transplantation

Between 1986 and 1993, the number of patients undergoing lung transplantation in the United States increased exponentially, but it has since leveled off at approximately 900 per year owing to a fixed number of donor organs. COPD has been by far the most common indication and currently accounts for about 40% of all lung transplants. In patients with COPD, transplantation has been shown to significantly improve pulmonary function, gas exchange, exercise tolerance and capacity, and quality of life. Major complications result primarily from long-term immunosuppression and chronic allograft rejection; the latter occurs in up to 40% of all transplant recipients. In patients with COPD, 2- and 5-year survival following transplantation is approximately 71 and 41%, respectively.

Given its associated morbidity and mortality, lung transplantation should be considered only in patients with severe disease who have symptoms unresponsive to optimal medical management and an estimated life expectancy of less than 2 years. Indications for referral to a transplant center as well as contraindications for transplantation are listed in Table 5 (see also Chap. 24).

Lung Volume Reduction Surgery

Although initially reported almost 40 years ago, lung volume reduction surgery (LVRS) has recently generated a tremendous resurgence of interest as a treatment for severe emphysema. This procedure involves stapled resection of severely diseased regions in both lungs in an effort to restore elastic recoil and thereby reduce airflow obstruction. LVRS may be performed through a median sternotomy or by using the much less invasive technique of bilateral video-assisted thoracoscopic surgery (VATS). Initial reports indicate that LVRS does, in fact, increase lung elastic recoil, reduce airflow obstruction, and decrease hyperinflation. These effects are reflected by improvements in pulmonary function (increased FVC and FEV_1; reduced TLC, FRC, and RV), gas exchange (increased P_{O_2} and reduced P_{CO_2}), exercise capacity, and quality of life. Despite these encouraging results, several questions must be answered before LVRS gains acceptance as a therapy for severe emphysema. For example: Are early improvements maintained over a long period of time? What is the best surgical approach (sternotomy vs. bilateral VATS)? Which patient characteristics predict both maximum benefits and low morbidity and mortality? A planned multicenter, prospective, randomized trial of LVRS sponsored by the National Institutes of Health will address these issues.

Table 5 Lung Transplantation in Patients
with COPD

Indications
   $FEV_1 < 25\%$ of predicted
   Arterial $P_{CO_2} > 50$ mmHg
   Moderate to severe pulmonary hypertension
   Rapidly declining lung function
Contraindications
   Continued cigarette smoking
   Significant extrapulmonary organ dysfunction
   Active pulmonary or extrapulmonary
     infection
   Malignancy
   Protein-calorie malnutrition
   Significant psychological impairment
   Lack of an adequate social support system

Elective Ventilatory Assistance

In theory, intermittent mechanical ventilation might have two beneficial effects in patients with severe, stable COPD. First, ventilatory assistance might reduce fatigue and increase the strength and endurance of the respiratory muscles, thereby reducing chronic hypercapnia and dyspnea and improving exercise tolerance. Second, since sleep-induced hypoventilation and hypoxemia are common in patients with severe COPD, positive-pressure ventilation might improve sleep quality and help to maintain adequate nocturnal oxygenation. Despite these potential benefits, the results of studies examining the elective use of both positive- and negative-pressure ventilation in patients with COPD have been largely disappointing. Most long-term, randomized trials of intermittent negative-pressure ventilation using a poncho or cuirass-type device have failed to show improvements in baseline respiratory muscle function, blood gases, dyspnea, or exercise tolerance. In addition, this form of ventilatory assistance can worsen upper airway obstruction during sleep and has a low level of patient compliance owing to the uncomfortable and cumbersome nature of the equipment. A number of studies have examined the effectiveness of noninvasive positive-pressure ventilation (NIPPV) using the BiPAP system. Although beneficial effects—such as decreased dyspnea, improved exercise tolerance, reduction of chronic hypercapnia, and improved sleep efficiency—have occasionally been documented, most studies have shown no improvement in any of these parameters. Furthermore, in the absence of obstructive sleep apnea, NIPPV, when combined with supplemental oxygen, is no more effective than oxygen alone in eliminating sleep-induced hypoxemia. Based on these findings, intermittent ventilatory assistance cannot be recommended in the routine management of patients with stable COPD.

EVALUATION AND MANAGEMENT OF COPD EXACERBATIONS

Most patients with COPD experience periodic worsening of their respiratory symptoms. These episodes are characterized by the development of increased dyspnea and are often accompanied by worsening cough and sputum production. Although often of little consequence in patients with mild disease, these episodes may lead to significant morbidity and mortality in patients with moderate to severe degrees of airflow obstruction.

Precipitating Factors

Despite their frequency and clinical importance, very little is known about the etiology of COPD exacerbations. Commonly cited causes are listed in Table 6, but there is virtually no information regarding the relative frequency of these disorders. Medication-induced respiratory depression and pneumothorax are usually readily apparent. The detection of other precipitating factors commonly presents a much greater diagnostic challenge.

Infection

Airway and parenchymal damage, often coupled with impaired secretion clearance, predisposes patients with COPD to a variety of pulmonary infections. Pneumonia, diagnosed by the presence of a parenchymal infiltrate and appropriate clinical findings, is an important, but relatively uncommon cause of disease exacerbations. *Streptococcus pneumoniae,*

Table 6 Disorders
Precipitating Exacerbations
of COPD

Infection
Pneumonia
Tracheobronchitis
Inflammation/bronchospasm
Pulmonary embolism
Left ventricular dysfunction
Use of sedatives or narcotics
Pneumothorax

Haemophilus influenzae, and *Branhamella catarrhalis* are the most common pathogens, but other organisms, particularly *Klebsiella pneumoniae* and *Staphylococcus aureus*, are also important.

In the absence of new radiographic abnormalities, COPD exacerbations, especially those characterized by increased sputum quantity and purulence, are commonly attributed to infectious tracheobronchitis. An association has, in fact, been established between the presence of viruses in lower respiratory tract secretions and worsening respiratory symptoms, and up to one-third of all COPD exacerbations may result from infection with influenza virus, parainfluenza virus, respiratory syncytial virus, coronavirus, or rhinovirus. Virus-induced exacerbations occur primarily during the winter and spring and are usually accompanied or preceded by pharyngitis, rhinorrhea, and nasal congestion.

Surprisingly, despite intensive investigation, the role of bacterial tracheobronchitis in the pathogenesis of COPD exacerbations remains unclear. This has resulted largely from the inability of sputum cultures to distinguish between colonization and infection, since potentially pathogenic bacteria are cultured with equal frequency during symptomatic exacerbations and periods of clinical stability. The importance of bacterial infection has been indirectly assessed by a number of randomized, placebo-controlled trials of antibiotic therapy in patients with increased dyspnea, cough, and sputum production. These studies have shown that antibiotics produce little or no *clinical* benefit even when a *statistically* significant effect can be demonstrated and suggest that bacterial tracheobronchitis is a relatively infrequent cause of respiratory decompensation in patients with COPD.

Airway Inflammation and Bronchoconstriction

Although a large percentage of patients with COPD demonstrate bronchial hyperresponsiveness to inhaled methacholine, only a small subset has a significant degree of reversible airflow obstruction during periods of clinical stability. Airway inflammation and bronchoconstriction are believed to play a much more important role during acute exacerbations and have been attributed to exposure to allergens and bronchial irritants such as cigarette smoke and air pollutants. The frequency with which bronchoconstriction precipitates an exacerbation of COPD, however, is unknown.

Pulmonary Embolism

The role of pulmonary embolism (PE) in acute exacerbations of COPD also remains unclear. Although patients frequently have one or more risk factors and often present with compatible clinical findings, the diagnosis of PE is only occasionally considered and even less commonly pursued. This probably results from two factors. First, the observation that most patients with COPD exacerbations improve without anticoagulant therapy has led to the widespread and perhaps incorrect belief that PE is rarely a precipitating factor. Second, the diagnosis of PE is difficult to make in this patient population. Clinical findings are of little help, since patients typically have many other reasons for dyspnea, tachypnea, tachycardia, and hypoxemia. Ventilation/perfusion ($\dot{V}/\dot{Q}$) lung scans are indeterminate, and therefore of no diagnostic value, in approximately 60% of patients. As in other populations, noninvasive studies of the lower extremities may be helpful if deep vein thrombosis is detected, but negative studies do not reliably exclude PE. Finally, pulmonary angiography, the ''gold standard'' for diagnosis, often carries an increased risk due to underlying renal insufficiency or pulmonary hypertension.

In the absence of published data, clinical experience suggests that the diagnosis of PE be considered in patients with dyspnea of sudden onset, pleuritic pain, or hemoptysis and in those who fail to improve with usual pharmacological therapy. Evaluation should begin with noninvasive leg studies and, if negative, proceed to $\dot{V}/\dot{Q}$ scanning. Since approximately 40% of patients will have high- or low-probability scans, this test remains useful even in patients with underlying lung disease. Finally, pulmonary angiography should be performed if PE cannot be diagnosed or excluded by the combination of clinical suspicion and $\dot{V}/\dot{Q}$ scan. With appropriate preparation and precautions, angiography can be performed safely in the vast majority of patients. Recently, spiral CT has been shown to be a sensitive method for detecting emboli in segmental and larger pulmonary arteries. In patients with decompensated COPD, the usefulness of this technique is limited by the requirement for a prolonged breath-hold and by its inability to detect peripheral (and potentially significant) emboli. Nevertheless, spiral CT may be useful in selected patients with indeterminate $\dot{V}/\dot{Q}$ scans, since a positive result may eliminate the need for pulmonary angiography.

Left Ventricular Dysfunction

Many patients with COPD have impaired cardiac function, most commonly from ischemic or hypertensive heart disease. In these patients, acute left ventricular (LV) dysfunction could lead to interstitial or alveolar edema and precipitate respiratory decompensation. Conversely, acute LV failure might be produced by a number of factors during a COPD exacerbation, thereby creating a vicious cycle leading to progressive respiratory failure. For example, increased myocardial oxygen requirements coupled with arterial hypoxemia could result in myocardial ischemia or infarction, and hypoxic pulmonary vasoconstriction could lead to an abrupt fall in LV compliance due to acute right ventricular (RV) dilatation.

Despite these plausible scenerios, no studies have attempted to determine the frequency with which LV dysfunction either precipitates or complicates an exacerbation of COPD. In practice, making the clinical diagnosis of LV failure is extremely difficult. Patients typically present with a nonspecific symptom complex that often includes orthopnea and paroxysmal nocturnal dyspnea. Physical findings—such as bibasilar rales and a third heart sound—are frequently undetectable because of pulmonary hyperinflation, wheezes, and rhonchi; elevated jugular venous pressures and edema may reflect isolated RV dysfunction. Finally, radiographic evidence of interstitial pulmonary edema or cardiac enlargement may be absent in patients with hyperinflation and parenchymal destruction from emphysema.

The following approach to the diagnosis of LV failure is recommended: A 12-lead electrocardiogram (ECG) should be performed in all patients presenting with a COPD

Table 7 Indications for Hospitalization of
Patients with a COPD Exacerbation

Inadequate response to outpatient management
Severe dyspnea that markedly impairs
   ambulation, eating, and sleep
Hypoxemia that cannot be corrected using home
   oxygen
Significant comorbid conditions (e.g.,
   myocardial ischemia, left ventricular failure,
   pulmonary embolism, pneumonia,
   pneumothorax)

exacerbation to evaluate the cardiac rhythm and screen for myocardial ischemia. A transthoracic and, if necessary, transesophageal echocardiogram is indicated in patients with physical findings or radiographic evidence of LV or RV dysfunction and in those who fail to improve with conventional therapy. Right heart catheterization is occasionally required to confirm or exclude LV failure in patients with COPD.

Management of COPD Exacerbations

The management of respiratory decompensation in patients with COPD must be based on the underlying cause. Obviously, specific therapy is indicated in patients with pneumonia, pneumothorax, PE, and LV failure; these disorders are not discussed further. In most cases, however, no definite precipitating factor can be identified, and patients are typically treated with bronchodilator and anti-inflammatory medications. Patients with mild exacerbations can usually be managed with outpatient therapy. Those with more severe respiratory impairment often require hospital admission for intensive pharmacotherapy, oxygen administration, and, when necessary, mechanical ventilation. Indications for hospitalization and intensive care unit admission are listed in Tables 7 and 8, respectively.

Pharmacological Therapy

Bronchodilators.   Increasing the frequency and/or dose of an inhaled beta agonist is the cornerstone of therapy for acute exacerbations of COPD. In outpatients, MDI use may be increased to three or four puffs every 4 h; inpatients may require even more frequent dosing. As in patients with stable disease, aerosol delivery via a jet nebulizer appears to offer no advantages over a MDI as long as proper technique and a spacer device are used. From a practical standpoint, however, patients who require hospital admission are often too dyspneic to use a MDI properly and nebulizer therapy is therefore preferred, at least initially.

Table 8 Indications for ICU Admission of
Patients with a COPD Exacerbation

Marked tachypnea with respiratory rate $> 30/min$
Hypoxemia requiring $F_{I_{O_2}} > 0.50$
New or worsening hypercapnia
Altered mental status

Ipratropium is as effective as beta agonists in producing subjective and objective improvements during acute exacerbations of COPD. Based on their differing mechanisms of action and on studies showing additive effects in patients with stable disease, combination therapy is often utilized in the acute setting. Studies during disease exacerbations, however, have failed to show any difference in the rate or degree of spirometric improvement, subjective response, or hospital length of stay when ipratropium is added to a beta agonist.

Although theophylline may be of benefit in patients with stable disease, there is very little evidence to support its use during acute exacerbations. Randomized, prospective trials have shown that intravenous aminophylline does not increase the rate of subjective or objective improvement when it is added to therapy with aerosolized bronchodilators.

Corticosteroids.   Although corticosteroids are effective in only a small subset of patients with stable COPD, two randomized, placebo-controlled trials indicate that they are of greater benefit during disease exacerbations. In outpatients, the addition of prednisone to inhaled bronchodilator therapy has been shown to produce a significantly greater improvement in FEV_1 and P_{O_2} and to reduce the number of patients eventually requiring hospitalization. Similarly, in hospitalized patients, a much more rapid improvement in FEV_1 and FVC has been demonstrated when intravenous solumedrol is added to standard therapy. Response to corticosteroids does not appear to correlate with either baseline lung function or bronchodilator responsiveness, but it remains unclear whether other factors, particularly the underlying disease process (i.e., chronic bronchitis vs. emphysema) is predictive of steroid responsiveness. Based on these studies, it seems reasonable to treat patients with a short course (i.e., 7–10 days) of corticosteroids. As discussed above, prolonged therapy must be avoided unless long-term, objective improvement can be demonstrated.

Antibiotics.   The role of empiric antibiotic therapy in the management of patients with acute COPD exacerbations remains unclear. As discussed above, antibiotics may have a small beneficial effect in patients with chronic bronchitis who present with increased sputum quantity and purulence. There is no evidence that antibiotics are beneficial in patients who lack these symptoms.

Oxygen Therapy

By reducing Sa_{O_2}, arterial hypoxemia decreases systemic oxygen delivery ($\dot{D}_{O_2}$) and may produce life-threatening tissue hypoxia. The correction of hypoxemia is, therefore, an essential component of the management of acute respiratory failure, regardless of the underlying cause. In patients with decompensated COPD, sufficient supplemental oxygen should be provided to increase the P_{O_2} to approximately 60–70 mmHg. Because of the sigmoidal shape of the oxygen-hemoglobin dissociation curve, higher levels do not significantly increase Sa_{O_2} or $\dot{D}_{O_2}$ and may increase the risk of acute hypercapneic respiratory failure (see below). Depending on the initial P_{O_2}, this can usually be accomplished by administering oxygen at a flow rate of 1–4 L/min via a nasal cannula or at an FI_{O_2} between 0.24 and 0.40 using a Venturi mask. Patients with intrapulmonary shunting resulting from pneumonia or pulmonary edema will often require higher oxygen concentrations delivered by a nonrebreather or high-flow aerosol mask.

It is well known that some patients with COPD develop an acute rise in P_{CO_2} when given supplemental oxygen. This appears to result primarily from worsening ventilation/perfusion imbalance and the subsequent increase in the ratio of dead space to tidal volume. Although frequently feared, acute hypercapnia and respiratory acidosis are, in fact, relatively uncommon and occur primarily in patients with both severe airflow obstruction and

Table 9   Indications for Endotracheal
Intubation in Patients with a COPD
Exacerbation

Acute respiratory acidosis, pH < 7.25
Respiratory slowing or apnea
Marked respiratory distress with air hunger
Refractory hypoxemia
Obtundation or coma

---

chronic CO_2 retention. Furthermore, a significant increase in P_{CO_2} is uncommon in the absence of excessive oxygen administration. In susceptible patients, therefore, it is prudent to initiate oxygen therapy at low levels (e.g., an F_{IO_2} of 0.28 or 1–2 L/min) and closely follow arterial blood gases. It is essential to remember, however, that hypoxemia must be corrected regardless of the effect on the P_{CO_2}. If necessary, mechanical ventilation can be used to correct severe hypercapnia and acute respiratory acidosis.

Mechanical Ventilation

Endotracheal intubation should be performed in patients with severe respiratory failure. Specific indications are listed in Table 9. Unfortunately, intubation is associated with a number of complications, including laryngeal and tracheal injury, barotrauma, and nosocomial pneumonia. In addition, although most patients are successfully extubated, a small minority will develop prolonged ventilator dependence. Recently, NIPPV, using devices that allow the independent selection of inspiratory (IPAP) and expiratory (EPAP) positive airway pressure (e.g., BiPAP), has been shown to significantly reduce the eventual need for endotracheal intubation in patients with milder forms of respiratory failure. By preventing intubation, NIPPV also decreases hospital stay, the overall rate of complications, and patient mortality; it has become an important adjunct to the therapy of patients with decompensated COPD. NIPPV should be initiated at an IPAP of 10 cmH_2O and an EPAP of 2.5 to 5.0 cmH_2O via a nasal mask. The IPAP is then gradually increased as needed based on arterial blood-gas measurements and clinical evidence of persistent respiratory distress. Supplemental oxygen is added via a mask port and adjusted to maintain Sa_{O_2} greater than 90%. An oronasal face mask is substituted when excessive air leakage occurs through the mouth. Initially, patients are maintained on continuous NIPPV with only short breaks for conversation and meals. As the patient's respiratory status improves, daily duration is gradually decreased until ventilatory support is no longer needed. Endotracheal intubation is required when patients fail to improve or worsen despite NIPPV.

CONCLUSION

Chronic obstructive pulmonary disease is an extremely common disorder and represents a major public health problem throughout the world. In addition to being a frequent cause of morbidity and mortality, COPD places a huge financial burden on society by increasing health care expenditures and reducing worker productivity. As reviewed in this chapter, a number of advances have been made in the management of patients with both stable and decompensated COPD, and these have led to decreased symptoms, improved quality of life, and even reduced mortality. It must be emphasized, however, that smoking cessation remains by far the most important intervention, since it can actually prevent the development of this disease. Physicians must play an active role in both the prevention and cessation of cigarette smoking and must not be content to simply diagnose and manage its consequences.

SUGGESTED READING

1. Albert RK, Martin TR, Lewis SW. Controlled clinical trial of methylprednisolone in patients with chronic bronchitis and acute respiratory insufficiency. Ann Intern Med 1980; 92:753–758.
2. American Thoracic Society. Standards for the diagnosis and care of patients with chronic obstructive pulmonary disease. Am J Respir Crit Care Med 1995; 152:S77–S120.
3. Anthonisen NR, Connett JE, Kiley JP, Altose MD, Bailey WC, Buist AS. Effects of smoking intervention and the use of an inhaled anticholinergic bronchodilator on the rate of decline of FEV_1: the lung health study. JAMA 1994; 272:1497–1505.
4. Callahan CM, Dittus RS, Katz BP. Oral corticosteroid therapy for patients with stable chronic obstructive pulmonary disease: a meta-analysis. Ann Intern Med 1991; 114:216–223.
5. European Respiratory Society. Optimal assessment and management of chronic obstructive pulmonary disease. Eur Respir J 1995; 8:1398–1420.
6. Gay PC, Hubmayr RD, Stroetz RW. Efficacy of nocturnal nasal ventilation in stable, severe chronic obstructive pulmonary disease during a 3-month controlled trial. Mayo Clin Proc 1996; 71:533–542.
7. Kramer N, Meyer TJ, Meharg J, Cece RD, Hill NS. Randomized, prospective trial of noninvasive positive pressure ventilation in acute respiratory failure. Am J Respir Crit Care Med 1995; 151:1799–1806.
8. Nocturnal Oxygen Therapy Trial Group. Continuous or nocturnal oxygen therapy in hypoxemic chronic obstructive lung disease. Ann Intern Med 1980; 93:391–398.
9. Thompson WH, Nielson CP, Carvalho P, Charan NB, Crowley JJ. Controlled trial of oral prednisone in outpatients with acute COPD exacerbation. Am J Respir Crit Care Med 1996; 154:407–412.
10. Sciurba FS, Rogers RM, Keenan RJ, Slivka WA, Gorcsan J, Ferson P. Improvement in pulmonary function and elastic recoil after lung reduction surgery for diffuse emphysema. N Engl J Med 1996; 334:1095–1099.
11. Vaz Fragoso CA, Miller MA. Review of the clinical efficacy of theophylline in the treatment of chronic obstructive pulmonary disease. Am Rev Respir Dis 1993; 147:S40–S47.

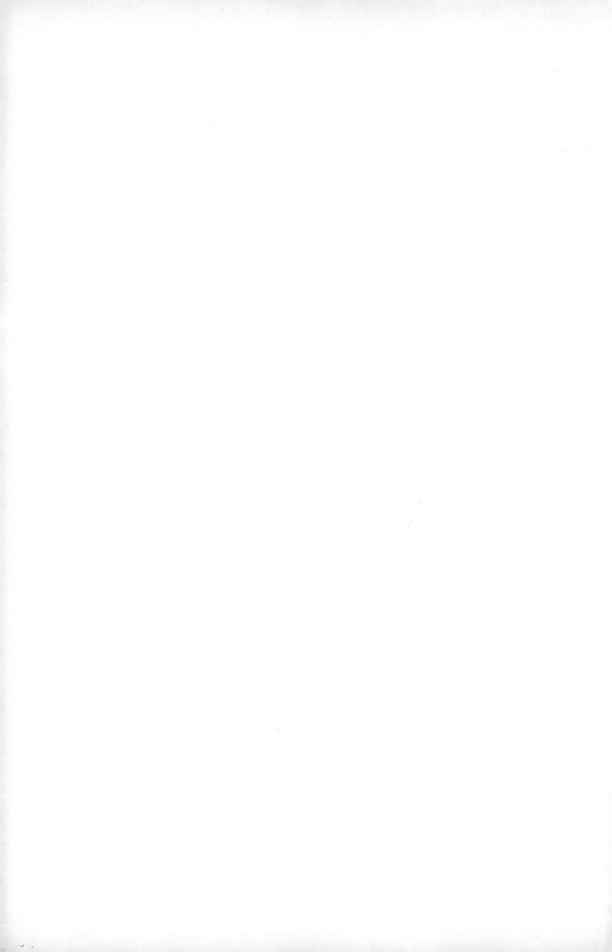

28
Sarcoidosis

Gunnar Gudmundsson
National University Hospital
Reykjavik, Iceland

Gary W. Hunninghake
University of Iowa
Iowa City, Iowa

INTRODUCTION

Sarcoidosis is a multisystem disease, characterized by formation of noncaseating granulomas in various organs but most often in the lungs and thoracic lymph nodes. The cause of sarcoidosis is unknown. It occurs worldwide and affects persons of both sexes, all races, and all ages. The prevalence of the disease has been estimated in several studies to range from 1 to 80 cases per 100,000 population. Certain ethnic groups and races are more prone to develop sarcoidosis. There are also differences in the severity of disease and patterns of organ involvement in these racial and ethnic groups. Scandinavians, Irish, and U.S. black populations have higher incidence rates of sarcoidosis than other groups. Caucasian patients frequently have a more benign form of the disease, while black patients often have a more severe form of sarcoidosis.

PATHOGENESIS

Since the cause of sarcoidosis is not known, its pathogenesis is not well understood. It is thought, however, that sarcoidosis occurs as a result of exposure to an unknown antigen. A schematic illustration of a possible pathogenesis is shown in Fig. 1. The early response of the lung in sarcoidosis is characterized by a mononuclear cell infiltrate that sets the stage for granuloma formation. This mononuclear cell response contains cells with the characteristics of antigen-specific T lymphocytes and antigen-presenting macrophages. Most of the T cells are of the T-helper 1 (Th1) phenotype; they secrete large amounts of interleukin-2 (IL-2) and interferon-γ. The macrophages are also activated to release the Th1-type cytokine, IL-12, and other cytokines, like tumor necrosis factor (TNF) and IL-1, that are necessary for granuloma formation. Some of the macrophages differentiate into the multinucleated giant cells and epithelioid cells that are characteristic of granulomas.

475

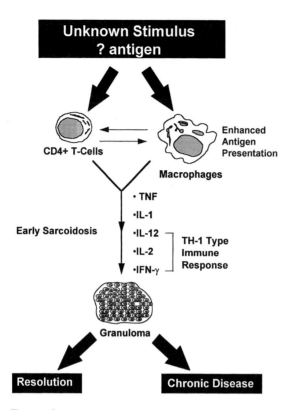

Figure 1 Pathogenesis of sarcoidosis. Schematic illustration of possible mechanism of pathogenesis in sarcoidosis. See text for details. (TNF, tumor necrosis factor; IL, interleukin; IFN-γ, interferon gamma.)

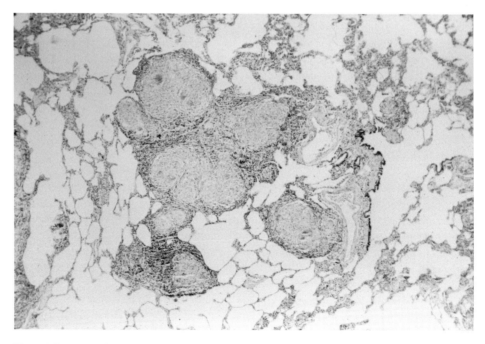

Figure 2 Photomicrograph of granuloma. Shown is a typical sarcoid granulomatous inflammatory response with surrounding fibrosis in lung tissue (hematoxylin and eosin, ×10).

T lymphocytes often form a rim around the granulomas. If this early response does not resolve, fibroblasts and mast cells surround the granuloma and produce collagen and proteoglycans, resulting in fibrosis. A photomicrograph of a sarcoid granuloma is illustrated in Fig. 2.

CLINICAL MANIFESTATIONS

Sarcoidosis can affect any organ of the body. The clinical manifestations depend on which organ is involved and the severity of organ involvement. As shown in Table 1, the lungs and lymphatics are most frequently affected, in greater than 90% of patients. The liver is affected in 40–70% of cases, but it is often asymptomatic. In about 30% of cases of sarcoidosis, there is involvement of the musculoskeletal system. Eyes and skin are affected in about one-quarter of patients with sarcoidosis, the endocrine system in 10% of patients, and the heart or nervous system in about 5%. Other organs are involved less frequently.

Patients with sarcoidosis may present in a number of different ways; however, a few types of presentations are most common. Some have no symptoms and their disease is discovered only during screening or workup for other reasons. Others present only with systemic symptoms, such as malaise, fever, weight loss, anorexia, and fatigue. Alternatively, patients may present with chronic involvement of an organ system, like the lung, with few systemic symptoms. With further evaluation, involvement of various organ systems is usually detected in these patients. Lofgren's syndrome is a common manifestation of acute disease, characterized by erythema nodosum, bilateral hilar adenopathy, and polyarthralgias.

The lungs are involved in almost all cases. Even when other organ systems account for most of the patient's symptoms or abnormal findings, subclinical lung disease is commonly present, and it may become important later on. The airways of the lungs can be involved, and these patients may present with dyspnea, airflow limitation, stridor, wheezing, or chronic cough. Diffuse lung disease is a common clinical presentation for acute sarcoidosis and is usually associated with hilar adenopathy. These patients present most often with dyspnea on exertion and sometimes with cough. Patients with hilar adenopathy

Table 1 Frequency of Organ Involvement

Organ	Frequency of involvement	Examples of presentation
Lungs	>90%	Asymptomatic, parenchymal lung disease, airway involvement
Lymphatic system	~90%	Lymphadenopathy, splenomegaly
Heart	~5–10%	Infiltrative cardiomyopathy, pericarditis, conduction defects, arrhythmias
Eyes	~25%	Anterior uveitis, corneal involvement
Nervous system	~5%	Nerve palsies, intracranial mass lesions, meningitis
Skin	~25%	Erythema nodosum, lupus pernio, plaques, and nodules
Musculoskeletal system	~30%	Polyarthritis, muscle weakness, myalgias
Endocrine system	~10%	Hypercalcemia, pituitary insufficiency
Liver	~40–70%	Granulomatous hepatitis

alone can be asymptomatic or may present with dyspnea with or without systemic symptoms. Lymphadenopathy, both intrathoracic (hilar or paratracheal) and peripheral nodes, can become symptomatic if the lymph nodes encroach on other organs or blood vessels. Atypical chest pain is often a manifestation of hilar adenopathy. Enlargement of the spleen can cause anemia, leukopenia, and/or thrombocytopenia and may lead to symptoms because of its size. Myocardial sarcoidosis can present in many ways, including sudden death. Other presentations include congestive heart failure, pericarditis, infiltrative cardiomyopathy, papillary muscle dysfunction, arrhythmias, and conduction abnormalities. Ocular sarcoidosis most commonly presents as anterior uveitis, with symptoms of lacrimation, photophobia, and blurry vision. Other eye lesions include conjunctival papules, retinal vasculitis, lacrimal gland involvement, and dacryocystitis. Among the presentations of neurosarcoidosis are cranial and peripheral neuropathies and space-occupying lesions. Hypothalamic and pituitary lesion also occur. Cutaneous manifestations can be divided into those characterized by noncaseating granulomas or erythema nodosum, which is a nongranulomatous, vasculitic type of lesion. Granulomatous skin lesions include plaques and papules. Involvement of the musculoskeletal system most commonly presents as arthralgias or arthritis, but muscle involvement is also seen. Hypercalcemia occurs less frequently than hypercalciuria. The liver can be enlarged and portal hypertension and other signs of hepatic failure can be seen. Abnormal liver function tests are common.

TREATMENT

The natural history and prognosis of sarcoidosis is highly variable, and many patients improve spontaneously. For this reason, it can be difficult to decide whom to treat and when. It is important to consider that treatment can cause more harm than the disease itself. Therapy is indicated, however, when the disease causes dysfunction of vital organs or when it is clearly worsening. For this reason, it is often prudent to observe the patient frequently for a period of time if there is no clear indication for treatment at the initial presentation—i.e., involvement of critical organs or clear evidence of a recent progression of the disease. The prognosis for complete resolution of intrathoracic disease can be estimated by the appearance of the disease on chest radiographs. A staging system that is based on chest radiographs is outlined in Table 2, and examples of these chest radiographs are shown in Fig. 3. Stage I disease is associated with a 60–80% rate of complete resolution of symptoms and radiographic findings. This increases to greater than 90% if it is associated with erythema nodosum and systemic symptoms. The complete remission rate in stage II disease is 50–60%, and stage III disease resolves in less than 30% of cases. It is important to note, however, that persistent symptoms and abnormal findings on chest radiographs do not necessarily imply active disease. Often patients with these findings

Table 2 Radiographic Staging in Thoracic Sarcoidosis

Stage	Findings
Stage 0	Normal chest radiograph
Stage I	Bilateral hilar lymphadenopathy (BHL)
Stage II	BHL and parenchymal infiltrates
Stage III	Parenchymal infiltrates alone

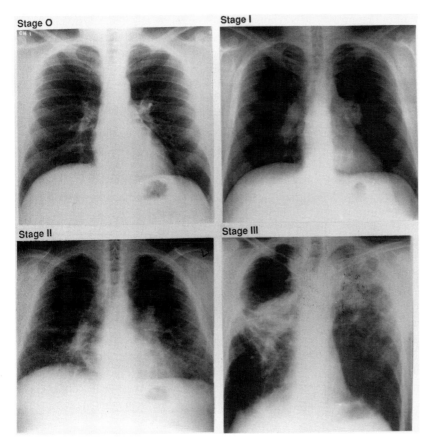

Figure 3 Radiographic stages of sarcoidosis. Shown are posteroanterior chest radiographs illustrating stages 0 through III of thoracic sarcoidosis.

have "burnt out" sarcoidosis, and they do not benefit from therapy. For those patients in whom it is not clear whether the disease is active, follow-up examinations to detect progression of the disease are the best means to determine need for therapy. Serial pulmonary function tests are a useful means to detect progression of pulmonary sarcoidosis.

Many tests other than chest radiographs or pulmonary function tests have been developed to predict the clinical course of sarcoidosis and response to therapy. Bronchoalveolar lavage fluid shows increased numbers of lymphocytes in the majority of patients, with a ratio of CD4+/CD8+ cells that is increased. These findings are not specific for sarcoidosis and have not been found to be helpful to predict prognosis or need for therapy. Serum angiotensin-converting enzyme is produced by activated macrophages and granulomas, and serum values are elevated in 60–70% of patients. However, this test can be abnormal in multiple other diseases, including pulmonary tuberculosis, idiopathic pulmonary fibrosis, and hypersensitivity pneumonitis. Most importantly, this test has not been shown to be a good indicator of the need for therapy in patients with sarcoidosis. In such patients, gallium 67 is taken up by activated macrophages and can detect sarcoid lesions. This uptake is not specific for sarcoidosis and can be seen in conditions such as pneumonia and tuberculosis. Most importantly, gallium 67 scanning has not been shown to predict need for therapy or prognosis. The best approach is close follow-up of patients. This should include a careful history and physical examination and tests targeted to organ systems that were determined to be involved at the time of the initial presentation. Routine tests can be used to monitor lung function. Serial chest radiographs should also be obtained. The frequency of radiographic exams and pulmonary function tests is determined by the extent of lung involvement and by changes in therapy. High-resolution computed tomography of the thorax is very sensitive in defining the extent and type of lung involvement. The findings of cystic air spaces and architectural distortion often indicate irreversible disease, while ground-glass changes, irregular linear and nodular opacities, and interlobular septal thickening are more likely to be reversible. Some of these changes are shown in Fig. 4. Another important finding on chest CT can be the presence of bronchiectasis. As many as one-third of patients with advanced radiographic changes will have this abnormality. The finding is important because symptoms in these patients often improve with antibiotic therapy, and they are often treated, inappropriately, with corticosteroid therapy. Exercise testing with measurement of gas-exchange abnormalities may be more sensitive than pulmonary function tests for detecting subtle lung disease. Bronchoscopy is usually performed to establish a diagnosis and it can be helpful to detect focal airway abnormalities. A variety of tests can be used to monitor cardiac sarcoidosis, depending on the manifestations of the disease. To assess myocardial involvement, echocardiography and thallium-201 radionuclide imaging can be used. Electrocardiograms and heart rhythm monitoring can be used to detect arrhythmias and heart block. For liver disease, ultrasound and biochemical markers can be helpful. For ocular sarcoidosis, serial slit-lamp examinations are commonly performed. Tests used to follow neurosarcoidosis depend on the presentation and type of disease. Magnetic resonance imaging and computed tomography are often used to monitor intracranial sarcoidosis. Nerve conduction studies and electromyographic studies help in

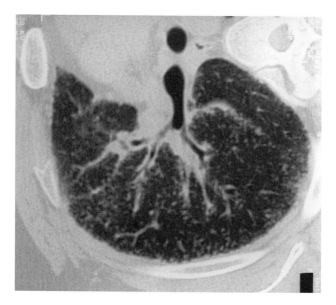

Figure 4   Example of a high-resolution computed tomography slide from a patient with stage II sarcoidosis. Shown are changes that are typical for sarcoidosis, such as accentuation of bronchovascular bundles and nodules.

evaluating involvement of peripheral nerves and muscle. Routine blood and urine tests can be used to detect and monitor hypercalcemia, hypercalciuria, and renal disease.

Corticosteroids

Corticosteroids have been the mainstay of therapy for sarcoidosis for a number of years. Studies have shown that they are effective for short-term stabilization of the disease, as manifested by regression of symptoms and improvement of abnormalities on tests, such as chest radiographic findings. However, there are no studies that have convincingly shown corticosteroids to affect long-term outcome. These agents also have the potential for serious side effects. For these reasons, they should be used only in patients who will benefit from the therapy, at the lowest possible dose, and for as short a time as possible. Particular attention should be given to preventing side effects from therapy. General guidelines for the treatment of sarcoidosis are shown in Fig. 5.

Pulmonary Sarcoidosis

Parenchymal Lung Disease

Overall, stage I disease will require treatment less frequently than stage II or III disease. Stage I disease most often resolves or stabilizes spontaneously. Corticosteroids are, therefore, seldom needed. If stage I disease is associated with fever, polyarthropathy, and/or erythema nodosum, nonsteroidal anti-inflammatory drugs can be used. If these agents are not effective, then a low dose of prednisone (20 mg/day) will usually result in improvement. In this instance, long-term treatment is not necessary. It is more common for stage II and III disease to need treatment with corticosteroids. A major reason to treat these forms of the disease is if there is evidence of a recent (within the past 3 months) deterioration in lung function at the initial presentation of the disease or if there is evidence of deterioration in lung function on follow-up examination. Often but not always, patients with stage III or IV disease have "burnt out" lung disease that does not benefit from therapy with corticosteroids.

Inhaled corticosteroid therapy has been used in patients with sarcoidosis with airway

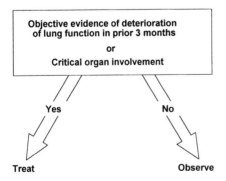

Figure 5 Treatment of sarcoidosis. Suggested scheme for making treatment decisions on initial evaluation of patients with sarcoidosis. Pulmonary sarcoidosis needs treatment only if there is objective evidence of deterioration in lung function. Critical organ involvement is discussed further in the text.

Management Decisions for Treatment of Extrapulmonary Sarcoidosis

- **Absolute indications for treatment**

  * Upper airway
  * Nervous system
  * Cardiac disease
  * Ocular sarcoidosis
  * Hypercalcemia

- **Possible indications for treatment**

  * Skin disease
  * Splenomegaly
  * Erythema nodosum
  * Lymphadenopathy
  * Constitutional symptoms
  * Abnormal liver function tests

Figure 6 Treatment of extrathoracic sarcoidosis. Critical organ involvement almost always calls for corticosteroid treatment and sometimes alternative treatment, as discussed in the text. In other instances, the need for treatment can be based on symptoms and signs and how disabling the disease is.

involvement, especially when asthma-like symptoms are present. Sarcoid lesions can cause stenosis of airways, resulting in chronic cough and collapse of airways; bronchoscopic interventions can been used to treat these complications. These procedures include placement of stents, balloon dilatation, and laser therapy.

Extrathoracic Sarcoidosis

Guidelines for the use of corticosteroids in extrathoracic disease are given in Fig. 6. Neurosarcoidosis, cardiac sarcoidosis, ocular sarcoidosis, hypercalcemia, and upper airway involvement with sarcoidosis almost always call for systemic corticosteroid therapy. With the exception of hypercalcemia (which responds well to therapy), a higher initial dose of corticosteroids (i.e., 60–80 mg of prednisone per day) is often used initially to treat these manifestations of sarcoidosis. Prolonged treatment of these manifestations of the disease is often needed. Skin involvement and lymph node, spleen, and parotid enlargement resulting in significant symptoms can often be treated with lower doses of corticosteroids, such as 20 mg daily, followed by tapering to 20 mg every other day. Mild, asymptomatic liver involvement does not require therapy.

Ocular Sarcoidosis

Topical steroids and cycloplegics are commonly used to treat anterior uveitis. Up to half of patients with anterior uveitis have an acute and self-limited inflammation, but the remaining patients can have chronic or recurrent disease. These patients often require systemic corticosteroid therapy. More extensive disease, such as infiltration of lacrimal glands, requires systemic steroid therapy. Periocular steroid injections are used in selected instances. Laser photocoagulation and surgery are also used. Glaucoma from chronic inflammation can be difficult to treat and often needs surgical intervention.

Cardiac Sarcoidosis

This form of sarcoidosis needs aggressive treatment, initially with systemic high-dose corticosteroid therapy, since it can be life-threatening. Other immunosuppressive agents may also be needed, and often other treatments are necessary, such as therapy for heart failure and antiarrhythmic agents. Permanent pacemakers and implantable cardioverter-defibrillator units may sometimes be needed. Surgical resection of ventricular aneurysms can help control ventricular arrhythmias. The role of heart transplantation is discussed further on.

Neurosarcoidosis

Systemic corticosteroids in doses of 60–80 mg daily are used as initial therapy for intracranial lesions and neuropathies, both peripheral and cranial. Cyclosporine has been used to treat cases refractory to corticosteroid therapy. The use of radiation therapy has been described for neurosarcoidosis but is rarely used today. Surgical treatment is sometimes necessary for mass lesions that cause increased intracranial pressure, especially if hydrocephalus is present. Medications to control seizures are sometimes needed.

Hypercalcemia

Sarcoid granulomas can produce 1,25-dihydroxyvitamin D. This causes increased intestinal absorption of calcium, bone resorption, and hypercalcemia. It usually responds well to low-dose corticosteroid therapy, using 10–20 mg of prednisone daily. Alternative agents are ketoconazole and hydroxychloroquine.

Dermatological Sarcoidosis

Large and/or disfiguring lesions often need systemic corticosteroid therapy. In other cases, intralesional injections of corticosteroids or their topical use may be effective. Methotrexate and hydroxychloroquine have been shown to be beneficial in treating dermatological manifestations. Erythema nodosum often responds to nonsteroidal anti-inflammatory drugs.

Liver Involvement

Mildly abnormal liver function tests do not need to be treated, but significant abnormalities require therapy with corticosteroids. Treatment often improves liver function but does not always normalize these abnormal findings.

Duration of Treatment with Corticosteroids

It is a common practice to maintain the initial dose of corticosteroids for 6–12 weeks and then gradually taper the dose to 5–10 mg daily or 10–20 mg every other day, as outlined in Fig. 7. Therapy is often continued at this lower dose for 6 months (except for erythema nodosum or systemic symptoms alone). After this period of time, therapy can be discontinued in many patients, but relapses may occur. With the exception of severe eye, heart, or neurological disease, an attempt should be made to taper patients off therapy after 6 months. If relapse occurs, therapy can be restarted and the patient usually responds to a second course of therapy.

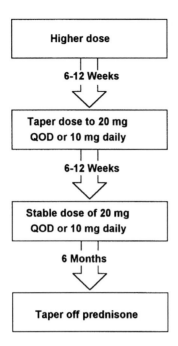

Figure 7 Treatment of pulmonary sarcoidosis. If the decision is made to treat the patient, prednisone is initiated at a dose of 0.5–1 mg/kg. The patient is then kept on this dose for 3 months. It is then tapered over the next 3 months. This dose is continued for 6 months and then discontinued.

Alternative Therapies for Sarcoidosis

Treatment modalities other than corticosteroids are needed in certain instances. Diabetic patients, in whom corticosteroid therapy is relatively contraindicated, would be candidates for alternative therapies. Also, patients who require high-dose corticosteroid therapy, could be treated instead with lower doses of corticosteroids in combination with cytotoxic agents. Alternative therapy can equally be used when the disease is resistant to corticosteroids and continues to progress despite treatment, and also when side effects from corticosteroids, even at low doses, are not tolerated or are not acceptable.

Cytotoxic Agents

Cytotoxic agents are most commonly used as corticosteroid-sparing agents or when corticosteroid therapy fails. Most reports of their use are in the form of uncontrolled studies or case reports. Methotrexate is the agent most commonly used, both as a steroid-sparing agent and when the disease is refractory to corticosteroids. Azathioprine has been used for therapy of chronic disease and may have efficacy similar to that of methotrexate. It is usually used in conjunction with prednisone. Cyclophosphamide and chlorambucil are usually used to treat refractory, chronic disease. The use of cytotoxic agents and their side effects is summarized in Table 3.

Other Agents

The antimalarials chloroquine and hydroxychloroquine have been used mainly to treat skin disease, such as lupus pernio. They have also been used for the treatment of hypercal-

Table 3 Cytotoxic Agents Used in the Treatment of Sarcoidosis

Drug	Dose	Examples of toxicity
Methotrexate	10–15 mg weekly	Hepatitis, pneumonitis
Azathioprine	50–200 mg daily	Myelosuppression
Chlorambucil	2–4 mg daily	Dermatitis, hepatitis
Cyclophosphamide	1–2 mg/kg daily	Cystitis, malignancy, leukopenia

cemia. The major side effects are gastrointestinal and ocular. All patients should have regular ophthalmological evaluation while being treated, and these medications should not be used in patients with active eye disease. The most commonly used dose for hydroxychloroquine is 200–400 mg per day.

Cyclosporine has been used to treat refractory, chronic disease, including neurosarcoidosis. The dose most commonly used is 5–10 mg/kg daily. It has multiple side effects, such as hypertension and renal insufficiency, that have limited its use.

Antibiotics are used to treat recurrent infections, which are often seen in patients with pulmonary sarcoidosis, especially those with bronchiectasis.

Nonsteroidal anti-inflammatory drugs are often used to treat fever, polyarthropathy, and/or erythema nodosum and may sometimes be the only treatment required.

Pulmonary Rehabilitation

Pulmonary sarcoidosis can lead to severe lung damage, with hypoxia and chronic symptoms such as dyspnea and cough that limit patients activity. This often leads to a sedentary lifestyle that results in deconditioning and a further increase in symptoms of dyspnea. Pulmonary rehabilitation can improve the quality of life in patients with such problems. The two main objectives of pulmonary rehabilitation, as defined by the American Thoracic Society, are to (1) control or alleviate as much as possible the symptoms that result from respiratory impairment and (2) teach the patient how to achieve optimal capacity for carrying out his or her activities of daily living. These goals can often be accomplished on an outpatient basis. Some of the components of such a program include exercise and education. Supplemental oxygen therapy is indicated in patents with hypoxia at rest and/or with exercise. Patients are encouraged to continue the program at home after supervision is finished.

Organ Transplantation

Chronic sarcoidosis can lead to severe irreversible organ damage and death. In some instances, the only treatment to prevent death is organ transplantation. The organs most commonly transplanted in patients with sarcoidosis are the lungs and heart, but liver transplantation has also been described. In general, the guidelines for recipient selection for transplantation are similar for sarcoidosis as for other diseases. A common problem in follow-up has been recurrence of sarcoidosis in the allograft. This is, however, often asymptomatic and does not compromise graft function.

SUGGESTED READING

1. Bresnitz EA, Strom BL. Epidemiology of sarcoidosis. Epidemiol Rev 1983; 5:124–156.
2. du Bois RM. Corticosteroids in sarcoidosis: friend of foe? Eur Respir J 1994; 7:1203–1209.
3. Elgart ML. Cutaneous sarcoidosis: Definition and types of lesions. Clin Dermatol 1986; 4:35–45.
4. Fleming HA. Cardiac sarcoidosis. Semin Respir Dis 1986; 8:65–71.
5. Hunninghake G, Crystal GR. Pulmonary sarcoidosis: a disorder mediated by excess helper T-lymphocytes at sites of disease activity. N Engl J Med 1981; 305:429–434.
6. Hutchinson J. Cases of Mortimer's malady. Arch Surg 1898; 9:307.
7. Hunninghake GW, Gilbert S, Pueringer R, Dayton C, Floerchinger C, Helmers R, Merchant R, Wilson J, Galvin J, Schwartz. Outcome of the treatment of sarcoidosis. Am J Respir Crit Care Med 1994; 149:893–898.
8. Lower EE, Baughman RP. The use of low dose methotrexate in refractory sarcoidosis. Am J Med Sci 1990; 299:153–157.
9. Mana J, Salazar A, Manresa F. Clinical factors predicting persistence of activity in sarcoidosis: a multivariate analysis of 193 cases. Respiration 1994; 61:219–225.
10. Muller NL, Miller RR. Computed tomography of chronic infiltrative lung disease: Part 2. Am Rev Respir Dis 1990; 142:1440–1448.
11. Selroos O. Treatment of sarcoidosis. Sarcoidosis 1994; 11:80–83.
12. Sharma OP, Sharma AM. Sarcoidosis of the nervous system: a clinical approach. Arch Intern Med 1991; 151:1317–1321.
13. Silver MR, Messner LV. Sarcoidosis and its ocular manifestations. J Am Optom Assoc 1994; 65:321–327.
14. Thomas PD, Hunninghake GW. Current concepts of the pathogenesis of sarcoidosis. Am Rev Respir Dis 1987; 135:747–760.
15. Weissler JC. Sarcoidosis: immunology and clinical management. Am J Med Sci 1994; 307:233–245.

29

Chronic Diffuse Parenchymal Lung Diseases

Talmadge E. King, Jr.
University of California
San Francisco General Hospital
San Francisco, California

Marvin I. Schwarz
University of Colorado
Denver, Colorado

INTRODUCTION

Definition and Epidemiology

The diffuse parenchymal lung diseases (DPLD), often collectively referred to as the interstitial lung diseases (ILDs), are a heterogeneous group of disorders classified together because of similar clinical, roentgenographic, physiological, or pathological manifestations. The most common known causes of DPLD are related to occupational and environmental exposures, especially to inorganic or organic dusts. Sarcoidosis, idiopathic pulmonary fibrosis (IPF), and pulmonary fibrosis associated with connective tissue diseases are the most common ILDs of unknown etiology. In this chapter, the illnesses of known cause are presented first, followed by diseases of unknown etiology.

It is not necessarily the clinical diagnosis that directs treatment and determines prognosis but rather the underlying histology. Different histological appearances can be responsible for the DPLD that appears in a single clinical entity. The DPLD that have underlying cellular interstitial responses are more apt to respond to treatment than those demonstrating interstitial fibrosis. A number of individual diseases have several potential underlying pathological appearances, and the histological pattern clearly affects outcome for the individual patient.

Population-based studies of the incidence and prevalence of interstitial lung diseases are few and the accuracy of the data is limited. A population-based study established in 1988 in Bernalillo County, New Mexico, showed that the prevalence of interstitial lung disease was higher in men (80.9 per 100,000) than in women (67.2 per 100,000). Similarly, the overall incidence of interstitial lung disease was slightly more common in men (31.5 per 100,000/year) than women (26.1 per 100,000/year). The prevalence and incidence of pulmonary fibrosis increased markedly with age; for example, among men and women 75 years of age or older, the prevalence of idiopathic pulmonary fibrosis was 250 per

100,000 and the incidence was 160 per 100,000/year. Vital statistics on pulmonary fibrosis are also scant and known to be of limited value. In 1988, there were an estimated 30,000 hospitalizations (compared to 665,000 hospitalizations for COPD and asthma) and 4851 deaths in the United States attributed to pulmonary fibrosis. The age-adjusted rate of pulmonary fibrosis among decedents in the United States increased from 48.6 per million in 1979 to 50.9 per million in 1991 among men and from 21.4 to 27.2 per million among women. Also, the frequency with which pulmonary fibrosis was listed as the underlying cause of death increased from 40% in 1979 to 56% in 1991. Importantly, the age-adjusted mortality rates varied by state, with the lowest rates in the Midwest and Northeast and the highest rates in the West and Southwest. Deaths from pulmonary fibrosis increase with increasing age.

Clinical Presentations of DPLD

Patients with DPLD have several recognizable clinical presentations. The most common is with progressive dyspnea and cough, usually present from days to several years, with an abnormal chest radiograph and physiological impairment of the lung. Other important symptoms and signs may include hemoptysis, wheezing, finger clubbing, and chest pain. A minority of patients with DPLD complain of the aforementioned symptoms but have normal chest radiographs. In this case, high-resolution computed tomography (HRCT), physiological testing, or bronchoalveolar lavage will often reveal abnormalities. However, in some cases, both HRCT and routine lung function testing (spirometry, lung volumes, DL_{CO_2}) are unrevealing. The most sensitive test for the determination of the presence of DPLD is formal exercise testing that measures rest and exercise arterial oxygen tensions, the alveolar-arterial oxygen gradients, and the dead-space ventilation. Rest followed by exercise oximetry demonstrating oxygen desaturation is adequate if the test is performed on a treadmill and according to an exercise protocol. However, less formal testing (walking up stairs, etc.) that demonstrates oxygen desaturation suggests the possibility of DPLD.

Patients may present with DPLD associated with another disease, such as a connective tissue disease. Importantly, clinical findings suggestive of a connective tissue disease (musculoskeletal pain, weakness, fatigue, fever, joint pains or swelling, photosensitivity, Raynaud's phenomenon, pleuritis, dry eyes, dry mouth) should be carefully elicited. The connective tissue diseases may be difficult to rule out, since the pulmonary manifestations occasionally precede the more typical systemic manifestations by months or years (particularly in rheumatoid arthritis, systemic lupus erythematosus, and polymyositis-dermatomyositis). Patients with DPLD associated with predominantly pulmonary vascular disease, particularly primary pulmonary hypertension and recurrent pulmonary thromboemboli, also present with dyspnea and normal chest radiographs. In this situation there will be an isolated reduction of the diffusing capacity for carbon monoxide, exercise-induced hypoxemia, and increased dead-space ventilation.

Asymptomatic individuals may have interstitial opacities discovered on a routine chest radiograph. This presentation is not unusual, and in this case, physiological testing, particularly gas-exchange measurements, will indicate abnormalities and hopefully prompt the physician to investigate further. Finally, a rare patient may be identified with lung function abnormalities on simple office spirometry, particularly a restrictive ventilatory pattern without other abnormalities.

Several major problems concerning the medical treatment of patients with DPLD exist. The first is a delay in diagnosis. For example, it is not unusual to see patients who are eventually diagnosed as having IPF who, 5–10 years prior, had abnormal chest radiographs demonstrating basilar interstitial infiltrates. Further radiographic, physiological, and histological evaluation may not have been carried out because the patient was relatively asymptomatic or because simple spirometric measurements were normal. It is in the early stages of an DPLD that improvement following treatment is most likely. In spite of relatively few or no symptoms and minimal physiological abnormalities, an aggressive approach to diagnosis that eventually includes lung biopsy is recommended. Another important issue is that there are few if any controlled treatment trials in this group of diseases. Therefore, many of the recommendations for management in this chapter are guided by anecdotal data and the personal experience of the authors. The final issue is the limited number of drugs presently available for the treatment of ILD. Although extensive efforts to develop new anti-inflammatory and antifibrotic agents are in progress, corticosteroids, several of the immunosuppressive agents, colchicine, and lung transplantation are today's potential therapies for ILD.

Initial Evaluation of DPLD

The initial evaluation should include a complete history and physical examination. The initial laboratory evaluation should include biochemical tests to evaluate liver and renal function and hematological tests to check for evidence of anemia, polycythemia, or leukocytosis. Serological studies should be obtained if clinically indicated by features suggestive of a connective tissue disease or vasculitis: sedimentation rate, antinuclear antibodies, rheumatoid factor, hypersensitivity panel, antineutrophil cytoplasmic antibodies, anti–basement membrane antibody. A recent chest x-ray should be obtained, and it also is important to review all old chest x-rays to assess tempo of change in disease activity. Complete lung function testing (spirometry, lung volumes, diffusing capacity) and resting room air arterial blood gases should be obtained. Common diseases—such as COPD, anemia, heart failure, and mycobacterial or fungal disease—can mimic DPLD, so they must be ruled out. In most cases, this initial evaluation will distinguish DPLD from other conditions.

Duration of Clinical Manifestations
Prior to Presentation

In the vast majority of DPLD the symptoms and signs are chronic, spanning months to years. This is typical in idiopathic pulmonary fibrosis, sarcoidosis, and pulmonary histiocytosis X (eosinophilic granuloma). Some DPLD may present with acute (days to weeks) or subacute (weeks to months) manifestations. These latter processes are often confused with atypical pneumonias, since many have diffuse radiographic opacities, fever, or relapses of disease activity. Examples include acute idiopathic interstitial pneumonia, acute eosinophilic pneumonia, hypersensitivity pneumonitis, bronchiolitis obliterans with organizing pneumonia, some drug-induced DPLD, the alveolar hemorrhage syndromes, and the acute immunological pneumonia that complicates either systemic lupus erythematosus or polymyositis.

Gender and Age

Gender is important in lymphangioleiomyomatosis, which occurs exclusively in premenopausal women. Also, DPLD in the connective tissue diseases is more common in women, the exception being DPLD in rheumatoid arthritis, which is more common in men. It is less likely to develop certain ILD, such as IPF, in patients under the age of 40. In patients under age 40 years, one is more likely to encounter sarcoidosis, eosinophilic granuloma, respiratory bronchiolitis, lymphangioleiomyomatosis, and desquamative interstitial pneumonia. In patients over 40 years, idiopathic pulmonary fibrosis and the pneumoconioses are more likely. The collagen vascular diseases, drug reactions, and hypersensitivity pneumonitis can occur at any age.

Environmental and Occupational History

The clinical evaluation of a patient with suspected DPLD includes a detailed review of potential environmental and occupational exposures for the purpose of excluding hypersensitivity pneumonitis or a pneumoconiosis. There is often a prolonged latent period between the pneumoconiotic exposure and the development of the ILD. Therefore it is important to obtain a lifelong work history. The environmental and occupational exposures that can lead to DPLD are discussed in Chaps. 39 and 40 of this text.

Drug Reaction

A drug reaction that results in DPLD can occur concomitantly with treatment or after the drug is withdrawn. Long latent periods (months to years) have been reported with certain cytotoxic chemotherapeutic agents. Moreover, chronic use of a drug—i.e., weekly methotrexate for rheumatoid arthritis or daily amiodarone for the prevention of potentially fatal cardiac arrhythmias—can result in a DPLD months to years after treatment is initiated. Drug-induced interstitial lung diseases are discussed below.

Collagen Vascular Disease

Interstitial pulmonary reactions that appear in an established collagen vascular disease do not usually present a problem in recognition. A variety of interstitial pneumonias with dissimilar responses to treatment and different outcomes can complicate these diseases. Moreover, drugs used for the treatment of these diseases (e.g., gold, methotrexate) can in themselves initiate a DPLD. Another potential problem in assigning DPLD to a specific collagen vascular disease is that the pulmonary component may precede the more typical manifestations of that particular disease by months or even years. There also are nonspecific increases in serum autoantibodies (antinuclear antibodies, rheumatoid factor, etc.) in a number of DPLDs, such as IPF, asbestosis, sarcoidosis, and hypersensitivity pneumonitis.

Family History

There are other issues to consider in evaluating a patient with suspected DPLD. Variants of IPF and unusual DPLDs such as Gaucher's disease or Hermansky-Pudlack syndrome have a genetic predisposition; therefore, familial cases appear. Sarcoidosis affects members of the same family, although it is unclear whether this is a genetic or an environmental propensity. A pneumoconiosis is occasionally reported in household contacts whose exposure to the mineral dust is obtained by handling the clothes of a worker. Asbestos-related diseases (asbestosis, mesothelioma) as well as berylliosis have been contracted in this manner.

Smoking History

Smoking exerts an influence on the development of some DPLD. Three entities—eosinophilic granuloma of the lung, respiratory bronchiolitis associated interstitial lung disease (RB-ILD), and desquamative interstitial pneumonia (DIP)—are considered to be smoking-related diseases. There is also evidence to suggest that tobacco usage increases the risk of developing IPF and asbestosis. In contrast, there is a low incidence of hypersensitivity pneumonitis from a variety of different antigens in those patients who smoke.

Physical Examination

The physical examination commonly shows tachypnea, reduced chest expansion, and bibasilar end-inspiratory dry crackles ("Velcro rales"). Crackles are less likely to be heard in the granulomatous lung diseases, especially sarcoidosis. Crackles may be present in the absence of radiographic abnormalities on the chest radiograph. Clubbing of the digits is common in some patients (idiopathic pulmonary fibrosis, asbestosis) and rare in others (sarcoidosis). Signs of pulmonary hypertension and cor pulmonale are generally secondary manifestations of advanced DPLD, although they may be primary manifestations of a connective tissue disorder (e.g., progressive systemic sclerosis).

Role of Diagnostic Studies in the Evaluation of DPLD

Routine Laboratory Studies

The routine laboratory evaluation is often not helpful in DPLD but should include biochemical tests to evaluate liver and renal function and hematological tests to check for evidence of anemia, polycythemia, or leukocytosis. An elevated erythrocyte sedimentation rate and hypergammaglobulinemia are commonly observed but entirely nonspecific. Antinuclear antibodies and anti-immunoglobulin antibodies (rheumatoid factors) are identified in many of these patients even in the absence of a defined connective tissue disorder. Elevation of the LDH may be noted but is a nonspecific finding common to pulmonary disorders (e.g., alveolar proteinosis, idiopathic pulmonary fibrosis). An increase in the angiotensin-converting enzyme (ACE) level may be observed in sarcoidosis but is nonspecific, as elevated ACE levels have been noted in several interstitial diseases including hypersensitivity pneumonitis. Antibodies to organic antigens may be helpful when hypersensitivity pneumonitis is suspected, although it is nondiagnostic, because many individuals with exposure will have antibodies without clinical disease. The electrocardiogram is usually normal in the absence of pulmonary hypertension or concurrent cardiac disease.

Lung Imaging Studies

Chest Roentgenogram. The diagnosis of DPLD will often be suspected initially on the basis of an abnormal chest roentgenogram. The most common radiographic abnormality is a reticular or nodular pattern; however, mixed patterns of alveolar filling and increased interstitial markings are not unusual. Most DPLD has a predilection for the lower lung zones. As the disease progresses, there is widespread infiltration associated with reductions in lung volume and the appearance of pulmonary hypertension. A subgroup of DPLD has a predilection for the upper lung zones and often produces nodular infiltrates that result in upward contraction of the pulmonary hilus. With progression of the disease, small cystic structures appear, representing fibrous replacement of the normal alveolar architecture, as does radiographic honeycombing.

Although the chest roentgenogram is useful in suggesting the presence of DPLD, the correlation between the roentgenographic pattern and the stage of disease (clinical or histopathological) is generally poor. Only the radiographic finding of honeycombing (small cystic spaces) correlates with pathological findings. When present, honeycombing portends a poor prognosis.

High-Resolution Computed Tomography (HRCT). HRCT is well suited for evaluation of diffuse pulmonary parenchymal disease. Chapter 11 discusses this technique in detail. Pattern recognition in diffuse lung disease is enhanced because HRCT avoids the problem of superimposition of structures and is relatively independent of film exposure variables. While still in the middle of extensive research, HRCT offers (1) more accuracy than conventional chest x-ray in distinguishing airspace from interstitial lung disease; (2) earlier detection and confirmation of suspected diffuse lung disease, especially in the investigation of a symptomatic patient with a normal chest radiograph; (3) better assessment of the extent and distribution of disease; (4) the ability to disclose coexisting disease, e.g., to discern occult mediastinal adenopathy, carcinoma, or emphysema; and (5) utility in more specifically selecting appropriate type and site for biopsy.

Gallium-67 Lung Scanning. Gallium-67 lung scanning has been tried as a means of evaluating the inflammatory component of DPLD, since gallium is not taken up by normal lung parenchyma. Uptake may be diffuse or patchy and is felt to reflect an increased accumulation of inflammatory cells in the lung. To date, gallium scans have not been proven useful in staging or follow-up of ILD.

Physiological Testing

Pulmonary function tests are an important aspect of the evaluation of any patient with suspected DPLD (see also Chap. 9). The finding of an obstructive or restrictive pattern is important in narrowing the number of possible diagnoses. Most of the interstitial disorders have a restrictive defect with reduced TLC, FRC, and RV. Flow rates are decreased (FEV_1 and FVC), but this is related to the decreased lung volumes. The FEV_1/FVC ratio is usually normal or increased. Smoking history must be considered in interpreting the functional studies. Reduction in lung compliance is also common. Importantly, in symptomatic patients with normal chest radiographs and minimal or no restrictive disease, measurement of elastic recoil (the pressure-volume curve) may be helpful by identifying lung stiffness. A few disorders produce interstitial infiltrates and obstructive airflow limitation—e.g., sarcoidosis, lymphangioleiomyomatosis, hypersensitivity pneumonitis, tuberous sclerosis, and COPD with superimposed ILD.

The assessment of gas transfer as measured by the diffusing capacity for CO (DL_{CO}) may also be useful. The decrease in DL_{CO} is due in part to effacement of the alveolar capillary units but more importantly to the extent of mismatching of ventilation and perfusion of the alveoli. Lung regions with reduced compliance due either to fibrosis or excessive cellularity may be poorly ventilated but still be well-perfused. The severity of the DL_{CO} reduction does not correlate well with disease stage. In some DPLD there can be considerable reduction in lung volumes and/or severe hypoxemia but normal or only slightly reduced DL_{CO}. The presence of moderate to severe reductions of DL_{CO} in the presence of normal lung volumes should suggest DPLD with associated emphysema, pulmonary vascular disease, pulmonary histiocytosis X, or lymphangioleiomyomatosis.

The resting arterial blood gas may be normal or may reveal hypoxemia (secondary to a mismatching of ventilation to perfusion) and respiratory alkalosis. Carbon dioxide retention is rare and usually a manifestation of far-advanced end-stage disease. Importantly, a normal resting Pao_2 (or O_2 saturation by oximetry) does not rule out significant hypoxemia during exercise or sleep). Further, although hypoxemia with exercise and sleep is very common, secondary erythrocytosis is rarely observed in uncomplicated DPLD. Because resting hypoxemia is not always evident and severe exercise-induced hypoxemia may go undetected, it is important to perform exercise testing with serial measurement of arterial blood gases or oximetry. Arterial oxygen desaturation, a failure to decrease dead space appropriately with exercise (i.e., a high $\dot{V}_D/\dot{V}_T$ ratio), and an excessive increase in respiratory rate with a lower than expected recruitment of tidal volume provide useful information regarding physiological abnormalities and extent of disease. There is increasing evidence that serial assessment of resting and exercise gas exchange are the best methods to identify disease activity and responsiveness to treatment.

Bronchoalveolar Lavage

Subsegmental lavage through the wedged bronchoscope has been used to retrieve and examine cells and soluble constituents of the lower respiratory airspaces. Bronchoalveolar lavage (BAL) studies have been performed on patients with many types of DPLD. As a result of these studies, numerous hypotheses have been advanced regarding the pathogenesis of the interstitial diseases. Differences in the quantity and distribution of BAL cells and other components among the interstitial disorders allows one to (1) narrow the differential diagnostic possibilities between various types of DPLD; (2) define the stage of disease; and (3) assess the progression of disease or response to therapy. However, the utility of BAL in the clinical assessment and management of DPLD patients remains to be established. Table 1 provides a list of the BAL findings that can confirm or suggest a specific diagnosis.

Lung Biopsy

The specific diagnosis of DPLD is often made only after histological examination of lung tissue. In a limited number of cases, either the bronchoalveolar lavage cellular distribution, HRCT appearance, specific laboratory results, or chest radiograph—all in conjunction with the clinical story—is sufficient to establish the diagnosis. However, examination of lung tissue not only confirms a diagnosis, but the prognosis may also be established depending on the relative amounts of cellularity versus fibrosis. A transbronchial biopsy that yields a specific diagnosis is sufficient. This is often the case for the alveolar filling disorders, such as alveolar proteinosis, or in other DPLD such as sarcoidosis and lymphangiitic

Table 1 Specific Findings in Bronchoalveolar Lavage Fluid That Assist Diagnosis

Condition	Lavage Finding
Lymphangiitic carcinomatosis, alveolar cell carcinoma, pulmonary lymphoma	Malignant cells
Diffuse alveolar bleeding	Hemosiderin-laden macrophages, red blood cells
Alveolar proteinosis	Lipoproteinaceous intraalveolar material
Lipoid pneumonia	Fat globules in macrophages
Eosinophilic granuloma	Monoclonal antibody-(T6) positive histiocytes, macrophage Birbeck granules by electron microscopy
Asbestos-related pulmonary disease	Asbestos fibers, ferruginous bodies
Silicosis, silica dust exposure	Particles by polarized light microscopy
Berylliosis	Immunoreactive lymphocytes (lymphocyte transformation test)

Source: Adapted from Schwarz MI. Approach to the patient with interstitial lung disease. In: Kelley W, ed. *Essentials of Internal Medicine*. Philadelphia: Lippincott, 1994:1893–1897.

carcinomatosis. However, a biopsy that is interpreted as showing only nonspecific in-flammation and/or fibrosis is not acceptable. In this case, video-assisted thoracoscopic lung biopsy by an experienced chest surgeon is recommended. In many centers, the biopsy sites are directed by HRCT findings and should include areas with reticular or nodular opacities, those with ground-glass density, and normal-appearing lung.

OCCUPATIONAL AND ENVIRONMENTAL CAUSES OF DPLD

Occupational or environmental exposures are among the most common and important causes of ILD. In order to establish a potential link to disease, it is critical that a careful history be obtained. This topic is discussed in detail in Chaps. 39 and 40 of this textbook.

DRUG-INDUCED INTERSTITIAL LUNG DISEASE

Many drugs are capable of causing interstitial lung reactions, as listed in Table 2. Most of the interstitial reactions occur concurrently with the administration of the drug or imme-diately following completion of a course of therapy. There are, however, delayed reactions. A group of individuals developed restrictive lung disease secondary to pulmonary fibrosis following carmustine treatment for brain malignancies when they were children. The fi-

Table 2 Drug-Induced Interstitial Lung Diseases

Acute onset
  Diffuse alveolar damage
    Amiodarone
    Any cytotoxic agent (bleomycin, carmustine, busulfan, methotrexate, etc.)
    Nitrofurantoin
    Crack cocaine
    Interleukin-2
  Acute noncardiogenic pulmonary edema (probably diffuse alveolar damage)
    Cytosine arabinoside
    Methotrexate (intrathecal)
    Aspirin and related compound
    Narcotics
    Terbutaline
    Hydrochlorothiazide
    Colchicine
  Diffuse alveolar hemorrhage
    Crack cocaine
    Penicillamine
    Phenytoin
    Anticoagulants
    Thrombolytic agents
    Retinoic acid
    Cytotoxic drugs which cause diffuse alveolar damage
    Propylthiouracil

Table 2 Continued

Acute or subacute onset
  Eosinophilic pneumonia
    Nonsteroidal anti-inflammatory agents
    Antibiotics (ampicillin, minocycline, sulfa, nitrofurantoin, sulfasalazine)
  Bronchiolitis obliterans organizing pneumonia
    Amiodarone
    Gold
    Methotrexate
    Sulfasalazine
    Tocainide
    Nitrofurantoin
    Bleomycin
    Mitomycin
  Desquamative interstitial pneumonia
    Nitrofurantoin
    Sulfasalazine
  Lymphocytic interstitial pneumonia
    Nitrofurantoin
    Phenytoin
  Pulmonary veno-occlusive disease
    Carmustine
    Bleomycin
Subacute or chronic onset
  Usual interstitial pneumonia
    Cytotoxic agents (see above)
    Nitrofurantoin
    Tocainide
    Amiodarone
    Gold
  Cellular or nonspecific interstitial pneumonia
    Cytotoxic agents
    Gold
    Amiodarone
    Sulfasalazine
    Cephalosporin
    Minocycline
    Nilutamide
    Tocainide
    Nitrofurantoin
    Carbamazine
  Bronchiolitis obliterans
    Penicillamine?
    Gold
  Alveolar proteinosis
    Busulfan (?)
    Cyclophosphamide
  Lipoid pneumonia
    Mineral oil

brosis was recognized up to 17 years posttreatment. Pulmonary reactions can occur acutely after a single dose of the drug—for example, nitrofurantoin or crack cocaine inhalation. The majority of drug reactions, however, occur during the therapeutic period or immediately thereafter.

Factors that affect the development of a drug-induced interstitial lung disease include the patient's age, the initial dosing, the cumulative dose, and associated conditions. For example, patients who receive cytotoxic chemotherapy for underlying malignancy with either bleomycin, busulfan, or carmustine are at risk of developing an acute interstitial pneumonitis with underlying diffuse alveolar damage after radiation therapy or treatment with high concentrations of oxygen. Further, the use of several cytotoxic drugs in combination also enhances the development of an interstitial lung reaction. Other conditions enhance the development of a drug-induced interstitial lung disease. Patients being treated with amiodarone, for example, who undergo a surgical procedure are at risk of developing a picture resembling that of acute respiratory distress syndrome (ARDS) owing to diffuse alveolar damage. This was first described in patients receiving chronic amiodarone therapy, who required cardiac surgery or underwent pneumonectomy. In systemic diseases, which in themselves are associated with an interstitial reaction (the collagen vascular diseases), it is often difficult to distinguish between a drug-induced pneumonitis and one that is due to the underlying disease. This is often the case in patients receiving weekly methotrexate therapy for the treatment of either rheumatoid arthritis or polymyositis or where gold therapy is used for the treatment of rheumatoid arthritis. Withdrawal of the drug followed by improvement and eventual resolution of the interstitial lung disease confirms the diagnosis of drug toxicity. Further proof of a drug-related interstitial lung disease is the return of the pneumonitis with reinstatement of the drug (not recommended).

Treatment depends on recognition of a potential problem followed by withdrawal of the suspected offending agent. In some cases the gas-exchange abnormalities are so severe as to require assisted mechanical ventilation. In this situation, corticosteroid medications are very effective. This is especially true for drug-induced eosinophilic pneumonia, bronchiolitis obliterans organizing pneumonia (BOOP), and some cellular (nonspecific) interstitial pneumonias. In some patients with diffuse alveolar damage secondary to cytotoxic drugs, corticosteroids can also have a beneficial effect. In others, drug-induced diffuse alveolar damage may progress to pulmonary fibrosis in spite of corticosteroid therapy. There is no rationale for the continued use of immunosuppressive medication in cases that do not respond to corticosteroids. However, failure to respond to discontinuation of the drug and the addition of corticosteroid medication should raise the possibility of another cause for the interstitial pulmonary reaction.

FIBROTIC DISEASES OF UNKNOWN ETIOLOGY

Idiopathic Pulmonary Fibrosis (IPF)

Clinical Manifestations

IPF (or cryptogenic fibrosing alveolitis, CFA) is one of the more commonly occurring interstitial lung diseases of unknown etiology. The clinical features and treatment strategies for IPF serve as an example for many similar conditions. The symptoms of IPF are dyspnea on exertion and nonproductive cough. High-pitched end-inspiratory ''Velcro''-type crackles are heard on chest examination. In advanced disease, signs of cor pulmonale, digital clubbing, and cyanosis may be noted on physical examination.

Laboratory Features

The routine laboratory is often not helpful. An elevated erythrocyte sedimentation rate and hypergammaglobulinemia are commonly observed. Antinuclear antibodies, rheumatoid factors, and circulating immune complexes are identified in many of these patients. The electrocardiogram is usually normal in the absence of pulmonary hypertension or concurrent cardiac disease.

Chest Imaging Studies

The chest roentgenogram typically reveals diffuse reticular opacities in the lower lung zones (Fig. 1A). Diffuse or patchy "ground-glass" haziness, small cystic lesions (honeycombing), evidence of reduced lung volumes, and signs of pulmonary hypertension may be seen. High-resolution computed tomography (HRCT) findings in IPF include (1) ground-glass opacification, patchy, predominantly peripheral, airspace opacities or a "hazy" increase in lung density (an increase in CT lung density that does not obscure the underlying lung parenchyma); (2) a lower lung zone–predominant reticular pattern consisting largely of thickened interlobular septa and intralobular lines (Fig. 1B); and (3) combined ground-glass and reticular patterns. Honeycombing, traction bronchiectasis, and subpleural fibrosis may also be present, depending on the stage of the disease (Fig. 2).

Physiological Studies

Pulmonary function studies often reveal a restrictive impairment (decreased static lung volumes). The coefficient of retraction (maximal static transpulmonary pressure/total lung capacity) is increased. The diffusing capacity for carbon monoxide (DL_{CO}) is reduced. Arterial blood gases show hypoxemia often exaggerated or elicited by exercise and a low Pa_{CO_2}, denoting hyperventilation.

Bronchoalveolar Lavage (BAL)

BAL has a limited role in the diagnosis of IPF. Active IPF is characterized by a several-fold increase in the total number of inflammatory cells recovered from the respiratory tract. It has been shown that there is no correlation between the percentage of various cell types found in the lavage fluid in patients with idiopathic pulmonary fibrosis and various clinical parameters, serum tests, or pulmonary function studies. However, BAL lymphocytosis is associated with moderate to severe alveolar septal inflammation and with a relative absence of histological honeycombing on the lung biopsy. On the other hand, BAL neutrophilia and eosinophilia are not correlated significantly with any of the histopathological abnormalities common to idiopathic pulmonary fibrosis.

The relationship between BAL cellular abnormalities and clinical response to therapy has not been defined. A strong correlation has been suggested between the percentage of neutrophils in lavage fluid and the prognosis of IPF, and it has been suggested that modification of therapy could be guided by the neutrophil percentage found in lavage fluid. Lavage eosinophilia has been reported to be associated with a poor response to corticosteroids. BAL lymphocytosis at the time of presentation appears to predict corticosteroid responsiveness, while neutrophilia or eosinophilia occasionally respond better to cyclophosphamide therapy. Consequently, these data suggest that the initial bronchoalveolar lavage cell counts can help to predict response to treatment. The role and value of serial bronchoalveolar lavage in assessment of the clinical progress of patients with idiopathic pulmonary fibrosis appear somewhat limited, although they have been studied incompletely. The quantity and composition of pulmonary surfactant phospholipids and the

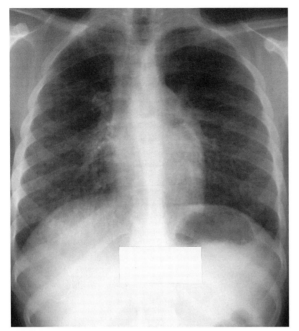

A

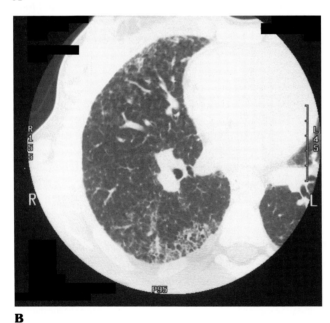

B

Figure 1   Idiopathic pulmonary fibrosis. A. Chest roentgenogram showing diffuse, reticular opacities in the middle to lower lung zones. B. High-resolution computed tomography (HRCT) scan of the right lung from the same patient shows diffuse subpleural reticular opacities. They appeared more extensive on HRCT than expected from the plain chest radiograph. Lung biopsy confirmed the presence of usual interstitial pneumonia.

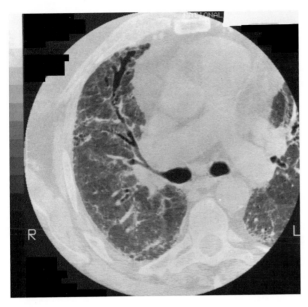

Figure 2 Idiopathic pulmonary fibrosis. High-resolution computed tomography scan of the right lung shows ground-glass opacities associated with traction bronchiectasis and subpleural fibrosis. These findings are consistent with a mainly fibrotic histology on lung biopsy. Honeycomb changes were seen in other regions of the lung. This patient died of progressive respiratory failure secondary to idiopathic pulmonary fibrosis.

associated protein secretory products of the alveolar type II cell [surfactant proteins A(SP-A), B(SP-B) and C(SP-C)] are abnormal in IPF. Several investigators have linked the patterns of abnormality in surfactant proteins and lipids to IPF course and response to therapy.

Lung Biopsy

The diagnosis of IPF (and many other DPLDs) generally requires open or thoracoscopic lung biopsy, since tissue obtained by transbronchial biopsy is usually insufficient. Lung biopsy is not indicated in the presence of extensive honeycombing on radiographic studies. The gross morphological findings in IPF range from a normal appearance in early cases to diffuse honeycombing in the later stages of the disease process. in the later stages of the disease process. Disease involvement is usually heterogeneous and worse in the lower lobes. Areas of mildly involved or even normal pulmonary parenchyma may be interspersed throughout a background of extensive fibrosis and honeycombing.

Usual interstitial pneumonia (UIP) is the histopathological pattern found on lung biopsy from patients with IPF. UIP is a specific pattern of interstitial pneumonia and should not be viewed as a pathological diagnosis of exclusion. At low magnification it has a heterogeneous appearance, with alternating areas of normal lung, interstitial inflammation, fibrosis, and honeycomb change. These changes affect the peripheral subpleural parenchyma most severely. The interstitial inflammation consists of an alveolar septal infiltrate of lymphocytes, plasma cells, and histiocytes associated with hyperplasia of type-2 pneumocytes. The fibrotic zones are composed mainly of dense acellular collagen, although scattered foci of proliferating fibroblasts (''fibroblastic foci''; the sites of early and active disease; usually in an intraalveolar location) may also be seen. Areas of honeycomb change are composed of cystic and fibrotic airspaces that are frequently lined by bronchiolar epithelium and filled with mucin. Other entities that resemble the pathological pattern of UIP include (1) desquamative interstitial pneumonia (DIP); (2) respiratory bronchiolitis–associated interstitial lung disease (RB-ILD); (3) nonclassifiable or nonspecific chronic interstitial pneumonias; (4) idiopathic bronchiolitis obliterans and organizing pneumonia; (5) hypersensitivity pneumonitis; and (6) pulmonary eosinophilic granuloma. Both adequate tissue and an experienced pathologist are needed to make these distinctions with confidence.

Rationale and Regimens for Treatment

The clinical course of IPF is variable, but the mean survival time is 4 to 6 years after diagnosis. The response to treatment is also variable, but patients with a more cellular biopsy are more likely to improve with corticosteroid and/or cytotoxic therapy. Table 3 summarizes a variety of factors that appear to influence the prognosis and response to treatment in IPF. Importantly, this disease will almost universally progress and do so in an often insidious fashion that may be difficult to detect based on commonly used parameters such as symptoms, chest x-ray findings, or spirometry. We recommend initiating treatment as early as possible in the disease process.

Corticosteroids.   Glucocorticoids are the main drugs used in the treatment of IPF. The optimal dose is not known. Our recommended starting regimen for patients with chronic progressive IPF is with prednisone (or equivalent dose of prednisolone) at 1–1.5 mg/kg in a once-daily oral dose (based on the patient's ideal body weight, but it should not exceed 100 mg/day). This dose is continued for 8–12 weeks, at which time the patient is reevaluated. If the patient's condition is felt to be stable or improved, the dose is tapered to 0.5–1 mg/kg and maintained at this level for an additional 12 weeks. If, at the end of the second 12 weeks, the patient continues to be stable or improved, the dose is again tapered to 0.25 mg/kg/day.

In some patients with rapidly progressive disease, we have used 3–5 days of high-dose intravenous corticosteroid therapy prior to initiating oral therapy. For this purpose we use methylprednisolone at 250 mg IV every 6 h. Once the course is stabilized, we continue therapy as outlined above for chronic disease. Intermittent high-dose parenteral corticosteroid treatment ("pulse therapy") has been used especially in patients with aggressive, severe disease. Treatment with intravenous methylprednisolone, 2 g once a week,

Table 3 Factors That Affect Outcome in Idiopathic Pulmonary Fibrosis

Factor	Adverse Risk for Progressive Disease	Favorable Risk for Treatment Response and Survival
Gender	Male	Female
Age	Older	Younger
Duration	Long history, gradual progression	Symptoms less than 1 year
Smoking	Extensive	None
Lung function	Severe impairment at presentation	Mild impairment at presentation
HRCT scan	Mixed or reticular; honeycombing	Ground-glass infiltrates
BAL cells	Neutrophils, eosinophils	Lymphocytes
Therapy	No initial response to steroids	Good initial response to steroids

Key: HRCT, high-resolution computed tomography; BAL, bronchoalveolar lavage.

plus oral prednisone, 0.25 mg/kg, suppresses the neutrophil component of the alveolitis but has not been clearly shown to improve the lung disease.

Many patients may have an initial positive response (within the first 6 weeks) but fail to sustain it after several more months of therapy. A favorable response to corticosteroid therapy is defined by a decrease in symptoms, especially dyspnea and cough; reduction or clearing of roentgenographic abnormalities; and physiological improvement (FVC, TLC, DL_{CO}, resting and exercise gas exchange). If the patient shows no further decline in lung function or other parameters of disease activity for prolonged periods of time (3–6 months), that should also be considered a positive response to treatment. Subjective decrease in symptoms without objective improvement occurs frequently (in up to 70% of treated patients) and should not be the only factor in determining whether to continue treatment. Objective improvement in physiological or radiographic abnormalities occurs in 20–30% of treated patients. Frequently, some parameters may improve while others show declines or no change.

The proper length of therapy for patients who respond to treatment is not known. We usually aim for a duration of therapy of at least 1 year. Some clinicians suggest that 2 years of treatment might be more effective in maintaining prolonged remission in corticosteroid-responsive patients. Lifelong treatment with low-dose therapy (prednisone 0.25 mg/kg/day) may be required by a small number of patients who respond to aggressive treatment. Importantly, premature discontinuation of treatment is a relatively frequent cause of relapse in a patient who has responded initially. Unfortunately, most patients experience decline in lung function and worsening exercise tolerance despite corticosteroid therapy. If the patient's condition continues to decline on corticosteroids, a second agent is often added and the prednisone is lowered to or maintained at 0.25 mg/kg.

Side effects are frequently encountered with corticosteroid therapy, and patients should be monitored carefully for their development. It is less frequent, however, that these side effects necessitate discontinuation of therapy. The numerous potential side effects of corticosteroids are well known and include hypertension, weight gain, abnormal fat deposition, peripheral edema, gastrointestinal discomfort, hyperglycemia, osteoporosis, cataracts, glaucoma, depression, anxiety, psychosis, insomnia, impaired wound healing, and easy bruising. Of particular importance is the potential for the development of a myopathy, which may affect the muscles of respiration. Respiratory muscle weakness as a result of corticosteroid treatment may be difficult to differentiate from progressive parenchymal lung disease. Because of the risk of osteoporosis in many older patients with IPF, we often institute treatment with calcium and vitamin D supplementation concurrently with prednisone therapy. Finally, it may be wise to apply a tuberculin skin test to patients prior to initiating high-dose steroids. Current recommendations are to institute isoniazid preventive therapy in persons who have a positive tuberculin skin test and will be receiving doses greater than 15 mg of prednisone daily for more than 3 weeks.

Cytotoxic Drugs   It is well known that only a minority of patients with IPF will respond to therapy with corticosteroids. Consequently, other agents have been sought to treat this condition. Cytotoxic drugs, particularly cyclophosphamide and azathioprine, have been the most commonly employed second-line drugs in the management of patients with IPF.

Cyclophosphamide.   Cyclophosphamide (Cytoxan) is a commonly used corticosteroid-sparing agent in the treatment of IPF. It is most often used as a second-line drug in patients whose condition is deteriorating despite corticosteroid therapy. Increasingly it is being used as first-line treatment in patients with contraindications to corticosteroids. Several reports suggest that cyclophosphamide (usually given with low-dose corticosteroid) may be beneficial in the treatment of IPF. A recent randomized, controlled trial comparing prednisolone alone with cyclophosphamide and low-dose prednisolone in combination showed a possible survival advantage for the group treated with cyclophosphamide and low-dose prednisolone. Cyclophosphamide is an alkylating agent of the nitrogen mustard group. It is an inactive drug that is metabolized by the cytochrome P450 system into active metabolites. These metabolites decrease lymphocyte numbers and function and may also have anti-inflammatory effects.

In patients with IPF, cyclophosphamide is usually administered orally as a once-daily dose. We usually begin dosing at 25–50 mg/day and increase gradually, by 25 mg increments in order to reduce and maintain the total count of white blood cells (WBC) between 4000 and 7000/mm^3 (we usually measure the WBC count biweekly for the first 6–12 weeks and then at least monthly thereafter). Occasionally the WBC count remains >7000 despite increases in the cyclophosphamide dose. In those instances we do not raise the dose above 150 mg/day. It is our clinical impression that cyclophosphamide responsiveness and reduced side effects occur at doses not exceeding 150 mg/day. Consequently, we do not exceed this dose even if the WBC count remains > 7000. In general, we do not expect to achieve a favorable response to cyclophosphamide therapy for at least 3–6 months after initiating treatment with this drug, with or without low-dose corticosteroid. Forced diuresis, eight glasses (8 oz each) of water daily and monthly monitoring of the urine for red blood cells or other abnormality is recommended in an attempt prevent clinically significant hemorrhagic cystitis.

There is little experience with the use of intermittent (''pulse'') intravenous cyclophosphamide therapy. It has been used occasionally in patients with rapidly progressive disease. The use of intermittent cyclophosphamide therapy is potentially valuable as a long-term treatment regimen because it is better tolerated, has less toxicity, and poses a lesser risk of malignancy than daily therapy. We have used a dose of 2 mg/kg ideal body weight administered over 30–60 min once daily for 3–5 days. Following this, oral daily therapy is initiated as detailed above. Other investigators have described an escalating regimen of intravenous cyclophosphamide beginning with a dose of 500 mg. The dose is increased by 100–200 mg every 2 weeks provided that the total WBC count remains > 3000/mm^3. The maximum single administered dose is 1000–1800 mg of cyclophosphamide. The patient is monitored for adverse side effects, as noted below.

Side effects include reductions in all hematological cell lines. We monitor the WBC count as above and adjust the cyclophosphamide dose if needed. As with most immunosuppressive therapies, patients on cyclophosphamide are at increased risk of infection. Hemorrhagic cystitis and carcinoma of the bladder have been associated with the use of cyclophosphamide, particularly when it is used in higher doses for cancer chemotherapy and in those patients who have persistent microscopic nonglomerular hematuria. These side effects are less common in the lower doses we use for IPF. The incidence of bladder cancer is 5% at 10 years and 16% at 15 years. Infertility may occur in both men and women. Cyclophosphamide may be teratogenic; therefore much caution should be used when it is prescribed for women of childbearing years. Gastrointestinal side effects include stomatitis, nausea, diarrhea, and, rarely, hepatotoxicity. Severe generalized fatigue has been reported by several of our patients. The risk of future cancer may be increased by cyclophosphamide.

Azathioprine. A recent small study suggested that the use of azathioprine (Imuran) with low-dose prednisone may be more effective in improving survival than prednisone alone. Azathioprine is converted to mercaptopurine, a purine analog that affects RNA and

DNA synthesis. In general, cellular immunity is suppressed to a greater degree than humoral immunity. The exact mechanism by which azathioprine affects autoimmune processes is not clear.

We recommend 2 mg/kg given as a once-daily oral dose. As with cyclophosphamide, we do not exceed 200 mg/day. However, the degree of leukopenia does not correlate with therapeutic efficacy in patients with rheumatoid arthritis and those with renal transplants. We do not require that the dose of azathioprine be adjusted if the WBC count falls below 4000/mm^3. A discernible response to therapy may not be evident until the patient has received 3–6 months of therapy.

The most common side effects—including nausea, vomiting, and diarrhea—are gastrointestinal. A small percentage of patients will demonstrate an increase in liver function tests; however, reports of severe hepatitis are rare. Hematological side effects include depression of all cell lines. An increased risk of subsequent malignancy has been reported in renal transplant patients who are treated with azathioprine and prednisone. Azathioprine may be a teratogen and therefore should be used with caution in women of childbearing age.

Colchicine. Limited clinical trials have suggested a benefit for IPF patients treated with colchicine. Colchicine has multiple effects, including the arrest of cell division, inhibition of granulocyte migration, and inhibition of the release of several proteins from cells. It may also interfere with the secretion of collagen from fibroblasts and may increase collagen degradation by enhancing the action of collagenase. We recommend a dose of 0.6 mg orally once or twice daily as tolerated. Colchicine is generally quite well tolerated. Side effects that may be encountered include nausea, vomiting, abdominal pain, and diarrhea.

Other Therapies for IPF. Several other drugs have been used in small numbers of patients with IPF, usually following therapeutic failure or toxicity of more common agents. The experience with each of these is limited and usually anecdotal. Methotrexate is a folic acid analog used for its immunosuppressive effects. Clinical experience with methotrexate in the treatment of interstitial lung disease is limited, except in sarcoidosis (see Chap. 28). We begin with an oral dose of 7.5 mg weekly, then gradually increase (e.g., increments of 2.5 mg every 2 weeks) until a dose of 15 mg per week is achieved. A trial of methotrexate therapy should last at least 4–6 months to assess effectiveness. The liver function tests and WBC count should be monitored monthly to assess for toxicity. The most serious side effects are hepatic fibrosis (in up to 10% of cases when the dose exceeds 5 g) and interstitial pneumonitis resulting in pulmonary fibrosis. In a patient with IPF being treated with methotrexate, it may be difficult to distinguish pulmonary drug toxicity from progression of the underlying disease. Because hepatic toxicity may be occult initially, some investigators have advocated liver biopsy when the total dose exceeds 1 g or after 18–24 months of therapy, even in the absence of signs of hepatic injury. Other toxicities include bone marrow suppression, nausea, alopecia, skin rash, transient gonadal suppression, teratogenic effects, and possible oncogenic potential.

Penicillamine plus prednisolone has been reported to be more effective than prednisolone alone or prednisolone plus azathioprine. Postulated mechanisms through which penicillamine may affect the progression of IPF include inhibition of collagen synthesis by interfering with collagen cross-linking and/or suppression of T-cell function. The dosage we recommend is that used for the management of rheumatoid arthritis. The initial dose is 125–250 mg daily given as an oral dose. After 4–8 weeks, the dose is increased weekly to a final dose of 500 mg daily. Doses as high as 1000 mg daily may be utilized if tolerated. A determination of effectiveness cannot be made before 3–6 months. Reported side effects include nausea, vomiting, diarrhea, dyspepsia, anorexia, transient loss of taste for sweet and salt, cutaneous lesions, hematological toxicity (leukopenia, aplastic anemia, agranulocytopenia), renal toxicity (reversible proteinuria and hematuria, nephrotic syndrome), myasthenia gravis, and bronchoalveolitis.

Cyclosporine is a potent immunosuppressive agent used widely to control graft rejection following solid-organ transplantation. There are a few anecdotal reports on the use of cyclosporine in interstitial lung disease, but the results have not been encouraging. The mechanisms of action and use of this drug are discussed in Chap. 24.

Transplantation of one or two cadaveric lungs is the ultimate definitive therapy for IPF. This treatment is described in detail in Chap. 24. Lung transplantation for IPF is effective when available but is often precluded by the age of most IPF patients and the upper age limit (60–65) imposed by most transplant programs. Limited availability of donor organs creates long waiting times (1–2 years) for patients with IPF who qualify for transplantation.

Desquamative Interstitial Pneumonia (DIP)

DIP is a distinct clinical and pathological entity that differs substantially from UIP. The incidence of the clinicopathological syndrome of DIP is quite rare (probably less than 3% of all DPLD cases). It affects cigarette smokers in the fourth or fifth decade of life. Most patients present with a subacute (weeks to months) illness characterized by dyspnea and cough. The chest x-ray shows less severe changes than IPF and may be normal in up to 20% of cases. The most characteristic chest x-ray pattern shows ground-glass opacities in the lower zones (Fig. 3A). HRCT scans show diffuse ground-glass opacity in the middle

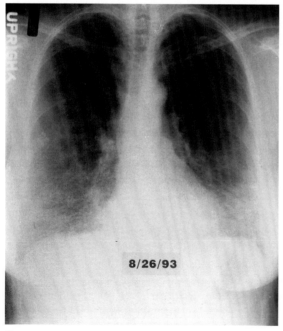

8/26/93

A

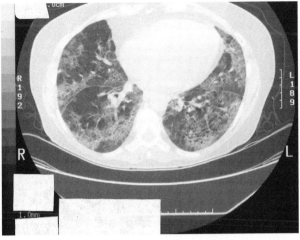

B

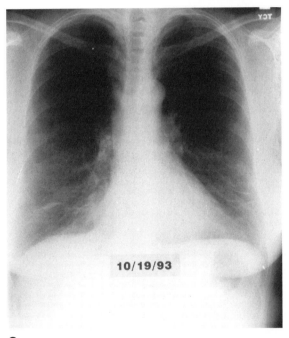

C

Figure 3 Desquamative interstitial pneumonitis. A. Chest radiograph showing diffuse ground-glass opacities in the lower lung zones. B. High-resolution computed tomography scan showing diffuse ground-glass opacification. C. Chest radiograph showing rapid improvement after treatment with high-dose corticosteroids.

and lower lung zones (Figure 3B). Lung function testing shows a restrictive pattern with reduced DL_{CO} and hypoxemia on blood-gas analysis. Lung biopsy is usually required to make the diagnosis. The pathology demonstrates a uniform, diffuse intraalveolar accumulation of macrophages and type II alveolar epithelial cells, with relative preservation of the underlying lung architecture. A DIP-like pattern can be seen in a number of other processes, but usually to only a minor degree: eosinophilic granuloma, drug reactions (e.g., amiodarone), chronic alveolar hemorrhage, eosinophilic pneumonia, pneumoconioses (e.g., talcosis, hard metal disease, asbestosis), obstructive pneumonias, and exogenous lipoid pneumonia. In fact, many cases previously called DIP are actually respiratory bronchiolitis–associated DPLD (see below). Clinical recognition of DIP is important because the process is associated with a better prognosis (overall survival is about 70% after 10 years) and a better response to smoking cessation and systemic corticosteroids. There is an estimated 5% mortality in 5 years.

Respiratory Bronchiolitis-Associated DPLD (RB-DPLD)

RB-DPLD is a distinct clinical syndrome found in current or former cigarette smokers. The clinical presentation resembles those of patients with other DPLDs: cough and breathlessness with exertion, crackles on chest examination. Routine laboratory studies are not helpful. Diffuse, fine reticular or nodular interstitial opacities are found on chest radiographs, usually with normal-appearing lung volumes. Other reported features include bronchial wall thickening, prominence of peribronchovascular interstitium, small regular and irregular opacities, and small peripheral ring shadows. HRCT scanning often reveals hazy opacities. A mixed obstructive-restrictive pattern is common on lung function testing. An isolated increase in RV may be found. Arterial blood gases show mild hypoxemia. The clinical course and prognosis of respiratory bronchiolitis is unknown. Smoking cessation is important in the resolution of these lesions. A favorable response to corticosteroids has been reported.

Acute Interstitial Pneumonia (Hamman-Rich Syndrome)

Acute interstitial pneumonia (AIP) is a rare fulminant form of lung injury that presents acutely (days to weeks from onset of symptoms), usually in a previously healthy individual. Most patients are over the age of 40 years (mean age 50 years, range 7–83 years). The onset is usually abrupt, although a prodromal illness usually lasting 7–14 days before presentation is common. The clinical signs and symptoms are most often fever, cough, and shortness of breath. There is no sexual predilection. AIP is similar in presentation to the acute respiratory distress syndrome (ARDS) and probably corresponds to the subset of cases of idiopathic ARDS.

Routine laboratory studies are nonspecific and generally not helpful. Diffuse, bilateral airspace opacification is seen on chest radiograph. CT scans show bilateral, patchy, symmetrical areas of ground-glass attenuation. Bilateral areas of airspace consolidation may also be present. A predominantly subpleural distribution may be seen. Mild honeycombing, usually involving <10% of the lung, may be seen on CT examination. These radiographic findings are similar to those seen in ARDS. Most patients have moderate to severe hypoxemia and develop respiratory failure. Mechanical ventilation is often required.

The diagnosis of AIP requires the presence of a clinical syndrome of ARDS without an obvious associated cause and pathological confirmation of organizing diffuse alveolar damage (DAD). Consequently, an open or thoracoscopic lung biopsy is required to confirm the diagnosis. The mortality from AIP is high (>60%), with the majority of patients dying within 6 months of presentation. However, those who recover usually do not have recurrence of the disease and most have substantial or complete recovery of lung function. It is not clear that corticosteroid therapy is effective in AIP. The main treatment is supportive care.

Nonspecific Interstitial Pneumonia (NSIP)

NSIP refers to a recently described histological appearance in DPLD that does not conform to the previously established pathology patterns. Whether this represents a separate disease entity or an earlier representation of an established histological pattern such as UIP (the underlying lesion of IPF) or other interstitial diseases remains to be seen. The clinical presentation is similar to that of IPF. Cough and dyspnea are present for months to years. Chest radiographic findings are nonspecific, demonstrating primarily lower-zone reticular opacities. Bilateral patchy opacities can also be seen. HRCT shows bilateral symmetrical ground-glass opacities or bilateral airspace consolidation.

The diagnosis of NSIP is established by thoracoscopic or open-lung biopsy. The main histological feature of NSIP is the homogeneous appearance of either inflammation or fibrosis as opposed to the heterogeneity seen in the other interstitial pneumonias. Honeycomb areas are rare. A similar histological pattern can occur in the collagen vascular diseases, hypersensitivity pneumonitis, and the nonspecific (noninfectious) interstitial pneumonia that occurs in some AIDS patients. It is likely that in the past many of the patients who are now being labeled NSIP were previously thought to be the more cellular (possibly more treatment-responsive) patients with IPF.

The response to corticosteroid medication was excellent in the one series of patients reported with non-AIDS NSIP. As expected, those patients with the cellular forms of NSIP demonstrated this therapeutic response versus those with primarily fibrosis. The only deaths occurred in the patients with a predominantly fibrotic pattern. After ruling out a collagen vascular disease or hypersensitivity pneumonitis, we treat patients with this histological pattern in a fashion similar to those patients with IPF. Please see the section on IPF, above, for the dosages and length of drug therapy. There is an estimated 15–20% mortality in 5 years for NSIP.

Cryptogenic Organizing Pneumonia (Idiopathic BOOP)

Cryptogenic organizing pneumonitis (COP) or idiopathic bronchiolitis obliterans with organizing pneumonia (idiopathic BOOP) is a specific clinicopathological syndrome of unknown etiology. The disease onset occurs usually in the fifth and sixth decades and affects men and women equally. Almost three-fourths of the patients have their symptoms for less than 2 months and few have symptoms for >6 months prior to diagnosis. A flu-like illness—characterized by cough, fever, malaise, fatigue, and weight loss—heralds the onset of COP in two-fifths of the patients. Inspiratory crackles are frequently present on chest examination. Routine laboratory studies are nonspecific. A leukocytosis without an increase in eosinophils is seen in approximately half the patients. The initial erythrocyte sedimentation rate (ESR) was frequently elevated in patients with COP. Pulmonary function is usually impaired, with a restrictive defect being most common. Resting and exercise arterial hypoxemia is common.

The roentgenographic manifestations of COP or BOOP are quite distinctive. Bilateral, diffuse alveolar opacities in the presence of normal lung volume constituted the characteristic radiographic appearance (Fig. 4). A peripheral distribution of the opacities, very similar to that thought to be ''virtually pathognomic'' for chronic eosinophilic pneumonia, is also seen in COP. Rarely, the alveolar opacities may be unilateral. Recurrent and migratory pulmonary opacities are common. Irregular linear or nodular interstitial opacities or honeycombing are rarely seen at presentation. HRCT scans of the lung reveal patchy airspace consolidation, ground-glass opacities, small nodular opacities, and bronchial wall thickening and dilation. These patchy opacities occur more frequently in the periphery of the lung and are often in the lower lung zone. The CT scan may reveal much more extensive disease than is expected by review of the plain chest x-ray.

BAL fluid recovery is lower in patients with COP than in healthy volunteers. However, the total cells recovered was greater in patients with COP. The proportion of macrophages is lower but the lymphocytes, neutrophils, and eosinophils are higher in COP than in normals. The patients with COP tended to have higher lymphocyte counts than those with patients with IPF. The ''mixed pattern'' of increased cellularity is thought to be characteristic of COP, especially in the right clinical setting, e.g., when associated with multiple alveolar opacities on the chest radiograph.

The histopathological lesions characteristic of COP include an excessive proliferation of granulation tissue within small airways (proliferative bronchiolitis) and alveolar ducts associated with chronic inflammation in the surrounding alveoli (Fig. 5). This or-

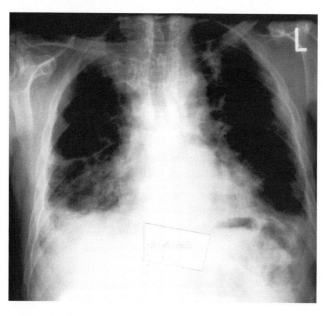

Figure 4 Cryptogenic organizing pneumonia (idiopathic bronchiolitis obliterans organizing pneumonia). This posteroanterior roentgenogram reveals volume loss with bilateral patchy alveolar opacities.

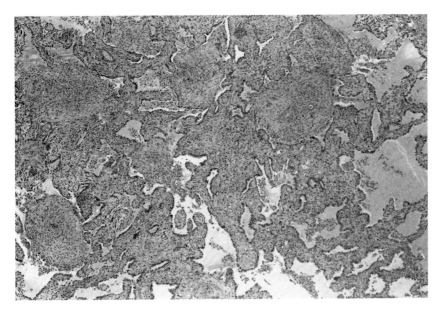

Figure 5 Cryptogenic organizing pneumonia (idiopathic bronchiolitis obliterans organizing pneumonia). Polypoid masses of granulation tissue fill the lumens of respiratory bronchioles and alveolar ducts. Adjacent alveolar interstices are broadened by a lymphoplasmacytic inflammatory infiltrate.

ganizing pneumonia is the most important process underlying the clinical and radiographic manifestations of COP. There are several other key features: there is a uniform appearance to the changes, suggesting they are recent and have all occurred at the same time; the lung architecture is not severely disrupted; the distribution is patchy and peribronchiolar; the lesions are usually located within the airspace; foamy macrophages are very common in the alveolar spaces, presumably secondary to the bronchiolar occlusion; the intraluminal buds of granulation tissue consist of loose collagen-embedding fibroblasts and myofibroblasts that extend from one alveolus to the adjacent one through the pores of Kohn, giving rise to the characteristic "butterfly" pattern; the bronchiolar lesions are secondary to intraluminal plugs of granulation tissue always in association with plugs in the alveolar ducts and alveolar spaces; severe fibrotic changes, such as honeycombing, is unusual at the time of diagnosis; giant cells are rare or absent; and no granuloma or vasculitis is present. Foci of organizing pneumonia (i.e., a "BOOP pattern") constitute a nonspecific reaction to lung injury and can occur as a secondary finding adjacent to other pathological processes or as a component of other primary pulmonary disorders (e.g., cryptococcosis, Wegener's granulomatosis, lymphoma, hypersensitivity pneumonitis, and eosinophilic pneumonia). Consequently, the clinician must carefully reevaluate any patient found to have this histopathological lesion to rule out these possibilities. Corticosteroid therapy is the most common treatment used; it results in clinical recovery in two-thirds of the patients.

Lymphocytic Interstitial Pneumonitis (LIP)

LIP is an uncommon cause of interstitial lung disease. It was first described in 1966 as a unique interstitial reaction that was distinguishable from the desquamative and usual interstitial pneumonias by the presence of monotonous sheets of lymphoplasmacytic cells that expand the interstitium. The majority of cases are associated with some form of dysproteinemia, either a monoclonal or polyclonal gammopathy. Most LIP are idiopathic, but the two most common known associations are with Sjögren's syndrome (primary or secondary) or with AIDS. LIP has also been described in other hypergammaglobulinemic states such as chronic hepatitis, primary biliary cirrhosis, myasthenia gravis, autoimmune thyroiditis, pernicious anemia, and autoimmune hemolytic anemia. It also manifests as chronic graft-versus-host disease following allogeneic bone marrow transplantation. LIP also accompanies common variable hypogammaglobulinemia in both adults and children. The types of LIP associated with common variable hypogammaglobulinemia or with AIDS have a higher incidence of conversion to lymphoma.

LIP is more common in women and usually appears between the fourth and seventh decades. The clinical symptoms are similar to those of other interstitial lung disorders and consist of nonproductive cough and dyspnea. Other findings depend upon the associated diseases.

The physical findings of LIP include bibasilar rales and clubbing in a small number of cases. The chest radiograph and HRCT are nonspecific, indicating bilateral, predominantly lower-zone mixed alveolar-interstitial opacities. Although this may represent benign disease, the possibility of a low-grade lymphoma should be considered if a pleural effusion or mediastinal lymphadenopathy is present. Other laboratory findings reflect the underlying disease state—for example, serum antinuclear antibody or rheumatoid factor in the secondary form of Sjögren's syndrome associated with a collagen vascular disease. Serum protein immunoelectrophoresis reveals either a mono- or polyclonal gammopathy or hypogammaglobulinemia.

There are four possible outcomes in LIP: (1) resolution following treatment with corticosteroid drugs alone or in combination with another immunosuppressive agent; (2) progression to pulmonary fibrosis and cor pulmonale; (3) recurrent superimposed pulmonary or systemic infection; and (4) the development of lymphoma. While there are no controlled data, there appears to be an excellent therapeutic response in certain patients. It is likely that up to 50% of patients with idiopathic LIP or that associated with primary or secondary Sjögren's syndrome will have complete resolution following corticosteroid therapy. In unresponsive or recurrent disease, chlorambucil has been recommended. In unresponsive patients, it is clear that progression to honeycomb lung can occur in spite of attempted therapeutic intervention. It is difficult to determine which patients will respond to therapy and which go on to respiratory failure.

Pulmonary Histiocytosis X (Eosinophilic Granuloma)

Pulmonary histiocytosis X of the lung is a rare, smoking-related, diffuse lung disease that primarily afflicts young adults between the ages 20 and 40. Pulmonary histiocytosis X occurs more commonly in men. The clinical presentation is variable, from an asymptomatic state (approximately 16%) to a rapidly progressive condition. The most common clinical manifestations at presentation are cough, dyspnea, chest pain, weight loss, and fever. Pneumothorax occurs in about 25% of patients and is occasionally the first manifestation of the illness. Hemoptysis and diabetes insipidus are rare manifestations. The physical examination is usually normal.

Routine laboratory studies are not helpful. The radiographic features vary depending on the stage of the disease. The combination of ill-defined or stellate nodules (2–10 mm

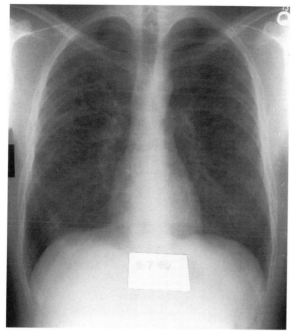

A

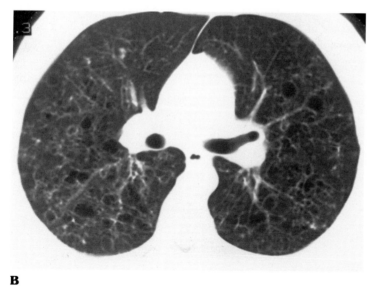

B

Figure 6 Pulmonary histiocytosis X (eosinophilic granuloma). A. Chest roentgenogram showing ill-defined reticular and nodular opacities with predominant upper zone cysts, preservation of lung volume, and sparing in the costophrenic angle. B. The CT lung scan in this patient shows thin-walled cysts of variable size.

in size), reticular or nodular opacities, upper-zone cysts or honeycombing, preservation of lung volume, and costophrenic angle sparing are felt to be highly specific for pulmonary histiocytosis X (Fig. 6A). However, the differentiation of pulmonary histiocytosis X from other fibrosing lung diseases by chest radiographic features alone can be difficult. CT lung scanning that reveals the combination of nodules and thin-walled cysts is virtually diagnostic of pulmonary histiocytosis X (Fig. 6B). Physiologically, the most prominent and frequent pulmonary function abnormality reported is a markedly reduced DL_{CO}, although varying degrees of restrictive disease, airflow limitation, and diminished exercise capacity are described. Discontinuance of smoking is the key treatment, resulting in clinical improvement in 33% of the subjects. Most patients with pulmonary histiocytosis X suffer persistent or progressive disease. Death due to respiratory failure occurs in about 10% of patients.

COLLAGEN VASCULAR DISEASES

Because of the systemic nature of the collagen vascular diseases (CVD) or connective tissue diseases, all components of the respiratory system can be involved. Any pulmonary complication of the CVD, including DPLD, may be the only manifestation of that particular systemic disorder. It also may occur simultaneously with the onset of the systemic disorder, or, as is usually the case, complicate a previously established CVD. Although infections and side effects of drug treatment are always possibilities, it is likely that at some point during the course of their illness most patients with CVD will have one or more of the pulmonary complications listed in Table 4.

Table 4 Relative Frequency of Respiratory Tract Involvement in the Collagen Vascular Diseases

	SLE	RA	Scl	PM-DM	MCTD	SS	AS
Primary pulmonary hypertension	+	+	+++	±	+	+	−
Vasculitis	+	±	±	−	±	−	−
Pleural disease	+++	+++	+	−	+	±	±
Bronchiolitis obliterans	±	++	+	+	±	+	−
Bronchiectasis	−	+	±	+	−	+	−
Follicular bronchitis	±	++	−	−	±	−	−
Aspiration pneumonia	−	−	++	+++	++	+	−
Diaphragmatic dysfunction	++	−	−	±	±	−	−
Lung nodules	−	++	−	−	−	+	−
Diffuse alveolar damage	+	±	±	+	+	−	−
BOOP	±	+	±	+	+	+	−
Usual interstitial pneumonia	+	++	+++	++	++	+	+
Pulmonary capillaritis	++	+	±	±	±	−	−
Lymphocytic interstitial pneumonia	+	+	+	±	±	++	−
Nonspecific interstitial pneumonia	+	++	+	++	++	+	−

Abbreviations: BOOP, Bronchiolitis obliterans organizing pneumonia; SLE, systemic lupus erythematosus; RA, rheumatoid arthritis; Scl, scleroderma; PM-DM, polymyositis-dermatomyositis; MCTD, mixed connective tissue disease; SS, Sjögren's syndrome; AS, ankylosing spondylitis.

Pulmonary Hypertension

Pulmonary hypertension must be differentiated from DPLD. It most frequently appears in patients with scleroderma, particularly those with the limited scleroderma or CREST syndrome (subcutaneous calcifications, Raynaud's phenomena, esophageal dysmotility, sclerodactyly, and cutaneous telangiectasis). Increased numbers of patients with rheumatoid arthritis (RA), systemic lupus erythematosus (SLE), and mixed connective tissue disease (MCTD) are being identified with pulmonary hypertension. This form of pulmonary hypertension is similar to the primary pulmonary hypertension (PPH) that occurs in young women with no associated CVD (see Chap. 33). Like PPH, pulmonary hypertension in CVD is also a fibroproliferative disorder (plexogenic arteriopathy). Pulmonary hypertension as a primary event should not be confused with the secondary forms of pulmonary hypertension resulting from hypoxic vasoconstriction produced by the gas-exchange abnormalities associated with the DPLD, which complicate CVD.

The characteristic presentation of pulmonary hypertension is a patient with gradually increasing dyspnea, fatigue, and a negative chest radiograph or one showing only enlarged pulmonary arteries. Pulmonary function tests reveal a low diffusing capacity but preserved lung volumes and flow rates. HRCT scan confirms the presence of enlarged pulmonary arteries without diffuse interstitial disease. With progressive obliteration of the pulmonary vascular bed, additional symptoms of worsening fatigue, syncope, peripheral edema, atrial arrhythmias, and overt cor pulmonale will appear. In scleroderma, the manifestations of the CREST syndrome accompany pulmonary hypertension. In RA and SLE, there is often accompanying Raynaud's phenomena and digital vasculitis. In SLE patients with suspected pulmonary hypertension, one should also consider recurrent pulmonary emboli due to the antiphospholipid syndrome.

Treatment for pulmonary hypertension in CVD is largely supportive, because corticosteroids and immunosuppressive agents are ineffective. Vasodilators, calcium-channel blocking agents, and supplemental oxygen improve symptoms temporarily but do not prolong survival, which is usually less that 24 months following diagnosis. For the primary pulmonary hypertension not associated with CVD, continuous prostacycline infusion via a subcutaneous pump has not only improved physical performance but significantly prolonged survival. A prostacycline trial of the pulmonary hypertension in CVD is under way and preliminary results are promising. The mechanism of action of prostacycline or its analog iloprost is poorly understood. Possibilities include pulmonary vasodilation, an increase in cardiac output, or anti-inflammatory action.

Vasculitis

Pulmonary vasculitis causing inflammation and fibrinoid necrosis of the walls of small and medium muscular pulmonary arteries is rare. It is seen most commonly in SLE. The features and treatment of vasculitis occurring in CVD are identical to those for the systemic vasculitides as detailed below (see "Systemic Vasculitis and Diffuse Alveolar Hemorrhage").

Bronchiolitis

There are several bronchiolar diseases that complicate the CVD. Bronchiolitis obliterans (BO) is a progressive obstructive lung disease that results from inflammation of the bronchiolar wall followed by concentric fibrosis, which causes obliteration of the bronchiolar lumen (Fig. 7). Although it is an infrequent complication of CVD, it appears most often in patients with RA. Follicular bronchitis and bronchiolitis (lymphocytic infiltration of airway walls) as well as bronchiectasis may also contribute to the obstructive lung disease seen in patients with RA. Whether follicular bronchiolitis predisposes to BO is unknown. It was once thought that the use of penicillamine for the treatment of RA was responsible for the development of BO. However, it is now clear that both men and women with rheumatoid arthritis who have never been treated with penicillamine can develop BO.

The physiological alterations include a progressive and eventually severe obstructive lung disease with hyperinflation. The diffusing capacity for carbon monoxide (DL_{CO}) is preserved until the condition is in its late stages. With advanced disease, hypoxia and hypoventilation appear. The chest radiograph may be normal or show evidence of hyperinflation. The HRCT demonstrates adjacent zones of increased and decreased opacity that coincide with areas of increased blood flow alternating with trapped air (see illustrations in Chap. 11). Bronchiectasis may be seen on HRCT as well. Although most cases of BO complicate an established case of RA, there are patients in whom BO develops prior to the joint manifestations.

There are reports of BO therapeutic responsiveness to prednisone and/or to immunosuppressive therapy with either azathioprine or cyclophosphamide, particularly in the early phases of this complication. It is here that the inflammatory as opposed to the concentric fibrotic component is present. Unfortunately, most patients do not present for medical care during this stage of their disease. However, it is recommended that both prednisone or one of the aforementioned immunosuppressive drugs be employed. Although there are no published data supporting this, there appears to be a period of stabilization after initia-

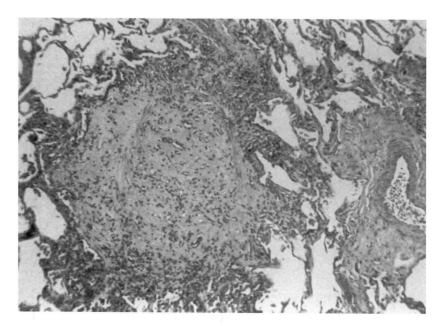

Figure 7   Bronchiolitis obliterans in rheumatoid arthritis. There is total obliteration of the membranous bronchiole. Note the accompanying small muscular pulmonary artery on the right.

tion of these drugs. Most cases will eventually progress to respiratory failure, and bilateral lung transplantation offers the only chance for survival.

Acute Interstitial Lung Disease in CVD

An acute presentation of DPLD is most likely to occur in systemic lupus erythematosus (SLE) and has occasionally been noted in the other CVD. The possible underlying histologies for this acute immunological pneumonia include bronchiolitis obliterans organizing pneumonia (BOOP); a cellular interstitial pneumonia (CIP), which may represent the cellular phase of non-specific interstitial pneumonia (NSIP) as described above; diffuse alveolar damage (DAD); and diffuse alveolar hemorrhage (DAH), either from pulmonary capillaritis or bland (noninflammatory) hemorrhage. Acute lupus pneumonitis may complicate an established case of SLE or can be the first and only manifestation of SLE. A similar immunological pneumonia has been reported in polymyositis-dermatomyositis, scleroderma, and MCTD. The presentation resembles an atypical viral pneumonia, with nonproductive cough, low-grade fever, diffuse alveolar infiltrates on x-ray, and severe hypoxemia, often requiring mechanical ventilation. It may coexist with serositis and nephritis. The underlying histology is most often DAD, but CIP and BOOP have been described. Bronchoalveolar lavage may help to exclude an infectious etiology but demonstrates nonspecific increases in inflammatory cell numbers. Thoracoscopic lung biopsy is recommended for any patient who presents in this manner, particularly those without a previously established CVD. If the histology demonstrates either DAD, BOOP, or CIP and no other cause is apparent, a CVD should be excluded, since there are also idiopathic acute interstitial pneumonias with similar underlying histologies.

The worst prognosis is for those patients who have underlying DAD. If it does not respond to treatment, DAD progresses to irreversible fibrosis and respiratory failure within weeks to months. In this case, it is similar to the Hamman-Rich syndrome. On the other hand, those patients with BOOP or CIP often demonstrate an excellent response to corticosteroid treatment. It is our practice to treat the acute immunological pneumonias with intravenous methylprednisolone (250–500 mg) every 6 h, followed over the next week by a gradual taper. The patient is then placed on 40–60 mg prednisone for 10–12 weeks tapered to 20 mg, which is maintained for an additional 6–8 months. In our experience, the addition of azathioprine or cyclophosphamide, particularly in those patients with DAD, has questionable if any benefit. Excessively rapid tapering of corticosteroid treatment or a shortened course prompts disease recurrence. Recurrent acute pneumonitis in SLE, even when responsive to treatment, has been reported to result in chronic fibrotic DPLD.

Chronic and Subacute Interstitial Pneumonias in CVD

This category of DPLD produces symptoms and/or radiographic abnormalities that are present from months to years. The possible underlying histologies include lymphocytic interstitial pneumonia (LIP), BOOP, CIP, and usual interstitial pneumonia (UIP). Unchecked, all of the aforementioned interstitial reactions can progress to end-stage honeycomb lung. Subacute BOOP is most commonly seen with RA or polymyositis-dermatomyositis. LIP may complicate primary Sjögren's syndrome or Sjögren's syndrome associated with RA. CIP and a UIP-like pattern can occur with any CVD. Overall, the highest incidence of DPLD is seen in scleroderma, followed by RA and polymyositis-dermatomyositis. The most frequent histological pattern is similar to UIP. Interestingly UIP, which is also the most common underlying lesion of IPF, is associated with a significantly longer survival in patients with scleroderma. Whether the same is true for other types of CVD is unknown.

In Sjögren's syndrome, other pulmonary complications are possible and related to the drying of secretions in the respiratory tract. This results in bronchitis, bronchiectasis, and recurrent pneumonias. Other primary lung complications of Sjögren's syndrome in addition to LIP and lymphoma are pulmonary vasculitis, pulmonary fibrosis, and bronchiolitis obliterans.

The radiographic features of both LIP and BOOP consist of diffuse or patchy bilateral mixed alveolar and interstitial opacities (Fig. 8). In UIP there are predominant lower-zone and peripheral reticular opacities with honeycomb change. In some asymptomatic patients with CVD who have negative chest radiographs, either HRCT, bronchoalveolar lavage, or exercise testing may indicate the presence of ILD. Whether a lung biopsy to prove the presence and type of DPLD is indicated or whether treatment at this very early stage will alter the course of the ILD remains unknown.

Response to treatment in LIP associated with CVD (see "Lymphocytic Interstitial Pneumonia," above) and BOOP (see "Cryptogenic Organizing Pneumonia," above) is generally good. However, compared to idiopathic BOOP, recurrences are common and can be followed by progression to UIP and end-stage fibrosis. In general, the BOOP associated with the CVD has a poorer prognosis than the idiopathic variety. Our impression is similar for LIP associated with CVD versus idiopathic LIP. The treatment of UIP in CVD is similar to that for IPF (see "Idiopathic Pulmonary Fibrosis," above).

Diffuse Alveolar Hemorrhage (DAH)

DAH is another form of acute DPLD that complicates CVD. Most cases occur in patients with SLE; it appears less commonly with RA, scleroderma, polymyositis-dermatomyositis,

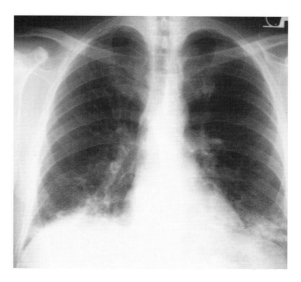

Figure 8   Lymphocytic interstitial pneumonia in Sjögren's syndrome. There are bilateral mixed alveolar and interstitial infiltrates in the lower zone. Bronchiolitis obliterans organizing pneumonia can produce a similar radiographic appearance.

or MCTD. DAH is discussed in detail in the following sections dealing with primary or unclassified syndromes of DPLD.

"PRIMARY" OR UNCLASSIFIED SYNDROMES

Sarcoidosis

Sarcoidosis is a multisystem disease of unknown etiology. It is one of the most important causes of DPLD and is described in detail in Chap. 28.

Diffuse Alveolar Hemorrhage And Vasculitis

Vasculitis

The vasculitides are clinicopathological processes characterized by pulmonary angiitis (i.e., inflammation and necrosis of blood vessels), with associated granuloma formation (i.e., infiltrates of lymphocytes, plasma cells, epithelioid cells, or histiocytes with or without the presence of multinucleated giant cells and with or without tissue necrosis). The lungs are virtually always involved, although any organ system may be affected. Wegener's granulomatosis, and allergic angiitis and granulomatosis (Churg-Strauss syndrome) primarily affect the lung but can be associated with a systemic vasculitis as well. Several of the granulomatous vasculitides are limited to the lung, including necrotizing sarcoid granulomatosis (NSG) and benign lymphocytic angiitis and granulomatosis (BLAG). Lymphomatoid granulomatosis and bronchocentric granulomatosis are no longer classified with pulmonary angiitis and granulomatosis group.

Granulomatous infection and pulmonary angiitis due to irritating embolic material (e.g., talc) are important causes of pulmonary vasculitis where the cause is known and must be considered in the differential diagnosis of patients with pulmonary vasculitis. In a number of the systemic vasculitides, pulmonary involvement can be a major manifestation and carries an unfavorable prognosis. These systemic vasculitides that may involve the lung include collagen vascular disease, hypersensitivity vasculitis, Behçet's syndrome, and disseminated or isolated giant-cell angiitis. Lung involvement is probably not a feature of classic polyarteritis nodosa.

Diffuse Alveolar Hemorrhage

Diffuse alveolar hemorrhage (DAH) is a clinical-pathological syndrome involving diffuse intraalveolar bleeding originating from the alveolar capillaries and occasionally the precapillary arterioles and postcapillary venules. The clinical syndrome is recognized by an acute onset of cough, increasing dyspnea, and hemoptysis. It should be realized that there can be significant alveolar bleeding without hemoptysis. Other features include patchy or diffuse radiographic alveolar opacities, a sequential hemorrhagic BAL, and an iron-deficiency anemia. Over 50% of DAH cases regardless of cause require mechanical ventilation. Furthermore, many of the causes of DAH are associated with recurrent episodes.

DAH is visualized as red blood cells that fill alveolar spaces. After several days or with recurrent alveolar bleeding, intraalveolar hemosiderin-laden macrophages and free interstitial hemosiderin appear. The most frequent underlying associated histology is pulmonary capillaritis. This involves an infiltration of neutrophils into the interstitium of the lung. Many of these neutrophils are fragmented and undergo cell death (apoptosis). Therefore, these cells appear pyknotic, and deposits of nuclear debris appear in the tissue. The interstitium becomes broad and edematous; eventually, fibrinoid necrosis and dissolution occur. Accompanying the red blood cells (DAH) into the alveolar spaces are the fragmented neutrophils. As shown in Table 5, the majority of cases of pulmonary capillaritis are associated with either a systemic vasculitis (most often isolated pulmonary capillaritis, Wegener's granulomatosis, or microscopic polyangiitis), a collagen vascular disease (particularly SLE), or Goodpasture's syndrome.

Conversely, there is no inflammation or destruction of the interstitium in bland pulmonary hemorrhage. Complications of anticoagulation or thrombolytic therapies, various coagulopathies, and mitral stenosis are examples of the bland form of DAH. Either bland hemorrhage or DAH secondary to pulmonary capillaritis can accompany Goodpasture's syndrome and SLE. Idiopathic pulmonary hemosiderosis (IPH), a disease most commonly seen in children, is another important cause of bland DAH. Currently, very few adult cases of IPH are being recognized. A possible explanation for this is that many of the previously described cases of IPH represent the newly described isolated pulmonary capillaritis (see below).

Patients with DAH will often have a previously recognized predisposing condition (systemic vasculitis, collagen vascular disease, mitral stenosis), but DAH may be the initial manifestation. Hemoptysis and progressive dyspnea typically are present for 2–14 days prior to presentation. If there is significant intraalveolar bleeding without hemoptysis, the patient will present with progressive dyspnea, nonproductive cough, diffuse alveolar opacities on chest x-ray, and possibly a low-grade fever. Other findings refer to the underlying systemic disease and may include the presence of a leukocytoclastic dermatological vasculitis, sinusitis, synovitis, myositis, and glomerulonephritis.

The evaluation of a patient with DAH includes a history of drug use, prior systemic or cardiac disease, the possibility of a coagulation disorder, or an occupational exposure. Smoking adversely affects the lung in patients with Goodpasture's syndrome, since almost 100% of patients who smoke develop DAH compared with 20% who do not. Physical examination reveals crackles and sometimes signs of consolidation. Physical findings such as Raynaud's phenomenon, raised purpura, conjunctivitis, iridocyclitis, myositis, or sinusitis point to a systemic disease. The chest radiograph is nonspecific, showing patchy focal or diffuse alveolar filling opacities. The patients are anemic and serial measurements of the hematocrit show further decreases. Most DAH patients show nonspecific elevations of the WBC and platelet counts, but severe drug-induced or idiopathic thrombocytopenia may in themselves induce DAH. Furthermore, patients with disseminated intravascular coagulation secondary to sepsis, patients with acute leukemia, or patients receiving anticoagulation or thrombolytic therapy can also present with DAH. Unexplained thrombocytopenia raises the possibility of the antiphospholipid syndrome, which either accompanies SLE or the primary antiphospholipid syndrome. Patients with DAH often have significant elevations of the erythrocyte sedimentation rate, signifying an accompanying vasculitis. Examination of the urine is particularly important to exclude active glomerulonephritis. A focal segmental necrotizing glomerulonephritis may accompany the systemic vasculitides, SLE, or Goodpasture's syndrome.

Bronchoalveolar lavage with hemorrhagic returns in all of several sequential syringes establishes the diagnosis of DAH, but not its underlying etiology or histology. Goodpasture's syndrome is confirmed by the presence of a circulating anti–basement membrane antibody as well as linear deposition of this antibody in kidney or lung. The DAH complicating SLE most often complicates a previously diagnosed case. However, DAH may be the presenting manifestation in 10–20% of SLE patients. In this situation, a low serum

Table 5   Causes of Diffuse Alveolar Hemorrhage

Pulmonary capillaritis
  Vasculitis
    Isolated pulmonary capillaritis
    Wegener's granulomatosis
    Microscopic polyangiitis
    Behçet's disease
    Henoch-Schönlein purpura
    Cryoglobulinemia
  Collagen vascular diseases
    Systemic lupus erythematosus
    Rheumatoid arthritis
    Scleroderma
    Polymyositis
    Mixed connective tissue disease
  Other autoimmune diseases
    Goodpasture's syndrome
    IgA nephropathy
    Antiphospholipid syndrome
    Idiopathic (pauci-immune) glomerulonephritis
    Lung allograft rejection
    Autologous bone marrow transplantation
    Ulcerative colitis
    Myasthenia gravis
  Drugs
    Diphenylhydantoin
    Retinoic acid
    Propylthiouracil
Without pulmonary capillaritis
  Autoimmune Disorders (BH)
    Goodpasture's syndrome[a]
    Systemic lupus erythematosus[a]
    Idiopathic pulmonary hemosiderosis
  Drugs
    Cytotoxic agents (DAD)
    Anticoagulants and fibrinolytic agents (BH)
    Penicillamine (BH)
    Crack cocaine (BH)
  Miscellaneous disorders
    Coagulopathies (BH)
    Trimellitic anhydride (?)
    Mitral stenosis (BH)
    Pulmonary veno-occlusive disease
    Lymphangioleiomyomatosis

Key: BH, bland hemorrhage; DAD, diffuse alveolar damage.
[a] Individual patients may show either underlying pulmonary capillaritis or bland alveolar hemorrhage.

complement level, positive antinuclear antibodies, and the presence of double-stranded anti–deoxyribonucleic antibodies in the serum points to the diagnosis. In the DAH associated with SLE, granular rather than linear deposition of immune complexes is found in the lung and kidney. In SLE, almost all cases of DAH are associated with nephritis. In isolated pulmonary capillaritis, Wegener's granulomatosis, and microscopic polyangiitis, tissue immunofluorescent studies are negative (pauciimmune). The presence of a serum antineutrophil cytoplasmic antibody (ANCA) is useful in confirming a diagnosis. Wegener's granulomatosis is characterized by the presence of c-ANCA (antiproteinase 3 antibody). The presence of serum p-ANCA (antimyeloperoxidase antibody) supports the possibility of microscopic polyangiitis or pauciimmune glomerulonephritis.

Diffuse Alveolar Damage (DAD)

Another lung injury that results in DAH is diffuse alveolar damage (DAD). DAD is the underlying lesion of the acute respiratory distress syndrome (ARDS), the Hamman-Rich syndrome, cytotoxic drug injury,and other forms of acute lung injury. DAH that follows DAD most commonly complicates cytotoxic drug therapy or inhalation of crack cocaine. The characteristic histology of DAD includes the presence of interstitial and intraalveolar edema, capillary congestion and microthrombi, and intraalveolar hyaline membrane formation.

Wegener's Granulomatosis

Wegener's granulomatosis is characterized by necrotizing granulomatous lesions in the lung and often in other organs as well. These patterns define individual cases as limited Wegener's granulomatosis or systemic disease. Pulmonary capillaritis with bleeding can be the initial pulmonary manifestation of Wegener's granulomatosis or can occur simultaneously with the more typical lesions, and DAH can exacerbate an established case. DAH due to pulmonary capillaritis and Wegener's granulomatosis is almost always associated with an active focal segmental necrotizing glomerulonephritis. In the patient presenting for the first time with DAH and glomerulonephritis, a positive c-ANCA points to the diagnosis of Wegener's granulomatosis.

Wegener's granulomatosis usually presents with underlying necrotizing granulomatous inflammation and small- and medium-vessel vasculitis involving both the airways and the lung parenchyma. This process is reflected on the chest radiograph as nodules or masses that undergo cavitation. If lesions appear only in the lung or upper airways, this is referred to as limited Wegener's granulomatosis. If this phase remains untreated, most patients will progress to a more generalized phase of the disease in which the kidneys are involved. The limited disease is associated with very few constitutional symptoms. Generalized disease, on the other hand, is usually associated with malaise, fevers, night sweats, weight loss, and sometimes migratory arthralgias. Pulmonary symptoms include cough, dyspnea, and hemoptysis. Because of tracheobronchial involvement, the symptoms may mimic asthma. The airway obstruction follows acute inflammation, mucosal ulceration, and eventually stenosis. It is most common in the subglottic area. Bronchial stenosis may cause lobar atelectasis and postobstructive pneumonia. Other manifestations include a leukocytoclastic vasculitis of the skin, which presents as palpable purpura, central or peripheral nervous system involvement, sinusitis, and glomerulonephritis. The presence of glomerulonephritis adversely affects outcome. The diagnosis of Wegener's granulomatosis is established by the presence of serum antiproteinase 3 antibody (c-ANCA) with a compatible clinical picture. If a biopsy is necessary, a lung biopsy is recommended. The renal biopsy rarely if ever shows necrotizing granulomatous inflammation.

Microscopic Polyangiitis

Microscopic polyangiitis is considered to be a microvascular variant of classical polyarteritis nodosa (PAN). The major difference is that in classic PAN there is involvement of small and medium vessels as opposed to the predominantly capillary focus in microscopic polyangiitis. The renal involvement is different as well. The renal lesion in classic PAN results in hypertension and microaneurysms, since it involves larger vessels. In microscopic polyangiitis, a focal segmental necrotizing glomerulonephritis occurs. Another important difference is that in approximately one-third of patients with microscopic polyangiitis, the lung is involved (pulmonary capillaritis and DAH); in classic PAN, lung disease is rare. Microscopic polyangiitis can be accompanied by leukocytoclastic vasculitis of the skin and by peripheral neuropathy. Glomerulonephritis is present in all cases. Serum antimyeloperoxidase antibody (p-ANCA) is present in over 80% of cases. The remainder are c-ANCA–positive. In the latter case, differentiation from Wegener's granulomatosis is difficult unless a granulomatous vasculitis eventually develops. Patients with microscopic polyangiitis who are c-ANCA–positive have a poorer outcome than the group as a whole.

Isolated Pulmonary Capillaritis

Isolated pulmonary capillaritis causes DAH but without systemic findings or serological manifestations of an associated disease. There are two types of isolated pulmonary capillaritis reported: a more common type in which serum ANCA is negative and a less common variety associated with the presence of serum p-ANCA. Long-term follow-up of the ANCA-negative patients indicates no further evolution into a systemic disease state. It is possible that adult cases of isolated pulmonary capillaritis were previously called idiopathic pulmonary hemosiderosis.

Other Forms of Systemic Vasculitis

Other causes of pulmonary capillaritis include Behçet's syndrome and Henoch-Schönlein purpura, IgA nephropathy, and idiopathic pauciimmune glomerulonephritis. Henoch-Schönlein purpura is characterized by circulating and tissue-bound IgA immune complexes. IgA nephropathy is a common form of glomerulonephritis with IgA immune complexes; it is sometimes associated with DAH and capillaritis.

Goodpasture's Syndrome (GPS)

GPS is characterized by an antibody common to glomerular and alveolar basement membranes. This antibody produces a distinct pattern of wavy, uninterrupted linear immunofluorescence when kidney or lung sections are stained with antibodies against IgG or complement (Fig. 9). This anti–glomerular basement membrane antibody (AGMB) appears in the serum. The antibody level seems to correlate with the severity of the renal disease. The antibody is directed against an antigen in the non-collagenous region of type IV collagen, the major component of basement membrane. In up to 80% of cases, the lung and renal disease occur simultaneously; in 10–30%, glomerulonephritis is the sole manifestation. Isolated renal disease is more likely to occur in older patients and in nonsmokers. Smoking is associated with a high incidence of DAH in GPS. Men (20–30 years) are more likely to develop this disease. In addition to the serum anti–basement membrane antibody, up to 40% of patients will have elevated serum ANCA levels (either pANCA or cANCA). There are cases in which it is difficult to distinguish between Goodpasture's syndrome and either Wegener's granulomatosis or microscopic polyangiitis. In 5–10% of patients with GPS, there is isolated lung involvement. In this case, differentiation from

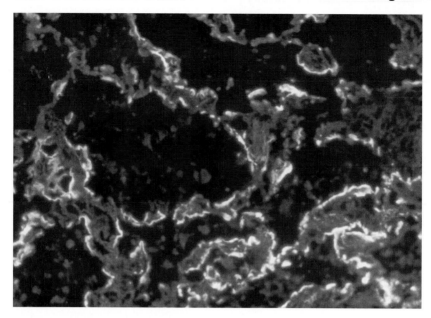

Figure 9 Goodpasture's syndrome. Immunofluorescent study demonstrating linear IgG staining of alveolar basement membranes.

isolated pulmonary capillaritis can be made only by immunofluorescent studies of the lung. In GPS, there is linear immunofluorescence, as opposed to no immune complex deposition in isolated pulmonary capillaritis.

Treatment of Diffuse Alveolar Hemorrhage and Vasculitis

The treatment of the systemic vasculitides is generally the same regardless of whether the disease is isolated to the lung or involves many systemic organs. Treatment usually includes both corticosteroids and cyclophosphamide. For patients with DAH secondary to pulmonary capillaritis and disease with a systemic vasculitis involving larger vessels, we initially treat with intravenous methylprednisolone (250–500 mg every 6 h for 3 days). Those patients with milder more limited forms of a systemic vasculitis and without capillaritis and DAH can be begun on oral prednisone, 1.5 mg/kg, not to exceed 100 mg daily. If renal dysfunction is present, treatment should be initiated before diagnostic studies are returned, since this is a rapidly progressive form of glomerulonephritis and permanent renal insufficiency may result. Patients on intravenous methylprednisolone are tapered over 1 week and switched to oral prednisone at 60–80 mg per day. Following this, prednisone is slowly tapered for as long as the patient remains in remission, and it is often possible to discontinue prednisone by 6–12 months.

Cyclophosphamide can be given initially as a single intravenous dose (1 g/m² body surface area). Alternatively, daily oral cyclophosphamide (2 mg/kg weight) may be chosen. Regardless of the route of administration, the effect of cyclophosphamide is delayed for approximately 2 weeks. The drug is continued for at least 1 year after the patient has achieved complete remission and then tapered by 25-mg decrements every 2–3 months until discontinuation. Patients who receive intravenous cyclophosphamide therapy initially can continue with monthly courses of cyclophosphamide until a remission is complete or alternatively oral cyclophosphamide can be started 1 month after the initial intravenous dose. The remission rate is somewhere between 75 and 90%. Since DAH has a tendency to recur, treatment with low doses of prednisone (10–20 mg/day) and oral cyclophosphamide should continue for a minimum of 18 months. Cyclophosphamide carries significant side effects, as presented in detail above, in the discussion of the treatment of IPF, and dosage should be adjusted as described there. Furthermore, a complicating *Pneumocystis carinii* pneumonia occurs in patients being treated for their vasculitis with prednisone and cyclophosphamide (5–20%). It is recommended that timethoprim-sulfamethoxazole prophylaxis be added to the therapeutic regimen. Alternatives for patients intolerant to cyclophosphamide include weekly methotrexate (10–20 mg) or daily azathioprine (2 mg/kg). Although methotrexate is effective in inducing remission, there are significant problems with *P. carinii* pneumonia and prophylaxis with trimethoprim sulfamethoxazole is again advised.

Trimethoprim-sulfamethoxazole has also been recommended as a primary therapeutic agent for Wegener's granulomatosis but not for the other vasculitides. When used in combination with standard immunosuppressive therapy and prednisone, there is a reduction in the incidence of relapse. Although there is some evidence suggesting that single therapy with this drug in patients with limited Wegener's granulomatosis is effective, it cannot be recommended at this time.

Plasmaphereses has a significant influence on the outcome of patients with Goodpasture's syndrome and probably with IgA nephropathy. This modality has little proven effect for any other cause of DAH, although one group of investigators reported improved early survival in microscopic polyangiitis with plasmapheresis. Plasmapheresis has been recommended for DAH in SLE; however, it has not been shown to improve the overall survival rate of about 50%. Intravenous immunoglobulin (IVIG) has been utilized for several patients with DAH who did not respond to immunosuppressive therapy, and a complete remission was achieved in a few cases of Wegener's granulomatosis. The use of IVIG should be reserved for patients who do not respond to standard therapy.

The Eosinophilic Pneumonias

The known causes of eosinophilic pneumonia include drug toxicity and parasitic infestations. Most eosinophilic infiltrations of the lung that occur in the United States are idiopathic disorders and are classified as follows: (1) acute eosinophilic pneumonia, (2) chronic eosinophilic pneumonia, (3) idiopathic hypereosinophilic syndrome, (4) allergic bronchopulmonary mycosis, and (5) allergic granulomatosis of Churg and Strauss. In these disorders the eosinophil is one of the predominant inflammatory cells and is present in both the interstitial compartment and the alveolar spaces. Additional histological features that are sometimes seen are diffuse alveolar damage and organizing pneumonia. In chronic persistent cases, inflammation and fibrosis can appear. Varying degrees of peripheral eosinophilia and BAL eosinophilia, usually exceeding 25% of the total lavaged cells, are common to all of the eosinophilic pneumonias.

Acute Eosinophilic Pneumonia (AEP)

AEP presents as a community-acquired pneumonia causing several days of dyspnea, nonproductive cough, and low-grade fever. It tends to appear in younger individuals. The chest radiograph shows diffuse bilateral alveolar opacities. The majority of AEP are idiopathic, but drug toxicity, particularly that due to nonsteroidal anti-inflammatory agents or to tetracycline and its related compounds can be responsible. AEP is not associated with allergies and is a one-time event, thereby differentiating it from chronic eosinophilic pneumonia (CEP). Both the acute and chronic forms involve peripheral and BAL eosinophilia. In AEP, however, the peripheral eosinophilia may be delayed. Both disorders respond excellently to corticosteroid medication. Another important difference between the two is that AEP does not result in pulmonary fibrosis.

Chronic Eosinophilic Pneumonia (CEP)

CEP is a recurrent disease, appearing intermittently over several years. Extensive lung fibrosis may occur in some cases. Most patients are between the fifth and eighth decades; the onset, as opposed to AEP, is subacute and gradual, with cough and dyspnea being present for weeks to months. Over half of the patients with CEP have a prominent background of asthma or allergy; therefore wheezing may be a prominent feature on physical examination. Another important finding is an increased serum IgE level in approximately two-thirds of the patients. The predominant physiological abnormality is a restrictive disorder, as with all DPLD. In patients with a background of asthma, there may be reversible airflow obstruction as well. The chest radiograph often shows a peripheral distribution to the opacities (Fig. 10). With recurrent disease, pulmonary fibrosis can develop, and this is most prominent in the upper lung zones. The response to corticosteroid therapy is prompt and often complete, but recurrences are to be expected with tapering of the drug. Maintenance therapy with low dosages of prednisone (5–20 mg) is often required for the prevention of recurrences.

Idiopathic Hypereosinophilic Syndrome (IHS)

IHS is a rare, often fatal disorder defined as unexplained peripheral eosinophilia exceeding 1500 cells per cubic millimeter lasting over 6 months and in the absence of any other

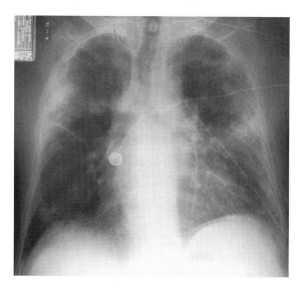

Figure 10   Chronic eosinophilic pneumonia. There is a peripheral distribution of the mixed alveolar interstitial infiltrates. Bronchiolitis obliterans organizing pneumonia can result in an identical radiographic pattern.

cause. IHS patients are usually young males. Since this is a systemic disease, night sweats, anorexia, weight loss, and fevers are reported. The bone marrow and peripheral blood examinations reveal excessive numbers of mature eosinophils as well as younger forms. The most serious complication of IHS is a restrictive cardiomyopathy secondary to endomyocardial fibrosis.

Eosinophilic infiltration of the lung occurs in 40%. Cough and dyspnea may result from either the lung or cardiac disease. The chest radiograph shows diffuse as well as localized opacities, and pleural effusions are common. Some of the surviving patients can develop pulmonary fibrosis. A response to corticosteroid medication occurs in 50%, particularly in those who have initially elevated levels of serum IgE. The responders also demonstrate a striking fall in the peripheral eosinophil count once corticosteroids are initiated. In the remaining corticosteroid-resistant patients, cyclophosphamide, alpha-interferon and cyclosporin A have occasioned remissions in some cases.

Allergic Bronchopulmonary Mycosis (ABPM)

ABPM refers to an eosinophilic infiltration of the airways and the lung parenchyma, which complicates asthma and cystic fibrosis. Most cases are associated with *Aspergillus* colonization, although other fungal species have been described. Thus the disease is often referred as allergic bronchopulmonary aspergillosis (ABPA). The criteria for diagnosis include the presence of asthma, peripheral eosinophilia, a positive prick test to the suspected fungal antigen, precipitating antibodies in serum or BAL, elevated serum IgE levels, and pulmonary infiltrates on chest radiograph. There is mucous plugging of the bronchi by fungal hyphae as well as an eosinophilic inflammatory bronchitis. Eosinophils also infiltrate the alveolar structures, producing eosinophilia pneumonia. As with CEP, this is a chronic disease which is recurrent and because of the asthmatic component; it is often difficult to treat and control. Because of this, upper-lung-zone proximal bronchiectasis and interstitial fibrosis can occur. The mainstay of therapy is corticosteroid medication. There are uncontrolled studies suggesting that chronic oral itraconazole therapy may have a corticosteroid-sparring effect. Inhaled amphotericin B is ineffective.

Allergic Granulomatosis of Churg and Strauss (Churg-Strauss Syndrome, CSS)

The Churg-Strauss syndrome (CSS) is a rare eosinophilic syndrome characterized by a systemic vasculitis that develops in a patient with a prior background of asthma. Several years separate the onset of asthma and the development of the systemic vasculitis. Skin involvement with nodules, purpura, and urticaria is common, along with small- and medium-vessel vasculitis involving the lung. The central nervous system is involved in 30%, mononeuritis multiplex in 66%, and cardiac involvement and glomerulonephritis in up to 50%. Other systemic manifestations include abdominal pain, diarrhea, and lower GI bleeding. Patients complain of cough, dyspnea, and hemoptysis. Histological features include a granulomatous eosinophilic vasculitis of the small and medium-sized pulmonary vessels, eosinophilic pulmonary effusions secondary to vasculitis of the pleural vessels, and eosinophilic pneumonia. IgE levels are elevated and the serum rheumatoid factor may be increased. Some patients demonstrate a serum antibody to neutrophil cytoplasmic myeloperoxidase (p-ANCA). Most patients respond to corticosteroid therapy alone; however, in resistant cases, cyclophosphamide or an alternative immunosuppressive agent is recommended (see ''Diffuse Alveolar Hemorrhage and Vasculitis'', above).

Lymphangioleiomyomatosis (LAM)

LAM is an uncommon disorder occurring almost exclusively in premenopausal women. It is recognized by an abnormal proliferation of smooth muscle cells that occurs primarily in the lung. Extra-pulmonary manifestations include a 40% incidence of angiomyolipomas of the kidney, abdominal lymphangioleiomyoma, and uterine and adrenal tumors. Patients become symptomatic between the ages of 17 and 47. Although cases have been reported in postmenopausal women, it is likely that the disease started prior to menopause. It does appear, however, that the older one is at the time of diagnosis, the more slowly the disease progresses. The salient histological feature of this disease is the proliferation of normal-appearing smooth muscle. In the lung, this results in lymphatic obstruction, causing chylous pleural effusions; bronchiolar obliteration, causing obstructive lung disease; interstitial deposition; and rupture of pulmonary veins, causing hemoptysis. Furthermore, the bronchiolar obstruction causes cystic lung disease, which results in physiological hyperinflation and airflow limitation and is complicated by spontaneous pneumothorax. The unexplained appearance of either a chylous pleural effusion, a benign renal tumor, unexplained obstructive lung disease, unexplained hemoptysis, or spontaneous pneumothorax in a young woman should raise the suspicion of LAM.

Chest radiographs indicate hyperinflation as well as interstitial opacities and sometimes Kerley B lines. In some cases, pneumothorax and pleural (chylous) effusions are present. The HRCT is often diagnostic (Fig. 11). Physiological testing demonstrates an obstructive lung disease with hyperinflation and a reduction in the diffusing capacity for carbon monoxide. This constellation of findings is similar to that for congenital emphysema in this age group.

Because of the occurrence of LAM in premenopausal women and its reported acceleration during pregnancy and following exogenous estrogen therapy in some cases, a hormonal influence is thought to be important in its pathogenesis. Therapy has been directed

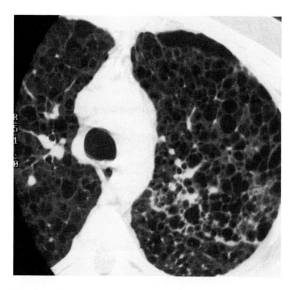

Figure 11 Lymphangioleiomyomatosis. This high-resolution computed tomography scan shows cystic replacement of the lung parenchyma and a loculated pneumothorax.

toward reducing estrogen activity and includes the use of medroxyprogesterone, oophorec-tomy, or a combination of the two. Tamoxifen, an antiestrogen agent, has also been recom-mended. Buserelin, a luteinizing hormone antagonist, has been tried in several patients. This agent produces a medical castration. It is difficult to determine whether any of the aforementioned medical therapies are effective. There are few cases, short follow-up pe-riods, and case reports as opposed to trials; most patients die of respiratory failure within 4–10 years of the onset of their symptoms. There is also a variable disease course, and older patients are known to have a prolonged survival. Lung transplantation is an alterna-tive for some of these women. There is one report of LAM recurring in the transplanted lung.

Pulmonary Alveolar Proteinosis

Pulmonary alveolar proteinosis (PAP), also known as pulmonary alveolar phospholipo-proteinosis, is a diffuse lung disease characterized by the accumulation of an amorphous, lipoproteinaceous material in the distal airspaces. This material stains positively in tissue sections with periodic acid–Schiff (PAS) stain. There is little or no lung inflammation, and the underlying lung architecture is preserved. Characterization of this lipoproteinaceous material shows it to be made up principally of the surfactant phospholipids and surfactant apoproteins. The etiology of PAP is unknown. Similar histopathological findings have been documented in acute silicosis (''silicoproteinosis''), aluminum dust exposure, tita-nium exposure, infections with *P. carinii*, and in various hematological malignancies and immunosuppression.

The clinical presentation of PAP usually is insidious. The typical age of presentation is 30–50 years, with a male:female ratio of 2:1. Approximately one-third of affected patients are asymptomatic despite infiltration of the alveolar airspaces. The major clinical manifestations are progressive dyspnea on exertion, fatigue, weight loss, and low-grade fever. A nonproductive cough is common but occasionally expectoration of ''chunky'' gelatinous material may occur. Physical examination is often normal. There is an increased risk of superinfection in PAP patients by opportunistic organisms such as *Nocardia*, myco-bacteria, and various fungi.

Nonspecific abnormalities in routine laboratory tests in PAP include polycythemia, hypergammaglobulinemia, and increased LDH levels. Pulmonary function tests show a restrictive ventilatory defect. An isolated decrease in DL_{CO} may be present and may be out of proportion to the degree of reduced lung volume. Hypoxemia and compensated respiratory alkalosis are common and frequently worsen with exercise. An elevated shunt fraction is usually present.

Radiographically, there are bilateral, symmetrical alveolar opacities located centrally in the mid- and lower-lung zones resulting in a ''batwing'' distribution. Air bronchograms are rare. A thin lucent band may sharply outline the diaphragm and the heart, consistent with sparing of the lung immediately adjacent to these structures. High-resolution com-puted tomography scanning (HRCT) shows ground-glass opacification, with thickened intralobular structures and interlobular septa in typical polygonal shapes called ''crazy-paving.''

The diagnosis of PAP frequently requires examination of tissue obtained by surgical lung biopsy. The normal alveolar architecture is usually preserved, although the alveolar septa may be slightly thickened due to type II epithelial cell hyperplasia. Typically, there is little or no inflammatory cell infiltration. The terminal bronchioles and alveoli are filled with a flocculent and granular lipoproteinaceous material that stains pink with PAS stain. Within this lipoproteinaceous material, there are macrophages ladened with PAS-positive material, scattered clefts of cholesterol crystals, and occasionally a histiocytic giant-cell reaction. Electron microscopy of BAL fluid or lung tissue shows concentrically laminated structures called lamellar bodies. The BAL fluid from patients with PAP is opaque rather than translucent, with a characteristic tan or cream color and suspended flocculent material. The BAL fluid's appearance is so distinctive that many clinicians believe a secure diagnosis can be made on these grounds alone.

Some patients with PAP are asymptomatic and have little or no physiological impairment despite extensive radiographic abnormalities; these patients do not require immediate treatment. In addition, up to 25% of patients may experience spontaneous remissions. Thus, treatment should be instituted when symptoms develop that are troublesome for the patient. The most widely accepted and effective form of treatment is therapeutic whole-lung lavage via a double-lumen endotracheal tube. This procedure is performed under general anesthesia, with one lung being ventilated while the other is washed by the repeated instillation and drainage of large volumes of normal saline solution. Patients often feel dramatically better after whole-lung lavage, with improvement in exertional dyspnea. The clinical course of PAP is variable; 30–40% of patients require only one lavage, while others may require repeat lung lavages at intervals of 6–12 months. There is no role for corticosteroids or other immunosuppressives; in fact, concern has been raised that corticosteroids may increase mortality.

SUGGESTED READING

1. Allen JN, Davis WB. Eosinophilic lung diseases. Am J Respir Crit Care Med 1994; 150: 1423–1438.
2. Bjoraker JA, Ryu JH, Edwin MK, Myers JL, Tazelaar HD, Schroeder DR, Offord KP. Prognostic significance of histopathologic subsets in idiopathic pulmonary fibrosis. Am J Respir Crit Care Med 1998; 157:199–203.
3. Camus P. Respiratory disease caused by drugs. Eur Respir J 1997; 10:260–264.
4. Cohen AJ, King TE Jr, Downey GP. Rapidly progressive bronchiolitis obliterans with organizing pneumonia. Am J Respir Crit Care Med 1994; 149:1670–1675.
5. Coultas DB, Zumwalt RE, Black WC, Sobonya RE. The epidemiology of interstitial lung disease. Am J Respir Crit Care Med 1994; 150:967–972.
6. Deheinzelin D, Capelozzi VL, Kairalba RA, et al. Interstitial lung disease in primary Sjögren's syndrome: clinical pathologic evaluation and response to treatment. Am J Respir Crit Care Med 1996; 154:794–799.
7. Johnston IDA, Prescott RJ, Chalmers JC, Rudd RM, for the Fibrosing Alveolitis Subcommittee of the Research Committee of the British Thoracic Society. British Thoracic Society study of cryptogenic fibrosing alveolitis: current presentation and initial management. Thorax 1997; 52:38–44.
8. Katsenstein ALA, Myers RL. Idiopathic pulmonary fibrosis: clinical relevance of pathologic classification. Am J Respir Crit Care Med 1998; 157:1301–1315.
9. Katzenstein ALA, Fiorellia RF. Nonspecific interstitial pneumonia/fibrosis: histologic features and clinical significance. Am J Pathol 1994; 18:136–147.
10. Kelly PT, Haponick EF. Goodpasture's syndrome: molecular and clinical advances, Medicine 1994; 73:171–185.
11. Kitaichi M, Nishimuta K, Itoh H, Isumi T. Pulmonary lymphangioleiomyomatosis: a report

of 46 patients including a clinicopathological study of prognostic factors. Am J Respir Crit Care Med 1995; 151:527–533.

12. Lynch JP III, McCune WJ. Immunosuppressive and cytotoxic pharmacotherapy for pulmonary disorders. Am J Respir Crit Care Med 1997; 155:395–420.

13. Muller NL, Muller RR. Computed tomography of chronic diffuse infiltrative lung disease. Am Rev Respir Dis 1990; 142:1206–1215.

14. Rosenow EC III, Myers JL, Swensen SJ, et al. Drug induced pulmonary disease: an update. Chest 1992; 102:239–250.

15. Schwarz MI, King TE, Jr. Interstitial Lung Diseases, 3rd ed. Hamilton, Ontario: Decker, 1998.

16. Taylor JR, Ryu J, Colby TV, et al. Lymphangioleiomyomatosis: clinical course in 32 patients. N Engl J Med 1990; 323:1254–1260.

17. Wade JF III, King TE Jr. Infiltrative and interstitial lung disease in the elderly. Clin Chest Med 1993; 14:501–521.

18. Wright L, King TE Jr. Cryptogenic organizing pheumonia (idiopathic bronchilolitis obliterans organizing pneumonia): an update. Clin Pulm Med 1997; 4:152–158.

30

Venous Thromboembolism

Roger H. Secker-Walker
University of Vermont College of Medicine
Burlington, Vermont

VENOUS THROMBOEMBOLISM

Etiology

The immediate causes of venous thrombosis relate to the triad of stasis, vessel wall trauma, and a hypercoaguable state described by Virchow more than 100 years ago. A fourth factor, genetic predisposition, operates in a variety of ways to increase the hypercoaguable state leading to thrombosis.

In symptomatic patients, most venous thromboses identified by objective tests are found in the proximal veins of the thigh and popliteal fossa and fewer in calf veins. However, in studies using radioactive fibrinogen to identify venous thrombosis prospectively in patients undergoing elective surgery, most thrombi formed in the soleal veins, unaccompanied by clinical signs or symptoms, and remained there. Such asymptomatic thromboses confined to the calf rarely embolized to the lungs; only about 20% extended into the popliteal vein or more proximally. The vast majority of pulmonary emboli originate as venous thromboses in the proximal veins of the legs, less commonly in the pelvic veins or inferior vena cava, and rarely in veins in the upper extremity.

Thrombi that break loose pass up the inferior vena cava and through the right heart, breaking up into smaller fragments during their passage through the right ventricle before entering to the pulmonary circulation and becoming impacted in the pulmonary arterial tree. In massive pulmonary embolism, usually defined as an obstruction of 50% or more of the pulmonary arterial bed, the thrombus lodges in the main, right, or left pulmonary artery. Smaller thrombi will embolize in the lobar, segmental, or subsegmental pulmonary arteries. After impaction in the larger arteries, emboli will often break up over the course of several hours or a day or two and then pass more peripherally, giving rise to pulmonary infarction. This more distal impaction associated with infarction is also accompanied by thrombosis in the pulmonary veins.

The hemodynamic effects accompanying pulmonary embolism are related to the extent of pulmonary arterial obstruction and the severity of preexisting cardiac or pulmonary disease; the greater the obstruction and the worse the preexisting cardiopulmonary situation, the more compromised the cardiac output. Hypoxemia, which in most patients

531

with pulmonary embolism is only mild to moderate, occurs from the failure to match ventilation with the diverted and relatively increased pulmonary blood flow to the nonembolized parts of the pulmonary arterial tree. With large emboli causing substantial elevation of the pulmonary artery pressure, hypoxemia may become unusually severe as the foramen ovale flaps open and allows blood to be shunted through to the left atrium. Rarely, fragments of thrombus may pass through the foramen ovale and embolize systemically.

Perfusion is restored to the lungs by both further fragmentation of the emboli and natural fibrinolysis. Most improvement occurs in the first 3 or 4 days, with the remainder taking place over the next 2 to 3 weeks. Little change is seen after 3 months. Subtle, clinically insignificant impairments in pulmonary capillary blood flow can be detected 1 year later. In a few patients with pulmonary embolism, little or no natural fibrinolysis takes place, leading to chronic thromboembolic pulmonary hypertension in the major vessels.

Because venous thrombosis and pulmonary embolism are both manifestations of the same underlying pathological process and their treatment has many features in common, they are best considered together as venous thromboembolism.

Risk Factors

Many risk factors have been identified for venous thromboembolism; these are summarized in Table 1. They include conditions associated with venous stasis, such as bed rest, immobility from stroke or paraplegia, congestive heart failure, and venous obstruction. A previous episode of venous thromboembolism increases the chances of a subsequent episode two- to threefold. Obesity (body mass index ≥ 29 kg/m^2); cancer, especially adenocarcinomas of the breast, lung, and colon; inflammatory bowel disease, the nephrotic syndrome; paroxysmal nocturnal hemoglobinuria; polycythemia rubra vera; erythrocytosis; and the presence of antiphospholipid antibodies (lupus anticoagulant) all increase the risk of venous thrombosis. Heavy cigarette smoking, ≥ 25 cigarettes per day, is an independent risk factor for pulmonary embolism in women.

Trauma is another major risk factor, and hip fractures in particular are associated with a high incidence of venous thrombosis, approaching 70%. Major orthopedic procedures, such as total hip replacement and total knee replacement, are also associated with a high rate of venous thrombosis, about 50%, without prophylaxis.

Other risk factors include type of anesthesia and operative time during surgery. There is a greater risk for general anesthesia than regional anesthesia. In the days before prophylaxis with low-dose heparin, the percentage of patients developing venous thrombosis postoperatively increased from 20% for operations lasting 1–2 h to 45% for those lasting 2–3 h to 65% for operations lasting more than 3 h.

Increasing age is a major risk factor. Venous thromboembolism is unusual below the age of 40, but the incidence increases rapidly after that, especially over the age of 60. For example, before the advent of prophylaxis with low-dose heparin in patients undergoing general surgery, the percent developing venous thrombosis postoperatively increased from 20% for those aged 40–60 years to 35% for those aged 60–70 years to 65% for those aged over 70 years.

Genetic factors play an important role by creating a hypercoaguable state, recently called thrombophilia (which also includes antiphospholipid antibodies). These factors include the relatively common factor V Leiden mutation, associated with resistance to activated protein C, and the substantially rarer congenital deficiencies of antithrombin III, protein C, and protein S; dysfibrinogenemia; disorders of plasminogen and plasminogen

Table 1 Risk Factors for Venous Thromboembolism

Age
  Rare below age 40
    Increases exponentially above that age
Hereditary factors
  Deficiencies
    Antithrombin III
    Protein C
    Protein S
  Disorders of
    Plasminogen
    Plasminogen activation
  Dysfibrinogenemia
  Factor V Leiden mutation
  Hyperhomocyteinemia
  Prothrombin polymorphism
Surgery
  Anesthesia: general > regional
  Operative time: the longer, the higher the risk
  Major orthopedic procedures
    Hip replacement
    Knee replacement
  Venous stasis
    Bed rest
    Immobility from stroke, paraplegia
    Congestive heart failure
    Venous obstruction
Previous venous thromboembolism
Obesity
Heavy cigarette smoking in women
Pregnancy and postpartum
  Oral contraceptives
Specific diseases
  Cancer, especially adenocarcinomas of breast, lung and colon
  Inflammatory bowel disease
  Nephrotic syndrome
  Paroxysmal nocturnal hemoglobinuria
  Polycythemia rubra vera, erythrocytosis
  Antiphospholipid antibodies, lupus anticoagulant
Trauma
  Hip fractures

activation; and hyperhomocysteinemia. There is also a newly recognized and relatively common prothrombin polymorphism associated with slightly raised prothrombin levels and an increased risk of venous thromboembolic disease. There is good evidence that in people with a tendency to thrombophilia, more than one gene is often involved.

As compared with nonpregnant women of childbearing age, in whom the risk is very low, the risk of venous thromboembolism during pregnancy is increased about five-fold, with an incidence of 1–2 per 1000 pregnancies. Increased venous stasis, venous compression by the gravid uterus, and alterations in the proteins of the coagulation and fibrinolytic systems all play a part in increasing the risk. The risk is spread throughout pregnancy and for several weeks postpartum, with venous thrombosis being more common before delivery and pulmonary embolism postpartum.

Oral contraceptives also increase the risk while they are being used, and the third generation of these agents, although they are associated with a lower risk of precipitating cardiovascular and cerebrovascular events than second- or first-generation compounds, pose a higher risk of venous thrombosis.

In spite of these known risk factors, none can be found at presentation in a substantial proportion—some 50–60%—of patients with venous thrombosis. These are, by exclusion, called idiopathic venous thromboses. The incidence of the subsequent development of cancer in patients with idiopathic venous thrombosis is about 7.5% in the 2 years following the initial venous thrombosis, compared with about 2% in patients with known noncancer risk factors. With recurrent idiopathic venous thrombosis during this time interval, the incidence is much higher, about 17%.

CLINICAL FEATURES

Venous Thrombosis

There is both autopsy and in vivo evidence from objective tests that extensive proximal and calf-vein thrombosis can be present in the lower extremities with neither symptoms nor signs. Thus their absence does not exclude a diagnosis of venous thrombosis. Typical symptoms are pain and/or swelling of a leg or, much less commonly, of an arm. Signs include edema, warmth, dilated veins, tenderness, and palpable cords. Homans's sign– pain in the calf or popliteal region on dorsiflexing the foot—is quite nonspecific. With an iliac vein thrombosis, the whole leg is involved, with marked swelling, discoloration, and dilated veins in the inguinal region; this is one of the few occasions when clinical examination may clinch the diagnosis. As a practical matter, when the diagnosis of deep vein thrombosis is suspected, objective confirmation is essential. Only 35–50% of patients with suspected venous thrombosis are found to have this condition on objective testing.

Venous thrombosis of the upper extremity is much less common than that of the lower extremity, although it is seen more now than earlier because of catheter-related venous injury. It occurs more often in men that in women and usually presents with swelling of the affected limb. Recognized causes include traumatic injury, malignancy, strenuous exertion of the arms held above the head, and central venous catheters and peripheral lines. The diagnosis may be confirmed by venography. Pulmonary embolism is uncommon in noncatheter-related upper extremity venous thrombosis but has been reported to be as high as 25% when associated with central venous catheters.

Pulmonary Embolism

The symptoms and signs of pulmonary embolism are well known to be nonspecific, but it is clinical suspicion that leads to the need for further investigation. Sudden shortness of breath, dyspnea on mild or moderate exertion, and pleuritic chest pain are most common; central chest pain and hemoptysis less common; and syncope unusual. Central chest pain, syncope, and sudden shortness of breath without pleuritic pain are more likely to occur with large emboli in the main or lobar pulmonary arteries. Pleuritic pain, dyspnea, and hemoptysis are more common with segmental pulmonary emboli, which are often accompanied by pulmonary infarction. The latter symptoms usually develop 2 or 3 days after the initial embolic episode, which may have been asymptomatic or perhaps accompanied by a fleeting episode of shortness of breath or dizziness.

Clinical signs are rarely helpful. Tachypnea is most common. Signs of pleural effusion, a pleural friction rub sometimes associated with skin tenderness, and crackles on auscultation are less common. There may be signs of deep vein thrombosis. Still less commonly seen are elevation of the jugular venous pressure or other signs of right heart failure. Central cyanosis, systolic or diastolic murmurs over the pulmonic area, or a left parasternal heave are rare. Tachypnea, tachycardia, hypotension, and collapse suggest massive pulmonary embolism.

Pulmonary embolism may be clinically silent. Approximately 40–50% of patients presenting with proxiaml vein thrombosis but without pulmonary symptoms have pulmonary embolism as judged by a high-probability ventilation/perfusion scan.

DIAGNOSIS

Venous Thrombosis

Whenever deep vein thrombosis is suspected, an objective test is indicated. These tests are summarized in Table 2. In experienced hands, compression ultrasonography of the legs, which is now widely available, has been shown to be highly sensitive, > 90% for proximal vein thrombosis—that is, thromboses in the femoral or popliteal veins and or at the calf trifurcation. Sensitivity for calf vein thrombosis is much lower, about 50%. Impedance plethysmography is not as accurate as compression ultrasonography in the diagnosis of proximal vein thrombosis but may have a role in distinguishing old from recurrent proximal vein thrombosis. A normal ultrasound examination should be followed by another about 7 days later to determine whether a previously undetected thrombosis in the calf has spread to the proximal veins.

Increasing experience with computed tomography and magnetic resonance imaging of the legs and abdomen looking for evidence of venous thrombosis indicates that these techniques, especially magnetic resonance imaging, are very promising. Thrombi in the proximal veins of the leg as well as in the iliac and pelvic veins and inferior vena cava

Table 2 Diagnostic Studies for Symptomatic Venous Thrombosis

Proximal vein thrombosis	Sensitivity %	Specificity %
Compression ultrasonography if normal, repeat on day 7	97	97
Impedance plethysmography	92	95
Magnetic resonance imaging	96	100
Calf-vein thrombosis		
Magnetic resonance imaging	87	97
Compression ultrasonography	50	—
Standard for confirmation		
Venography—ascending phlebography		

can all be identified. Magnetic resonance imaging has been shown to have 100% sensitivity and 96% specificity for proximal vein thrombosis and 87% sensitivity and 97% specificity for calf vein thrombosis. This would be an ideal technique were it not so expensive and its availability somewhat limited.

The standard for comparison remains venography, which has the advantage of visualizing calf veins as well as veins in the thigh. Thrombi, which are seen as filling defects, should be identified in two views. The radiographic appearance of old organized thrombi with their associated collateral vessels is characteristic. Although widely available even in small hospitals, venography is not an ideal standard. Approximately 20% of venograms are technically unsatisfactory, legs in casts cannot be examined, and, in a few patients, previous contrast reactions preclude their use. In addition, the passage of the dye up the leg, which can be most uncomfortable, causes contrast medium–induced thrombosis in 2–3% of patients, which then requires treatment.

Clinical Judgment and the Probability of Venous Thrombosis

By combining risk factors for venous thrombosis and clinical signs, the clinical probability of venous thrombosis can be rated as either high, moderate, or low. The frequency of deep vein thrombosis diagnosed by venography is 85% for high, 33% for moderate, and 5% for low pretest probabilities. Major points in this model include the following risk factors: active cancer being treated or within 6 months of treatment, paralysis, paresis, or recent immobilization of the lower extremities in plaster, recent confinement to bed for more than 3 days or major surgery within 4 weeks, and a family history of deep vein thrombosis in two or more first-degree relatives. Other major points are localized tenderness along the deep venous system and measurable swelling of the thigh and calf. Minor points include a history of recent trauma, pitting edema, dilated nonvaricose superficial veins each involving only the symptomatic leg, erythema, and hospitalization within the previous 6 months. A scoring system—involving combinations of major and minor points and also whether or not there is an alternative diagnosis—completed using a checklist, is used to categorize the probability of venous thrombosis as either high, moderate, or low. Estimating pretest probabilities in this fashion, which takes less than 2 min once the relevant data have been collected, may be most useful when the pretest probability and noninvasive test results are discordant. This should lead to the use of venography to resolve the issue and when the noninvasive test is normal in patients with a low pretest probability, in whom serial noninvasive tests can then be safely avoided.

Pulmonary Embolism

Diagnostic tests for pulmonary embolism are listed in Table 3. Whenever pulmonary embolism is suspected, compression ultrasonography of the legs, a ventilation perfusion lung scan, and a chest x-ray should be arranged. The ultrasound examination will indicate whether or not there is proximal vein thrombosis. The chest x-ray may indicate other causes for shortness of breath or pleuritic chest pain and is also essential in the interpretation of the ventilation perfusion scan.

Interpretations of ventilation/perfusion scans fall into two clinically useful categories: normal and high probability; but these account for only about 25% of interpretations (10% normal and 15% high probability). There is a third nondiagnostic category that includes all other interpretations—intermediate, indeterminate, and low probability—con-

Table 3 Diagnostic Studies for Pulmonary Embolism

Initial investigations
   Ventilation perfusion lung scan and chest x-ray
   Compression ultrasonography looking for proximal venous
      thrombosis
   D-dimer level measured by enzyme-linked immunosorbent assay
Standard for confirmation
   Pulmonary angiography
Supplemental tests
   Arterial blood gases
   Electrocardiogram

stituting the remaining 75%. Between one-third and one-half of patients with nondiagnostic lung scan interpretations have venous thromboembolism. The PIOPED (Prospective Investigation of Pulmonary Embolism Diagnosis) study (see ''Suggested Reading'') showed quite clearly that agreement between radiologists was excellent for normal and high-probability interpretations but less satisfactory for the other categories, so that, for clinical decision making, lumping these other categories together as nondiagnostic is pragmatic and indicates the need for further investigation.

   In patients with suspected pulmonary embolism, the other tests usually ordered are an electrocardiogram (ECG) and arterial blood gases. These are of more use for management than diagnosis. Only rarely will the ECG show signs of acute right heart strain, but other cardiac conditions, such as arrhythmias or evidence of ischemia or infarction, may be identified. The usual arterial blood-gas findings in pulmonary embolism—of mild to moderate hypoxemia and respiratory alkalosis—are seen in many other pulmonary conditions. An arterial P_{O_2} in the normal range is seen in about 15% of patients with acute pulmonary embolism, as it takes embolization of two lung segments before the P_{O_2} falls below the normal range. A normal alveolar-arterial oxygen tension difference, once thought to exclude the diagnosis, is also seen in 10–15% of patients with acute pulmonary embolism.

   The most reliable technique for the diagnosis of pulmonary embolism short of autopsy is pulmonary angiography, the standard by which the other techniques are judged. With selective injection of contrast medium, pulmonary angiography can be performed with reasonable safety in patients with pulmonary hypertension. However, it is not an ideal standard because it is an invasive procedure involving catheterization of the right heart, which carries a mortality rate of about 0.5%. It also requires a highly experienced radiologist and meticulous technique if the results are to be reliable. In almost 30% of patients with suspected pulmonary embolism, pulmonary angiography may not be practical or the results are uninterpretable.

   Pulmonary angiography is not available in many smaller hospitals; in centers where it is available, however, it is of most use in patients with nondiagnostic lung scans and no evidence of proximal venous thrombosis in whom a decision to treat or not treat needs to be made swiftly.

   In the last few years, computed tomography and magnetic resonance imaging of the lungs have been used to look for pulmonary emboli. (Pulmonary embolism demonstrated by helical CT scan is illustrated in Chap. 11, Fig. 5.) As with venous thrombosis, both show much promise and can reliably visualize central, lobar, and segmental emboli. Resolution of both techniques is not fine enough to visualize subsegmental emboli. Whether missing such small emboli as the only manifestation venous thromboembolic disease has any clinical relevance remains to be determined. The fact that previous venous thrombo-embolism is an important risk factor for future venous thromboembolism suggests that long-term clinical trials will be needed to settle this issue.

Postphlebitic Syndrome

The postphlebitic syndrome, which can become quite disabling, is due to incompetent venous valves whose function has been impaired usually by thrombi obstructing valves even transiently. In symptomatic, venographically confirmed venous thrombosis, symptoms and signs of the postphlebitic syndrome develop in about one-quarter of patients. Most become symptomatic in the first year, but the incidence continues to increase for at least 5 years and probably longer. About one-third of these patients develop severe postphlebitic manifestations.

Symptoms in the leg include pain, cramps, heaviness, pruritus, and paresthesia. Clinical signs include pretibial edema, induration of the skin, hyperpigmentation, new venous ectasia, redness, pain during calf compression, and venous ulcers. Only the development of ipsilateral recurrent deep venous thrombosis clearly increases the risk of developing the postphlebitic syndrome. Surprisingly, features of the initial venous thrombosis—such as thrombi in the popliteal vein, occlusive thrombi, or the extent of thrombosis—are not significant risk factors when they are included in analyses with recurrent ipsilateral deep venous thrombosis.

MANAGEMENT

Prevention

The prevention of venous thromboembolism is summarized in Tables 4, 5, and 6 and can be thought of in two ways. First from a public health perspective, the incidence of venous

Table 4   Prevention of Venous Thromboembolism

Lifestyle modification
   Sedentary to regular physical activity
   Inappropriate caloric intake to appropriate caloric intake
   Smoking to no smoking
   Excess alcohol consumption to two drinks a day or less
   No seat belt use to regular seat belt use
Surgery
   Regional anesthesia whenever practical
   As short an operative time as possible
   As swift a postoperative mobilization as possible
Prophylaxis
   Low-dose unfractionated heparin
   Low-molecular-weight heparin
   Warfarin
   External pneumatic compression
   Made-to-measure graduated compression stockings
   Aspirin

Table 5 Venous Thromboembolism Prophylaxis for Elective Abdominal and Thoracic Surgery

Low-risk procedures	**Risk**
Calf-vein thrombosis	<3%
Proximal vein thrombosis	<1%
Fatal pulmonary embolism	<0.01%

Age < 40 years and an uncomplicated surgical procedure
    ≥ 40 years and a minor surgical procedure
Prophylaxis: Early ambulation, graduated compression stockings

Moderate-risk procedures	**Risk**
Calf-vein thrombosis	<10–40%
Proximal vein thrombosis	<2–8%
Fatal pulmonary embolism	<0.1–0.7%

Abdominal or thoracic prcedures under general anesthesia for >30 min
Prophylaxis (one of the following)
    Low-dose-heparin 5000 U subcutaneously every 12 h
    Low-molecular-weight heparin[a] subcutaneously every 12 h
    External pneumatic compression
Risk increases with age, heart disease, obesity, estrogen treatment, varicose veins, and prolonged bed rest

High-risk procedures	**Risk**
Calf-vein thrombosis	<40–80%
Proximal vein thrombosis	<10–20%
Fatal pulmonary embolism	<1–5%

History of previous venous thrombosis or pulmonary embolism
Extensive pelvic or abdominal surgery for malignant disease
Extensive hip or knee surgery, extensive soft tissue injury
Major fractures, multiple trauma
Risk increases with age, heart disease, obesity, estrogen treatment, varicose veins, and prolonged bed rest
Prophylaxis (one of the following)
    Low-dose heparin 5000 U subcutaneously every 8 h
    Low-molecular-weight heparin[a] subcutaneously every 12 h
    External pneumatic compression
    Warfarin, aiming for INR of 2.0 by fourth postoperative day

[a] The dose of low-molecular-weight heparin is fixed; the amount given depends on which product is used.

Table 6 Venous Thromboembolism Prophylaxis for High-Risk Medical Patients

High-risk medical conditions
    Myocardial infarction, stroke, congestive heart failure
    Prophylaxis (one of the following)
       Low-dose heparin 5000 U subcutaneously every 12 h
       Low-molecular-weight heparin[a] subcutaneously every 12 h
       External pneumatic compression

[a] The dose of low-molecular-weight heparin is fixed; but the amount given depends on which product is used.

thromboembolism would tend to be postponed into old age if the behavioral risk factors—such as a sedentary lifestyle and inappropriate caloric intake (leading to obesity), smoking (causing lung cancer and other cancers and contributing to cardiovascular and cerebrovascular disease as well as osteoporosis), excess alcohol consumption, and lack of seat belt use (causing serious injuries)—could be influenced effectively through individual, health professional, and public health measures. Shorter times for surgery, use of regional anesthesia, and early postoperative mobilization would all contribute to a lower incidence.

Second, from the perspective of clinicians and patients, the incidence of venous thromboembolism is markedly reduced through the prophylactic use of low-dose unfractionated heparin, which prevents thrombus formation by inhibiting thrombin activity via cofactor antithrombin III; low-molecular-weight heparin, which prevents thrombus formation primarily by inhibition of factor Xa; or warfarin, which inhibits the proper synthesis of vitamin K–dependent coagulation factors II, VII, IX, and X. Aspirin is much less effective. Mechanical measures—such as intermittent external pneumatic compression devices for the calf or leg, which prevents venous stasis and activates fibrinolysis, or made-to-measure elastic compression stockings—have also been shown to be effective. The evidence favoring these prophylactic measures is more extensive for patients with surgical problems than for those with medical ones.

For elective abdominal and thoracic surgery, the level of risk for developing postoperative venous thrombosis has been categorized as low, medium, and high based on age and type of surgery. In the low-risk category are patients under the age of 40 having an uncomplicated surgical procedure and those over the age of 40 having a minor surgical procedure. Such patients have < 3% risk of calf vein thrombosis, <1% risk of proximal vein thrombosis, and <0.01% risk of fatal pulmonary embolism. Early ambulation or graduated compression stockings are recommended.

In the medium-risk category are patients over the age of 40 having abdominal or thoracic procedures under general anesthesia lasting more than 30 min. Such patients have a 10–40% risk of calf vein thrombosis, 2–8% risk of proximal vein thrombosis, and 0.1–0.7% risk of fatal pulmonary embolism. Within this category, risk increases with age, the presence of malignant disease, extensive dissection, large-bowel surgery, varicose veins, inflammatory disease, heart disease, obesity, estrogen treatment, and prolonged bed rest. Either low-dose heparin (5000 U subcutaneously every 12 h), low-molecular-weight heparin, or external pneumatic compression provide effective prophylaxis.

In the high-risk category are patients with a history of previous venous thromboembolism undergoing extensive pelvic or abdominal surgery for advanced malignant disease or elective hip or knee surgery or who have sustained extensive soft-tissue injury, major fractures, and multiple trauma. Such patients have a 40–80% risk of calf vein thrombosis, 10–20% risk of proximal vein thrombosis, and 1–5% risk of fatal pulmonary embolism. Within this high-risk category, risk also increase with age, heart disease, obesity, estrogen treatment, and prolonged bed rest. Low-dose heparin (5000 U subcutaneously every 8 h), low-molecular-weight heparin, external pneumatic compression, or oral anticoagulation with warfarin to prolong the prothrombin time to an International Normalized Ratio (INR) of 2.0 by postoperative day 4 have all been shown to reduce the incidence of postoperative venous thrombosis.

External pneumatic compression provides effective prophylaxis for genitourinary surgery, neurosurgery, and major knee surgery. For hip replacement surgery, low-dose heparin, low-molecular-weight heparin, and recently hirudin—a specific thrombin inhibitor, have all been used to prevent thromboembolic complications. Hirudin has been shown to be more effective than either heparin preparation but with a similar safety profile.

For high-risk medical patients, low-dose heparin or low-molecular-weight heparin provide effective prophylaxis after myocardial infarction, stroke, and in a number of other chronic diseases including congestive heart failure. For transmural myocardial infarction, full anticoagulation is recommended. External pneumatic compression may also be used for stroke.

Pregnant women requiring prophylaxis are those at risk for venous thromboembolism—for example, those with a previous history of this condition; antithrombin III, protein C, or protein S deficiencies; other causes of thrombophilia; the antiphospholipid antibody syndrome; valvular heart disease; or a mechanical heart valve. A greater degree of anticoagulation than used for prophylaxis in surgical patients is recommended, although firm guidelines are not well established. For conditions normally requiring long-term anticoagulation—such as antithrombin III deficiency, the antiphospholipid antibody syndrome with a prior history of venous thromboembolism, valvular heart disease, or the presence of a mechanical heart valve—adjusted-dose subcutaneous heparin to prolong the activated partial thromboplastin time to $1\frac{1}{2}$ to 2 times the control value during pregnancy is recommended, followed by warfarin postpartum. For other risks—such as previous venous thromboembolism, protein C or protein S deficiency, and the antiphospholipid antibody syndrome without a prior history of venous thromboembolism—either 7500 to 10,000 IU of subcutaneous heparin twice daily or adjusted-dose heparin to maintain plasma heparin levels between 0.1 and 0.2 IU/mL are recommended. Warfarin should be given for 6 weeks postpartum.

Treatment Decisions

Venous Thrombosis

In symptomatic patients with venous thrombosis in the lower extremity, the crucial question is to determine whether the thrombosis is proximal or solely confined to the calf. Proximal vein thromboses are threatening; thromboses confined to the calf are not. If the thrombus is confined to the calf and does not extend into the popliteal fossa over the next 7–10 days, the risk of subsequent pulmonary embolism is negligible and anticoagulant treatment is unnecessary. However, if the thrombus is in the popliteal fossa or more proximally or if a calf vein thrombosis extends into the popliteal fossa, as occurs in about 2% of such cases, treatment is necessary, as the risk of pulmonary embolism approaches 50%. Compression ultrasonography is the method of choice in making this determination as it is less invasive than venography, the reference standard, and more accurate than impedance plethysmography. After an initial negative study, it should be repeated on day 7, looking for extension into the proximal veins. In patients with initially normal compression ultrasonography and a history of previous venous thrombosis and also in those with persisting symptoms, venography should be considered, as such patients with calf vein thrombosis have been found to have a high rate of recurrence of venous thromboembolism. If a calf vein thrombosis is found in these circumstances, the patient should receive anticoagulant treatment.

Pulmonary Embolism

For pulmonary embolism, if the lung scan is normal and there is no objective evidence of venous thrombosis, anticoagulation is unnecessary. Long-term follow-up of such patients has shown no excess incidence of subsequent thromboembolic episodes. If the lung scan is interpreted as showing a high probability for pulmonary embolism (sensitivity approximately 90%), anticoagulation can be started. If the lung scan is nondiagnostic but proximal venous thrombosis is present, anticoagulation is clearly in order.

In ambulatory patients with adequate cardiopulmonary reserve, if the lung scan is nondiagnostic and proximal venous thrombosis is not present and does not appear during 14 days of serial observations, anticoagulation may be safely withheld or withdrawn. The risk of subsequent venous thromboembolism in this situation is slightly but not significantly higher than that seen after a normal lung scan, but it is significantly lower than that which occurs in patients treated appropriately for pulmonary embolism. It is important to remember that this noninvasive approach to the management of patients with suspected pulmonary embolism should be used only in patients with adequate cardiopulmonary reserve in whom it has been shown to be safe. Adequate cardiopulmonary reserve is defined as the absence of pulmonary edema, right ventricular failure, hypotension (systolic blood pressure < 90 mmHg), acute tachyarrhythmias, or respiratory failure as shown by severely abnormal spirometry (forced expiratory volume in 1 s, < 1 L or vital capacity < 1.5 L) or arterial blood gases with a P_{O_2} < 50 mmHg or P_{CO_2} > 45 mmHg on room air. These are listed in Table 7.

The major drawback of this noninvasive approach is the time required to ensure that an unrecognized calf vein thrombosis does not extend proximally. Pulmonary angiography, when available, is the best way to resolve this issue. The part that computed tomography or magnetic resonance imaging can play in this situation has yet to be clearly defined.

In patients with nondiagnostic lung scans, no evidence of proximal vein thrombosis, but poor cardiopulmonary reserve, the safety of not treating has not been established; therefore pulmonary angiography should be considered. In experienced hands, the results of pulmonary angiography may be used to guide treatment. If pulmonary angiography is not available, clinical judgment must dictate the need for anticoagulation, weighing up the risks and benefits for each individual patient.

Table 7 Definition of Adequate Cardiorespiratory Reserve

Adequate cardiopulmonary reserve is:
the absence of
pulmonary edema
right ventricular failure
hypotension (systolic blood pressure <90 mmHg)
acute tachyarrhythmias
or the absence of
respiratory failure as shown by severely abnormal spirometry:
forced expiratory volume in 1 s < 1 L or vital capacity
<1.5 L or by arterial blood gases on room air:
P_{O_2} < 50 mmHg
P_{CO_2} > 45 mmHg

Source: Hull RD, Raskob GE, Ginsberg JS, Panju AA, Brill-Edwards P, Coates G, Pineo GF. A noninvasive strategy for the treatment of patients with suspected pulmonary embolism. Arch Intern Med 1994; 154:289–297.

There has been a resurgence of interest in the role that measurement of plasma D-dimer, a degradation product of cross-linked fibrin, can play in this decision-making process. The method used to measure plasma D-dimer levels is important if they are to be used for this purpose. When measured by latex agglutination, normal plasma D-dimer levels are unreliable in excluding pulmonary embolism. However, when measured by the enzyme-linked immunosorbent assay in patients with suspected pulmonary embolism, plasma D-dimer levels in the normal range exclude the presence of venous thromboembolism in all but 5–10% of patients. Normal D-dimer levels have been used to supplement negative initial ultrasound results in patients with nondiagnostic ventilation/perfusion scans, thus reducing the need for pulmonary angiography.

Several schemes, ranging from clinical judgment based on experience to strict data-collection protocols, have been devised to assess the pretest probability of pulmonary embolism. These schemes are based on clinical history, including risk factors for venous thromboembolism, clinical signs and the results of arterial blood gases, the chest x-ray, and, in one scheme, impedance plethysmography. Using this latter scheme, 78% of patients with a high pretest probability, 58% of patients with an intermediate pretest probability, and 33% of patients with a low pretest probability had objective evidence of venous thromboembolism. For clinicians familiar with such schemes, they are most useful in the face of a nondiagnostic ventilation/perfusion lung scan. If the clinical pretest probability is low in a patient with a nondiagnostic lung scan, the likelihood of pulmonary embolism is sufficiently low that further investigation is unnecessary. If the clinical pretest probability is high with such a nondiagnostic lung scan result, pulmonary angiography is unnecessary and treatment for pulmonary embolism can be initiated.

Anticoagulation

Heparin

Heparin and warfarin remain the cornerstones of treatment for venous thromboembolism. Once the diagnosis has been made, unfractionated heparin (subsequently referred to as heparin) is given for 4–7 days and warfarin is started on the second day. Heparin works best when given as a continuous infusion. Use of intermittent intravenous heparin is accompanied by excessive bleeding. Until recently, standard heparin therapy started with a bolus of 5000 U, followed by 1000 U/h, with adjustment of the dose as needed based on the activated partial thromboplastin time (APTT) and aiming for a value 1.5–2.5 times control. Alternatively, plasma heparin levels can be used to guide therapy, aiming for plasma concentrations of 0.2–0.4 U/mL. Several schemes for heparin infusion rates and their adjustment have been described. One of these is shown in Table 8.

There is now good evidence that with use of a weight-based dosing scheme, anticoagulation can be achieved more rapidly and the risk of recurrent thromboembolism is also reduced. The initial bolus is 80 U/kg body weight, followed by 18 U/kg/h by continuous intravenous infusion. Heparin therapy is monitored every 6 h by measurement of the APTT, which should be kept between 1.5 and 2.3 times the control value. Using this weight-based adjustment scheme, a combination of bolus and increase in infusion rate is used when the APTT is below the desired range, no change when it is within the range, and reductions or stopping of the infusion when it is above the range. Details of this weight-based scheme are shown in Table 9.

Table 8 Intravenous Dose Titration Scheme for Unfractionated Heparin[a]

APPT, s	Intravenous Infusion		Additional Action
	Rate of Change, mL/h	Change in Dose U/24 h	
≤ 45	+ 6	+ 5760	Repeat APTT in 4–6 h
46–54	+ 3	+ 2880	Repeat APTT in 4–6 h
55–85	0	0	In first 24 h, repeat APPT in 4–6 h, after that no action; do APPT daily
86–110	− 3	− 2880	Stop heparin for 1 h, repeat APTT 4–6 h after restarting heparin
>110	− 6	− 5760	Stop heparin for 1 h, repeat APTT 4–6 h after restarting heparin

[a] Starting dose is 5000-U bolus, followed by 40,000 U/24 h if patient is at low risk of bleeding or 30,000 U/24 h if there is a high risk of bleeding.
APPT, activated partial thromboplastin time; S, seconds.
Sources: Hull RD, Raskob GE, Rosenbloom D, et al. Optimal therapeutic level of heparin therapy in patients with venous thrombosis. Arch Intern Med 1992; 152:1589–1595. Ginsberg JS. Management of venous thromboembolism. N Engl J Med 1996; 335:1816–1828.

Although the relationship between plasma heparin concentration and APTT is approximately linear over the therapeutic range, the reagents used to measure APTT vary from one laboratory to another, so that the same concentration of heparin can be associated with different APTT values. Ideally, the range of APTT values corresponding to 0.2–0.4 U/mL of heparin for each laboratory should be used to monitor therapy.

Low-Molecular-Weight Heparin.   The days of unfractionated heparin as the initial treatment of venous thromboembolism may be numbered. Low-molecular-weight heparin preparations, although substantially more expensive than unfractionated heparin, are at

Table 9 Weight-Based Dosing Scheme for Unfractionated Heparin

Initial bolus of 80 U/kg of body weight, followed by an infusion starting at the rate of 18 U/kg/h. The APTT is measured every 6 h and the heparin dose adjusted as follows:

Measured Value	Adjustment
PPT < 35 s (<1.2 × control)	80 U/kg bolus, then increase infusion rate by 4 U/kg/h
APTT 35–45 s (1.2 − 1.5 × control)	40 U/kg bolus, then increase infusion rate by 2 U/kg/h
APTT 46–70 s (>1.5 − 2.3 × control)	No change
APTT 71–90 s (>2.3 − 3 × control)	Decrease infusion rate by 2 U/kg/h
APTT >90 s (>3 × control)	Stop infusion for 1 h, then decrease infusion rate by 3 U/kg/h

PPT, partial thromboplastin time; APPT, activated partial thromboplastin time.
Sources: Raschke RA, Reilly BM, Guidry JR, Fontana JR, Srinivas S. The weight-based heparin dosing nomogram compared with "standard care" nomogram: a randomized controlled trial. Ann Intern Med 1993; 119:874–881. Ginsberg JS. Management of venous thromboembolism. N Engl J Med 1996; 335:1816–1828.

least as safe and effective and may, in fact, be both safer and more effective. In randomized trials comparing low-molecular-weight heparin preparations and unfractionated heparin for the initial treatment of venous thrombosis, recurrence rates and episodes of major bleeding were both reduced to between one-third and two-thirds the rates seen with unfractionated heparin.

Low-moleuclar-weight heparin preparations have several other advantages compared with unfractionated heparin. They have longer half-lives; the dose response is more predictable, so that they can be given in fixed doses without laboratory monitoring; and they can be self-administered subcutaneously. The last two features mean that patients trained to give their own injections can be treated at home, leading to substantial cost savings because less time is spent in hospital.

Warfarin

Warfarin should be started within 24 h of the initiation of heparin and the dose adjusted according to an INR of 2.0–3.0. Keeping the INR in this range effectively prevents the formation or extension of venous thromboses, with minimal risk of bleeding. INR values above 3.0 are no more effective than those in the range of 2.0–3.0, but the incidence of bleeding is substantially greater. Because warfarin causes the levels of factor VII and protein C to fall rapidly before those of prothrombin and other clotting factors have fallen much, thus inducing a transient prothrombotic state, it is important to continue heparin therapy for 2 full days after the INR has been in the therapeutic range.

Warfarin therapy must be monitored carefully and the dose adjusted as necessary based on regular assessment of the INR. Different patients have different requirements, and within the same patient, requirements may change over time. Numerous drugs interact with warfarin, so that the frequency of INR assessment needs to be increased when starting, stopping, or changing the dose of drugs that interact with warfarin or perhaps any drug.

In the last decade, the optimal length of time that warfarin should be administered to patients with pulmonary embolism or venous thrombosis has been the subject of both cohort studies and randomized controlled trials. Clear guidelines have emerged for several situations but not for all; these are summarized in Table 10. Patients whose thrombotic episodes occurred in relation to an acute transient risk factor—such as surgery, pregnancy, trauma, or prolonged bed rest—can be safely treated for 6 weeks after the risk factor is no longer present. The rate of recurrence after that time is very low. For patients presenting for the first time with continued risk factors that tend to be medical rather than surgical— such as cancer, chronic inflammatory conditions, or prolonged immobilization—6 months of maintenance treatment with warfarin is recommended. Patients with idiopathic venous thrombosis should also be treated for this length of time.

Lifelong warfarin treatment is indicated for patients with a second episode of venous thrombosis. Although hemorrhagic complications are more common than with a 6-month course, the rate of recurrent venous thromboembolism is about eightfold less and the balance of complications is clearly in favor of indefinite treatment. Lifelong therapy should also be considered for persons with thrombophilia and other continuing risk factors, such as metastatic cancer.

Pregnancy

Venous thromboembolism occurring during pregnancy should be treated with unfractionated heparin because heparin does not cross the placenta. Warfarin, which is teratogenic, also causes fetal hemorrhage, so its use is absolutely contraindicated. Anticoagulation is

Table 10 Length of Time for Warfarin Treatment for Venous Thromboembolism

Clinical Situation	Recommendation

For acute transient risk factors:
  Surgery
  Pregnancy
  Trauma
  Prolonged bed rest
	Continue warfarin for 6 weeks after the risk factor is no longer present

For continued risk factors:
  Chronic medical conditions
    Cancer
    Chronic inflammatory disease
    Prolonged immobilization
    Thrombophilia[a]
  Idiopathic venous thromboembolism
	Continue warfarin for 3 to 6 months

Second episode of venous thromboembolism Metastatic cancer	Continue warfarin indefinitely

[a] For people with thrombophilia, some recommend lifelong anticoagulation. However, the risks and benefits of long-term anticoagulation have yet to be clearly defined for people with the various types of thrombophilia.

started with 5 days of intravenous heparin, followed by subcutaneous heparin every 12 h adjusted to prolong the activated partial thromboplastin time—measured 6 h after the injection—to $1\frac{1}{2}$ times the control value until delivery. Supplemental calcium should be also given because of the risk of osteoporosis with prolonged administration of heparin. Low-molecular-weight heparin can probably be substituted for unfractionated heparin. Although it is substantially more expensive, no laboratory monitoring is required and the risks of bleeding and osteoporosis may be less.

Complications of Anticoagulation

The major complication of anticoagulation is bleeding. Other side effects include thrombocytopenia and osteoporosis with heparin and, rarely, skin necrosis with warfarin. With heparin, recent surgery, liver disease, severe thrombocytopenia, and concurrent antiplatelet therapy are stronger predictors of bleeding than a prolonged APTT. With warfarin, excessive prolongation of the prothrombin time is the leading cause of bleeding. Other risk factors include age over 65 years, previous gastrointestinal bleeding, stroke, atrial fibrillation, renal or hepatic failure, and concurrent use of antiplatelet medication. When bleeding occurs with an INR of less than 3.0, another underlying cause should be sought.

For patients on heparin with a prolonged APTT and also for those who bleed while on low-molecular-weight heparin or who have life-threatening bleeding, protamine should be given by slow intravenous injection over the course of 10 min. This drug is markedly basic and combines with and neutralizes heparin, 1 mg protamine per 100 U of heparin. A dose of 50 mg will neutralize 10,000 U of heparin given 30 min earlier; 25 mg will neutralize 10,000 U of heparin given 60 min earlier; and 12.5 mg will neutralize 10,000 U of heparin given 120 min earlier.

For bleeding in otherwise asymptomatic patients on warfarin, the drug should be stopped and return of the INR to the therapeutic range used to begin therapy again. With more serious bleeding, local measures to control bleeding should be instituted and vitamin

K given orally, subcutaneously, or intravenously. Plasma or factor IX concentrates may need to be given in urgent circumstances.

Thrombocytopenia associated with heparin therapy may be early, transient, and benign. The more serious immune thrombocytopenia, mediated by IgG, tends to occur later, usually 5 or more days after initiating unfractionated heparin; however, it may occur earlier in patients who have been given heparin recently. It is seen in about 3% of patients and is often accompanied by extension of existing thrombi or emboli; arterial thrombosis may also occur. Treatment is difficult. Heparin should be stopped and low-molecular-weight heparin should not be used as a substitute. Warfarin may be given, but it takes several days to become effective. With threatening venous thrombosis, an inferior vena caval filter should be considered. Other rapid-acting anticoagulant drugs—such as danaparoid sodium, ancrod (from snake venom), and hirudin (from leeches)—although not readily available, are all effective. With the early introduction of warfarin and the use of low-molecular-weight heparin, this immune-mediated complication should be seen less often.

Thrombolytic Therapy

Although streptokinase and tissue plasminogen activator are approved for the treatment of venous thromboembolism, their use is severely limited by contraindications in many patients and also the serious risk of major bleeding. There is no doubt that both venous thrombi and pulmonary emboli are lysed much more rapidly with these agents than occurs naturally during treatment with heparin and warfarin. However, in patients with venous thrombosis, the evidence that thrombolytic therapy can reduce the incidence of the postphlebitic syndrome is conflicting. Therefore, in cases of venous thrombosis, thrombolytic therapy should be reserved for those patients with extensive iliofemoral thrombosis. In patients with pulmonary embolism, thrombolytic therapy should be reserved for those who are hemodynamically unstable. The recommended dosage for streptokinase in the treatment of venous thrombosis is a 250,000-U bolus intravenously followed by 100,000-U/h for up to 72 h. For pulmonary embolism, 100 mg of tissue plasminogen activator is given intravenously over the course of 2 h.

Compression Stockings

Use of made-to-measure graded compression elastic stockings, worn during the day for up to 2 years, more than halves the development of the postphlebitic syndrome after the first episode of symptomatic proximal vein thrombosis, whether assessed as mild to moderate postthrombotic syndrome (20% with made-to-measure graded compression stockings vs. 47% without stockings) or severe (11% with made-to-measure graded compression stockings vs. 23% without stockings). Most cases develop in the first 24 months.

Inferior Vena Caval Filters

In patients with proximal vein thrombosis, there are many circumstances in which the use of anticoagulation is too dangerous and the risk of fatal pulmonary embolism (about 20%) too high to ignore; then the insertion of a vena caval filter is clearly indicated. These circumstances include neurological problems such as stroke, cerebral malignancy, spinal injury or disease, and after neurosurgery. Other conditions in which the risk of anticoagulation is too great to ignore and the insertion of a vena caval filter is indicated are malignant hypertension, gastrointestinal hemorrhage, and frank hematuria.

Insertion of an inferior vena caval filter is also indicated in several other situations. One of these is failed anticoagulant therapy, which is rarely seen nowadays. The others are after massive pulmonary embolism and at the time of embolectomy, when there is urgent need to prevent any more emboli from reaching the lungs.

The insertion of filters into the inferior vena cava has supplanted surgical approaches to prevent emboli from reaching the lungs, such as ligation, plication, or placement of a clip. Inferior vena caval filters are placed percutaneously. The most popular device is the Greenfield filter, which is associated with postinsertion caval patency rates exceeding 95% and a low rate of swelling of the legs. Misplacement and migration of the filter or perforation of the wall of the inferior vena cava are infrequent events. Except in patients with massive pulmonary embolism or those few undergoing pulmonary embolectomy, evidence of deep vein thrombosis should be established before insertion. In the absence of a contraindication, it is customary to anticoagulate patients after insertion of an inferior vena caval filter, although there is no good evidence to support this.

Although there are no randomized controlled trials testing the efficacy of vena caval filters, low rates of pulmonary embolization are consistently found after their insertion. In patients in whom there are relative contraindications for antithrombotic therapy but who are at high risk for deep vein thrombosis and pulmonary embolism, the apparent success of vena caval filters has also led to their prophylactic use in multiple trauma, severe head injury, spinal cord injury, and long-bone fractures.

Surgical Approaches to Venous Thromboembolism

Venous patency may be restored by surgical thrombectomy, but in most cases, because of incomplete removal of the thrombus and damage to the vascular endothelium, the vein reoccludes. Because of disappointing long-term results, surgical thrombectomy is not recommended in the management of venous thrombosis except for extensive venous occlusion with compromised arterial circulation, when even a small improvement in venous blood flow could save the limb.

Patients with massive pulmonary embolism can be treated by emergency pulmonary embolectomy, but such an approach requires all the facilities for major cardiothoracic surgery to be at hand on very short notice. With the advent of thrombolytic therapy, causing rapid clot dissolution and some restoration of pulmonary blood flow, there is little need for emergency pulmonary embolectomy.

Pulmonary emboli have been extracted using transvenous catheter techniques; this has met with moderate success and has been accompanied by mortality rates similar to those associated with emergency pulmonary embolectomy. In centers where catheter embolectomies have been done, the indications—in addition to hemodynamic instability—have been absolute contraindications to thrombolytic therapy and failed lytic therapy. The sooner the procedure can be undertaken, the greater the likelihood of success.

In patients with pulmonary hypertension due to chronic major vessel thromboembolic disease, a condition that may be commoner than previously suspected, thromboendarterectomy is in order and results in marked sustained reductions in pulmonary artery pressure and pulmonary vascular resistance as well as an increase in cardiac output.

SUMMARY

Prospective studies and randomized controlled trials have led to substantial progress in defining the appropriate management strategies for venous thromboembolism prophylactically, diagnostically, and therapeutically and also in understanding the natural history of the postphlebitic syndrome. Indications for the use of low-dose heparin and external pneumatic compression for prophylaxis among surgical patients with different levels of risk for venous thromboembolism are well defined.

The use of compression ultrasound to identify proximal vein thrombosis in suspected venous thrombosis has been clearly established. When proximal vein thrombosis is present, anticoagulant treatment is indicated; but when compression ultrasonography is normal and remains so at 7 days, anticoagulation can safely be withheld.

In ambulatory patients with suspected pulmonary embolism who have adequate cardiopulmonary reserve and a nondiagnostic ventilation/perfusion scan, anticoagulation can be safely withheld when noninvasive studies of the legs remain normal over 14 days, indicating the absence of proximal vein thrombosis and hence the risk of further pulmonary embolism. In addition, assessing the clinical likelihood of pulmonary embolism or D-dimer concentration measured by the enzyme-linked immunosorbent assay can each be used to indicate when it is safe to withhold anticoagulation and when pulmonary angiography is needed to establish the diagnosis.

The sensitivity and specificity of magnetic resonance imaging for segmental or larger emboli in the lungs and for thrombi in the abdomen, pelvis, and lower extremities makes it an ideal diagnostic test for venous thromboembolism. However, although more clinical experience with the use of magnetic resonance imaging is needed, its lack of availability and high cost may limit its widespread adoption.

Treatment for venous thromboembolism is with continuous intravenous unfractionated heparin, in doses determined by weight and activated partial thromboplastin time, or with low-molecular-weight heparin subcutaneously in fixed doses for about 5 days, with warfarin started after the first day. Low-molecular-weight heparin can be self-administered, requires no laboratory tests; it is probably safer than unfractionated heparin and may replace it as the initial treatment of choice.

For venous thromboembolism with transient risk factors, warfarin treatment may be discontinued 6 weeks after the risk has disappeared. For idiopathic venous thrombosis and initial episodes of venous thromboembolism in the presence of lasting risk factors, up to 6 months of warfarin therapy is recommended. For recurrent episodes, lifelong anticoagulation is required.

When anticoagulation is contraindicated or fails, a vena caval filter provides excellent protection from pulmonary embolism. Thrombolytic therapy has a place in the treatment of massive pulmonary embolism and also in extensive iliac vein thrombosis. Thromboendarterectomy is effective in chronic thromboembolic disease of a major vessel.

SUGGESTED READING

1. Becker DM, Philbrick JT, Selby JB. Inferior vena cava filters: indications, safety, effectiveness. Arch Intern Med 1992; 152:1985–1994.
2. Brandjes DPM, Buller HR, Heijboer H, Huisman MV, de Rijk M, Jagt H, ten Cate JW. Randomized trial of effect of compression stockings in patients with symptomatic proximal-vein thrombosis. Lancet 1997; 349:759–762.

3. Cogo A, Lensing AWA, Koopman MMW, Piovella F, Siragusa S, Wells PS, Villata S, Buller HR, Turpie AGG, Prandoni P. Compression ultrasonography for diagnostic management of patients with clinically suspected deep vein thrombosis: prospective cohort study. BMJ 1998; 316:17–20.

4. Consensus conference. Prevention of venous thrombosis and pulmonary embolism. JAMA 1986; 256:744–749.

5. den Heijer M, Blom HJ, Gerrits WB, Rosendaal FR, Haak HL, Wijermans PW, Bos GM. Is hyperhomocysteinaemia a risk factor for recurrent venous thrombosis? Lancet 1995; 345:882–885.

6. Ginsberg JS. Management of venous thromboembolism. N Engl J Med 1996; 335:1816–1828.

7. Hull RD, Hirsh J, Carter CJ, Jay RM, Dodd PE, Ockelford PA, Coates G, Gill GJ, Turpie AG, Doyle DJ, Buller HR, Raskob GE. Pulmonary angiography, ventilation lung scanning, and venography for clinically suspected pulmonary embolism with abnormal perfusion lung scan. Ann Intern Med 1983; 98:891–899.

8. Hull RD, Raskob GE, Ginsberg JS, Panju AA, Brill-Edwards P, Coates G, Pineo GF. A noninvasive strategy for the treatment of patients with suspected pulmonary embolism. Arch Intern Med 1994; 154:289–297.

9. Hull RD, Raskob GE, Rosenbloom D, Lemaire J, Pineo GF, Baylis B, Ginsberg JS, Panju AA, Brill-Edwards P, Brant R. Optimal therapeutic level of heparin therapy in patients with venous thrombosis. Arch Intern Med 1992; 152:1589–1595.

10. Hyers TM, Hull RD, Weg JG. Antithrombotic therapy for venous thromboembolic disease. Chest 1995; 108(suppl):335S–351S.

11. Koch A, Bouges S, Ziegler S, Dinkel H, Daures JP, Victor N. Low molecular weight heparin and unfractionated heparin in throbosis prophylaxis after major surgical intervention: update of previous meta-analyses. Br J Surg 1997; 84:750–759.

12. Monreal M, Lafoz E, Ruiz J, Valls R, Alastrue A. Upper-extremity deep venous thrombosis and pulmonary embolism: a prospective study. Chest 1991; 99:280–283.

13. Moser KM, Daily PO, Peterson K, Dembitsky W, Vapnek JM, Shure D, Utley J, Archibald C. Thromboendartectomy for chronic, major-vessel thromboembolic pulmonary hypertension. Ann Intern Med 1987; 107:560–565.

14. Perrier A, Bounameaux H, Morabia A, de Moerloose P, Slosman D, Didier D, Unger P-F, Junod A. Diagnosis of pulmonary embolism by a decision analysis-based strategy including clinical probability, D-dimer levels, and ultrasonography: a management study. Arch Intern Med 1996; 156:531–536.

15. Prandoni P, Lensing AWA, Buller HR, Cogo A, Prins MH, Cattelan AM, Cuppini S, Noventa F, ten Cate JW. Deep-vein thrombosis and the incidence of subsequent symptomatic cancer. N Engl J Med 1992; 327:1128–1133.

16. Prandoni P, Lensing AWA, Cogo A, Cuppini S, Villata S, Carta M, Cattelan AM, Polistena P, Bernardi E, Prins MH. The long-term clinical course of acute deep venous thrombosis. Ann Intern Med 1996; 125:1–7.

17. Raschke RA, Reilly BM, Guidry JR, Fontana JR, Srinivas S. The weight-based heparin dosing nomogram compared with ''standard care'' nomogram: a randomized controlled trial. Ann Intern Med 1993; 119:874–881.

18. Ridker PM, Miletich JP, Hennekins CH, Buring JE. Ethnic distribution of factor V Leiden in 4047 men and women. JAMA 1997; 277:1305–1307.

19. The PIOPED Investigators. Value of the ventilation/perfusion scan in acute pulmonary embolism: results of the Prospective Investigation of Pulmonary Embolism Diagnosis. JAMA 1990; 263:2753–2759.

20. Toglia MR, Weg JG. Venous thromboembolism during pregnancy. N Engl J Med 1996; 335:108–114.

21. Weinmann EE, Salzman EW. Deep-vein thrombosis. N Engl J Med 1994; 331:1631–1641.

22. Wells PS, Hirsh J, Anderson DR, Lensing AW, Foster G, Kearon C, Weitz J, D'Ovidio R, Cogo A, Prandoni P, Girlami A, Ginsberg JS. Accuracy of clinical assessment of deep-vein thrombosis. Lancet 1995; 345:1326–1330.

31
Sleep-Disordered Breathing

David E. Gannon
University of Vermont College of Medicine
Fletcher Allen Health Care
Burlington, Vermont

INTRODUCTION

Sleep-associated breathing disorders have been recognized for centuries and colorful descriptions can be found in historical texts, yet little attention was paid to these disorders until recently. Most physicians practicing today did not learn about sleep disorders during their clinical training in medical school or residency. Fortunately, extensive work to gain a better understanding of this long-neglected group of diseases has led to recognition of how common, debilitating, and potentially fatal they can be. Sleep disorders are receiving increasing attention in the medical literature and in the popular press, and patients often raise concerns about sleep disorders, including sleep-disordered breathing, during visits to their primary care physicians. Sleep-disordered breathing has become an important clinical problem for primary care physicians.

Recent epidemiological studies estimate that 9 to 24% of adults have sleep-disordered breathing in some form and that 2 to 4% of adults have sleep apnea syndrome. Despite this high prevalence, sleep apnea syndrome is underrecognized, and the vast majority of people with sleep apnea syndrome remain undiagnosed. Untreated sleep apnea is a serious problem that can cause disabling daytime fatigue and somnolence, significant medical complications, and even death. With proper treatment, sleep apnea can be controlled and the morbidity and mortality can be prevented.

PHYSIOLOGY OF SLEEP AND SLEEP-DISORDERED BREATHING
Physiology of Normal Sleep

Sleep can be divided into two distinct states: rapid eye movement (REM) sleep and non–rapid eye movement (non-REM) sleep. Non-REM sleep can be further divided into four stages. Stages 1 and 2 are often referred to as light sleep. Stages 3 and 4 are often referred to as slow-wave sleep or delta sleep. The waking state, the REM sleep state, and the various stages of non-REM sleep can be identified (and are defined) by electrophysiologi-

551

cal criteria using electroencephalogram (EEG), electro-oculogram (EOG), and electromyelogram (EMG) waveform patterns. At the beginning of a normal night of sleep, the sleeper will start in the waking state, progress through non-REM stages 1 through 4, and finally reach the first REM state after 60–120 min of sleep. After the first period of REM, the normal sleeper will cycle through the various stages of non-REM sleep and REM, with the episodes of REM becoming more frequent and more prolonged as the night progresses. The timing and duration of these stages during a typical night are illustrated in Fig. 1.

Automatic functions, skeletal muscle tone, and control of breathing are different in the various states of sleep. Non-REM sleep is a state of low cortical activity, with a low level of brain oxygen consumption. Heart rate, respiratory rate, and blood pressure are regular during non-REM sleep. Skeletal muscle tone is somewhat diminished during non-REM sleep as compared with the waking state. In non-REM sleep, the ventilatory response to hypercarbia is similar to the response during the waking state.

In contrast, REM sleep is a state of high cortical activity, with brain oxygen consumption similar to that in the waking state. Heart rate, respiratory rate, and blood pressure are irregular during REM sleep and can vary from minute to minute; periods of breath-holding are common. Skeletal muscle tone is markedly decreased during REM sleep, and the generalized hypotonia affects all skeletal muscles except the diaphragm and the extraocular muscles (which are active in REM sleep). The ventilatory response to hypercarbia is blunted in REM sleep.

Pathophysiology of Upper Airway Obstruction

The patency of the upper airway can be viewed as a balance between the forces that open the upper airway and factors that compromise it. The defining event in obstructive sleep apnea is the collapse of the upper airway (nasopharynx, oropharynx, larynx) during inspiration, which leads to obstruction of the airway and cessation of airflow. This collapse of the upper airway occurs when the negative pressure in the lumen of the pharynx exceeds the ability of the walls of the pharynx to resist collapse.

When any space-occupying lesion intrudes into the lumen of the upper airway enough to reduce its cross-sectional area, a greater inspiratory force will have to be generated to move the same quantity of air (tidal volume) through the narrowed airway. This

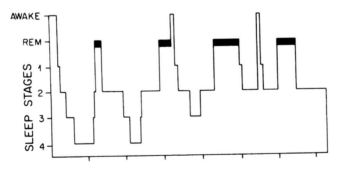

Figure 1 Histogram showing a night of normal sleep in a young adult. REM (shown by darkened horizontal bars) occurs cyclically throughout the night. The first REM period usually occurs 60–120 min after sleep onset. As sleep continues, subsequent REM periods become progressively more prolonged and less time is spent in non-REM sleep between the REM periods. (From Baker TL. Introduction to sleep and sleep disorders. Med Clin N Am 1985; 69:1123–1152.)

higher inspiratory force will result in a greater negative pressure in the pharynx, which can lead to collapse of the pharyngeal walls and obstruction to airflow. Structural lesions that compromise the patency of the upper airway and predispose to obstructive apneas include lesions that narrow the airway through the nose, such as allergic rhinitis, nasal polyps, and deviated nasal septum; lesions that narrow the lumen of the pharynx directly, such as enlarged tonsils or enlarged uvula; and lesions that cause soft tissue normally contained in the oral cavity to shift posteriorly and crowd into the pharynx, such as macroglossia, micrognathia, retrognathia, and the supine position itself (in which gravity causes the jaw and tongue to fall posteriorly into the pharynx when muscle tone is reduced).

The genioglossus muscle and other pharyngeal muscles move the tongue and jaw forward and open the upper airway, counterbalancing the factors that may compromise airway patency. In order to be effective, these muscle actions must occur with sufficient strength, must be coordinated together, and must occur at the same time that the respiratory muscles initiate inhalation. When there are positional factors (supine position) or structural lesions that narrow the pharynx, more assertive action on the part of the oropharyngeal musculature will be required in order to achieve adequate opening of the pharynx during inhalation. Factors that adversely affect the strength or coordination of the upper airway muscles will predispose to obstructive apneas. Upper airway muscle function is diminished during sleep, and is especially diminished during REM. Upper airway muscle function can be further impaired by drugs that affect skeletal muscle tone and coordination, such as alcohol, benzodiazepines, and other sedating medications.

DEFINITIONS

Snoring is caused by partial obstruction of the pharynx.

An *apnea* is defined as complete cessation of airflow for at least 10 s.

Central apnea occurs when there is a cessation of respiratory effort and thus also cessation of airflow; central apneas represent a problem with control of respiration and respiratory drive.

Obstructive apnea occurs when there is a cessation of airflow despite continued respiratory efforts; obstructive apneas are caused by obstruction of the upper airway (not by lack of respiratory effort) and represent a problem of upper airway structure or function.

Mixed apnea has features of both central and obstructive apnea; clinically, mixed apneas have the same implications as do obstructive apneas.

Hypopneas are defined as episodes of shallow breathing lasting for at least 10 s and accompanied by oxygen desaturation of at least 4% from baseline. Hypopneas may contain periods when airflow stops altogether, but if the cessation of airflow is not of sufficient degree or duration to meet the definition of an apnea, the event is classified as a hypopnea. Hypopneas may be caused by obstructive or central mechanisms.

During a sleep test, respiratory events are tabulated and summed to yield the apnea-hypopnea index or *respiratory disturbance index (RDI)*, which is defined as the number of respiratory events (apneas plus hypopneas) per hour.

The episodes of apneas and hypopneas may be associated with episodes of *oxygen desaturation*, during which the oxygen saturation falls by more than 4% from baseline. These episodes of low oxygen may be mild and transient, or they

may be profound and prolonged and result in nocturnal hypoxemia severe
    enough to cause medical complications such as pulmonary hypertension and
    cor pulmonale.
The recurrent respiratory events often cause the patient to repeatedly *arouse* to
    lighter stages of sleep in order to start breathing again; these arousals may not
    lead to full awakenings, but they disrupt the sleep and can lead to symptoms of
    sleep deprivation, such as daytime fatigue and somnolence.
Sleep-disordered breathing is defined as recurrent respiratory events during sleep
    occurring at least 30 times per night or at least 5 times per hour (an RDI $\geq$5).
Sleep apnea syndrome is defined as the combination of sleep-disordered breathing
    plus waking symptoms such as daytime fatigue and somnolence.

RISK FACTORS

Structural lesions that cause narrowing of the upper airway lumen and conditions that
impair the function of the upper airway muscles predispose to upper airway obstruction
and obstructive sleep apnea syndrome. In addition to these factors, some groups appear
more susceptible to developing obstructive sleep apnea syndrome.

People who are overweight are at greater risk for developing obstructive sleep apnea
syndrome. Some 60–90% of patients with obstructive sleep apnea syndrome are obese,
and the prevalence of sleep apnea in population groups increases with greater degrees of
overweight.

The prevalence of obstructive sleep apnea syndrome appears to increase with age.
Although the largest epidemiological studies on the prevalence of obstructive sleep apnea
syndrome have been conducted in middle-aged adults, other studies have shown a higher
prevalence of obstructive sleep apnea syndrome among patients over the age of 65.

Men are more likely to develop obstructive sleep apnea syndrome than are women,
and there appears to be a male:female ratio of 2–3:1 in the general population. This
gender difference is less pronounced among the elderly owing to the increased prevalence
in postmenopausal women as compared with premenopausal women.

Certain minority populations—including African Americans, Mexican Americans,
and Pacific Islanders—appear to have a higher prevalence of obstructive sleep apnea syndrome. Comorbid factors are also more prevalent in these populations. Race as an independent risk factor for obstructive sleep apnea syndrome has been difficult to establish with
certainty.

CLINICAL PRESENTATION

The typical patient with sleep apnea is an older male who is obese, manifests loud snoring
at night, and has daytime fatigue and somnolence. This profile should not be relied upon
too heavily, however. Although the majority of patients with sleep apnea are overweight,
obesity is not a universal trait, and many patients with normal body weight also have
sleep apnea. In fact, sleep apnea affects people of either gender at any age and with any
body habitus.

The presence of loud snoring and excessive daytime sleepiness (as assessed objectively by a spouse or physician) is enough to suggest the presence of sleep apnea syndrome.

People with sleep apnea may also manifest a variety of behaviors during their sleep which can be reported by their bed partners. These include observed apneas, nocturnal gasping or choking, restless sleep, excessive movement during sleep, and waking up confused or disoriented. In addition, the daytime fatigue and somnolence can be severe, and patients can experience cognitive impairment (poor concentration, impaired memory), mood changes (depression, irritability), and sexual dysfunction (loss of libido, impotence).

The disruptive sleeping behaviors at night and the neuropsychiatric symptoms during the day can have serious consequences and can lead to disruption of family life and difficulties on the job. Many spouses have resigned themselves to sleeping in a separate room owing to the loud snoring and active movements manifested by the patient with obstructive sleep apnea syndrome. Many patients have been laid off from work for inattentiveness to details or for falling asleep on the job. Their excessive daytime sleepiness can also lead to industrial mishaps and automobile accidents. Patients with obstructive sleep apnea are at a two- to sevenfold increased risk for motor vehicle accidents.

Patients with obstructive sleep apnea have a twofold higher prevalence of systemic hypertension compared with the general population. The mechanism of this is unclear but may have to do with increased sympathetic nervous system activity, which has been noted in patients with untreated obstructive sleep apnea syndrome. Reductions in blood pressure

Table 1 Common Clinical Manifestations of Obstructive Sleep Apnea Syndrome

Sleep behaviors
  Loud snoring
  Observed apneas
  Gasping or choking
  Restless sleep
  Awakening with confusion or disorientation
  Morning headaches
Neuropsychiatric symptoms
  Fatigue
  Excessive daytime sleepiness
  Cognitive impairment (poor concentration, impaired
    memory)
  Mood changes (depression, irritability)
  Sexual dysfunction (loss of libido, impotence)
Medical sequelae
  Systemic hypertension
  Pulmonary hypertension
  Cor pulmonale
  Erythrocytosis
  Cardiac hypertrophy
  Cardiac arrhythmias
  Myocardial infarction (MI)
  Cerebrovascular accident (CVA)
  Motor vehicle accident (MVA)
Social consequences
  Marital difficulties
  Disruption of family life
  Loss of employment

over the months after initiating successful treatment of the obstructive sleep apnea syndrome have been reported in many studies.

The recurrent episodes of oxygen desaturation that occur during the night in patients with obstructive sleep apnea syndrome can lead to medical complications including pulmonary hypertension, cor pulmonale, erythrocytosis, and right and left ventricular hypertrophy. These episodes of oxygen desaturation are also thought to exacerbate preexistent ischemic heart disease, cardiac arrhythmias, and cerebrovascular disease; moreover, the incidence of myocardial infarction and stroke may be increased in patients who have untreated obstructive sleep apnea syndrome.

The common clinical manifestations of obstructive sleep apnea syndrome are shown in Table 1.

Despite the plethora of symptoms and signs, it is often difficult for clinicians to recognize patients who have sleep apnea syndrome. The onset of symptoms is usually quite insidious, often occurring gradually over years. The patients themselves do not always recognize something being ''wrong'' and therefore tend to underreport their symptoms. Compounding this problem is the fact that the symptoms of sleep apnea syndrome are nonspecific. Because emotional stress and excessive work schedules are integral features of modern American culture, daytime fatigue and somnolence are common, and these symptoms are often not viewed as abnormal either by patients or their physicians. The challenge for all health care workers is to recognize patients with sleep apnea syndrome and to expedite their diagnosis and treatment.

CLINICAL EVALUATION OF PATIENTS

History and Physical Examination

Patients who have sleep disorders are recognized primarily on the basis of the symptoms they or their bed partners report during the medical history. It is not practical for a primary care practitioner to conduct a complete and detailed history of all the sleeping and waking symptoms typical of sleep apnea syndrome and other sleep disorders on every patient. However, a few strategic screening questions may help the physician to decide whether a more detailed history should be obtained (see Table 2).

If the answers to the screening questions suggest the possibility of sleep apnea syndrome, a more detailed history of sleeping and waking behaviors should be undertaken. The goal of this detailed and somewhat specialized history is to determine whether testing should be carried out to investigate the possibility of a sleep disorder. A referral to a sleep specialist at this point can be helpful in obtaining an appropriate sleep-specific history and making that determination. A referral to a recognized sleep disorders center can be particularly useful. A well-equipped sleep center should be able to provide a broad range of services, including consultative services with a sleep specialist to provide advice on

Table 2   Screening Questions for Sleep Apnea

1. Do you snore?
2. Has anyone seen you stop breathing during sleep?
3. Do you fall asleep easily during the day?
4. What medications do you take?

the need for objective testing, a complete array of tests to evaluate patients with sleeping and waking disorders, and treatments appropriate for patients with a variety of sleep disorders.

Sleep habits and behaviors can be strongly suggestive of certain sleep disorders. Because patients are not conscious during sleep and are therefore not aware of their behavior, much of the history of sleep and sleep behaviors must be obtained from the patient's bed partner. The quantity and consistency of uninterrupted sleep time should be assessed in order to evaluate sleep hygiene and rule out simple sleep deprivation. If the patient experiences nocturnal awakenings, the frequency of the awakenings should be assessed and the reason for them established if possible (e.g., noises in the house, waking up gasping and short of breath, waking up with heartburn symptoms, waking up with pain from arthritic joints). The presence of snoring should be established. The loudness of the snoring can be quantified by asking who complains about the patient's snoring, how far away people are who are inconvenienced by the patient's snoring (e.g., same room, same house, neighbors), and what accommodations have been made by the patient's spouse or house mates as a result of the noise level. Patients should be asked if anyone has observed apneas, and if so, the frequency and duration of the apneas. Gasping or snorting at the end of the apneas is particularly suggestive of upper airway obstruction as a cause. The presence of excessive movements during the night can be assessed directly (history from the bed partner) or indirectly (disrupted bedclothes) and is consistent with sleep apnea (patients often move when they arouse at the end of the apneic episode) or periodic limb movement syndrome; the presence of excessive movements but not snoring should strongly suggest the possibility of periodic limb movement syndrome.

Daytime symptoms and waking behaviors can be helpful in evaluating the impact of the patient's sleep disorder on the patient's life. Daytime fatigue and somnolence are the primary symptoms experienced by patients with sleep disorders and should be carefully quantified according to the level of importance of the activities affected (sitting and waiting, watching television to pass the time, watching television program in which the patient is really interested, reading, talking, eating). The degree to which daytime fatigue and somnolence interfere with ability to function should also be explored in order to evaluate the level of disability and risk of adverse events. The presence of somnolence while driving or a history of motor vehicle accidents due to falling asleep at the wheel are particularly important symptoms and should always be part of the detailed history. Some states have requirements for reporting obstructive sleep apnea syndrome as one of the disabilities that affects driving; practitioners should be aware of the requirements in their own state. At the very least, clinicians should caution any patient who reports somnolence while driving that he or she should abstain from driving until the cause of the excessive daytime sleepiness is identified, treatment is initiated, and success of the treatment assured. The presence of morning headaches or lower extremity swelling (as a symptom of cor pulmonale) can signal significant nocturnal hypoxemia from a variety of causes. Other questions about cognitive impairment, mood changes, impotence, and loss of libido will help establish the full extent of impairment being experienced by the patient.

The remainder of the history and physical examination can help identify factors that predispose to obstructive sleep apnea syndrome or may suggest alternative diagnoses that are responsible for the patient's symptoms, such as nocturnal hypoxemia due to cardiac or pulmonary disease or sleep disruption due to discomfort or other external factors. For patients who turn out to have sleep apnea, the weight history will help to establish whether the onset of symptoms correlated with a period of weight gain and will thereby help to determine the likelihood that weight loss will result in an improvement. The history and physical relevance to the nose, throat, and upper airway will help to establish the presence of nasal obstructions, pharyngeal obstructions, or other craniofacial abnormalities that may predispose to sleep apnea. A history of pedal edema or other signs of cor pulmonale may suggest the presence of medical complications due to nocturnal hypoxemia. Symptoms or signs of hypothyroidism, acromegaly, or other endocrine abnormalities will influence the laboratory workup. The list of current medications can give clues to pharmacological reasons for daytime fatigue and somnolence.

Laboratory Evaluation

Decisions to obtain specific testing to evaluate patients for the presence of sleep disorders is based largely on the medical history and the physical examination. The laboratory evaluation of patients suspected of having sleep disorders should be brief and focused.

Patients who have severe daytime fatigue and somnolence or who have signs of cor pulmonale should be screened for the presence of daytime hypoventilation by obtaining a resting arterial blood gas while awake. An elevated carbon dioxide level during the day may signify the presence of obesity-hypoventilation syndrome in those who are obese and have no other explanation for their chronic hypoventilation (such as lung disease or neuromuscular disorders). Patients who have symptoms or signs of lung disease (and who may therefore have nocturnal hypoxemia as a result) should be evaluated for the presence of pulmonary dysfunction, which may be contributing to their problem, by obtaining pulmonary function tests and a resting arterial blood gas while awake.

A measurement of hemoglobin or hematocrit should be obtained in any patient who has severe daytime fatigue and somnolence, symptoms of nocturnal hypoxemia such as morning headaches or cor pulmonale, or symptoms or signs of lung disease that may be causing nocturnal hypoxemia. The presence of erythrocytosis suggests that the patient is having a significant degree and duration of hypoxemia. The hemoglobin or hematocrit can be followed during treatment as a parameter indicating the efficacy of the therapy.

Cardiac testing may be needed in patients who have symptoms or signs of ischemic heart disease or congestive heart failure. Thyroid function tests or other endocrinological evaluation should be done if the history and physical suggest the possibility of hypothyroidism, acromegaly, or other endocrine disorders.

Diagnosis

The symptoms and signs of sleep apnea syndrome are nonspecific: obesity is an increasingly common condition; 25% of people are at least occasional snorers and 15% are habitual snorers; many people feel tired during the daytime due to stress, anxiety, and overwork. Yet only some of the people who suffer these common symptoms have sleep apnea. Moreover, there are many disorders that can cause excessive daytime sleepiness and may have presentations clinically similar to that of sleep apnea (see Table 3). Attempts to devise clinical scales that accurately predict the presence of sleep apnea syndrome based solely on history and physical examination have been unsuccessful. Consequently, treatment based on clinical impression alone and involving costly medical devices or surgery would be inappropriate. Objective testing is required to accurately identify people who have sleep apnea syndrome or to diagnose other sleep disorders so that appropriate treatment can be undertaken.

Table 3 Causes of Excessive Daytime Sleepiness

Obstructive sleep apnea syndrome (OSAS)
Central sleep apnea syndrome (Ondine's curse)
COPD with nocturnal hypoxemia
CHF with nocturnal hypoxemia
CHF with Cheyne-Stokes respiration
Restless legs syndrome
Periodic limb movement syndrome (PLMS)
Narcolepsy
Hypothyroidism
Depression
Insomnia
Sedating medications
Poor sleep hygiene
Overwork, lack of sleep

The conventional method for diagnosing sleep disorders is with a laboratory polysomnogram. This test requires that the patient sleep overnight in a sleep laboratory, where numerous parameters can be monitored simultaneously (see Table 4). Laboratory polysomnograms are conducted under the constant supervision of sleep technologists, so that malposition of leads or other problems with data acquisition can be corrected as the problems arise. Occasionally a second night of testing is required if the patient does not sleep adequately during the first night.

The objective of a laboratory polysomnogram is to monitor during a night of normal sleep all of the relevant physiological parameters necessary to make a definitive diagnosis of the patient's sleep disorder. When patients undergo laboratory polysomnography, they are asked to arrive at the sleep laboratory in the late evening after a day of typical working and eating patterns and after having taken their usual medications. Some modifications may need to be made if a patient is in the habit of taking significant amounts of alcohol or sedating medications or if he or she does shift work and sleeps during the day. When the patient arrives for the sleep test, technologists explain the test, attach and connect the leads that will transmit the data to the recording device, make sure the patient is comfortable in bed with the leads connected, and then turn the lights out and allow the patient to sleep. The technologists then oversee the test from a control room, where they can monitor the acquisition of data and observe the sleeping patient directly through a one-way mirror or indirectly by video monitor. As the patient sleeps, data are acquired and recorded by the electronic equipment and the sleep behavior is observed and recorded by the technologists. If leads fall off or become disconnected during the test or if other problems with patient comfort arise during the night, the technologists can correct the situation so that the integrity of the data acquisition is restored. When the patient wakes up in the morning, the test is terminated. After this, the data are scored (events are identified and quantitated) by a computer and then reviewed and interpreted by a sleep specialist.

Since sleep technologists are present as the laboratory polysomnogram is being recorded, there is an opportunity to carry out trials of various treatments once sufficient data have been gathered to establish a diagnosis. These ''split-night studies'' can streamline patient management by obtaining the diagnosis and evaluating the efficacy of a treatment all during the same test. For patients with sleep apnea syndrome, nasal continuous

Table 4 Components of Laboratory Polysomnography

Polysomnogram channels	Physiological parameters
Electrophysiological parameters	
Electroencephalogram (EEG)	Presence of sleep
Electro-oculogram (EOG)	Sleep stages
Submental electromyelogram (EMG)	Sleep architecture
Eyelid electromotor activity[a]	Presence of arousals
Respiratory parameters	
Airflow at nose[a]	Apneas
Airflow at mouth[a]	Hypopneas
Chest wall motion[a]	Oxygen saturation
Abdominal wall motion[a]	
Oximetry[a]	
Microphone for breath sounds and snoring[a]	
Cardiovascular parameters	
Electrocardiogram (ECG)	Arrhythmias
Pulse counter[a]	Heart rate
Musculoskeletal parameters	
Body position sensors[a]	Body position
Limb electromyelogram (EMG)[a]	Limb movements
Behavioral parameters	
Observation by technologist	Parasomnias

[a] Measured by some portable sleep testing systems.

positive airway pressure (CPAP) can be titrated during the second half of the study. For patients with nocturnal hypoxemia due to causes other than sleep apnea syndrome, supplemental oxygen can be titrated during the second half of the study.

Although they represent the "gold standard" for diagnosing sleep disorders, laboratory polysomnograms are no longer the only method by which an overnight sleep test can be obtained. The technology of data acquisition and storage has improved to the extent that portable equipment is now available for performing unattended sleep tests in patients' homes. These home sleep tests are abbreviated versions of the more comprehensive laboratory polysomnograms; the portable equipment that is currently available is able to collect only a limited amount of data, and the data are focused on parameters of breathing and oxygen level (see Table 4). Moreover, home sleep tests are unattended (no technologist is present during the test), leads can fall off or become disconnected as the patient sleeps, and data can be lost. Nevertheless, home sleep tests can establish the diagnosis of obstructive sleep apnea syndrome in many cases. Occasionally a second night of testing is required if the patient does not sleep adequately during the first night or if leads become disconnected and inadequate data are acquired.

The objective of a home sleep test is to monitor during a night of normal sleep the relevant physiological parameters necessary to make a diagnosis of obstructive sleep apnea syndrome. When a patient undergoes a home sleep test, a technologist usually comes to the patient's house, explains the test, helps the patient attach and connect the leads that will transmit the data to the recording device, and explains how to disconnect and reconnect the wiring harness if the patient needs to get up during the night. Alternatively, the patient

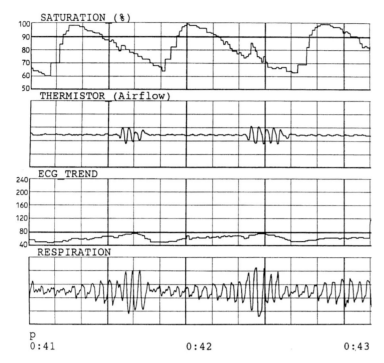

Figure 2 Home sleep test of a 49-year-old female with obstructive sleep apnea syndrome. Parameters displayed are oxygen saturation measured by a pulse oximeter, airflow measured by an oral thermistor and a nasal thermistor and combined into one tracing, heart rate measured by chest ECG leads, respiratory effort measured by chest impedance and abdominal impedance and combined into one tracing, and time shown in military time. The patient is having recurrent obstructive apneas signified by periods with no airflow despite continued respiratory efforts. As the oxygen saturation falls during each apnea, respiratory efforts progressively increase until the upper airway obstruction is overcome and airflow is achieved; oxygen saturation subsequently increases after several deep breaths are taken.

can go to a sleep center where a technologist explains the test, explains how to attach and connect the leads and the wiring harness, and then gives the patient the device to take home and set up on his or her own. On the morning after the test, the device can be picked up at the patient's home by a technologist or the patient can bring the device back to the sleep center. After the device is received at the sleep center, the data are downloaded into a computer, where they can be scored; then they are reviewed and interpreted by a sleep specialist. If significant data are missing (leads connected improperly or leads disconnected and not reconnected during the night), arrangements are made for the test to be repeated on another night. Data from a typical home sleep test are shown in Fig. 2.

The advantages and disadvantages of laboratory polysomnograms and home sleep tests are outlined in Table 5. The laboratory polysomnogram can be used to diagnose all types of sleep disorders. During a laboratory polysomnogram, a full data set is obtained and technologists are present to ensure that the data acquisition is uninterrupted. However, laboratory polysomnograms are expensive (usually costing $1200–$2000), personnel-intensive, and inconvenient for patients who have to travel to a sleep center and sleep over-

Table 5 Comparison Between Laboratory Polysomnograms and Home Sleep Tests

Laboratory polysomnogram	Home sleep test
Pro	Pro
Full data set is obtained.	Cost is lower.
Test is witnessed by technologist:	More convenient for patient.
Equipment problems can be corrected.	Patient sleeps at home.
Patient problems can be addressed.	
Therapeutic interventions can be tried	
and titrated (split-night studies).	
Con	Con
Cost is higher:	Data set is focused on diagnosis
Sophisticated equipment.	of sleep apnea.
Space requirements.	Data is lost if leads become dis-
Personnel-intensive.	connected.
Patient must travel to sleep laboratory.	Limited data variables are moni-
Patient sleeps in different environment.	tored.

night in a sleep laboratory in order to have the test. Home sleep tests are less costly (usually $600–$800) and more convenient for patients, but the data set acquired during a home sleep test is limited and usually focused on making the diagnosis of sleep apnea syndrome.

The indications for obtaining an overnight sleep test are outlined in Table 6. Any patient who snores loudly and experiences excessive daytime sleepiness should undergo an overnight sleep test. Since daytime fatigue and somnolence are often underreported, any patient who has loud snoring and exhibits sleep behaviors suggestive of sleep apnea (observed apneas, episodes of waking up, gasping, or choking) should also undergo an overnight sleep test. In addition, patients who have some of the symptoms or some of the medical complications of sleep apnea syndrome may need to undergo an overnight sleep

Table 6 Indications for Overnight Sleep Test

Obtain *overnight sleep test* for:
   Loud snoring *plus* excessive daytime sleepiness
   Loud snoring *plus* sleep behaviors characteristic of obstructive
      sleep apnea (observed apneas, awakening with gasping or
      choking, etc.)
Consider *home sleep test* when evaluating patients with:
   Symptoms and signs characteristic of obstructive sleep apnea
      syndrome
   No significant heart disease
   No significant lung disease
Laboratory *polysomnogram* may need to be obtained at some point
      during the workup of patients with:
   Excessive daytime sleepiness
   Pulmonary hypertension
   Cor pulmonale
   Polycythemia

test at some point during their evaluation if other testing fails to identify the etiology of their problem.

The decision whether to obtain a laboratory polysomnogram or a home sleep test will depend upon the local availability of diagnostic facilities and testing equipment; relative costs of the two types of tests; a complete understanding of the advantages, disadvantages, and limitations of the testing alternatives available; and specific patient factors. Overall, it must be recognized that home sleep tests are less sensitive than laboratory polysomnograms for diagnosing sleep disorders in general, including sleep apnea. Portable devices will be unsuccessful in picking up sleep apnea in a number of cases (false negatives), and most devices are not able to evaluate patients for the presence of other sleep disorders. Because of these limitations, the indications for doing a sleep test in a patient's home using portable equipment are more focused, and only a subset of patients who need to undergo an overnight sleep test are candidates for a home sleep test. In addition, some patients who undergo a home sleep test may need to undergo a laboratory polysomnogram later on. Laboratory and home portable polysomnography—and reimbursement for them—are evolving fields. Some insurance carriers will pay only for a portable test as an initial evaluation, while other payers will reimburse only for a laboratory study. Many payers require prior approval before a test is carried out.

Patients who appear to have the classic symptoms and signs of obstructive sleep apnea syndrome and who have no other significant medical problems may be considered for a home sleep test. If this fails to establish the cause of the patient's symptoms, a laboratory polysomnogram should then be undertaken to define the etiology of the patient's sleep problem. Patients with significant cardiac or pulmonary problems (who may have nocturnal hypoxemia for reasons other than sleep apnea syndrome) should not be evaluated with a home sleep test; these patients should undergo a laboratory polysomnogram in order to differentiate between the multiple possible causes of nocturnal hypoxemia. In addition, any patient whose history and physical examination suggests the possibility of a sleep disorder other than sleep apnea syndrome (see Table 3) should undergo a laboratory polysomnogram to resolve this issue.

Once the diagnosis of a specific sleep disorder has been established, effective treatment can be undertaken.

MANAGEMENT OF OBSTRUCTIVE SLEEP APNEA SYNDROME

Assessment of Severity

A number of options are available to treat patients with sleep apnea syndrome (see Table 7). The urgency of treatment and the type of treatment chosen will depend upon the severity of the disease and the immediacy and degree of the risk to the patient. Factors to consider in assessing the severity of sleep apnea syndrome include the following:

1. Severity of excessive daytime sleepiness, especially the level of impairment at work (employment difficulties, work disability) or the presence of somnolence while driving (risk of trauma)
2. Degree of nocturnal hypoxemia (especially when the patient has ischemic heart disease)

3. Presence of medical complications caused by the nocturnal hypoxemia, such as pulmonary hypertension, cor pulmonale, or erythrocytosis

Goals of Treatment

A number of medications have been tried for the treatment of obstructive sleep apnea syndrome, but pharmacological approaches have been disappointing. Fundamentally, obstructive sleep apnea is a mechanical problem of upper airway obstruction, and treatment usually requires a mechanical approach, such as a mechanical device or a surgical intervention. The goals of treatment are to prevent apneas and hypopneas, maintain normal oxygenation throughout the night, and restore normal sleep architecture, thereby eliminating the symptoms of excessive daytime sleepiness. These goals are achievable in most cases, but different patients will require different approaches.

Treatment Options

All patients with sleep apnea should be encouraged to have good sleep hygiene and should strive for adequate sleep time taken on a regular schedule. Medications that impair skeletal muscle function, such as alcohol or sedatives, will worsen sleep apnea. Patients with obstructive sleep apnea syndrome should avoid taking these substances, especially around bedtime. Sleep apnea is often worse in the supine position, and some patients with mild sleep apnea will manifest the problem only when lying supine. For them, position therapies

Table 7 Options for Treatment of Obstructive Sleep Apnea Syndrome

General measures
  Good sleep hygiene
  Avoidance of alcohol and sedatives
  Weight loss
Positive airway pressure
  Nasal continuous positive airway pressure (nasal CPAP)
  Nasal bilevel positive airway pressure (nasal BiPAP)
Oral appliances
  Tongue-retaining devices
  Mandibular advancement devices
Maxillofacial surgeries
  Chin advancement
  Mandibular advancement
  Maxillary advancement
  Genioglossus advancement ± hyoid suspension
ENT surgeries
  Septoplasty
  Nasal polypectomy
  Tosillectomy and adenoidectomy (T&A)
  Uvulopalatopharyngoplasty (UPPP or UVPP)
  Laser-assisted uvulopalatoplasty (LAUP)
Tracheostomy

can be attempted to encourage sleep in the prone or decubitus positions. These measures are rarely satisfactory, however, and rarely serve to eliminate the problem. Weight loss should be encouraged in all patients with sleep apnea who are overweight; this is especially true in those who experienced the onset or the worsening of their symptoms as they gained weight. However, significant weight loss, even when successful, may take a considerable amount of time, so other methods of treatment are often needed until sufficient weight loss is achieved. Surgical procedures to encourage a more rapid and reliable weight loss (bariatric surgery) are undertaken in some patients who are markedly impaired or disabled by morbid obesity. Even in these cases, the treatment of sleep apnea should be implemented first in order to resolve the sleep-disordered breathing and decrease the risk of complications during and after surgery.

The definitive treatment for obstructive sleep apnea syndrome is tracheostomy. Since a tracheostomy bypasses the upper airway (and therefore any upper airway obstructions), this treatment always works. With a tracheostomy in place, the patient can breathe through the tracheostomy and bypass the upper airway at night, precluding the possibility of having apneas due to upper airway obstruction. During the daytime, the patient can occlude the tracheostomy with a plug, and can talk normally. Tracheostomy is the gold standard of treatment and that with which other treatments are compared. However, it is not accepted eagerly by patients. Tracheostomies affect a patient's appearance, require maintenance and cleaning, and limit a patient's activities. The presence of a tube in the front of the neck can be difficult to conceal. Moreover, since the tracheostomy bypasses the upper airway, where inhaled air is humidified and sputum that is expectorated can be swallowed, most patients develop some degree of chronic bronchitis and expectorate sputum from the tracheostomy tube and from the site around the tube. The tracheostomy tube and tracheostomy site need to be cleaned and cared for regularly. Patients with tracheostomies need to be vigilant in keeping their tracheostomies covered to prevent aspiration of foreign bodies; also, they cannot swim or become submerged while bathing. Fortunately, alternatives to this extreme form of treatment have been developed, and few patients require tracheostomies for treatment of sleep apnea. Nevertheless, tracheostomy is still an option when other forms of treatment are ineffective or not feasible.

The most widely used treatment for obstructive sleep apnea syndrome is continuous positive airway pressure (CPAP) delivered through a nasal device. A nasal CPAP machine blows air through the nose and into the throat, providing a pneumatic splint that helps hold the pharynx open and prevents upper airway collapse. Nasal CPAP is almost always effective when the patient is able to wear the device, and patients usually notice a dramatic improvement in their symptoms within a day or two after starting to use it. Nasal CPAP is not trouble-free, however. The hoses and apparatus required to connect to the nasal delivery devices can be cumbersome, and the devices themselves can irritate the skin or cause discomfort. These problems can usually be overcome with appropriate local skin care, a change of nasal delivery devices, or topical measures to alleviate dryness or nasal congestion. For patients who report difficulty breathing while using the machine, it is important to ask if the difficulty is felt while trying to breathe in or while trying to breathe out. If the patient is having difficulty breathing in while using the CPAP machine, the machine may not be delivering sufficient airflow or pressure to overcome the patient's upper airway obstruction, and an increase in the CPAP setting may alleviate this sensation. If the patient is having difficulty breathing out against the pressure being delivered by their CPAP machine, a decrease in the CPAP setting may allow for more comfortable exhalation. For patients who continue to have difficulty exhaling against the CPAP level that is required to overcome the upper airway obstruction during inhalation, more sophisticated machines are available. Bilevel constant positive airway pressure (BiPAP) devices cycle airway pressure with inhalation and exhalation and are usually set with a higher inhalation pressure and a lower exhalation pressure. Machines that detect airway obstruction and adjust CPAP in real time as the device is used can also help to alleviate some of the discomfort of exhaling against positive pressure.

The success of positive airway pressure machines in treating patients with obstructive sleep apnea is directly related to patient compliance. Long-term compliance, and therefore the success of the treatment, is strongly influenced by the experience the patient has during the first few days of treatment. Positive airway pressure machines and delivery devices are cumbersome and awkward to use, and patients can have difficulty adjusting to these devices while sleeping. It is up to the clinician to help the patient through the initial adjustment period by maximizing the comfort of the device and providing motivation for the patient to use it. Care should be taken to choose a nasal delivery device that fits the patient and is comfortable enough to allow the patient to sleep with it in place. An ill-fitting device will frustrate the patient and sabotage the effort to create a positive experience. The best motivator for getting patients to make a sincere and concerted effort to use their positive airway pressure machine is a full understanding of the seriousness of their disease. Patients should be told how abnormal their overnight sleep test is (how many episodes they had where they stopped breathing, how many times their oxygen went low, how low their oxygen went), which of their symptoms are due to their sleep apnea syndrome, what the major health risks of untreated sleep apnea are (heart attacks, strokes, motor vehicle accidents), and what the goals of treatment are (full resolution of symptoms, return to a normal lifestyle). For most patients, the positive effects experienced from using the positive airway pressure machine (resolution of symptoms, improved sense of well-being) become the primary reinforcement for long-term compliance.

With appropriate strategies to maximize comfort, provide motivation, and reinforce the positive effects and benefits, most patients with obstructive sleep apnea syndrome adapt well to using nasal CPAP. But if discomfort continues or if the patient is unable to sleep while wearing a nasal delivery device connected to a positive airway pressure machine, another form of treatment needs to be sought.

A variety of oral appliances have been developed to treat obstructive sleep apnea syndrome. The most successful of these are the mandibular advancement devices that reposition the lower jaw slightly down and forward to improve the patency of the pharynx. Although these devices may not cause enough improvement in upper airway patency to treat patients with severe sleep apnea, they can be useful for treating patients with less severe disease. The best candidates for treatment with an oral appliance are patients with mild to moderate sleep apnea who have solid dentition (on which to anchor the device) and who have micrognathia or retrognathia contributing to their sleep apnea. Many patients wear these devices successfully for years, but some have difficulty with temporomandibular joint pain and are not able to continue wearing the device. A variety of maxillofacial and orthognathic surgeries have been used to treat patients with sleep apnea syndrome, including chin advancement, mandibular advancement, maxillary advancement, and genioglossal advancement with or without hyoid bone suspension. Patients with specific craniofacial abnormalities that are contributing to their sleep apnea syndrome are most likely to benefit from these procedures. Patients who benefit from an oral appliance such as a mandibular advancement device but who are unable to continue wearing the device due to discomfort are particularly good candidates for these types of surgical treatments.

A variety of surgical procedures have been used for patients with sleep apnea syndrome. Septoplasty, nasal polypectomy, tonsillectomy, and adenoidectomy can all be useful when a patient has specific lesions that are obstructing the upper airway and contributing to the sleep apnea syndrome. These procedures can also be useful adjuncts for treating patients who have difficulty using nasal CPAP and who have structural lesions compromising the patency of the upper airway. Removal of upper airway lesions from such patients may not result in resolution of the sleep apnea syndrome, but the improvement in upper airway patency may improve the patient's ability to use the nasal CPAP and thereby improve the device's efficacy. Uvulopalatopharyngoplasty (UPPP or UVPP) can be very effective for reducing snoring in many patients and can improve sleep apnea in some. Unfortunately, accurate identification of the patients with obstructive sleep apnea who will benefit from this operation has not been possible, and even those who do benefit may not experience full resolution of their apneas. UVPP can be an effective treatment for some patients with mild to moderate sleep apnea syndrome and can also be a useful adjunct to nasal CPAP in those who have difficulty using the device. A variation on the conventional UVPP is the laser-assisted uvulopalatoplasty (LAUP), which employs a YAG laser to modify the uvula and palate and improve the patency of the pharynx. The advantage of the LAUP is that it can be performed in the outpatient setting. The indications for LAUP in the treatment of sleep apnea syndrome are not fully established, but it is likely that selected patients may benefit from these approaches alone or in conjunction with other treatments.

CONCLUSION

Obstructive sleep apnea syndrome is a common problem that affects as many as one in twenty-five adults and can lead to significant morbidity and mortality. When recognized, this disorder can be treated and the morbidity and mortality can be prevented. Because the symptoms are nonspecific, sleep apnea syndrome is underrecognized and many patients who are symptomatic continue to be undiagnosed and untreated. The challenge for health care providers is to recognize patients with sleep apnea syndrome, diagnose the problem with appropriate testing, institute treatment that is effective, and allow the patient to return to a normal lifestyle and function.

SUGGESTED READING

1. American Sleep Disorders Association Standards of Practice Committee. Practice parameters for the treatment of snoring and obstructive sleep apnea with oral appliances. Sleep 1995; 18: 511–513.
2. Engleman HM, Martin SE, Deary IJ, Douglas NJ. Effect of continuous positive airway pressure treatment on daytime function in sleep apnoea/hypopnoea syndrome. Lancet 1994; 343:572–575.
3. Findley LJ, Levinson MP, Bonnie RJ. Driving performance and automobile accidents in patients with sleep apnea. Clin Chest Med 1992; 13:427–435.
4. Hudgel DW. Mechanisms of obstructive sleep apnea. Chest 1992; 101:541–549.
5. Kuna ST. Pathophysiology of upper airway closure during sleep. JAMA 1991; 266:1384–1389.

6. Schmidt-Nowara W, Lowe A, Wiegand L, Cartwright R, Perez-Guerra F, Menn S. Oral appliances for the treatment of snoring and obstructive sleep apnea: a review. Sleep 1995; 18:501–510.

7. Shepard JW. Hypertension, cardiac arrhythmias, myocardial infarction, and stroke in relation to obstructive sleep apnea. Clin Chest Med 1992; 13:437–458.

8. Strohl KP, Redline S. Recognition of obstructive sleep apnea. Am J Respir Crit Care Med 1996; 154:279–289.

9. Strollo PJ, Rogers RM. Obstructive sleep apnea. N Engl J Med 1996; 334:99–104.

10. Young T, Palta M, Dempsey J, Skatrud J, Weber S, Badr S. The occurrence of sleep-disordered breathing among middle-aged adults. N Engl J Med 1993; 328:1230–1235.

32

Lung Cancer

M. Patricia Rivera
University of North Carolina
Chapel Hill, North Carolina

Diane E. Stover
Cornell University
Memorial Sloan-Kettering Cancer Center
New York, New York

EPIDEMIOLOGY

Lung cancer is one of the most prevalent and lethal cancers in the United States. While the incidence appears to have leveled off to approximately 70/100,000 in white men, it continues to rise in nonwhite men. A sharp rise in the incidence of lung cancer has occurred in women (6/100,000 in 1960 to 28/100,000 in 1987). The estimated overall incidence of lung cancer in the United States for 1998 is 171,000 cases.

Although lung cancer accounts for only 14% of all cancers, it accounts for approximately 33% of all cancer deaths. Lung cancer is the leading cause of cancer deaths among males and has surpassed breast cancer as the leading cause of cancer deaths among females.

Despite attempts at creating effective early detection and smoking cessation programs, the survival of lung cancer victims has not changed over the past 30 years, and lung cancer mortality in the 1990s is expected to rise to a rate of 53.2 deaths per year per 100,000.

RISK FACTORS/ETIOLOGY

Cigarette Smoke

Approximately 85% of lung cancer cases are attributed to smoking. *N*-nitrosamines and polycyclic hydrocarbons are the two major classes of tobacco-related inhaled carcinogens. The risk of developing lung cancer in nonsmokers exposed to cigarette smoke is approximately 1.35 times the risk of unexposed nonsmokers.

Occupational Factors

Asbestos, radon, cadmium, uranium, arsenic, nickel, and polycyclic hydrocarbons have been associated with an increase risk of lung cancer.

Most likely asbestos acts as a tumor promoter. The relative risk of lung cancer in asbestos workers is 1.4–2.6 times the risk of unexposed nonsmokers. When smoking is combined with asbestos exposure, the relative risk of lung cancer is increased to 28.8.

Genetic Factors

Because only a fraction of individuals who smoke and only a portion of individuals exposed to occupational carcinogens develop cancer, cancer susceptibility may have a genetic basis. Several findings seem to support this theory. First, there is an increased risk of lung cancer in individuals with chronic obstructive pulmonary disease (COPD)—i.e., studies have shown that smokers with COPD have higher rates of lung cancer than smokers without COPD. Since the development of COPD appears to have a familial association, the increased risk of lung cancer may also involve a genetic risk. Second, lung cancer is more common in first-degree relatives. Third, increased metabolism of the antihypertensive drug debrisoquine has been associated with an increased risk of lung cancer. It is suggested that individuals with increased oxidative activity may be at risk for developing cancer because of their increased level of activated carcinogens.

Gender Factors

Recent reports suggest that smoking women are more vulnerable to the development of lung cancer than their male counterparts.

MOLECULAR BIOLOGY

Chromosomal Abnormalities

Cytogenetic analysis of lung cancer has shown multiple nonrandom breaks involving chromosomes 1,3,7,15, and 17. Most consistent in lung cancer has been deletion of chromosome 3p, which is observed in about 50% of patients with non-small-cell lung cancer (NSCLC). The gene on 3p has not yet been identified, but it appears to be a tumor suppressor gene; once it is deleted, carcinogenesis occurs.

Lesions in Dominant Oncogenes

The *ras* oncogene codes for a protein that mediates signal transduction pathways. Mutations in the *ras* oncogene occur in about 35% of lung adenocarcinomas. Activation almost always involves point mutations at codons 12 or 13. The *myc* oncogene family appears to play a role in the pathogenesis of small-cell lung cancer.

Tumor Suppressor Genes

Under normal conditions, the production of p53 protein is increased when DNA damage occurs. The p53 protein induces arrest of cellular differentiation, thereby allowing time for DNA repair. Mutations or deletions in the p53 gene allow abnormal cellular differentiation. Abnormalities in the p53 gene occur in approximately 45% of NSCLC tumors.

Prognostic Significance of Molecular Markers

A significant decrease in both disease-free and overall survival has been observed in patients with NSCLC whose tumors have k-*ras* mutations. The presence of p53 mutations in both early and late stages of NSCLC is reported to be associated with decreased survival. Overexpression of p53 has been reported to correlate with disease progression to lymph nodes.

HISTOLOGY

The distinction between NSCLC and small cell lung cancer (SCLC) is of major clinical importance because it significantly alters treatment options. Of new lung cancer cases, approximately 80% will be NSCLC. Although NSCLC is divided into different histological types, they are clinically staged and treated in the same way (Table 1).

CLINICAL PRESENTATION

Approximately 15% of patients with NSCLC have no symptoms at the time of diagnosis; the rest have symptoms related to the primary tumor and/or to metastatic disease.

Common signs and symptoms at presentation include cough, dyspnea, hemoptysis, wheezing, and pneumonia. The last three findings are generally related to endobronchial growth, as seen with squamous- and small-cell carcinoma. More peripheral growth, which

Table 1 Histological Classification of Lung Cancer

Non-Small-Cell Lung Cancer[a]
  Adenocarcinoma (50%)
    Bronchogenic
      Acinar
      Papillary
  Squamous cell (30%)
  Large cell (20%)
    Solid tumor with mucin
    Solid tumor without mucin
    Giant cell
    Clear cell

Small-Cell Lung Cancer

[a] It should be noted that some NSCLC have histological characteristics of both adenocarcinoma and squamous cell carcinoma.

occurs with adenocarcinoma, can result in pain due to pleural, chest wall, or rib involvement. Other symptoms include weight loss, hoarseness, and fever.

Pancoast syndrome, characterized by shoulder pain radiating to the arm in an ulnar distribution, is caused by tumor invasion of the eighth cervical and first thoracic nerves in the superior sulcus. Horner's syndrome—which consists of enophthalmos, ptosis, meiosis, and ipsilateral dyshidrosis—may be caused by extension of the tumor into the paravertebral sympathetic nerves.

The most common sites for metastatic spread are hilar and mediastinal lymph nodes, bone, brain, contralateral lung, pleura, liver, and adrenal glands. About one-third of patients present with symptoms associated with distant metastasis, bone pain being the most common.

PARANEOPLASTIC SYNDROMES

The production of ectopic hormones or hormone-like substances is not uncommon in lung cancer. Most paraneoplastic syndromes are associated with SCLC. The most common paraneoplastic syndromes in SCLC include hyponatremia [the syndrome of inappropriate antidiuretic hormone (SIADH)], caused by production of argenine vasopressin, and Cushing's syndrome, caused by excessive production of the precursor peptides of ACTH. The development of autoantibodies to normal neuronal antigens in patients with SCLC can lead to Eaton-Lambert syndrome, cerebral and cerebellar degeneration, and sensory neuropathy. Anorexia and weight loss occur in nearly one-third of patients with SCLC and may be caused by the actions of various cytokines including interleukin-1, interleukin-6, and tumor necrosis factor. Hypercalcemia due to release of a PTH-related peptide is the most frequent paraneoplastic syndrome in NSCLC and is commonly associated with squamous-cell carcinoma. Hypertrophic pulmonary osteoarthropathy, characterized by painful periostitis of the long bones and clubbing of the fingers and toes, is most commonly seen with adenocarcinoma.

DIAGNOSIS

Sputum Cytology

In the case of a central lesion, sputum cytology is an appropriate first step. Sputum can be collected spontaneously, or it can be induced by saline inhalation in patients unable to provide a sample spontaneously.

Fiberoptic Bronchoscopy (FOB)

Fiberoptic bronchoscopy has a twofold role in the management of patients with suspected lung cancer: diagnosis and local staging. For suspected central lung cancers that are not diagnosed on sputum cytology, FOB is the next step. FOB can visualize endobronchial tumors, document their exact position, and add useful information about staging. For lesions that are visualized endoscopically, the diagnostic yield is up to 97% with the combination of bronchial brushings and endobronchial biopsies. The role of FOB in the diagnosis of peripheral lung cancers is controversial. The size of the lesion is the best determinant of yield: lesions less than 4 cm have a yield of only 30–60%, whereas lesions greater than 4 cm are reported to have a diagnostic yield of between 70 and 80%.

Transthoracic Fine Needle Aspiration (TFNA)

Because fluoroscopic TFNA has a diagnostic yield in the range of 80–95%, TFNA is the most efficacious means of diagnosing peripheral lung lesions, particularly those less than 4 cm in diameter. However, the risk of pneumothorax following TFNA is about 30%, with 5–8% requiring chest tube insertion.

Solitary Pulmonary Nodule (SPN)

A widely accepted approach to the patient with a SPN (a single well-demarcated lesion <3 cm within the lung parenchyma) of unknown etiology is surgical removal unless benignity is highly likely or there are absolute contraindications to surgery. Clinical criteria for benignity include popcorn, laminated, and diffuse calcification; detection of fat within the lesion on computed tomography; stability (i.e., no growth) of the nodule over a 2-year period from review of prior chest radiographs; and/or a low probability of malignancy based on age and lack of risk factors for lung cancer (see Chapter 20).

Occult Lung Cancer

Occult lung cancer is defined as the detection of cancer cells on analysis of sputum cytology in patients with no chest radiographic abnormalities. The diagnostic approach to these patients include direct visualization of the upper respiratory tract by an ear, nose, and throat specialist, a chest CT, and careful visualization of the tracheobronchial tree with FOB. If a lesion is found and/or cytology is positive for carcinoma, surgical intervention is recommended once the location of malignancy is documented.

An autofluorescent imaging system has been developed to detect early lung cancer. Clinical trials have found the fluorescent FOB to have a 50% greater sensitivity than white-light FOB in the detection of dysplasia and carcinoma in situ. The clinical utility of the fluorescent FOB at present is unproved.

Evaluation of Pleural Effusion in Patients with NSCLC

Although some experts believe that the mere presence of a pleural effusion in association with NSCL portends a poor prognosis, not all effusions indicate pleural metastases. We feel that proof of malignancy is important, since it significantly changes the therapeutic options for the patient. Cytological examination of pleural fluid is the preferred diagnostic approach. Of patients with malignant pleural effusions, 65% will have malignant cells present on cytological examination. A repeat thoracentesis can increase the yield by 30%. In a study comparing cytological analysis with pleural biopsy, the yield from the latter was much lower. Therefore, a second thoracentesis is preferred over needle biopsy if the initial pleural tap is negative for malignant cells. If these manuvers do not yield a diagnosis of malignancy, video-assisted thoracoscopic surgery (VATS) should be done at the time of the planned surgical resection. If there is no evidence of pleural metastases on VATS, surgical resection should be undertaken. If there is evidence of metastatic disease, any attempt at surgical resection should be aborted.

PREOPERATIVE ASSESSMENT OF NSCLC

Physiological Assessment of Lung Function

All potentially operable NSCLC patients should undergo physiological evaluation of their lung function. In our experience, measurement of the FEV_1 by spirometry is the single best test to assess postoperative lung function. If the FEV_1 is greater than 2 L or 60% of the predicted value, a pneumonectomy or lesser resection is likely to be tolerated. Measurement of the diffusing capacity (DL_{CO}) is also helpful to predict a patient's ability to tolerate surgical resection. A diffusing capacity greater than 60% of the predicted value is considered acceptable for a pneumonectomy or lesser resection. Although hypercapnea (P_{CO_2} greater than 45 mmHg) has traditionally been considered a relative contraindication to surgery, this has never been proved. In two recent studies, no significant difference in the overall complication rate following surgical resection was noted for patients with a preoperative P_{CO_2} greater than or equal to 45 mmHg. In our experience, however, COPD patients whose P_{CO_2} remains 45 mmHg on maximal therapy usually have significant impairment of pulmonary function tests. Preoperative hypoxemia (i.e., Pa_{O_2} less than 60 mmHg) is difficult to evaluate since ventilation/perfusion imbalance created by some tumors can cause a decrease in the Pa_{O_2}, which improves after resection.

If the preoperative FEV_1 and DL_{CO} are less than 60% of the predicted value, a quantitative radionuclide perfusion scan should be obtained to assess regional lung function. The product of the preoperative FEV_1 and the percentage perfusion to the lung that remains after surgery has been shown to reliably predict postoperative FEV_1. If the predicted postoperative FEV_1 is greater than or equal to 40% of the predicted value, a pneumonectomy or lobectomy is considered acceptable.

Exercise testing stresses the entire cardiopulmonary and oxygen delivery systems and assesses the reserve that can be expected after lung resection. Several studies have found a significant relationship between maximal oxygen consumption ($\dot{V}_{O_2 \, max}$) and postoperative mortality. If the $\dot{V}_{O_2}$ max is less than or equal to 15mL/kg/min, the risk of surgery is unacceptably high. Exercise testing is recommended in patients who have a predicted postoperative FEV_1 of less than 40% of their predicted value but otherwise are good candidates for surgical resection.

Balloon occlusion of the pulmonary artery on the side to be resected with measurement of the contralateral pulmonary artery pressure has been shown to provide additional information in evaluating operative risks. In our experience, this test is infrequently used.

Staging NSCLC

A detailed history and physical examination remain the most important steps in assessing a patient with lung cancer. Symptoms suggesting local spread include chest pain, hoarseness, or superior vena caval obstruction. Symptoms suggestive of metastatic disease include headache, mental status changes, bone pain, or weight loss.

After an accurate history, physical examination, and chest radiograph, routine studies should include a hematological survey and specific biochemical markers such as serum calcium, alkaline phosphatase, and liver enzymes (AST, ALT).

Role of Chest Computed Tomography (CT) and
Magnetic Resonance Imaging (MRI) in Staging NSCLC

Chest CT with intravenous contrast and chest MRI are equivalent for staging the mediastinum with a sensitivity of 70–80% and a specificity of 60–80%. Of course, chest CT is less expensive. Lymph nodes greater than 1.0 cm in transverse diameter suggests lymphadenopathy and should be further investigated. The false-negative rate of chest CT in the staging of mediastinal lymph nodes is 15%; the false-positive rate when lymph nodes are >3 cm in size is about 25%. CT imaging is not only helpful for staging but can also detect parenchymal nodules, pleural effusions, local invasion to the chest wall, and abnormal vertebral or mediastinal structures not visualized on plain films. CT of the chest is recommended in the evaluation of all patients who are suspected of having lung cancer. MRI is better in the assessment of superior sulcus tumors and tumors suspected of invading major blood vessels, such as the superior vena cava. When these conditions are under consideration, an MRI may need to be performed in addition to a chest CT.

Role of Mediastinoscopy in Staging NSCLC

Mediastinoscopy is the most accurate way to stage the mediastinum prior to surgery. The procedure is safe, with an overall complication rate of < 3%. Mediastinoscopy is essential to define the extent of disease, predict prognosis, and guide treatment. Absolute indications for performing mediastinoscopy include enlarged lymph nodes on chest CT (>1 cm), and intent to use neoadjuvant therapy prior to surgery or radiation if mediastinal nodal metastasis is present. Relative indications include the presence of a T2 primary lesion or a potentially resectable T3 lesion and/or the presence of a central primary lesion. The false-negative rate is about 3% and is mostly due to inaccessible nodes.

Table 2 International Staging System for Non-Small-Cell Lung Cancer—TNM Definitions

T—primary tumor	
TX	Malignant cells in sputum or bronchial washings but tumor not visualized by imaging or bronchoscopy
T0	No evidence of primary tumor
Tis	Carcinoma in situ
T1	No greater than 3 cm in size
	Surrounded by lung or visceral pleura
	No evidence of invasion proximal to a lobar bronchus
T2	Greater than 3 cm in size
	Involves main bronchus, 2 cm or more distal to carina
	Invades visceral but not parietal pleura
	Associated atelectasis or obstructive pneumonia
T3	Tumor of any size that invades any of the following: chest wall, diaphragm, mediastinal pleura, or pericardium
	Extends within 2 cm of the carina but without involvement of carina
T4	Associated with a malignant pleural effusion
	Invades the mediastinum, trachea, heart, great vessels, esophagus, or carina
	Satellite nodule(s) within the primary bearing lobe
N—regional lymph nodes	
N0	No nodes involved
N1	Peribronchial or ipsilateral hilar node
N2	Ipsilateral mediastinal, or subcarinal nodes
N3	Contralateral mediastinal, contralateral hilar, scalene, or supraclavicular nodes
M—distant metastases	
M0	No distant metastases
M1	Distant metastases

Source: Adapted from Mountain CF. The new lung cancer staging system. Chest 1997; 111: 1710–1717.

Table 3   Revised International Stage Grouping

Stage 0	Tis
Stage IA	$T_1N_0M_0$
Stage IB	$T_2N_0M_0$
Stage IIA	$T_1N_1M_0$
Stage IIB	$T_2N_1M_0$
	$T_3N_0M_0$
Stage IIIA	$T_3N_1M_0$
	$T_1N_2M_0$
	$T_2N_2M_0$
	$T_3N_2M_0$
Stage IIIB	Any T N_3M_0
	T_4 any N M_0
Stage IV	Any T any N M_1

Source: Adapted from Mountain CF. The new lung cancer staging system. Chest 1997; 111: 1710–1717.

Extent of Disease Evaluation

Approximately 15% of patients with clinically operable NSCLC have distant metastases present at the time of diagnosis. All patients considered for curative treatment of lung cancer should undergo CT scanning with contrast of the chest and upper abdomen to evaluate the mediastinum and detect unsuspected liver and adrenal metastases. (CT scanning reveals adrenal abnormalities in 10–20% of patients, but only one-third of these will have metastases.) In the absence of clinical symptoms and biochemical abnormalities, the routine use of bone scans in the staging of NSCLC is not necessary. Similarly, the routine use of CT or MRI scanning of the brain to detect asymptomatic cerebral metastasis is not cost-effective in the evaluation of the asymptomatic patient. The present recommendation is to perform head CT only in patients with positive findings, such as headaches, seizures, or new-onset of neurological signs or in patients who have findings compatible with widespread disease (e.g., cachexia, anemia, anorexia).

Following completion of a staging workup, the disease is assigned a TNM stage (see Tables 2 and 3). The international staging system was revised in 1996. Some aspects of the new staging system include (1) a category for noninvasive tumors, defined as carcinoma in situ; (2) stages I and II are subdivided into stage IA and IB and stage IIA and IIB based on the size of the primary tumor, because smaller tumors have a better prognosis; (3) T3N0 tumors that invade contiguous structures but are surgically resectable are moved from stage IIIA to stage IIB owing to the better survival of these patients.

STAGING OF SCLC

Just as with NSCLC, a detailed history and physical examination remain the most important steps in assessing a patient with SCLC. The initial survey of a patient with SCLC should include a chest radiograph and hematological and biochemical profiles

(AST, ALT, alkaline phosphatase). A CT scan of the chest and abdomen is necessary to evaluate local disease as well as intrabdominal organ involvement. All patients diagnosed with SCLC should have a bone scan and a brain CT scan or MRI as part of the staging workup.

The TNM staging system has not been prognostically significant in SCLC. An alternative staging system classifies into *limited disease* and *extensive disease*. Limited disease includes disease confined to a hemithorax as well as supraclavicular nodes and ipsilateral pleural effusion. Extensive disease is tumor beyond these limits and usually accounts for 60–70% of patients with SCLC.

NATURAL HISTORY OF LUNG CANCER

Lung cancer is a lethal disease if left untreated. Median survival for NSCLC ranges from 2–5 months, and 1-year survival is approximately 15%. All patients are dead within 3 years without treatment. Median survival for untreated SCLC is 12 weeks in patients with disease confined to the hemithorax and 5–7 weeks in patients with clinically apparent metastatic disease.

TREATMENT OF NSCLC

Stage I NSCLC

Surgery is the most effective method for curing stage I NSCLC. Patients should undergo lobectomy if their cardiopulmonary status permits, as lobectomy is associated with decreased local recurrence rate compared with segmentectomy or wedge resection. Five-year survival after surgery is affected by the T status (i.e., size) of the primary tumor: stage IA patients (T1 N0 tumor) have a 70–80% 5-year survival. Stage IB patients (T2 N0 tumor) have a 50–60% 5-year survival. New strategies under investigation for stage I NSCLC include (1) chemoprevention with *cis*-retinoic acid for patients with stage IA disease (i.e., after potentially curative surgery), which may decrease the incidence of a second primary cancer, and (2) adjuvant (postoperative) chemotherapy for patients with stage IB disease. If patients cannot medically tolerate surgery, high-dose radiation therapy (3D) with intent to cure is usually recommended.

Stage II NSCLC

Surgery is the treatment of choice for patients with stage II NSCLC. Adequate surgery consists of a lobectomy, bilobectomy, pneumonectomy, or en bloc resection of a T3 tumor and adjacent invaded structure. A mediastinoscopy sampling five nodal stations should be performed on all patients with clinical stage II disease prior to surgery. As in stage I disease, 5-year survival is affected by the T status of the tumor. Five-year survival for stage IIA (T1 N1 tumor) is about 54%; for stage IIB (T2 N1 tumor), it is 35–40%. Five-year survival for stage IIB (T3 N0 tumors) ranges between 20 and 40%. Currently ongoing clinical trials are randomizing patients with stage IIA and IIB disease to receive postoperative radiation therapy plus chemotherapy vs. radiation therapy alone or postoperative chemotherapy vs. no treatment.

Stage III NSCLC

The use of combined-modality therapy in stage III NSCLC is an area of considerable investigation. Ideally, patients with stage III disease should be referred to a multidisciplinary thoracic oncology program with input from a pulmonologist, thoracic surgeon, medical oncologist, and radiation oncologist. Although stage IIIA can be considered potentially resectable, surgery should not be considered primary therapy for stage IIIB disease.

Management of Stage IIIA NSCLC (N2 Disease)

The treatment of patients with N2 disease is controversial. The use of neoadjuvant chemotherapy prior to surgery or radiation therapy in patients with N2 disease has been extensively investigated. The rationale for using neoadjuvant chemotherapy is based on the fact that micrometastatic disease is usually present at the time of diagnosis. Several studies have demonstrated long-term disease-free survival rates of 17–30% in patients treated with preoperative chemotherapy. Two trials that randomized patients to receive cisplatin-based chemotherapy prior to surgery versus surgery alone confirmed these results. Patients who achieve a complete pathological response following chemotherapy (that is, no evidence of cancer in the primary site or in the mediastinal lymph nodes) have the best chance for long-term survival.

Several clinical trials have shown improved median and 5-year survival in patients treated with combined cisplatin-based chemotherapy and thoracic radiotherapy compared with thoracic radiotherapy alone.

At present it is not known whether surgery is superior to radiation therapy in terms of local control following neoadjuvant chemotherapy in patients with stage IIIA NSCLC. Several trials are currently being conducted in order to answer this question.

Management of Stage IIIB NSCLC

Stage IIIB patients are also candidates for multimodality therapy. A number of clinical trials have been conducted comparing thoracic radiotherapy with or without chemotherapy in patients with stage IIIB disease. Four large randomized trials have reached the same conclusion—that combined modality therapy is superior to radiotherapy alone.

Newer agents like topoisomerase 1 inhibitors, navelbine, and gemcitabine and combination of the taxanes with radiation to treat locally advanced NSCLC are undergoing evaluation in large randomized trials.

Stage IV NSCLC

Five large, randomized trials have compared best supportive care to chemotherapy in patients with metastatic disease. All five trials showed a reduction in mortality at 6 months and increased 1-year survival with chemotherapy, but a statistical significance was only attained in two of the five trials. Patients likely to respond to chemotherapy are those with good performance status, weight loss of < 5%, and no bone or liver metastases. In this group of patients, chemotherapy has been found to be more cost-effective and to improve quality of life compared with best supportive care (see Fig. 1).

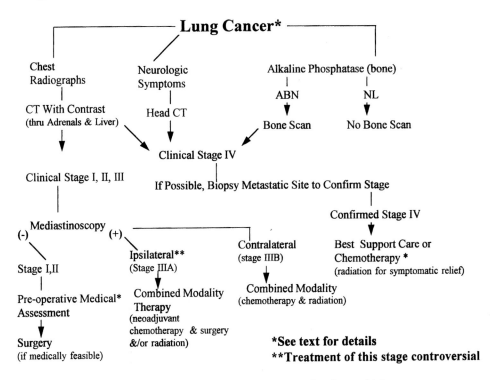

Figure 1   Outline for diagnostic evaluation and treatment of patients with lung cancer.

TREATMENT OF SCLC

Limited Disease

Combination chemotherapy with etoposide (VP-16) and cisplatin with concurrent thoracic radiotherapy significantly improves median and 2-year survival. Approximately 60% of patients will have a complete response, and median survival is 12 to 18 months. The 2-year survival is about 20% in SCLC, and the 5-year survival rate is about 10%.

Brain metastases are a significant problem in patients with initially diagnosed limited disease, occurring in up to 80% of those surviving 2 years or longer. Elective brain irradiation for patients with limited disease remains controversial. Several randomized trials have demonstrated a significant reduction in SCLC relapse rates in the brain, from 22% without elective brain irradiation to 8%. Although none of the randomized trials have demonstrated an improvement in overall survival, there are data that suggest a survival benefit for the subgroup of patients with a complete response to chemotherapy.

Extensive Disease

The response to chemotherapy is lower than in limited disease. There is no survival advantage with concurrent thoracic radiotherapy. Palliative radiotherapy should be administered to sites of metastatic disease (brain, bone). Median survival in extensive disease is about 9 months. Only a small number of patients (1–3%) survive 5 years.

PREVENTION

Patients who are cured of lung cancer are at increased risk to develop second primary tumors of the upper and lower respiratory tracts. Several prospective studies have shown that patients who continue to smoke after therapy of their initial cancer (including lung and head-and-neck neoplasms) have a higher risk of developing second primary tumors than do the patients who stop smoking. Epidemiological studies suggest that people who consume large amounts of fruit and vegetables have a lower risk of cancer. A possible explanation is that antioxidant vitamins contained in fruits and vegetables interfere with oxidative damage to DNA and lipoproteins, thereby preventing carcinogenesis. To date, however, the use of antioxidants has not been shown to lower the incidence of lung cancer.

Cis-retinoic acid, an analog of vitamin A, shows promise as a tumor preventive agent. In a placebo-controlled trial, patients with cured squamous cell head-and-neck cancer randomized to receive *cis*-retinoic acid demonstrated a significant decrease in the rate of second primary tumors of the head and neck regions when compared with those receiving placebo. Similar trials are now taking place in patients with ''cured'' primary lung cancer. The usefulness of these drugs in high-risk patients without a prior cancer history is unknown. To date, the most effective way to prevent lung cancer is not to smoke, and if you do smoke, to stop. Additionally, lots of fruits and vegetables cannot hurt.

THE FUTURE

In addition to new chemotherapeutic agents, novel treatment modalities—such as antiangiogenesis factors and photodynamic therapy—are being considered to treat lung cancer. Even if these modalities are effective, they are likely to have little success in the treatment of advanced lung cancer. The best way to affect lung cancer survival beneficially is to detect the disease early. The usefulness of induced sputum monoclonal antibodies and flow cytometry to detect malignant cells early in the disease is being investigated. For now, the best recommendation is to screen high-risk populations with yearly chest radiographs and to educate the public, particularly the young, on the risks of smoking.

SUGGESTED READING

1. Clinical practice guidelines for the treatment of unresectable non-small cell lung in cancer. J Clin Oncol 1997; 15:2996–3018.
2. Diamandidis D, Huber M, Pisters K. Non-small cell lung cancer. In: Pazdur R, ed. Medical Oncology: A Comprehensive Review. Huntington, NY: PRR, Inc., 1995:181–203.
3. Ginsberg R, Vokes EE, Raben A. Non-small cell lung cancer. In: DeVita VT, Hellman S, Rosenber SA, eds. Cancer: Principles and Practice of Oncology. Philadelphia: Lippincott, 1996: 858–910.
4. Greco FA, Hainsworth JD. Multidisciplinary approach to potentially curable non-small cell carcinoma of the lung. Oncology 1997; 11:27–49.
5. Marshall MC, Olsen GN. The physiologic evaluation of the lung resection candidate. Clin Chest Med 1993; 14:305–320.
6. Mountain CF. The new lung cancer staging system. Chest 1997; 111:1710–1717.
7. Pretreatment evaluation of non-small cell lung cancer. Official statement of the American Thoracic Society and European Respiratory Society. Am J Respir Crit Care Med 1997; 156:320–332.

33

Heart Disease Caused by Lung Disease

William E. Hopkins
University of Vermont College of Medicine
Fletcher Allen Health Care
Burlington, Vermont

INTRODUCTION

The heart can be adversely affected by both parenchymal lung disease and disease processes that primarily affect the pulmonary vasculature. While hypoxemia secondary to lung disease can adversely affect left ventricular function, lung disease that causes heart disease invariably does so through an increase in pulmonary artery pressure, which then causes right heart dysfunction. The pathophysiology and clinical manifestations of pulmonary hypertension are often poorly understood. Since pulmonary hypertension is central to the pathophysiology of heart disease caused by lung disease, this chapter focuses primarily on pulmonary hypertension with an emphasis on pathophysiology and clinical manifestations. This chapter does not focus on the specifics of interstitial or airway lung disease. Instead, the reader is referred to other chapters in this book for discussions of the pathophysiology of specific parenchymal lung diseases. Thromboembolism should be considered in all patients with pulmonary artery hypertension. For a detailed review, the reader is referred to Chap. 30, on thromboembolism.

PULMONARY HYPERTENSION

Definition

Under normal circumstances the pulmonary circulation is a high-capacitance, low-resistance circulation and pulmonary artery pressure and right ventricular wall thickness represent a fraction of systemic blood pressure and left ventricular wall thickness. The normal pulmonary vascular resistance is about one-tenth the normal systemic vascular resistance. Because the pulmonary vasculature is so compliant, pulmonary artery pressure increases only minimally with exercise in normal individuals less than 50 years of age.

Pulmonary vascular resistance is quantified as the ratio of pressure drop across the pulmonary bed to flow across the bed. Specifically, pulmonary vascular resistance (PVR) is calculated as:

$$PVR = (\text{mean pulmonary artery pressure} - \text{mean left atrial pressure})/\text{pulmonary flow}$$

The result is a value in Wood units (mmHg/l/min). Pulmonary vascular resistance can also be expressed in metric units (dynes-sec-cm^{-5}). To convert to metric units, the pulmonary vascular resistance expressed in Wood units is multiplied by 79.9. The normal pulmonary vascular resistance is up to 1.5 Wood units or 120 dynes-sec-cm^{-5}.

Pulmonary artery hypertension results when there is an increase in one or more of the following: pulmonary vascular resistance, pulmonary flow, or pulmonary venous pressure. Pulmonary hypertension has been defined by some as a mean pulmonary artery pressure of greater than 20 mmHg at rest and by others as a mean pulmonary artery pressure greater than 25 mmHg at rest or greater than 30 mmHg with exercise. The normal resting pulmonary artery systolic pressure should be less than 30–35 mmHg. There are no references that differentiate pulmonary hypertension as mild, moderate, or severe. Some have defined severe pulmonary hypertension as a pulmonary artery systolic pressure greater than 75% the systemic blood pressure in normotensive individuals. However, one must keep in mind that even lower pulmonary artery pressures may cause significant right heart dysfunction and marked symptomatology. From a practical standpoint, one could label pulmonary artery hypertension as severe if the patient has end-organ damage—i.e., right heart dilatation and dysfunction (Fig. 1A).

Like systemic pressure and resistance, pulmonary artery pressure and resistance increase with age. It has been reported that pulmonary hypertension (mean pulmonary artery pressure >20 mmHg as defined above) may be as common as 28% of individuals in their seventies.

Symptoms

Symptoms related to pulmonary hypertension are secondary to reduced cardiac output and/or elevated right heart filling pressures. As pulmonary hypertension worsens, the right ventricle becomes hypertrophied, dilated, and dysfunctional. The response of the right ventricle depends on the acuity of the rise in resistance and pressure. With rare exception (to be discussed below), severe pulmonary hypertension in adults results in marked dilatation and dysfunction of the right ventricle (Fig. 1B). As right ventricular systolic function worsens, cardiac output falls. Reduced cardiac output can lead to symptoms of chronic fatigue. During exercise, pulmonary artery pressure increases secondary to the fixed pulmonary vascular resistance. Patients are unable to adequately increase their cardiac output with exertion, if they are able to increase it at all, and experience exertional dyspnea. Tricuspid regurgitation, which can be significant in the setting of severe pulmonary hypertension, leads to a further decrease in cardiac output and exacerbates the exertional dyspnea and fatigue. Patients with pulmonary hypertension commonly experience exertional dyspnea and fatigue prior to any physical evidence of right atrial hypertension (see below).

It should be noted that the lack of significant resting pulmonary hypertension in individuals with lung disease or primary pulmonary hypertension does not exclude pulmonary hypertension as a cause of exertional dyspnea. Significant pulmonary hypertension may be noted only with exercise in some individuals. The exercise-induced pulmonary

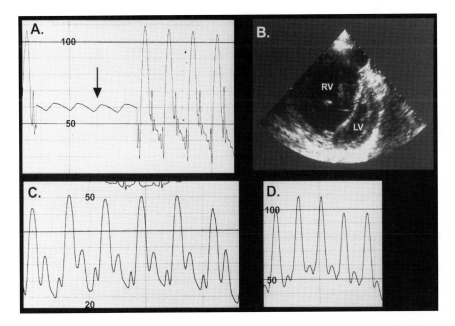

Figure 1 A. Pulmonary artery pressure tracing from an individual with severe primary pulmonary hypertension. The arrow depicts the mean pulmonary artery pressure. Note that pulmonary artery systolic pressure is greater than 100 mmHg. B. Echocardiographic parasternal short-axis image depicting the right ventricle (RV) and left ventricle (LV) of an individual with severe pulmonary artery hypertension. Note the marked dilatation of the right ventricle and the reverse curvature of the interventricular septum. C. Pulmonary artery pressure tracing from an individual with primary pulmonary hypertension. The pulmonary artery pressure is mild to moderately increased. The pressure was recorded with the patient at rest. D. Pulmonary artery pressure tracing from the same individual depicted in panel C. The pressure was recorded during exercise (alternating leg lifts). The pulmonary artery systolic pressure has increased to more than 100 mmHg.

hypertension in these individuals can result in right heart dysfunction and an inadequate rise in cardiac output, as noted above (Fig. 1C and D; see also ''Evaluation,'' below).

The normal mean right atrial pressure is less than or equal to 10 mmHg (Fig. 2A). As right ventricular systolic function worsens, right heart filling pressure invariably increases, resulting in right atrial hypertension and right-sided congestion (Fig. 2B). Edema begins in the most dependent portion of the body, which, in ambulatory individuals, is the feet. As right atrial pressure increases further, the edema ascends from the feet to the lower legs, thighs, and abdomen. Patients can develop hepatic congestion and ascites. The pleura and pericardium are drained via systemic veins. Consequently, significant right atrial hypertension can lead to both pleural and pericardial effusions. Like patients with left heart failure, patients with significant pleural effusions and/or ascites commonly experience orthopnea. Angina-like chest pain and syncope can also occur in patients with severe pulmonary hypertension. In most cases, syncope appears to be related to poor flow rather than arrhythmias.

It is important to keep in mind that symptoms related to pulmonary hypertension may also depend on the severity of associated lung or heart disease. For instance, the symptoms in individuals with primary pulmonary hypertension are related entirely to the

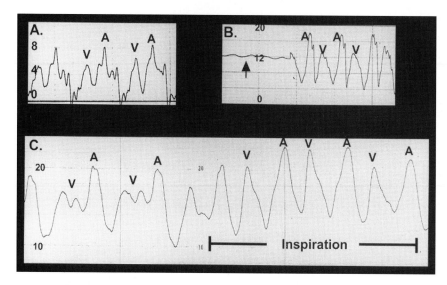

Figure 2   A. Normal right atrial pressure trace. ÒAÓ and ÒVÓ denote A and V waves respectively. B. Elevated right atrial pressure. The arrow depicts the mean right atrial pressure (12 mmHg). ÒAÓ and ÒVÓ denote A and V waves respectively. C. Kussmaul's sign. Right atrial pressure trace depicting an increase in right atrial pressure with inspiration. Note the increased V wave with inspiration as well. ÒAÓ and ÒVÓ denote A and V waves respectively.

consequences of the pulmonary hypertension. In contrast, individuals with pulmonary artery hypertension secondary to chronic obstructive lung disease may be limited more from the parenchymal lung disease and/or associated coronary artery disease than the elevated pulmonary artery pressure. Similarly, individuals with pulmonary artery hypertension secondary to elevated pulmonary venous pressure may be symptomatic more from pulmonary edema than from the elevated pulmonary artery pressure.

Signs

A thorough cardiovascular examination in patients with pulmonary hypertension provides important information about right atrial pressure, right-sided valvular function, right ventricular function, and cardiac output. A thorough examination involves inspection of the jugular veins, palpation of the peripheral pulses and heart, and auscultation.

Venous Pulsations

The jugular venous pulse reflects right atrial pressure. The normal jugular venous pulse should not exceed a total of 9 cmH$_2$O, or 4 cm above the sternal angle. The A wave amplitude exceeds the V wave amplitude in normal subjects (Fig. 2A). Elevation of the jugular venous pulse implies right atrial hypertension (Fig. 2B). The initial finding in patients with pulmonary hypertension may be an elevated A wave secondary to right ventricular hypertrophy. With progressive right heart dysfunction and dilatation, tricuspid regurgitation may result in an increase in the amplitude of the V wave. The jugular venous pulse normally falls with inspiration due to a fall in intrathoracic pressure. Elevation of the jugular venous pressure with inspiration (Kussmaul's sign) occurs in patients with pericardial constriction, restrictive myopathies, and significant right heart dysfunction

(Fig. 2C). Although some texts state that the most common cause of a Kussmaul's sign is pericardial constriction, clinical experience suggests that the most common cause is right heart dysfunction.

Arterial Pulsations

More information than the heart rate can be obtained from careful examination of the peripheral pulse. The volume and contour of the arterial pulse are determined by a combination of factors including vascular elasticity, left ventricular stroke volume, and ejection velocity. The carotid pulse provides the most accurate representation of the central aortic pulse. The normal carotid pulse rises rapidly to a smooth, rounded peak. Its descending limb is less steep than its ascending limb. The most common abnormality noted in the arterial pulsations of patients with pulmonary hypertension is a diminished pulse. Diminished pulsations are secondary to a decreased pulse pressure and occur in patients with decreased stroke volume, which, as noted above, is common in patients with severe pulmonary hypertension (Fig. 3A). Pulsus paradoxus can occur in patients with obstruction to airflow and, therefore, may be present in patients with pulmonary hypertension secondary to chronic obstructive lung disease (Fig. 3B). It is characterized by a decrease of 10 mmHg or more in systolic pressure with inspiration. It is often palpable in those patients who have a fall of at least a 20 mmHg in pressure with inspiration. The other cause of pulsus paradoxus is pericardial tamponade and should at least be considered in anyone with a paradox. Though pericardial effusions are common in patients with severe pulmonary hypertension, tamponade is rare.

Precordial Palpation

The presence of a parasternal lift suggests right ventricular dilatation and/or hypertrophy. In patients with significant pulmonary artery hypertension, the second heart sound is often

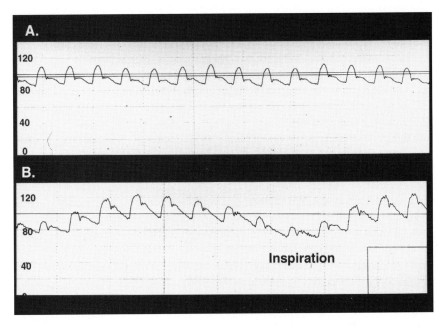

Figure 3   A. Arterial pressure tracing depicting a reduced pulse pressure. B. Arterial pressure tracing depicting pulsus paradoxus. This individual had severe chronic obstructive lung disease.

palpable along the upper left sternal border (pulmonic area), as is the pulmonary artery itself (pulmonary artery tap).

Auscultation

The most reproducible auscultatory finding in pulmonary hypertension is a loud pulmonic component of the second heart sound (P_2). With progressive pulmonary hypertension, the intensity of P_2 increases. The duration of splitting of the second heart sound decreases in patients with pulmonary hypertension without right ventricular dysfunction because of decreased compliance of the pulmonary arteries. However, as the right ventricle fails, the duration of splitting increases and patients develop wide, persistent splitting of the second heart sound. Wide, persistent splitting of the second heart sound also occurs secondary to right bundle branch block even in patients with normal pulmonary artery pressure and right ventricular function. A blowing holosystolic murmur at the lower left sternal border that increases with inspiration suggests tricuspid regurgitation. Patients may also develop a decrescendo diastolic murmur of pulmonic insufficiency. This is the so called Graham Steell murmur. The murmur of pulmonic insufficiency in patients with significant pulmonary hypertension is typically a high-frequency, holodiastolic murmur very similar in quality to the murmur of aortic insufficiency. In contrast, the murmur of pulmonic insufficiency in patients with normal pulmonary artery pressure or minimal pulmonary hypertension is lower in frequency and shorter in duration, typically terminating in mid-diastole.

Natural History

The natural history or prognosis of patients with severe pulmonary hypertension is very poor. The best available data are from patients with primary pulmonary hypertension. The National Institutes of Health registry on primary pulmonary hypertension included the long-term follow-up of 194 adults with well-established primary pulmonary hypertension (see references). The median survival of that group was 2.8 years from the time of enrollment. Importantly, the study revealed that survival of patients with primary pulmonary hypertension could be estimated based on three hemodynamic factors: mean right atrial pressure, mean pulmonary artery pressure, and cardiac index. These hemodynamic measures can be used in a regression analysis to determine the likelihood of survival at specific time points. The most common cause of death was right heart failure (47%) and sudden death (26%). Median survival of patients with a mean right atrial pressure of greater than or equal to 20 mmHg was 1 month.

While there are virtually no data regarding the life expectancy of patients with pulmonary hypertension caused by other pulmonary vascular or parenchymal lung disorders, it's my feeling that, for a given set of hemodynamic factors, their prognosis is as bad or even worse than that of primary pulmonary hypertension. In addition to the pulmonary hypertension, these patients also have to contend with their primary abnormality, such as interstial lung disease, collagen vascular disease, sarcoidosis, or obstructive lung disease.

Patients with Eisenmenger syndrome (defined and discussed below) are unique in that they often do not develop right heart failure despite severe pulmonary hypertension. The prognosis of patients with Eisenmenger syndrome appears to be more favorable than that of patients with pulmonary hypertension from other causes.

Evaluation

This section focuses exclusively on the evaluation of pulmonary artery hypertension. The reader is referred to appropriate chapters for the evaluation of parenchymal lung disease, pulmonary function testing, and thromboembolic disease.

An echocardiogram with Doppler should be performed in patients suspected of having pulmonary artery hypertension. The pulmonary artery systolic pressure can be determined based on the Doppler velocity of the tricuspid regurgitant jet, utilizing the following equation:

$$\text{Pulmonary artery systolic pressure} = 4(\text{velocity of the TR jet})^2 + \text{right atrial pressure}$$

The right atrial pressure can be estimated from the neck vein evaluation or size of the inferior vena cava (see below), or a value of 10 mmHg can be substituted into the equation. This equation has been extensively validated and there is excellent correlation between Doppler-derived measures of pulmonary artery pressure and catheter-derived measures of pulmonary artery pressure. Echocardiographic evaluation also provides information on the size of the right atrium and ventricle and right ventricular function. Right atrial pressure can be estimated based on the diameter of the inferior vena cava. If the inferior vena cava is greater than 2 cm in diameter and does not decrease at least 50% in diameter with inspiration, then the mean right atrial pressure is generally greater than 10 mmHg. It is important to note that patients with lung disease may have poor echocardiographic images secondary to interposed air between the heart and chest wall. This will limit the diagnostic utility and accuracy of the test.

Contrast or bubble echocardiography should be considered in patients with significant pulmonary artery hypertension and hypoxia. This is performed by an intravenous injection of agitated sterile saline. Right-to-left shunt at the atrial level suggests a patent foreman ovale or atrial septal defect. Delayed appearance of microbubbles in the left heart suggests the presence of pulmonary arteriovenous malformations, which can occur in patients with hereditary hemmorrhagic telangiectasia or hepatic cirrhosis. Transesophageal echocardiography should be considered in selected patients with pulmonary artery hypertension. It is the diagnostic test of choice to assess for congenital cardiac malformations at the atrial level—such as atrial septal defect, sinus venosus defect, or anomalous pulmonary venous connection—all of which can cause pulmonary hypertension in adults. Contrast echocardiography and transesophageal echocardiography are discussed further below, under ''Pulmonary Vascular Occlusive Disease with Right Heart Failure.''

As noted above, a subset of patients are characterized by exertional pulmonary artery hypertension with minimal resting pulmonary artery hypertension (Fig. 1C and D). An exercise echocardiogram can be useful in the initial assessment of individuals suspected of primarily having exercise-induced pulmonary artery hypertension. Echocardiographic images may reveal right heart dilatation and dysfunction and flattening of the interventricular septum with exercise (see Fig. 1B). An increase in the volume of tricuspid regurgitation can be detected by color-flow Doppler. Resting and exercise pulmonary artery systolic pressure can be measured with Doppler, as discussed above.

Invasive hemodynamic assessment should be considered in selected patients with pulmonary artery hypertension. This is discussed further below, under ''Pulmonary Vascular Occlusive Disease with Right Heart Failure.''

PARENCHYMAL LUNG DISEASE AND HYPOXIA

Pulmonary hypertension and right heart dysfunction are often associated with both interstitial and airway parenchymal lung disease. The primary mechanisms are vasoconstriction secondary to hypoxemia and acidosis and vascular destruction. In patients with both parenchymal lung disease and pulmonary hypertension, it is often very difficult or even impossible to determine if dyspnea or fatigue are primarily due to the parenchymal lung disease, pulmonary hypertension, or both. Even after thorough cardiopulmonary evaluation, it may not be possible to differentiate. The focus of treatment should be on potentially reversible or correctable factors that may be contributing to the patient's symptoms, such as hypoxia, bronchoconstriction, or peripheral edema. For those patients who have persistent severe pulmonary artery hypertension despite oxygen therapy, there are no data to suggest that vasodilator therapy will be beneficial. It should be kept in mind that pulmonary hypertension in patients with parenchymal lung disease is often due predominantly to vascular destruction. Thus, vasodilators would not be expected to be of benefit. This section does not focus on the specifics of the various interstitial and airway disorders but rather on the mechanisms responsible for cardiac dysfunction.

Hypoxemia

Left Ventricular Dysfunction

Hyoxpemia secondary to lung disease can cause left ventricular dysfunction. With severe lung disease (interstitial or airway disease), I found that a subset of patients have evidence of diastolic dysfunction manifest as an increased left ventricular end-diastolic pressure. A small subset ($< 5\%$) have significant left ventricular systolic dysfunction as well. These patients usually do not have other forms of heart disease, including coronary artery disease. Importantly, left ventricular function usually improves with supplemental oxygen in those patients with left ventricular systolic dysfunction. It is important to keep in mind that left ventricular dysfunction may further impair the functional status of a patient with significant lung disease. Patients may also be excluded from lung transplantion if left ventricular dysfunction is present. Assumptions that the left ventricular dysfunction is irreversible may be erroneous.

Pulmonary Vasoconstriction

Parenchymal lung disease that causes heart disease invariably does so through an increase in pulmonary artery pressure, which then results in right heart dysfunction. Central to this process is hypoxia-induced pulmonary artery vasoconstriction. The magnitude of the vasoconstrictor response appears to be more profound in younger individuals, especially infants, and differs from individual to individual. It appears that small pulmonary arteries and arterioles are the major sites of hypoxia-induced vasoconstriction. The exact mechanism of the vasoconstriction is not known. It has been speculated that the vascular endothelium plays a pivotal role in hypoxia-induced vasoconstriction. Whether the response is related to excess endothelin, reduced endothelium-derived relaxing factor, or both is currently unknown. It appears that alveolar hypoxia causes vasoconstriction secondary to reduced diffusion of oxygen into the blood of small pulmonary arteries and arterioles. This is evidenced by the fact that hypoxia without lung disease can result in potent vasoconstriction, as may be seen in patients with sleep apnea or neuromuscular abnormalities. The oxygen tension in mixed venous blood may also play a role, as patients with hypoxemia who do not have alveolar hypoxia, such as infants with cyanotic congenital heart disease, can also experience pulmonary vasoconstriction.

Supplemental oxygen should be prescribed for those patients with pulmonary hypertension secondary to alveolar hypoxia, as the pulmonary vasoconstriction is often reversible. Keep in mind that in patients with significant vascular destruction, such as those with severe idiopathic pulmonary fibrosis, the pulmonary hypertension may not improve even with correction of hypoxia.

PULMONARY VASCULAR OCCLUSIVE DISEASE WITH RIGHT HEART FAILURE

Primary Pulmonary Hypertension

Lung disease that causes heart disease does not have to involve the lung parenchyma. Pulmonary vascular occlusive disease without parenchymal lung disease can occur secondary to a variety of pathological processes. The end result is pulmonary hypertension and right heart dysfunction.

The classic cause of pulmonary vascular occlusive disease is primary pulmonary hypertension. Primary pulmonary hypertension is a rare disorder occurring in only 1 to 2 per million people in the general population, yet it has been well studied owing to the efforts of a small group of persistent individuals. It is rarely familial. The mean age of individuals in the National Institutes of Health registry referred to above was 36 ± 15 years, and 63% were women. The diagnosis of primary pulmonary hypertension is one of exclusion. All patients suspected of having primary pulmonary hypertension should undergo a thorough evaluation to exclude parenchymal lung disease, pulmonary thrombo-embolic disease, pulmonary vasculitis, collagen vascular disease, liver disease, congenital heart disease, and left ventricular myocardial or structural abnormalities as the cause of their pulmonary hypertension. Patients should also be questioned thoroughly about past or present use of appetite suppressant medications. Use of these medications for even very brief periods can still result in significant pathology (see below).

The pulmonary hypertension in primary pulmonary hypertension is most commonly due to vasoconstriction, intimal and medial hypertrophy and hyperplasia, and plexiform and other more advanced vascular lesions. Pathologically, this is often referred to as plexogenic pulmonary hypertension. The most common classification system used to describe these changes is that of Heath and Edwards (Fig. 4). Less commonly, the pulmonary hypertension is due to veno-occlusive disease, pulmonary hemangiomatosis, or marked in situ thrombosis of the small pulmonary arteries.

The pathogenesis of primary pulmonary hypertension is not known. Studies suggest multiple possible etiologies, including growth factor and cytokine stimulation of cell growth and division in the vascular intima and media, abnormalities in endothelial and smooth muscle cell function secondary to endothelin and/or endothelium-derived relaxing factor, abnormal platelet and coagulation function, and apoptosis of normal vascular cells.

Primary pulmonary hypertension is a fatal disorder. Though little is known of the pathogenesis, the symptoms and natural history of patients with primary pulmonary hypertension are well known (see above). A subset of patients with primary pulmonary hypertension (about 25–30%) are said to respond favorably to therapy with oral vasodilators. The vasodilator most often used has been nifedipine. Invasive hemodynamic monitoring (by pulmonary artery catheter) should be used to assess patients and to determine their responsiveness to vasodilators. For those patients who do respond with both a decrease in pulmonary artery pressure and an increase in cardiac output, symptoms and survival markedly improve. Limited data suggest that survival may be somewhat prolonged by chronic anti-coagulation with warfarin. More recently, continuous infusion of intravenous prostacyclin

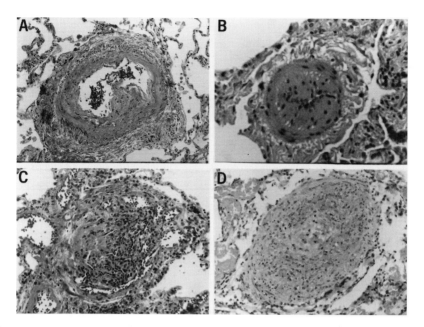

Figure 4   Pulmonary artery histopathology from an individual with plexogenic pulmonary artery hypertension. Heath and Edwards classification. A. Medial hyperplasia and hypertrophy and intimal proliferation (grade II). B. Medial hyperplasia and hypertrophy, intimal proliferation, and subendothelial fibrosis (grade III). C. Plexiform lesion (grade IV). Note the multiple thin walled, irregular vascular dilatations. D. Fibrinoid necrosis (grade VI). (From Ref. 3, with permission.)

has been shown to improve functional status and may prolong survival of patients with primary pulmonary hypertension. Patients require continuous infusions and may rapidly decompensate if the infusion is terminated for any reason. Infection remains a constant threat and may lead to acute decompensation in patients with little if any functional reserve. For patients who do not respond to oral vasodilators, lung transplantation (either single or bilateral) can be considered. The 1-year posttransplant survival of patients with primary pulmonary hypertension is about 60–65%. Atrial septostomy (creation of an atrial septal defect) to decompress the right atrium and increase cardiac output has been performed in selected patients with severe primary pulmonary hypertension. The positive hemodynamic benefits of reduced right atrial pressure, increased left heart filling, and increased cardiac output occur at the expense of hypoxemia secondary to right-to-left shunt.

Hypoxia is common in patients with primary pulmonary hypertension. The proposed mechanisms are right-to-left shunt through a patent foreman ovale and ventilation/perfusion abnormalities secondary to the vascular changes noted above. A contrast bubble study to determine the presence or absence of a right-to-left intracardiac shunt can be performed at the time of echocardiographic evaluation. Patients with evidence of right-to-left shunt should undergo transesophageal echocardiographic evaluation to exclude the presence of an atrial septal defect with Eisenmenger physiology (see below).

Invasive hemodynamic assessment should be used to determine right heart hemodynamics (right atrial pressure, pulmonary artery pressure, pulmonary vascular resistance) and cardiac output and to exclude left atrial hypertension in patients suspected of having primary pulmonary hypertension. In fact, invasive hemodynamic assessment should be considered in the assessment of all patients with significant pulmonary hypertension irrespective of the cause. As noted above, the data provide important diagnostic and prognostic information. It should be noted that right heart catheterization can be very difficult in patients with severe pulmonary hypertension owing to the size of the right atrium and ventricle, tricuspid regurgitation, and pulmonary insufficiency. The risk in these patients is increased as well owing to their extremely limited reserve. Further, tricuspid regurgitation and low cardiac output reduce the accuracy and reproducibility of thermodilution as a measure of cardiac output. One should utilize the Fick technique to measure cardiac output in this patient cohort. A pulmonary catheter wedge pressure can be very difficult to obtain because of the marked dilatation of the large pulmonary arteries. Elevation of the pulmonary capillary wedge pressure should be confirmed with a wedged oxygen saturation.

The reader is referred to the references below for more detailed information on primary pulmonary hypertension.

Appetite Suppressant Drugs

In the late 1960s and early 1970s in Europe, there was a marked increase in the number of patients diagnosed with primary pulmonary hypertension. The outbreak was attributed to the appetite suppressant drug aminorex. More recently, considerable focus has centered on the role of Redux (dexfenfluramine) and Fen-phen (fenfluramine-phentermine) in cardiopulmonary disease. In addition to valvular heart disease, both have been noted to occasionally cause severe pulmonary artery hypertension. The pulmonary vascular pathology appears identical to that seen in plexogenic primary pulmonary hypertension. Severe pulmonary artery hypertension or valvular heart disease can occur in people who have taken the medications for less than 1 month. It is important to consider appetite suppressant medications when seeing an individual with possible primary pulmonary hypertension. It has been suggested that these medications may worsen or accelerate preexisting pulmonary vascular pathology.

Other

Patients with portal hypertension rarely develop a similar pulmonary vascular occlusive process as that seen in primary pulmonary hypertension. Interestingly, some patients with AIDS develop pulmonary vascular occlusive disease. The incidence in these individuals may be as high as 1–2%. Patients with collagen vascular disorders such as scleroderma, systemic lupus erythematosus, and mixed connective tissue disease can have similar pulmonary vascular pathological changes as those seen in primary pulmonary hypertension. However, the pulmonary artery pathology is dominated by intimal and medial hyperplasia, hypertrophy, and fibrotic occlusion rather than by plexogenic lesions or fibrinoid necrosis. As with primary pulmonary hypertension, the pathogenesis of the pulmonary vascular occlusive process is unknown.

Pulmonary vasculitis may involve the lung primarily or as part of a more systemic process. For example, the vasculitis of Wegener's granulomatosis or Churg-Strauss syndrome may be confined to the lung. The vasculitis of polyarteritis nodosa, Takayasu's disease, and the collagen vascular diseases may involve the pulmonary blood vessels in the setting of a more systemic process. These processes can result in significant vascular pathology and lead to severe pulmonary hypertension, with the clinical manifestations and natural history discussed above. As one would expect, the primary site of vascular pathology within the lung may differ in the various vasculitides. When it occurs in the lung, Takayasu's disease primarily involves the larger, more central pulmonary arteries, sparing the medium-sized and smaller arteries and thus allowing for possible revascularization through bypass conduits or angioplasty. Most pulmonary vasculitis occurs primarily in the smaller arteries and is therefore not amenable to mechanical procedures.

PULMONARY VASCULAR OCCLUSIVE DISEASE WITHOUT RIGHT HEART FAILURE

Eisenmenger Syndrome

Patients with Eisenmenger syndrome do not have lung disease that causes heart disease but heart disease that causes lung disease. The pulmonary vascular pathology found in patients with Eisenmenger syndrome is essentially the same as that of patients with plexogenic primary pulmonary hypertension. For that reason a brief discussion of Eisenmenger syndrome is included in this chapter.

Eisenmenger syndrome occurs with diverse congenital cardiac anomalies and is manifest by severe, irreversible pulmonary artery hypertension with dilatation of the central pulmonary arteries and reversal of a previous left-to-right shunt at the atrial, ventricular, or aortopulmonary level. The resultant right-to-left or bidirectional shunt leads to clinical cyanosis and the secondary manifestations of chronic hypoxemia. Eisenmenger syndrome occurs only in patients with hemodynamically nonrestrictive cardiac defects. Nonrestrictive defects or communications are those that are large enough that there is no pressure difference from one side of the defect or communication to the other (Fig. 5A). These individuals are unique in that they have cyanosis and severe pulmonary artery hypertension yet often have preserved right heart function and normal right atrial pressure (Fig. 5B). Further, the natural history of Eisenmenger syndrome appears far superior to that of primary pulmonary hypertension despite similar pulmonary vascular resistance, pulmo-

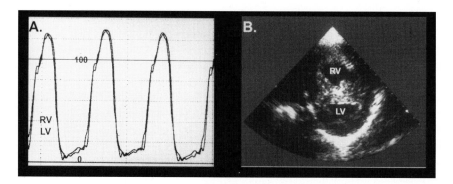

Figure 5 A. Simultaneous tracings of right and left ventricular pressure from a patient with a nonrestrictive ventricular septal defect and Eisenmenger syndrome. Note the equalization of right and left ventricular pressure. B. Echocardiographic parasternal short-axis image depicting the right ventricle (RV) and left ventricle (LV) of an individual with severe pulmonary artery hypertension. This individual has a nonrestrictive ventricular septal defect and Eisenmenger syndrome. Note the difference compared with the case shown in Fig. 1B.

nary artery pressure, and pulmonary vascular pathology. Importantly, the natural survival of patients with Eisenmenger syndrome appears superior to survival after lung or heart-lung transplant. For more information, the reader is referred to the reference on Eisenmenger syndrome, below.

SUGGESTED READING

1. Curfman GD. Diet pills redux (editorial). N Engl J Med 1997; 337:629–630.
2. D'Alonzo GE, Barst RJ, Ayres SM, Bergofsky EH, Brundage BH, Detre KM, Fishman AP, Goldring RM, Groves BM, Kernis JI, Levy PS, Pietra GG, Reid LM, Reeves JT, Rich S, Vreim CE, Williams GW, Wu M. Survival in patients with primary pulmonary hypertension: results from a national prospective registry. Ann Intern Med 1991; 115:343–349.
3. Hopkins WE. Severe Pulmonary hypertension in congenital heart disease: a review of Eisenmenger syndrome. Curr Opin Cardiol 1995; 10:517–523.
4. Perloff JK, Braunwald E. Physical examination of the heart and circulation. In: Braunwald E, ed. Heart Disease: A Textbook of Cardiovascular Medicine, 5th ed. Philadelphia: Saunders, 1997:15–52.
5. Rich S, Braunwald E, Grossman W. Pulmonary hypertension. In: Braunwald E, ed. Heart Disease: A Textbook of Cardiovascular Medicine, 5th ed. Philadelphia: Saunders, 1997:780–806.
6. Rubin LJ. Primary pulmonary hypertension. N Engl J Med 1997; 336:111–117.

34

Cystic Fibrosis

William P. Sexauer and Stanley B. Fiel

*Medical College of Pennsylvania
and Hahnemann University School of Medicine
Philadelphia, Pennsylvania*

INTRODUCTION

Cystic Fibrosis (CF) is the most common fatal genetic disease of Caucasians. The last several decades have seen a dramatic increase in survival of the CF patient. In 1960, the median survival age for CF patients was less than 5 years. Today CF patients can expect to live 30 years or more. The reasons for this dramatically improved outlook are protean. Included among the many contributing factors are new and more potent antibiotics, improved nutritional support, more efficacious pancreatic enzyme formulations, and more effective airway clearance techniques.

Cystic fibrosis has historically been considered a disease of childhood. The marked improvement in survival, however, has led to increasing numbers of patients living into adulthood, many leading active and productive lives. As of 1995, about 35% of the CF population was ≥18 years of age. This chapter describes today's approach to the comprehensive care of pulmonary disease in the adult cystic fibrosis patient. However, many of the principles of care are similar to those in the pediatric population, especially for adolescents. The "team" approach to the care of the CF patient in a modern CF center is discussed. A review of the major principles of therapy, including antimicrobial therapy, airway clearance techniques, bronchodilators, and mucolytics follows. More recent therapeutic advances, such as lung transplantation and anti-inflammatory medications are discussed. Finally, an approach to some of the more common pulmonary complications of CF is outlined.

PATHOPHYSIOLOGY

Knowledge of the pathophysiology underlying the physical abnormalities in CF is essential to understand the approach to and treatment of CF. This is a genetic disease, caused by mutations at a single gene locus on the long arm of chromosome seven. This gene codes for a protein called cystic fibrosis transmembrane conduction regulator (CFTR), which

595

governs chloride conductance across epithelial cell membranes. CF patients have mutations in both alleles of the gene, resulting in an absent, malfunctioning, or underfunctioning CFTR. The most common mutation is designated ΔF508, but to date over 650 different mutations have been identified. The large number of possible genotype combinations is at least in part responsible for the wide variability in phenotypic presentations seen in CF. Heterozygotes with only one abnormal (mutant) allele are clinically asymptomatic. The resulting abnormalities in electrolyte and fluid transport across a variety of epithelial cell membranes are felt to be the cause of the multisystem disorder characteristic of CF.

The organ of greatest concern with regard to morbidity and mortality is the lung. Airway epithelial cells have an impaired ability to secrete chloride to the epithelial cell surface (airway lumen) in response to cyclic-AMP stimulation, coupled with an increased absorption of sodium from the airway surface fluid (Fig. 1). This results in an abnormal, desiccated airway surface fluid of abnormal ion content that, for reasons that are still poorly elucidated, becomes readily colonized with a variety of bacterial pathogens. This bacterial colonization and infection, once established, is almost impossible to eradicate and results in a chronic suppurative state in the lower airways leading to progressive airway destruction over time. The hallmark pathological change in CF is bronchiectasis, but with progressive disease, interstitial fibrosis and patchy areas of emphysema also occur. Pulmonary function studies typically show an obstructive pattern with a normal diffusing capacity.

The abnormalities of electrolyte and fluid transport are also responsible for the extrapulmonary manifestations of CF. The presence of abnormal pancreatic secretions leads to the occlusion of pancreatic ductules, resulting in destruction and fibrosis of the gland and ultimately pancreatic insufficiency (93% of cases). Males are almost universally sterile; this is thought to be secondary to resorption of the vas deferens due to its occlusion with secretions during fetal life. A functional bowel obstruction can occur due to abnormal secretions in the small bowel, leading to a disorder known as distal intestinal obstruction syndrome (DIOS). Other common CF manifestations that relate directly or indirectly to the basic molecular defect include obstructive cirrhosis, decreased female fertility due to

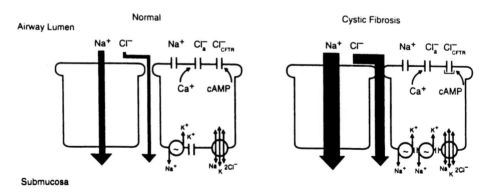

Figure 1 Ion transport across airway epithelia in normal and cystic fibrosis patients. In the normal airway, chloride may be secreted to the airway lumen both by cAMP-mediated CFTR and alternative calcium-activated chloride channels. In CF, chloride secretion via CFTR is impaired, accompanied by increased sodium ion reabsorption from the airway lumen. Chloride reabsorption from the airway lumen follows sodium passively, leading to abnormal airway surface fluid ion and water content. (From Knowles MR, Olivier K, Noone P, Boucher RC. Am J Respir Crit Care Med 1995; 151:S66.)

abnormal cervical mucus, and excess salt and fluid loss due to sweating. In fact, the abnormally high chloride content of the sweat in CF patients forms the basis for the diagnostic test for CF, the ''sweat test.''

APPROACH TO THE PATIENT

About 87% of CF patients in the United States are cared for in CF centers, accredited and partially funded by the Cystic Fibrosis Foundation. Within a center, a team of health care professionals coordinates the care of the CF patient. The team will typically consist of one or more physicians, including the CF center's director; a nurse; a dietitian or nutritional specialist; a respiratory therapist; and a social worker. In some centers, physical therapists also contribute on a regular basis.

The vast majority of CF patients are diagnosed in infancy or early childhood, and thus grow up with CF as part of their everyday lives. By adolescence and young adulthood, they are usually very knowledgeable of their condition and the care involved, though coming to grips with the implications of their disease as they enter the adult world is a challenge in its own right. The transition to independent living from the relatively secure haven of parental care can be a difficult and frightening experience. However, approximately 7–8% of patients are diagnosed after 10 years of age, and 3–4% are diagnosed ≥18 years of age. For these patients, education about the disease and its treatment must occur simultaneously with adaptation to life with a newly identified chronic disease state.

The main goal of all therapy for the CF patient is to preserve the highest level of health and functioning while attempting to minimize the adverse effects of the disease and its treatment on the patient's daily life. Obviously, the success of this approach will vary depending on an individual's health status and rate of disease progression, especially with regard to pulmonary function. Patients are typically seen at least four times a year for an outpatient evaluation, even if stable. Patients are seen more frequently if they have advanced disease, are ''active'' in the sense of more frequent exacerbations, or are experiencing a rapid rate of decline.

Evaluation at each visit consists of a history to assess new or changing symptoms, physical examination, weight, and spirometry. Once a year, patients will undergo a more extensive ''annual'' evaluation consisting of full pulmonary function studies (spirometry pre- and postbronchodilators, lung volumes, diffusing capacity), chest x-ray, sputum Gram stain and culture, routine blood studies (CBC, electrolytes, BUN and creatinine, liver function studies, lipid profile, and vitamin E and A levels). Some centers also do a maximal exercise study, which provides prognostic information and is useful to detect exercise-induced hypoxemia. All patients should receive the influenza vaccine yearly in the fall.

As mentioned earlier, CF is a systemic disease involving multiple organ systems. Though the focus of this chapter is CF pulmonary disease, the importance of maintaining optimal nutritional status cannot be overstated. Patients with CF are predisposed to malnutrition via several mechanisms. The most obvious is that of exocrine pancreatic insufficiency, which predisposes to malabsorption of fat, bile salts and acids, and the fat-soluble vitamins. Less appreciated is a strong correlation between nutritional status and lung function. As lung function worsens, metabolic rate increases and energy requirements rise. This is most pronounced during periods of infectious exacerbations, where the common occurrence of anorexia aggravates an acute rise in caloric requirements. This is observed clinically as an acute and often precipitous weight loss that must be promptly addressed if the patient is to optimally overcome the exacerbation. Diabetes mellitus and cholestatic liver disease are two relatively common complications in adult patients that may further aggravate an individual's nutritional status. The importance of nutrition in CF is illustrated by studies showing that patients with pancreatic insufficiency have a shorter life expectancy than pancreatic-sufficient patients.

Nutritional status must be monitored closely and interventions made early if there are signs of worsening status. As mentioned, monitoring of weight and vitamin levels is performed at regular intervals. All pancreatic-insufficient patients should receive supplemental pancreatic enzymes, usually in the range of 1000 to 2500 U of lipase/kg per meal. Dosage should be individualized and optimized in consultation with a dietitian. Dosages greater than 2500 U of lipase/kg per meal should be avoided because of the association between high doses of lipase and the occurrence of colonic strictures. In addition, the patient should receive regular vitamin supplementation, especially the fat-soluble vitamins D (400 IU/day) and A (5000 IU/day) in addition to a standard multivitamin. It is recommended that all patients receive a liberal, unrestricted diet unless certain complications or comorbidities (e.g., diabetes mellitus) exist.

For patients who are unable to maintain adequate nutrition despite optimization of the above interventions, a variety of high-calorie supplemental nutritional formulas are available. These can be used intermittently for the exacerbated patient until nutrition returns to normal or chronically for the patient with advanced lung disease who is unable to maintain sufficient weight. During exacerbations, when anorexia can be a major problem, supplemental intravenous nutrition in the form of peripheral parenteral nutrition is sometimes administered. Total parenteral nutrition is rarely indicated. In cases of refractory malnutrition, supplemental enteral feedings via gastrostomy, jejunostomy, or intermittent (e.g., nocturnal) nasogastric tube placement may be indicated.

ANTIMICROBIAL THERAPY

Maybe the single most important factor contributing to the increased survival of CF patients has been the development of effective antimicrobials against the most common airway pathogen—*Pseudomonas aeruginosa*. A variety of other pathogens occur less commonly, either alone or in combination with *Pseudomonas* species. These include *Staphylococcus aureus*, *Haemophilus influenzae*, *Burkholderia cepacia*, and *Stenotrophomonas* (formerly *Xanthomonas*) *maltophilia*. The antimicrobial choice in a given patient is governed by the results of sputum cultures and sensitivities, which are routinely obtained at the time of an exacerbation or annually in the very stable patient. In the occasional individual who cannot or does not produce sputum, a culture of a throat swab has been shown to correlate with cultures of the lower respiratory tract and may be used as a substitute for sputum.

Acute Exacerbations

CF lung disease is characterized by chronic low-grade infection punctuated by periodic exacerbations. An exacerbation is usually heralded by an increase in cough, quantity and viscosity of sputum, dyspnea, lethargy, and weight loss. Fever is often absent or low-grade. Hemoptysis may be present and is most often small in quantity or consists of blood-streaked sputum, but occasionally it may be large in quantity and persistent. Other symptoms that may be present include chest pain and wheezing.

Pulmonary function, as measured by spirometry, invariably falls during an exacerbation and is the single most important objective marker of the severity of an exacerbation and response to therapy. Spirometry is routinely checked at presentation and at the midpoint and end of a course of antimicrobial therapy in the exacerbated patient.

Despite substantial drops in FVC and FEV_1, the chest x-ray is often unchanged during an exacerbation. Changes, if they occur, most often consist of increased interstitial markings, peribronchial thickening, and mucous plugging. Frank pneumonic infiltrates occur only occasionally, and pleural effusions are rare.

If symptoms, signs, and pulmonary function decrements are mild, the exacerbation may be treated on an outpatient basis with oral antibiotics, assuming that the patient has an organism sensitive to an oral agent. Commonly used oral agents and their recommended doses are given in Table 1. Antibiotic courses are commonly administered for 2 weeks, or longer if the patient has had an incomplete response at 14 days. With outpatient therapy, it is essential that the patient be followed closely to ascertain that there is clinical improvement and that pulmonary function has returned toward baseline. Patients are instructed to notify the care team promptly if there is a clear worsening trend while they are on therapy.

For more severe exacerbations, or if the sputum reveals no susceptibility to available oral agents, intravenous (IV) antibiotics are employed. This is done most commonly in the hospital, though there is an increasing trend toward administration of IV antibiotics at home. A common practice is to admit the more severely exacerbated patients to initiate therapy; if there is a good initial response, they are discharged home after 7–10 days to complete the balance of the IV antibiotic course. Initial in-hospital care ensures regular

Table 1 Oral Antibiotics Commonly Used in Cystic Fibrosis

Antibiotic	Usual Adult Dose	Targeted Organism(s)
Dicloxacillin	500 mg every 6 h	*S. aureus*
Amoxicillin/clavulanate	500 mg amoxicillin every 8 h or 875 mg amoxicillin every 12 h	*S. aureus, H. flu*
Cephalexin	500 mg every 6 h	*S. aureus*
Cefuroxime	500 mg every 12 h	*S. aureus, H. flu*
Cefaclor	500 mg every 8 h	*S. aureus, H. flu*
Erythromycin	500 mg every 6–8 h	*S. aureus*
Clarithromycin	500 mg every 12 h	*S. aureus*
Azithromycin	500 mg on day 1; then 250 mg daily for 4 days	*S. aureus, H. flu*
Trimethoprim/sulfamethoxazole	160 mg trimethoprim/800 mg sulfamethoxazole every 12 h	*S. aureus, H. flu, B. cepacia*
Ciprofloxacin[a]	500–750 mg every 12 h	*P. aerug, S. aureus, H. flu*
Ofloxacin	400 mg every 12 h	*P. aerug, S. aureus, H. flu*
Levafloxacin	500 mg once daily	*S. aureus, H. flu, P. aerug*
Chloramphenicol	500 mg every 6 h	*B. cepacia, H. flu*

P. aerug, Pseudomonas aeruginosa; H. flu, Haemophilus influenzae; S. aureus, Staphylococcus aureus; B. cepacia, Burkholderia cepacia.
[a] Not approved for patients < 18 years of age.

chest physiotherapy, aerosol therapy, and more aggressive attention to nutritional issues as well as relieving the patient of home-related responsibilities and pressures. Patients with milder exacerbations requiring IV antibiotics can be treated initially at home provided that close follow-up can be arranged, as outlined above.

As stated earlier the choice of antibiotics in a given individual is guided by sputum cultures and sensitivities. *Pseudomonas* species and other commonly resistant organisms such as *B. cepacia* or *S. maltophilia* are best treated with at least two different agents from different classes. This is to improve the efficiency of bacterial killing through a synergistic or additive effect while decreasing the risk of resistant organisms that could result in failure of therapy. Table 2 lists commonly used IV antimicrobials—their dosages, frequencies, and targeted microorganisms.

Among the most commonly used agents are the antipseudomonal penicillins (pipera-cillin, ticarcillin), antipseudomonal cephalosporins (e.g., ceftazidime), and the aminogly-cosides. All of these agents have altered pharmacokinetics in the CF population compared with non-CF patients. For poorly understood reasons, CF patients have a higher volume of distribution and an increased renal clearance of beta-lactam antibiotics and aminoglyco-sides and thus require a higher than standard dosage to obtain optimal therapeutic affect. Beta-lactam antibiotics are usually given at the highest recommended (nonmeningitis)

Table 2 Intravenous Antibiotics Commonly Used for Cystic Fibrosis Exacerbations

Antibiotic	Usual Adult Dose	Targeted Organism(s)
Nafcillin	1–2 g every 6 h	*S. aureus*
Vancomycin	1 g every 2 h	*S. aureus*
Clindamycin	600–900 mg every 8 h	*S. aureus*
Piperacillin, piperacillin/ tazobactam	3–4 g every 4–6 h	*P. aerug, H. flu*
Ticarcillin, ticarcillin/ clavulanate	3 g every 4–6 h	*P. aerug, H. flu*
Ceftazidime	2 g every 8 h	*P. aerug, H. flu*
Aztreonam	1–2 g every 6–8 h	*P. aerug, H. flu*
Imipenem/cilastin	0.5–1.0 g every 6 h	*S. aureus, H. flu, P. aerug*
Tobramycin	10 mg/kg/day in 3–4 divided doses[a]	*P. aerug, H. flu*
Amikacin	20–30 mg/kg/day in 3 divided doses[a]	*P. aerug, H. flu*
Ciprofloxacin[b]	400 mg every 12 h	*P. aerug, H. flu, S. aureus*
Trimethoprim/ sulfamethoxazole	5 mg trimethoprim/25 mg sulfamethoxazole/kg every 6 h	*S. aureus, H. flu, B. cepacia*
Chloramphenicol	50 mg/kg/day in 4 divided doses	*B. cepacia, H. flu*

Key: P. aerug = Pseudomonas aeruginosa; H. flu, Haemophilus influenzae; S. aureus, Staphylococcus aureus; B. cepacia, Burkholderia cepacia.

[a] Dosages given are starting doses; dosages are adjusted based in serum levels as follows: Tobramycin peak = 8–12 µg/mL, trough <2 µg/mL; amikacin peak, 25–30 µg/mL; trough <5 µg/mL.

[b] Not approved for patients <18 years of age.

doses. Aminoglycoside dosages are adjusted according to peak and trough levels. Tobramycin is the preferred aminoglycoside because of better penetration of the drug into the airway. Optimal peak serum levels of tobramycin are in the range of 8–12 µg/mL, with trough levels maintained < 2 µg/mL to minimize toxicity.

Factors other than susceptibility testing may have a bearing on the choice of antimicrobial agent in a given patient. For example, aminoglycosides may be avoided in a patient with a history of toxicity to this class of drugs. Patients with a severe penicillin allergy may be more safely treated with a fluoroquinolone or aztreonam as an alternative to desensitization. Agents such as ceftazidime or aztreonam, which are optimally administered every 8 h, may more readily facilitate home IV therapy than agents that require more frequent (e.g., q4–6h) dosing.

A commonly encountered clinical dilemma is the patient with a multidrug or pan-resistant organism. One option in this scenario is to send the isolate to a reference lab for synergy testing. This may reveal combinations of drugs with particular activity against an organism that shows no sensitivity to individual agents. Even if these results are not available, patients will often show in vivo response (albeit slow) to combinations of high doses of antimicrobial agents.

Patients with *B. cepacia* require special attention and treatment. Infection or colonization with this organism is associated with a more rapid decline in pulmonary function and higher mortality. It has been well established that *B. cepacia* is spread by patient-to-patient contact. It is therefore recommended that patients colonized with *B. cepacia* be physically separated from noncolonized patients during hospitalization, in the outpatient clinic, and any other areas where the two groups may come into contact (for example, physical therapy, educational/support groups, etc.). Hospitalized patients are usually admitted to a private room to minimize transmission of organisms of different susceptibilities between patients and for the protection of non-CF patients, especially those who may be immunocompromised.

Antimicrobial treatment of *B. cepacia* also presents unique problems as this organism tends to be resistant to many of the commonly used antibiotics and is sometimes found to be resistant to all antibiotics tested individually in vitro. Even in this setting, combinations of high doses of antibiotics given over a prolonged course (21–28 days) will often result in clinical improvement. Commonly used agents in this scenario include ceftazidime, trimethoprim/sulfamethoxazole, chloramphenicol, and tobramycin. *Stenotrophomonas maltophilia* is another organism commonly found to be multiresistant; doxycycline and some of the newer quinolones have been found to have activity against some strains of this organism.

Chronic Suppressive Oral Antibiotics

The practice of chronic administration of oral antibiotics to suppress airway infection is common. This practice differs from antibiotic administration during an exacerbation in that the patient is at or near baseline with respect to symptoms and pulmonary function. The usual practice is to rotate two antibiotics of different classes at 2-week intervals on an indefinite basis, with periodic changes made individually. The choice of antibiotics is often empiric and not necessarily guided by culture-proven susceptibility. The agents used are the same ones listed in Table 1.

This practice, though commonplace, is controversial and suffers from a lack of objective data to support its efficacy. Disadvantages include the added cost of therapy, side effects of the antibiotics themselves, and the paucity of available oral antibiotics with effective antipseudomonal activity. Some of the oral flouroquinolones have very good antipseudomonal activity, but the relatively rapid emergence of resistance has made these drugs a poor choice for prophylactic use.

Inhaled Antibiotics

The administration of inhaled antibiotics is an old idea that has recently become common practice in the CF population. It offers the advantage of allowing administration of high doses of drug directly to the lower airways while minimizing systemic side effects that would otherwise be dose-limiting.

The agents most commonly used in the United States and for which there is the greatest supporting data are the aminoglycosides, especially tobramycin. Aerosolized tobramycin in high doses (600 mg three times daily) was shown in a multicenter, placebo-controlled study to result in a significant improvement in pulmonary function and a decreased sputum density of *P. aeruginosa* as compared with placebo.* Most importantly, the well-known side effects of ototoxicity and nephrotoxicity were not seen, and inhaled tobramycin did not appear to hasten the emergence of resistant organisms.

Administration of such high doses of tobramycin has several disadvantages, including high cost and prolonged administration time. Practical delivery of these doses requires the use of a high-output ultrasonic nebulizer. Use of lower doses or less frequent administration is commonplace, though there are less data to support this. In a stable patient, many clinicians initiate therapy with doses ranging from 80–400 mg two or three times daily. The dosage can be gradually increased as tolerated to achieve the desired effect.

As of this writing there is no tobramycin solution specifically formulated for inhalation. The most cost-effective approach is to administer preservative-containing injectable tobramycin solution, but this is associated with bronchospastic airway reactions in a minority of subjects. At initiation of inhaled tobramycin therapy, we administer the first dose under direct observation in our outpatient clinic. The few subjects who develop bronchospasm can then be promptly treated with an inhaled bronchodilator and switched to the more expensive preservative-free solution.

A new tobramycin solution specifically formulated for inhalation has recently completed clinical trials. Preliminary results from a large multicenter trial showed that inhalation of 300 mg of this preparation twice daily resulted in a 12% improvement in FEV_1 compared to placebo. FDA approval of this promising new agent is expected within the year.

There are few data on the use of inhaled antibiotics in the setting of an acute exacerbation. Mild exacerbations can be treated with inhaled tobramycin, often in conjunction with an oral antibiotic. More severe exacerbations should be treated with intravenous antibiotics, as outlined above.

Other antibiotics are sometimes administered as aerosols, but with much less information to support their efficacy. These include colistin sulfate, ceftazidime, and gentamicin.

---

* Ramsey BW, Dorkin HL, Eisenberg JD, et al. Efficacy of aerosolized tobramycin in patients with cystic fibrosis. N Engl J Med 1993; 328:1740–1746.

CHEST PHYSIOTHERAPY AND
MUCOCILIARY CLEARANCE

Maneuvers that promote clearance of mucus are routinely employed in patients with CF. The "gold standard" has been manual chest percussion with postural drainage. This is usually performed two to four times daily, often preceded by aerosol inhalation therapy and followed by vigorous coughing. During childhood, this is usually performed on a regular basis by a parent. For many patients, compliance tends to wane during adolescence and adulthood for a variety of reasons: it is time-consuming, boring, sometimes painful, and usually requires the assistance of another person.

A variety of other techniques have been shown to be efficacious in promoting clearance of mucus while overcoming some of the problems associated with traditional chest physiotherapy. The force expiratory technique (FET) consists of a series of forced expirations through an open glottis ("huffs") at different lung volumes to gradually move secretions from distal to more central airways, with final expectoration facilitated by a cough. Autogenic drainage is another technique that utilizes controlled breathing at a variety of lung volumes to promote gradual clearance of mucus. The "active cycle of breathing" technique uses a combination of controlled breathing, forced expiration, and thoracic expansion to promote mucus clearance. All require teaching and practice and all have an associated learning curve; but once mastered, all can be performed independently.

Several devices are also available to assist with mucus clearance, either alone or in combination with the techniques outlined above. The flutter is a hand-held device consisting of a hard plastic shell, slightly larger than a metered-dose inhaler, that encloses a movable metal ball. Exhalation through this device causes the ball to oscillate, sending vibratory waveforms down the tracheobronchial tree and thereby loosening secretions. Advantages include simplicity, low cost, portability, and lack of need for an assistant. One small study showed that the flutter resulted in expectoration of more than three times the amount of mucus as compared with either traditional chest percussion with postural drainage or vigorous voluntary coughing.*

High-frequency chest compression consists of delivery of oscillating compressions to the chest wall via an inflatable vest, creating forceful expiratory airflow that mimics cough. Another device used in conjunction with manual airway clearance techniques is the positive-expiratory-pressure (PEP) mask. This device is placed over the mouth and delivers 10–20 cm of water pressure to the airways to prevent airway collapse during expiratory clearance maneuvers. In general, data on the efficacy of these two devices are limited and they suffer the disadvantages of high cost and cumbersome size.

There is some evidence that physical exercise may promote mucus clearance, though clear evidence of efficacy comparable to that of the above techniques has not been established. Exercise offers several additional advantages, including increased exercise tolerance, improved cardiopulmonary fitness, and an improved sense of well-being. There is strong evidence that diminished exercise tolerance is associated with higher mortality in the CF population. Whether improving exercise tolerance with a regular regimen of aerobic exercise improves prognosis remains to be determined.

Regular aerobic exercise is advised to all patients who are able and willing to partici-

---

* Konstan MW, Stern RC, Doershuk CF. Efficacy of the flutter device for airway mucus clearance in patients with cystic fibrosis. J Pediatr 1994; 124:689–693.

pate. Patients with advanced lung disease should first be evaluated for the presence of exercise-induced oxygen desaturation. This can be accomplished by a formal exercise study or by performing at least the first few sessions in a supervised setting where oximetry monitoring is available. Exercise conditioning programs are best initiated while the patient is in a stable state. Careful attention should be paid to the patient's weight and nutritional status and replenishment of the excess calories expended during exercise sessions.

BRONCHODILATORS AND AEROSOLS

The regular inhalation of beta-agonist and/or anticholinergic bronchodilators is common in patients with CF. Airway hyperreactivity, as determined by bronchoprovacation testing, is more common in CF patients than in the general population. This may be related to airway inflammation and infection, as suggested by the finding that bronchodilator response tends to increase during pulmonary exacerbations. For those with clearly demonstrable airway hyperreactivity, inhaled bronchodilators are administered three to four times daily. These agents may be combined with inhaled tobramycin by patients who are taking both aerosols. Short-acting beta agonists (e.g., albuterol) are the most commonly used agents, in doses similar to those used in other obstructive lung diseases. Atropine derivatives (e.g., ipratropium bromide) and long-acting beta agonists (salmeterol) are less commonly used but appear to be efficacious. Salmeterol may be particularly useful for patients in whom wheezing is chronic and nocturnal symptoms are troublesome.

The use of inhaled bronchodilators in patients without demonstrable airway hyperreactivity or a significant response to bronchodilators on pulmonary function testing is more controversial. In this setting, these agents may still provide benefit by inducing cough and perhaps improving mucociliary clearance. It is because of these last two properties that inhaled beta agonists are often administered just prior to chest physiotherapy. Inhaled bronchodilators should be avoided in the small minority of patients who demonstrate a clear worsening of lung function after inhalation.

Cromolyn sodium and nedocromil, inhaled agents with anti-inflammatory properties, are sometimes used in atopic CF patients with reactive airways disease. Small studies have not demonstrated clear efficacy for these agents in the CF population as a whole, but select individuals may benefit from a therapeutic trial.

Oral bronchodilators are rarely indicated in the older CF population. Oral formulations of beta agonists have a much higher incidence of systemic side effects than their inhaled counterparts and are primarily used in very young children who are unable to use inhaled agents. Likewise, theophylline is a weak bronchodilator with an unfavorable risk: benefit profile that adds little additional bronchodilation when used in conjunction with inhaled agents. Other disadvantages of theophylline include variable GI absorption in the setting of pancreatic insufficiency and possible interactions with other drugs that interfere with its metabolism. It is usually reserved for those patients with clear-cut reactive airways disease uncontrolled by inhaled bronchodilators.

MUCOLYTICS AND DNase

The exceptionally thick, viscous mucus that is characteristic of CF lung disease prompted decades of search for effective mucolytics. One of the earlier mucolytics examined was

N-acetylcysteine, which was felt to thin mucus by cleavage of disulfide bonds in airway mucus. This agent has fallen into disuse, however, because of unproven efficacy, adverse reactions (especially bronchospasm), and the availability of more effective agents.

Most of the viscosity of purulent sputum is due to the polymerization of large quantities of DNA released from dead and dying inflammatory cells within the airways. Deoxyribonuclease (DNase) is a naturally occurring enzyme capable of cleaving this high-molecular-weight DNA; if administered to the airway, it could theoretically thin mucus and facilitate expectoration. This was first attempted with bovine DNase in the 1960s. Though found to be effective, it was abandoned owing to adverse respiratory reactions felt to be due to allergy to the foreign enzyme.

Interest in DNase was revived with the isolation and cloning of the human DNase gene, leading to the production of large quantities of recombinant human DNase (rhDNase). A large randomized, placebo-controlled study in over 900 CF patients showed that inhalation of rhDNase resulted in a significant improvement in pulmonary function and a reduced frequency of pulmonary exacerbations requiring parenteral antibiotics compared to placebo.* The recommended dosage for most patients is 2.5 mg once daily via nebulizer, though some patients with more advanced disease appear to benefit from twice-daily administration. Because pulmonary function rapidly falls to baseline when the drug is stopped, continued daily dosing is required for sustained benefit. DNase is generally well tolerated, with a mild pharyngitis and a self-limited alteration in voice being the most common adverse effects.

Common practice is to use rhDNase in patients with moderate or severe lung disease or mild lung disease with significant respiratory symptoms or sputum production. Patients should be given a trial period to determine if they demonstrate either subjective or objective improvement. The optimal duration of a therapeutic "trial" is unknown. Even patients who show no pulmonary function improvement initially may benefit if they experience a reduction in pulmonary exacerbations. Thus a trial of up to 6 months may be necessary to fully assess efficacy. Use of this agent may be limited in some patients by the cost involved.

Gelsolin is an investigational agent that has been shown to decrease the viscosity of CF sputum in vitro. It is a protein that is thought to work by cleaving polymerized actin filaments released into the sputum from airway leukocytes. Because actin appears to have an inhibitory effect on the activity of DNase in vitro, gelsolin and DNase may act synergistically to reduce sputum viscosity. Further studies are necessary to determine if these promising findings will translate into improved mucus clearance in vivo.

ANTI-INFLAMMATORY THERAPIES

The rationale for anti-inflammatory therapy in CF derives from the fact that much of the lung destruction in CF is a result of the host's inflammatory response to endobronchial infection. Neutrophils recruited to the airway release cytokines, oxygen free radicals, and a variety of proteases. These neutrophil products may directly cause local airway destruc-

---

* Fuchs HJ, Borowitz DS, Christiansen DH, Morris EM, Nash ML, Ramsey BW, Rosenstein BJ, Smith AL, Wohl ME. Effect of aerosolized recombinant human DNase on exacerbations of respiratory symptoms and on pulmonary function in patients with cystic fibrosis. N Engl J Med 1994; 331:637–642.

tion or contribute to lung injury by increasing mucus secretion, interfering with antibody and complement-mediated phagocytosis of *P. aeruginosa*, and acting as chemoattractants that perpetuate the inflammatory cycle. Therapies that limit or control the inflammatory response with the goal of preserving lung function have recently been investigated.

The broad anti-inflammatory properties of corticosteroids make this class of agents an intuitively attractive therapy. Most of the studies available on the utility of corticosteroids in CF have been performed on the pediatric population. One study on 45 children of ages 1–12 years with mild to moderate lung disease randomized patients to prednisone (2 mg/kg on alternating days) versus placebo for over 4 years.* The prednisone group was found to have better pulmonary function, fewer hospitalizations, and lower serum IgG levels than the placebo group. No short-term adverse events were reported, but long-term follow-up revealed a higher incidence of growth retardation in the prednisone-treated group.

A larger study on 285 patients ages 6–14 years compared two different doses of prednisone over a 4-year study period.[†] Patients were randomized to receive high-dose prednisone (2 mg/kg), low-dose prednisone (1 mg/kg), or placebo on alternate days. The high-dose arm of the study was terminated early because of a high incidence of adverse effects including glucose intolerance, cataracts, and growth retardation. The low-dose prednisone group was found to have a small but significant improvement in pulmonary function as compared with the placebo group at the end of the 4-year study period. However, the low-dose prednisone group was found to have growth retardation beginning at about 24 months into therapy. Any beneficial effects of long-term systemic corticosteroids must therefore be weighed against concomitant adverse effects in children. There are no good data on the use of long-term corticosteroids in CF lung disease in adults. Given the beneficial effects that have been demonstrated in children, however, short courses administered during an acute exacerbation or for periods of 6 months or less may be beneficial in select cases. In such cases, close monitoring to detect early evidence of corticosteroid-related side effects is recommended.

Only recently has information become available on the use of inhaled corticosteroids in CF. A crossover study on 12 CF patients with documented bronchial hyperresponsiveness showed that inhaled budesonide (1600 µg/day) improved cough, dyspnea, and bronchial hyperresponsiveness, though there was no significant change in spirometry.[‡] A separate study using inhaled beclomethasone in 26 patients with CF over 4 months showed no significant change in pulmonary function or sputum inflammatory markers.[§] The results of larger controlled studies are necessary to determine if inhaled corticosteroids are effica-

---

* Auerbach HS, Kirkpatrick JA, Williams M, Colten HR. Alternate-day prednisone reduces morbidity and improves pulmonary function in cystic fibrosis. Lancet 1985; 2:686–688.

† Eigen H, Rosenstein BJ, Fitzsimmons S, Schidlow DV. A multicenter study of alternate-day prednisone therapy in patients with cystic fibrosis. J Pediatr 1995; 126:515–523.

‡ Van Haren EHJ, Lammers JWJ, Festen J, Heijerman HGM, Groot CAR, van Herwaarden CLA. The effects of the inhaled corticosteroid budesonide on lung function and bronchial hyperresponsiveness in adult patients with cystic fibrosis. Respir Med 1995; 89:209–214.

§ Schiotz PO, Jorgensen M, Flensborg EW, Faero O, Husby S, Hoiby N, Jacobsen SV, Nielsen H, Svehag SE. Chronic *Pseudomonas aeruginosa* lung infection in cystic fibrosis. A longitudinal study of immune complex activity and inflammatory response in sputum sol-phase of cystic fibrosis patients with chronic *Pseudomonas aeruginosa* lung infections: influence of local steroid treatment. Acta Paediatr Scand 1983; 72:283–287.

cious in the general CF population. At this time it seems reasonable to recommend these agents for patients that clearly have bronchial hyperreactivity.

Nonsteriodal anti-inflammatory drugs have also demonstrated activity that may ameliorate airway inflammation in CF. Ibuprofen in high doses has been shown to inhibit neutrophil migration, adherence, and the release of lysosomal enzymes. A randomized placebo-controlled study in 85 CF patients with mild lung disease showed that ibuprofen-treated patients had a significantly slower rate of decline in pulmonary function, body weight, and chest radiographic abnormalities at the end of the 4-year study period.* The study was performed on both adults and children ≥5 years of age but the majority of the beneficial effects were seen in the 5- to 13-year age group. The group of patients aged 13–39 years demonstrated no significant change in pulmonary function. There was no significant difference in overall or gastrointestinal side effects between the ibuprofen and placebo groups, though two patients in the ibuprofen group withdrew, one due to epistaxsis and the other due to conjunctivitis.

Ibuprofen thus appears to be a therapeutic option for CF patients 5–13 years of age with mild lung disease. In this group, ibuprofen is effective, with a superior side-effect profile as compared with systemic corticosteroids. The recommended starting dose is 20–30 mg/kg/day in two divided doses. Monitoring and adjustment of dosage as necessary to maintain plasma levels between 50–100 μg/mL is strongly recommended, as levels less than this may paradoxically result in increased lung inflammation. Ibuprofen therapy in patients above 13 years of age cannot be recommended at this time.

LUNG TRANSPLANTATION

For those CF patients who progress to end-stage lung disease, the option of lung transplantation should be considered and discussed with the patient and his or her family. Since the first lung transplant was attempted in a CF patient in 1984, surgical techniques, perioperative care, and patient selection have improved to where CF is now the third leading indication for lung transplant worldwide. For those patients who survive the initial surgical hospitalization, there is a marked improvement in pulmonary function, functional capacity, and lifestyle. Survival is also improved in these patients: though there is intercenter variation, overall 1-year survival is about 70%, and 3-year survival is in the range of 50–70%.

Lung transplantation, however, is far from a panacea for the CF patient. A major problem is the scarcity of donor organs relative to the number of patients who need them. Many patients will die while on the transplant list, and waiting periods greater than 18 months are not unusual. Patients require lifelong immunosuppression after transplant with drugs that may pose particular problems in CF patients. Chronic corticosteroid therapy may aggravate preexisting diabetes mellitus or osteopenia. Cyclosporine pharmacokinetics are altered in the CF patient, making attainment of therapeutic serum levels more difficult. Most patients require higher-than-normal cyclosporine dosages, which may aggravate the economic burden on the patient. Chronic immunosuppression places the patient at continued risk for bacterial and opportunistic infection. Acute rejection can usually be controlled,

---

* Konstan MW, Byard PJ, Hoppel CL, Davis PB. Effect of high-dose ibuprofen in patients with cystic fibrosis. N Engl J Med 1995; 332:848–854.

but the risk of chronic rejection in the form of bronchiolitis obliterans increases steadily with time after transplantation and is much more difficult to reverse or control.

Not all patients will be candidates for lung transplantation. As the demand/supply ratio of donor organs continues to worsen, patient selection criteria have become more stringent. Patients with advanced liver disease, malnutrition, and debility (often defined as an inability to perform rehabilitative exercise) are often excluded. Many patients with *B. cepacia* or other multiresistant organisms are excluded, as these patients have been shown to have a higher posttransplant morbidity and mortality. Prior thoracic surgical procedures resulting in pleural adhesions and scarring make transplantation more difficult or prolonged, but this is not usually a contraindication to transplantation. Invasive mechanical ventilation in and of itself does not prohibit transplant in most centers, but the debility, deconditioning, and other complications of prolonged mechanical ventilation often do.

The optimal timing for referral of an individual patient can be difficult to judge. The significant risk of transplantation must be weighed against the potential for a prolonged wait for available donor organs; at the end of the waiting period, the patient must still be in sufficiently good condition to withstand the significant rigors of this major surgical procedure. Probably the best guideline for timing of referral derives from a retrospective study undertaken in 673 CF patients to determine which variables best predict 2-year mortality.* An FEV_1 of less than 30% predicted was the single best predictor of 2-year survival and is currently the most commonly used guideline determining timing for transplant referral. A P_{O_2} less than 55 torr and a P_{CO_2} greater than 50 torr are less significant predictors of 2-year mortality. For a given lung function, female patients and patients less than 18 years of age have a higher mortality rate than the population as a whole. Earlier referral for these patients should be considered.

COMPLICATIONS

CF patients are at risk for a number of pulmonary complications resulting from their underlying lung disease. These may occur singularly, repeatedly, or never in a given individual. When they do occur, however, prompt and appropriate intervention can be lifesaving.

Pneumothorax

Pneumothorax occurs when a subpleural bleb ruptures through the visceral pleura. The frequency of pneumothorax rises with increasing age and severity of lung disease; 5–8% of all patients and greater than 18% of all adult patients experience a pneumothorax at least once. The initial diagnostic and therapeutic approach to the patient is similar to that of other patients with a spontaneous pneumothorax. Abrupt onset of pain, dyspnea, and tachypnea are the usual presenting symptoms. The chest radiograph establishes the diagnosis and rules out other causes for the symptoms. All patients, even if asymptomatic, should be admitted to the hospital.

A large (>20%) or symptomatic pneumothorax should be treated with chest-tube

---

* Kerem E, Reisman J, Corey M, Canny GJ, Levison H. Prediction of mortality in patients with cystic fibrosis. N Engl J Med 1992; 326:1187–1191.

thoracostomy. In the past, because spontaneous pneumothorax in CF has been associated with an increased mortality and a single episode is associated with a high (>50%) recurrence rate, some have advocated an aggressive approach to treatment, including early chemical pleurodesis or surgery. However, with the possibility of future lung transplantation, which is a real prospect for many patients, a more conservative approach is now usually employed, because pleurodesis results in more technically difficult surgery at the time of transplantation. Most transplant centers will still list such a patient, but in some instances a prior pleurodesis may result in exclusion from transplantation.

After a first episode of pneumothorax, if the pneumothorax resolves and the air leak ceases, the chest tube is simply withdrawn and no other therapy is administered. If an air leak persists for more than 5–7 days, surgical pleurodesis will likely be necessary. Chemical pleurodesis is employed in appropriate patients who are poor surgical candidates or refuse surgery. Recurrent ipsilateral pneumothorax after a first episode is best treated with early surgical intervention.

Hemoptysis

Hemoptysis in CF is categorized into minor and major hemoptysis. Minor hemoptysis, usually blood-streaked sputum, is common, may be indicative of an infectious exacerbation, and is often an indication for more aggressive antimicrobial therapy. Occasional, intermittent blood streaking in a patient with no other signs or symptoms and stable pulmonary function may require no change in therapy.

Major hemoptysis is less frequent but may be life-threatening. Defined by the Cystic Fibrosis Foundation Registry as greater than 240 mL of hemoptysis in 24 h or the need for a blood transfusion, major hemoptysis occurs in 1.0% of patients per year. The incidence of major hemoptysis increases with age. In 1995, 81% of the reported instances of major hemoptysis occurred in patients ≥18 years of age. Major bleeding places the patient at risk for respiratory compromise, asphyxiation, and anemia. An aggressive approach is thus warranted.

Patients with major hemoptysis should be admitted to the hospital, sputum cultures obtained, and IV antibiotics begun. A chest radiograph may help localize the site of bleeding if a new focal infiltrate is present. Coagulation studies should be obtained; if these are abnormal, attempts at correction should be initiated. Any medications that may contribute to impaired coagulation, such as aspirin or NSAIDs, should be discontinued. Many clinicians believe that continued percussive chest physiotherapy may aggravate the bleeding and recommend a temporary discontinuation of these measures. Blood transfusions should be considered for those patients in whom a significant anemia develops.

Most episodes of major hemoptysis occur in association with an infectious pulmonary exacerbation and resolve with conservative antibiotic treatment and the measures outlined above. Patients with hemoptysis that continues after the above measures are initiated will require more invasive interventions. For most patients, bronchial artery emobilization is the initial procedure of choice. Most major bleeds in CF arise from very dilated, tortuous bronchial arteries that can be readily visualized by angiography. In this setting, embolization of all large tortuous vessels is performed. Successful embolization results in abrupt cessation of bleeding. Recurrent bleeding is not uncommon and may be treated with repeat emobilization.

Bronchoscopy is not routinely employed in the setting of major hemoptysis, especially if the bleeding ceases after antibiotic administration or bronchial artery embolization. The main utility of bronchoscopy is to localize the site of bleeding in a patient who rebleeds after an initial embolization or if surgery is being considered. Bronchoscopy will be helpful only if the patient is actively bleeding and the rate of bleeding does not obscure visualization of the lower airway. Rarely, bronchoscopy may be used as a therapeutic measure in patients with severe, life-threatening bleeds. Such measures include endobronchial balloon tamponade and topical therapy with thrombin or vasocontrictors. In the setting of ongoing major bleeding, rigid bronchoscopy may be preferable to flexible bronchoscopy.

Despite its efficacy, bronchial artery embolization is associated with a number of severe, even catastrophic complications. Chief among these are spinal cord infarction and paralysis, which may occur in the 5% of patients who have spinal arteries rising from the bronchial vascular tree. Other, less commonly reported complications, include embolic infarction of other organs (e.g., stroke, ischemic colitis), increased bleeding from collateral vessels, and death. Because of the hazards involved, the procedure should be performed by experienced operators. If an experienced interventional radiologist is not readily available, the patient should be transferred to an institution where this service is available.

Major bleeding usually occurs in the setting of advanced lung disease. In order to preserve lung function to the greatest extent possible, surgical lung resection is considered a therapy of last resort. Rare instances occur where all lesser measures have failed and surgery becomes the only option for control of bleeding. In this setting it is essential that the site of bleeding be localized and the patient have adequate pulmonary reserve to allow independent respiration after surgery.

Respiratory Failure

Respiratory failure will ultimately occur in the majority of CF patients unless lung transplantation takes place. Initially, patients will usually develop hypoxemic respiratory failure, defined as a P_{O_2} less than or equal to 55 torr. With disease progression, most patients will also develop hypercapnic respiratory failure. The initial and most fundamental approach to the patient with early respiratory failure is intensification of standard medical therapy as outlined previously in this chapter. This may include IV antibiotics, increased frequency of chest physiotherapy and aerosol administration, nutritional supplementation, and possibly administration of anti-inflammatory agents (e.g., corticosteroids). The latter may be particularly useful in the subset of patients with reactive airways disease and bronchospasm.

In hypoxemic patients, if the above measures do not result in adequate improvement in hypoxemia, chronic supplemental oxygen therapy is initiated. There are very few data on the use of chronic oxygen supplementation specifically for CF. Most of the information regarding efficacy, indications, and guidelines for use are extrapolated from the population with chronic obstructive pulmonary disease (COPD). For COPD patients with a $P_{O_2} \leq$ to 55 torr, chronic oxygen therapy has been shown to limit or reverse pulmonary hypertension, improve neuropsychological functioning, and decrease dyspnea. Oxygen delivery should be adjusted to the lowest level that will produce a P_{O_2} greater than 60 torr. Monitoring of P_{CO_2} and pH levels will be necessary in hypercapnic patients who are administered oxygen.

Some patients may develop significant oxygen desaturation while sleeping and/or while exercising despite adequate daytime resting oxygenation. It is recommended that these patients receive supplemental oxygen during these times because of the risk of progressive pulmonary hypertension and cor pulmonale.

The treatment of hypercapnic respiratory failure in patients who have not responded to intensified medical therapy is more problematic. Augmentation of CO_2 elimination requires mechanically assisted ventilation. The options include invasive positive-pressure ventilation via endotracheal tube, noninvasive ventilation via nasal mask (positive pressure), or negative-pressure ventilation. Negative-pressure ventilation is rarely, if ever, used in CF because of the potential for induction of obstructive apneas and interference with chest physiotherapy.

The "gold standard" for assisted ventilation is positive-pressure ventilation via an endotracheal tube. The decision to proceed with this option depends in large part on the clinical circumstances at the time severe respiratory failure occurs. The patients who will benefit the most are those who have an identifiable, acute, reversible cause of respiratory failure. Such entities include pneumothorax, hemoptysis, acute bronchospasm, acute pneumonia, and respiratory failure in the setting of clearly suboptimal medical therapy, especially if previous lung function can be identified as better than "end-stage." In this setting, the precipitating process should be corrected and mechanical ventilation discontinued as quickly as possible. While a patient is on mechanical ventilation, mucociliary clearance maneuvers, nutritional supplementation, and physical therapy should be vigilantly administered.

In general, patients whose respiratory status has deteriorated to end stage despite aggressive medical therapy and who have no obvious reversible precipitating insult do not benefit from invasive mechanical ventilation. These patients rarely are successfully weaned off the ventilator, and if they are, survival is usually short term. Frank discussion with the patient and family is advised about the limited benefits of mechanical ventilation as the patient is approaching end-stage lung disease.

An exception to the above recommendation may apply to the terminal patient who has accrued substantial time on a transplant waiting list. Some transplant centers will consider transplantation of mechanically ventilated patients provided that they have not progressed to an advanced stage of debility. Practices and recommendations in this setting will vary regionally and should be discussed with the transplant center on a case-by-case basis.

There is an increasing volume of data regarding the utility of noninvasive positive-pressure ventilation via nasal or face mask in cystic fibrosis. This procedure benefits primarily the hypercapnic patient by assisting carbon dioxide elimination and may provide partial "rest" for weak or fatigued respiratory muscles. Assisted ventilation may be applied continuously, with brief periods of removal for chest physiotherapy and cough; more optimally, it may provide part-time ventilatory assistance with nocturnal use. This technique is often applied to patients awaiting transplant as a "bridge" until donor organs become available.

SUMMARY

CF is a complex disease whose pathophysiological basis mystified clinicians and researchers for decades since its initial description in the 1930s. The ensuing years, and in particular the last decade, have seen a tremendous growth in our knowledge and understanding of the pathology underlying this deadly disease. The knowledge is paying off—the life expectancy of CF patients has increased dramatically and continues to improve. Given the dedication and coordinated efforts of the entire CF community, it is anticipated that this progress will continue.

Despite these advances, many pieces of the CF puzzle are still missing. One key question that is the subject of intense investigation is how and why the basic defect in epithelial ion transport predisposes to airway infection. Delineation of this pathological step may suggest therapies not yet anticipated. As therapies improve and patients live longer, new problems may be encountered, either secondary to CF and its treatment or simply due to aging.

This chapter outlines a comprehensive approach to the care of lung disease in the older CF patient. Continued refinements in antibiotics, nutritional support, and mucociliary clearance—coupled with ongoing development of new therapies—holds promise for improving the length and quality of life of CF patients for the foreseeable future. The ultimate goal—a cure for CF—was not even a realistic dream only 10 years ago. Now the potential for a cure in the form of gene therapy is tangible, though still possibly a long way off. Preserving our patients' health and function to the greatest extent possible until a cure becomes a reality should be every clinician's aim.

SUGGESTED READING

1. Clinical Practice Guidelines for Cystic Fibrosis. Cystic Fibrosis Foundation, Bethesda, Maryland, 1997.
2. Cystic Fibrosis Foundation, Patient Registry 1995. Annual Data Report, Bethesda, Maryland, August 1996.
3. Davis PB, Drumm Mitchell, Konstan MW. State of the art: cystic fibrosis. Am J Respir Crit Care Med 1996; 154:1229–1256.
4. Rosenfeld MA, Collins FS. Gene therapy for cystic fibrosis. Chest 1996; 109:241–252.
5. Ramsey BW. Management of pulmonary disease in patients with cystic fibrosis. N Engl J Med 1996; 335:179–188.
6. Schidlow DV, Taussig LM, Knowles MR. Cystic Fibrosis Foundation Consensus Conference Report on Pulmonary Complications of Cystic Fibrosis, Pediatr Pulmonal 1993; 15:187–198.
7. Kotloff RM, Zuckerman JB. Lung transplantation for cystic fibrosis: special considerations. Chest 1996; 109:787–798.
8. Ramsey BW, Dorkin HL, Eisenberg, Gibson RL, Harwood IR, Kravitz KM, Schidlow DV, Wilmott RW, Astley SJ, McBurney M, Wentz K, Smith AL. Efficacy of aerosolized tobramycin in patients with cystic fibrosis. N Engl J Med 1993; 328:1740–1746.
9. Fuchs HJ, Borowitz DS, Christiansen DH, Morris EM, Nash ML, Ramsey BW, Rosenstein BJ, Smith AL, Wohl ME. Effect of aerosolized recombinant human DNase on exacerbations of respiratory symptoms and on pulmonary function in patients with cystic fibrosis. N Engl J Med 1994; 331:637–642.
10. Eigen H, Rosenstein BJ, Fitzsimmons S, Schidlow DV. A multicenter study of alternate-day prednisone therapy in patients with cystic fibrosis. J Pediatr 1995; 126:515–523.
11. Konstan MW, Byard PJ, Hoppel CL, Davis PB. Effect of high-dose ibuprofen in patients with cystic fibrosis. N Engl J Med 1995; 332:848–854.

35
Tuberculosis

Jeffrey D. Edelman and Milton D. Rossman
University of Pennsylvania
Philadelphia, Pennsylvania

INTRODUCTION

Tuberculosis (TB) is an infection in humans due to either *Mycobacterium tuberculosis* (MTB) or *Mycobacterium bovis*. This disease has afflicted the human population since prehistoric times. In 1882, the tubercle bacillus was first described by Koch. At the turn of the century, TB was the leading cause of death in the United States. The history of tuberculosis in the twentieth century is notable for an initial decline in incidence due to improved living standards and isolation of infected patients, followed by the development of effective medical therapy in the late 1940s. In the mid 1980s, the incidence of TB infection in the United States began to rise after declining nearly 75% over the previous four decades. This rise was attributed to coinfection with HIV, decreased resources for TB control, immigration from high-prevalence countries, and outbreaks of TB in congregative facilities (homeless shelters, correctional facilities, crack houses, hospitals, nursing homes, and residential facilities for AIDS patients). Coupled with the rise in incidence of TB has been the emergence of multiple drug-resistant strains. The recent resurgence of TB in the mid-1980s led to increased efforts aimed at prevention of transmission, early diagnosis, and effective therapy, resulting in a gradual decline in TB incidence since 1992. In 1996, there were 21,337 reported TB cases in the United States, reflecting nearly a 20% decline since 1992 (Fig. 1).

In order to maintain this trend, it is imperative that health care workers be familiar with the clinical manifestations, diagnostic evaluation, prophylaxis, treatment, and prevention of transmission of tuberculosis infection. These topics are all addressed in this chapter.

CLINICAL PRESENTATION OF TUBERCULOSIS

Pathogenesis of Tuberculosis Infection

Primary infection with TB generally occurs through inhalation of organisms suspended in aerosolized droplets 1–5 μm in size. Inhalation of small numbers of viable organisms can establish infection. Once in the lung, organisms are ingested by alveolar macrophages.

613

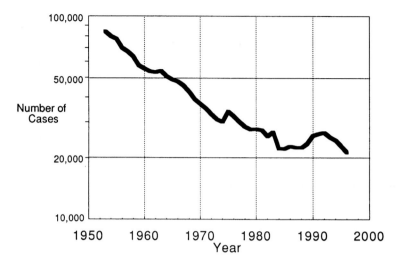

Figure 1   Reported cases of tuberculosis in the United States, 1953–1996.

MTB is able to evade the microbicidal mechanisms of the alveolar macrophages and multiplies slowly within these cells. Specific cell-mediated immunity to MTB develops approximately 4–8 weeks after exposure. During this time, the organisms may disseminate through the lymphatics and the bloodstream. The development of cell-mediated immunity is characterized by granuloma formation with collections of activated T cells and macrophages surrounding MTB bacilli. TB granulomas are loosely organized with central necrosis (caseation). Multinucleated giant cells formed by the fusion of tissue macrophages are present. The combination of primary site of infection within the lung (Ghon focus) and involvement of the regional draining lymph nodes is called the Ranke Complex.

In most individuals, the initial infection is arrested after the development of cell-mediated immunity, although viable bacilli may persist within granulomas at sites of dissemination. Individuals with TB infection without active disease generally have reactive tuberculin skin tests but are not infectious. In this setting, with normal immune function, the risk of developing active tuberculosis is approximately 5% over the first 2 years and 10% over a lifetime.

When cell-mediated immunity fails to contain MTB infection, active disease develops. Manifestations of active TB are characterized as primary, miliary, reactivation, or extrapulmonary. Systemic symptoms of active disease may include fever, night sweats, weakness, fatigue, anorexia, and weight loss. Pulmonary symptoms include cough, hemoptysis, and chest pain. Dyspnea is unusual and usually suggests advanced disease or other underlying lung disease.

Primary Tuberculosis

Historically, primary tuberculosis was considered to be a disease of infancy and childhood. In developed countries, where most adults have not previously been infected, primary TB may occur at any age. Primary TB involves infection at the site of initial inoculation in the lung. The most common radiographic manifestation is an ill-defined homogeneous infiltrate, often in the middle or lower lung zones. As primary TB generally occurs prior to the development of significant cell-mediated immunity, cavitation is usually not present. Hilar or paratracheal adenopathy may occur in the presence or absence of an infiltrate. Approximately 10% of patients may present with a pleural effusion, which results from seeding of the pleura through rupture of a granuloma into the pleural space. These patients present with cough, fever, and pleuritic chest pain. Although TB pleuritis will usually resolve spontaneously, 50% of patients will ultimately develop active pulmonary TB.

Miliary Tuberculosis

Miliary or disseminated TB occurs when large numbers of bacilli spread throughout the bloodstream and establish sites of active disease, resulting in small (approximately 2-mm) granulomatous lesions throughout the body. In general, miliary TB occurs in the setting of inadequate cell-mediated immunity. Risk factors include age below 5 years, malignancy, poor nutritional status, alcoholism, HIV infection, and immunosuppressive therapy.

Reactivation Tuberculosis

Reactivation TB may occur months to years after initial infection. The upper lung zones, particularly the apical and posterior segments of the upper lobes or the superior segment of the lower lobes, are most frequently involved. Although hematogenous dissemination of organisms at the time of initial infection is systemic and widespread, these regions of the lung provide a richly oxygenated environment ideal for the growth of TB organisms. Reactivation TB is characterized by inflammation with airspace consolidation. Caseation with granuloma rupture, endobronchial spread, and ongoing tissue destruction leads to radiographic findings of cavitation. Rarely, cavities may rupture into the pleural space producing a TB empyema and associated bronchopleural fistula. Pleural fluid in this setting is loaded with organisms and always requires drainage procedures. In chronic disease, fibrosis and calcification may be present. The radiographic findings of apical fibrosis or calcification may be seen in the setting of active or inactive disease and should therefore never be assumed to represent "inactive TB." In advanced HIV infection, where cell-mediated immunity is severely impaired, caseation and cavitation may not occur.

Extrapulmonary Tuberculosis

At the time of initial infection, hematogenously disseminated organisms can establish foci of asymptomatic infection anywhere in the body. These foci are established preferentially in well-oxygenated, highly vascular areas, most commonly the kidneys, meninges, spine, and growing ends of long bones. Gastric TB may result from the swallowing of infectious sputum. Laryngeal TB, which is highly infectious due to aerosolization of large numbers of organisms, results from direct extension along the tracheobronchial tree. Approximately 15% of people with reactivation may present with extrapulmonary disease.

DIAGNOSIS OF TB INFECTION

Specimen Collection

The "gold standard" for the diagnosis of TB is a positive culture. Freshly expectorated sputum is the best sample to stain and culture for MTB. A minimum of three specimens should be collected on successive days, preferably in the early mornings. The volume of sputum collected should be 5–10 mL. Smaller volumes will reduce the yield of cultures and smears. In patients who are not spontaneously producing sputum, sputum may be induced by the administration of inhaled hypertonic saline solution.

When sputum is unobtainable, samples for culture may be obtained via gastric aspiration early in the morning after instillation of 20–50 mL of sterile distilled water. Laryngeal swabbing may also provide specimens for stain and culture. Bronchoscopy can be used to obtain brushings, washings, and biopsy specimens for stains and culture. As washings obtained during bronchoscopy lead to dilution of the organisms present in airway and alveolar secretions, direct examination of this fluid for organisms has a lower yield in comparison to that for expectorated sputum. Given the significant exposure risks associated with bronchoscopy in the setting of active TB, it is advisable to attempt to obtain and evaluate adequate sputum samples before proceeding to bronchoscopy. If TB infection is suspected, biopsy specimens should be sent for both mycobacterial culture and histological examination. Postbronchoscopy sputum should also be sent for culture and staining.

In the setting of TB pleuritis, pleural fluid is almost always exudative, with elevated protein and lactate dehydrogenase and low or normal glucose. Large numbers of lymphocytes are usually present, although a predominance of neutrophils may occur in acute presentations. Mesothelial cells are rarely present. Direct staining of pleural fluid almost never reveals organisms, and culture is positive in only 25% of cases. Pleural biopsy is required for diagnosis and may be performed "blindly" using a Cope or Abrams needle or under visualization by pleuroscopy or video thoracoscopy. When multiple (three or more) samples are obtained and sent for both histological examination and culture, a diagnosis of TB may be made in approximately 90% of cases.

Organisms may also be cultured from samples obtained from extrapulmonary sites of infection, including urine, cerebrospinal fluid, synovial fluid, or bone marrow. Consultation with the mycobacterial laboratory to ensure proper collection and handling of these specimens should be considered prior to obtaining samples.

Laboratory Diagnosis

Smear examination (usually by Ziehl-Nielson or direct auramine staining) provides a means for rapidly detecting acid-fast bacilli (AFB) in a clinical specimen. AFB smears are not very sensitive and are not specific for MTB. A positive smear generally implies that organisms are present at a concentration greater than or equal to 10,000/mL of specimen. Therefore, patients with positive sputum smears are generally highly infectious. However, 50% of patients with active pulmonary TB diagnosed by culture may have negative smears. Although a positive smear or high clinical suspicion may be sufficient for initiation of medical therapy, ongoing treatment should be based upon culture and sensitivity results.

Conventional culture techniques using Lowenstein-Jensen medium or Middlebrook agar generally require 4–8 weeks. The BACTEC system for radiometric detection of mycobacteria allows for detection in 1–2 weeks. Both conventional and radiometric techniques permit sensitivity testing. The use of nucleic acid probes can shorten the time for identification of MTB once growth is detected by culture. The commercially available AccuProbe system is based upon hybridization of known labeled DNA with ribosomal RNA in the cultured organisms. This test is nearly 100% sensitive and specific for MTB.

Direct amplification techniques for rapid detection of MTB have recently become available. These tests are based upon amplification of mycobacterial DNA by polymerase chain reaction (PCR) or amplification of ribosomal RNA. The exact role of these tests in the clinical mycobacteriology laboratory and in directing therapeutic decisions has not yet been established. However, these tests may be useful in determining whether a positive AFB smear is due to nontuberculous *Mycobacterium*.

TUBERCULIN SKIN TESTING AND PROPHYLAXIS

Tuberculin skin testing uses a standardized purified protein derivative (PPD) from MTB. Two forms of tuberculin testing are used in the United States. The Mantoux test involves the intracutaneous injection of 0.1 mL (5 tuberculin units) of PPD into the volar surface of the forearm. The multiple puncture test (MPT) uses a multipronged applicator to introduce PPD into the skin. Although the MPT is easier to administer, the results of this test may be less reliable. Tuberculin skin tests should be read after 48–72 h by persons proficient in measuring responses. Patients should not be permitted to read their own skin-test results. Results should be reported as millimeters of induration and not as positive or negative.

Reactivity to PPD generally occurs within 2–10 weeks after primary infection and persists for years but may wane with advancing age. Reactivity to PPD is neither sensitive nor specific for MTB. Up to 10% of patients with active disease may be nonreactive to PPD. Patients with HIV infection, poor nutritional status, or other superimposed chronic or acute medical illness may exhibit anergy. When anergy is suspected, PPD testing should be performed in conjunction with testing to at least two other antigens (usually tetanus toxoid, mumps, or *Candida*). Contrary to common belief, PPD reactivity does not vary significantly during pregnancy. False reactivity may occur in patients infected with nontuberculous mycobacteria or in patients who have received vaccination with bacille Calmette-Guérin (BCG). In general, reactivity due to BCG vaccination is unlikely to persist for more than 10 years after vaccination.

A booster response may be observed in patients who have experienced waning sensitivity to PPD after remote exposure to TB or BCG vaccination. If these patients receive serial testing, an initial test may fail to demonstrate reactivity but may increase the memory response to a subsequent test. This may be falsely interpreted as representing recent infection. To rule out booster responses in serially screened adult populations (such as health care workers), a two-step approach should be considered, with repeat testing of all initial nonresponders several weeks after the initial test (booster testing).

The size of reaction that defines a ''positive'' test depends upon the age, immunological status, and TB exposure history of the individuals being tested. In the setting of HIV infection, fibrotic changes on chest radiographs, or close contact with known infectious individuals, a reaction of greater than or equal to 5 mm is considered positive. For other at-risk adults and children, a reaction of greater than or equal to 10 mm is considered positive. Testing is not indicated for individuals without risk factors for TB infection. If testing is performed in this setting, however, a reaction of greater than or equal to 15 mm is considered to be positive. In certain instances, prophylaxis may also be considered in patients without a significant PPD response. Specific indications for prophylaxis are outlined in Table 1. All patients being considered for prophylactic therapy should have a chest radiograph to screen for evidence of active disease.

Isoniazid (INH) treatment for 6–12 months is effective in reducing the risk of future TB in individuals with positive PPD reactivity. Standard INH dosage is 300 mg/day for

Table 1 Indications for Prophylaxis Based on PPD Reactivity and Risk Factors

<5 mm	≥5 mm	≥10 mm	Patients without risk factors
1. Children who are recent close contacts of infectious TB cases 2. Anergic HIV-infected adults 3. HIV-infected recent close contacts of infectious TB cases	1. Close contacts of sputum-positive cases 2. HIV-infected persons 3. IV drug users of unknown HIV status 4. Fibrotic changes on chest x-ray	Age under 35: 1. Foreign-born from high-prevalence countries 2. Long-term-care facility residents (i.e., correctional institution or nursing home residents) 3. Medically underserved, high-prevalence populations 4. Infants and children <4 years of age All ages: 1. Risks for HIV infection with unknown HIV status 2. HIV-negative IV drug users 3. Health care workers or mycobacteriology lab workers 4. Other medical conditions (diabetes, steroid or other immunosuppressive drug treatment, silicosis, conditions associated with rapid weight loss or chronic malnutrition, end-stage renal disease, hematological and reticuloendothelial malignancies)	Age under 35: 1. Consider treatment if reactivity ≥15 mm 2. Recent converters: ≥10 mm increase within 2 years Age 35 and over: 1. Recent converters: ≥15 mm increase within 2 years

adults and 10–15 mg/kg/day up to a maximum of 300 mg for children. For most adults, 6 months of treatment is felt to represent adequate therapy; 9 months of prophylaxis is recommended for children. Children with PPD reactivity less than 5 mm who have had close contact with infectious individuals within 3 months are candidates for INH prophylaxis until repeat PPD testing is performed 12 weeks after their last contact. Adults and children with HIV infection and other conditions associated with immunosuppression should be treated for 12 months. Patients with silicosis or fibrotic lesions suggesting prior TB infection and no evidence of active disease should receive either 4 months of combined therapy of INH plus rifampin or 12 months of INH provided that drug-resistant infection is felt to be unlikely. In the setting of pregnancy, preventive therapy is generally delayed until after delivery unless recent infection is suspected or high-risk medical conditions such as HIV infection are present.

Persons presumed to be infected with INH-resistant organisms should be treated with rifampin in place of INH. Some clinicians advocate adding a second drug (such as ethambutol) to which the organism is believed to be sensitive in this setting. If infection with multidrug-resistant organisms is likely, observation without preventive therapy is usually recommended. In high-risk patients (i.e., HIV-infected), 6 months of ethambutol plus pyrazinamide (PZA) may be considered. If resistance to ethambutol is also likely, a quinolone may be substituted for ethambutol in this regimen.

The relative risks of developing TB must be weighed against the risks of INH therapy. All patients should be monitored for both compliance with therapy and adverse effects. Patients should be informed to notify their health care provider immediately for prompt evaluation if they experience symptoms suggestive of INH toxicity (anorexia, nausea, vomiting, dark urine, icterus, rash, paresthesias, persistent fatigue, weakness, abdominal tenderness, or fever of greater than 3 days duration). Factors associated with increased risk of INH-induced hepatitis include advancing age, daily alcohol use, chronic liver disease, injection drug use, and concurrent therapy with medications with additional risks of hepatotoxicity. Postpubertal black and Hispanic women may also be at increased risk. In the absence of risk factors for INH toxicity, patients under 35 years of age should be evaluated monthly for signs and symptoms of toxicity. Patients over age 35 and those with other risk factors for INH toxicity should have hepatic enzymes measured prior to starting therapy and then monthly throughout treatment in addition to monthly clinical evaluation. INH should be discontinued if liver enzymes rise above three times normal values. Fatalities associated with INH-induced hepatitis are rare and are usually associated with continued administration of INH after the onset of drug-induced hepatitis. INH therapy also carries a risk of peripheral neuropathy through interference with pyridoxine metabolism. Although this is an uncommon side effect, patients with conditions associated with increased risk for neuropathy (diabetes, uremia, alcoholism, and malnutrition) as well as persons with seizure disorders and pregnant women should receive pyridoxine with INH. INH may also interfere with metabolism of certain drugs. Concurrent use with phenytoin leads to elevation of the levels of both INH and phenytoin, necessitating close monitoring of phenytoin levels and dosage adjustment.

TREATMENT OF ACTIVE TUBERCULOSIS

Successful treatment of active TB is based upon the use of multiple drugs to which the organism is susceptible, compliance with drug therapy, and sufficient duration of therapy. Prior to initiation of therapy, adequate specimens for culture and sensitivity should be obtained. Patients with active TB or suspected active TB should be reported to the local department of public health. Promoting and monitoring compliance is essential and consideration should be given to treating all patients with directly observed therapy (DOT). Dosages and side effects of commonly used first-line agents are shown in Table 2. Discussion of therapy in this section is limited to first-line agents. Additional drugs of potential use in the treatment of TB are shown in Table 3.

Therapy for Uncomplicated Tuberculosis

The current minimal acceptable treatment duration for culture-positive adults and children is 6 months. Acceptable drug regimens are shown in Table 4. If the resistance rate in the

Table 2 Dosages and Toxicities of First-Line Antituberculosis Agents

Drug	Daily dosage, mg/kg (max) Children	Adults	2 × weekly dosage, mg/kg (max) Children	Adults	3 × weekly dosage, mg/kg (max) Children	Adults	Common toxicities and side effects
Isoniazid	10–20 (300 mg)	5 (300 mg)	20–40 (900 mg)	15 (900 mg)	20–40 (900 mg)	15 (900 mg)	Hepatitis, peripheral neuritis, hypersensitivity
Rifampin	10–20 (600 mg)	10 (600 mg)	10–20 (600 mg)	10 (600 mg)	10–20 (600 mg)	10 (600 mg)	Hepatitis, GI upset, orange coloration of urine and secretions
Pyrazinamide	15–30 (2000 mg)	15–30 (2000 mg)	50–70 (4000 mg)	50–70 (4000 mg)	50–70 (3000 mg)	50–70 (3000 mg)	Hyperuricemia, hepatitis
Ethambutol	15–25	15–25	50	50	25–30	25–30	Optic neuritis
Streptomycin	20–40 (1000 mg)	15 (1000 mg)	25–30 (1500 mg)	25–30 (1500 mg)	25–30 (1500 mg)	25–30 (1500 mg)	Eighth-nerve damage, nephrotoxicity

Table 3 Additional Agents with Documented or Potential Activity Against *Mycobacterium tuberculosis*

Drugs in current use as second-line agents for treatment of MTB	Drugs with potential activity against MTB
Para-aminosalicylic acid	Amikacin
Ethionamide	Ofloxacin
Cycloserine	Ciprofloxacin
Capreomycin	Clofazamine
Kanamycin	Rifambutin
Thiacetazone	Amoxicillin + clavulanic acid

community is known to be less than 4% and the patient has no prior history of treatment with anti-TB drugs, is not from a country with a high rate of drug resistance, and has no known exposure to a drug-resistant case, a three-drug regimen may be used. This consists of INH, rifampin, and PZA for the first 2 months, followed by an additional 4 months of INH and rifampin. If a potential for drug resistance exists, ethambutol or streptomycin should be added to the initial regimen until sensitivities are known. Ethambutol cannot be used in young children where visual assessment is not possible. Nine-month regimens using only INH and rifampin are also effective in adults and children when organisms are known to be fully drug-susceptible. Treatment for less than 6 months for culture-positive TB is generally not recommended. However, in adults with uncomplicated sputum culture–negative pulmonary TB, treatment may be shortened to 4 months.

Table 4 Preferred Regimens for Initial Treatment of Adults and Children

Option 1	Option 2	Option 3
Daily isoniazid, rifampin, and pyrazinamide for 8 weeks followed by 16 weeks of isoniazid and rifampin daily or 2–3 times/week.[a] In areas where the isoniazid resistance is not documented to be less than 4%, ethambutol or streptomycin should be added to the initial regimen until susceptibility to isoniazid and rifampin is demonstrated. Consult a TB medical expert if the patient is symptomatic or smear- or culture-positive after 3 months.	Daily isoniazid, rifampin, pyrazinamide, and streptomycin or ethambutol for 2 weeks followed by 2-times-per-week[a] administration of the same drugs for 6 weeks, and subsequently, with 2-times-per-week administration of isoniazid and rifampin for 16 weeks. Consult a TB medical expert if the patient is symptomatic or smear- or culture-positive after 3 months.	3 times/wk[a] treatment with isoniazid, rifampin, pyrazinamide, and ethambutol or streptomycin for 6 months. Consult a TB medical expert if the patient is symptomatic or smear- or culture-positive after 3 months.

[a] All regimens administered 2 or 3 times per week should be monitored by directly observed therapy.

Monitoring for Adverse Drug Reactions

Patients should be monitored for adverse reactions related to antituberculous therapy and they should be instructed to watch for the common symptoms associated with adverse reactions to their specific medications. Frequent medical follow-up (monthly at least) is required. Baseline studies for all adults should include hepatic enzymes, bilirubin, creatinine, and complete blood count with platelet count. Serum uric acid measurement should be obtained if PZA is used. If ethambutol is used, baseline measurement of visual acuity and red-green color perception is necessary. When baseline studies are normal and no risk factors for toxicity exist, routine laboratory monitoring is not required. Additional testing may be necessary, however, to evaluate signs and symptoms of drug toxicity.

Response to Therapy

Patients receiving treatment should have monthly sputum examinations until negative smears and cultures (sputum conversion) are documented. Most patients treated with adequate regimens containing both INH and rifampin will have negative sputum cultures after 2 months of treatment. These patients should have at least one more sputum smear and culture performed at the completion of therapy. A follow-up chest x-ray should also be obtained at completion of therapy.

Persistent positive smears or cultures after 2 months of therapy mandate reevaluation with repeat susceptibility testing and the institution of DOT. Drug regimens should not be altered unless resistance is documented. If drug resistance is noted, therapy should be modified to include at least two new drugs to which the organism is sensitive.

Patients with negative pretreatment sputum who receive treatment because of radiographic findings suggestive of TB should be followed with serial chest x-rays and clinical evaluation. The failure of these findings to improve after 3 months of therapy suggests that they may be due to either inactive disease or an alternative process. In this setting, if the PPD is reactive and other diagnoses have been excluded, therapy may be discontinued after 4 months.

Special Considerations

Extrapulmonary TB

Regimens of 6 to 9 months may be effective in treating extrapulmonary TB. However, because of insufficient data, 12-month therapy is recommended in the setting of miliary TB, bone/joint TB, and TB meningitis. The use of adjunctive corticosteroid therapy should be considered in tuberculous pericarditis to prevent constrictive pericarditis and in TB meningitis to prevent neurological sequelae.

Pregnancy and Lactation

Active TB during pregnancy requires treatment. The risk of untreated disease to the mother and fetus far outweighs the risk of therapy. Initial therapy should consist of INH and rifampin. Ethambutol should also be used unless INH resistance is unlikely. Although these drugs do cross the placenta, teratogenic effects have not been demonstrated. Although routine use of PZA has been recommended by international TB organizations, teratogenicity data for this drug are inadequate and therefore recommendations for routine use in the United States cannot be made. Streptomycin should not be used in pregnancy because it interferes with development of the ear and may cause congenital deafness. The presence of small concentrations of antituberculous drugs in breast milk does not pose a contraindication to breast feeding and has no therapeutic effects in treatment of nursing infants.

HIV Infection

Treatment regimens for TB in the setting of concurrent HIV infection do not require significant modification. However, these patients must be closely monitored for toxicity and compliance. Therapy should be continued for at least 9 months and for 6 months after sputum conversion. Monitoring of drug levels may be necessary in HIV patients with chronic diarrhea where poor drug absorption has been reported as a cause of treatment failure.

Treatment Failure or Relapse

Patients who remain smear- or culture-positive after 5 to 6 months of therapy are considered to have failed treatment. Repeat susceptibility testing must be performed on a recently obtained sputum. Current therapy may be continued until sensitivities are known or may be augmented by the addition of at least three new drugs. The regimen should be adjusted when susceptibility results are known. DOT is required in patients who have failed treatment.

Patients who experience relapse also require repeat susceptibility testing and DOT. If relapse occurs after completion of treatment for sensitive organisms with regimens containing INH and rifampin, organisms often remain susceptible to these agents and treatment often consists of reinstitution of the previous regimen. Patients who relapse after treatment with regimens not containing both INH and rifampin should be assumed to have organisms resistant to the previously used agents and treated with at least two new agents.

Drug-Resistant TB

The frequency of resistance is predominantly a function of the adequacy of tuberculosis treatment programs. Initial drug resistance occurs when patients with no history of previous antimycobacterial therapy become infected with resistant organisms. Secondary resistance occurs in patients who have had previous treatment. Treatment of patients with resistant organisms requires administration of at least two drugs to which there is documented susceptibility. When INH resistance is detected after institution of standard four-drug therapy, INH should be discontinued and PZA continued for the total 6-month duration of therapy.

Organisms that are resistant to both INH and rifampin often exhibit resistance to other first-line agents as well. Detailed sensitivity testing to multiple agents is required. Treatment with three or more drugs to which the organism is sensitive is required and should be continued until the patient is culture-negative, followed by an additional 12 months of therapy with at least two drugs. Surgery may be of significant benefit in patients in whom the bulk of diseased tissue can be resected.

PREVENTION OF TRANSMISSION

Identification of patients with active tuberculosis, isolation from susceptible individuals, and prompt initiation of therapy are required to prevent the transmission of tuberculosis. Failure to recognize active tuberculosis cases can lead to inadvertent exposure of other patients and health care workers. All patients entering a health care facility should be promptly questioned for symptoms of cough at the time of registration. Masks should be placed upon patients with a productive cough of more than 2 weeks duration. These patients should be placed in an isolation room, and anyone entering this room should wear a TB mask. If TB remains a concern after further evaluation, including assessment for additional symptoms suggestive of active TB and risk factors for TB infection, a chest x-ray should be performed.

Hospital admission is not always required for patients with active or suspected tuberculosis. Patients who are not severely ill and can be relied upon to take medications and avoid unexposed persons may be evaluated and treated at home. Patients who are sicker, felt to be potentially unreliable, or whose living situation places others at risk require hospitalization. Inpatient management ensures prompt evaluation and treatment and provides an opportunity to educate patients with reference to the importance of compliance with therapy.

Inpatients suspected of having active TB require isolation until three adequate sputum samples with negative smears have been obtained. Inpatients with active TB require isolation until they are no longer deemed to be contagious. Patients receiving appropriate therapy will usually be noninfectious within 2–3 weeks after treatment is initiated. The decision to discontinue isolation and discharge a patient should be based upon improvement in clinical signs and symptoms with decreasing sputum AFB. Patients with multi-drug-resistant (MDR) TB require isolation until sputum smears are negative.

AFB isolation requires a private, negative-pressure room capable of at least six air exchanges per hour, with exhaust directed to the outside environment. Windows and doors should be kept closed. In clinics and emergency departments, where immediate AFB isolation and effective ventilation may not be feasible, secondary environmental controls such as high efficiency particulate air (HEPA) filtration and ultraviolet lighting should be employed.

The proper mask for worker protection is a subject of ongoing debate. Standard surgical masks may not provide adequate protection. The use of particulate respirators (PR), form-fitting devices worn over the face capable of filtering submicron particles from the air, has been advocated by the Occupational Safety and Health Administration (OSHA) and the Centers for Disease Control (CDC). These agencies presently have different standards for the type of PRs required. The CDC currently recommends the use of a dust-mist respirator, which resembles a cupped surgical mask. OSHA requires a dust-mist fume respirator—a reusable mask that straps behind the head, has a separate exhalation valve, and maintains a tighter seal. Employee fit-testing, training in proper use, and assessment of ability to breathe while wearing this mask are required. In areas of high MDR TB prevalence, OSHA requires the use of powered HEPA-filtered air pressure respirators.

Routine screening of hospital workers is important for identification of newly infected individuals to prevent the development of active TB and transmission to other workers or patients. All employees should be screened at least annually. Workers with PPD reactivity ≥10 mm should receive prophylaxis. Booster testing (described previously) should be considered when screening is initiated.

SUGGESTED READING

1. American Thoracic Society/Centers for Disease Control and Prevention. Treatment of tuberculosis and tuberculosis infection in adults and children. Am J Respir Crit Care Med 1994; 149: 1359–1374.

2. American Thoracic Society. Rapid diagnostic tests for tuberculosis: what is the appropriate use? Am J Respir Crit Care Med 1997; 155:1804–1814.
3. Barnes PF, Barrows SA. Tuberculosis in the 1990s. Ann Intern Med 1993; 119:400–410.
4. Dunlap NE, Briles DE. Immunology of tuberculosis. Med Clin North Am 1993; 77:1235–1248.
5. Heifets L. Mycobacteriology laboratory. Clin Chest Med 1997; 18:35–53.
6. Iseman MD. Treatment of multidrug-resistant tuberculosis. N Engl J Med 1993; 329:784–791.
7. McCray E, Weinbaum CM, Braden CR, Onorato IM. The epidemiology of tuberculosis in the United States. Clin Chest Med 1997; 18:99–113.
8. Rossman MD, MacGregor RR. Tuberculosis: Clinical Management and New Challenges. New York: McGraw-Hill, 1995.

36

Infections Due to Nontuberculous Mycobacteria

Michael D. Iseman

University of Colorado School of Medicine
National Jewish Medical and Research Center
Denver, Colorado

INTRODUCTION

''Nontuberculous'' mycobacteria (NTM) include species of the genus *Mycobacterium* that are associated with human infection and disease (excluding *Mycobacterium tuberculosis*, *Mycobacterium bovis*, and *Mycobacterium leprae*). Semantically, this terminology may not be wholly accurate, since these mycobacteria do produce ''tuberculous'' lesions. However, the usage NTM has gained preference over the more accurate reference, mycobacteria other than tuberculosis (MOTT), and is used herein to refer to these organisms.

The NTM are variably distributed in nature. Hence, their presence in nonsterile spaces or tissues of the human body means that they *may* be there as colonizing or saprophytic microorganisms. Hence, when we refer to *disease*, we are talking about cases in which there are not only significant numbers of mycobacteria in the tissues but where the tissues are sufficiently inflamed or damaged to be characterized as diseased.

VARIOUS FORMS OF PULMONARY DISEASE

The NTM can involve human lung tissue in both a primary invasive capacity and as a secondary invader of previously damaged or abnormal lung parenchyma. These illnesses may present as a tuberculosis-like disease with rapidly progressive symptoms and extensive fibronodular infiltration with typical cavitation, most often in the upper lung zones. Such cases are usually not clinically subtle or diagnostically elusive. Most of such cases involve males with underlying lung disorders such as chronic obstructive pulmonary disease (COPD) or inorganic dust pneumoconioses. More problematic are the less dramatic presentations, such as the nodular bronchiectatic variety of disease. Over the past decade, there has been increasing recognition that a substantial portion if not the majority of NTM pulmonary disease cases represent the latter variation. In these cases the illness primarily manifests itself as a coughing and spitting disorder rather than the dramatic wasting or consumptive features of the TB-like illness. Epidemiologically, NTM pulmonary disease

627

of this variety appears to be substantially more frequent among women than men. Notably, these persons typically do not suffer from the classic underlying disorders noted above and, over the past two decades, the NTM seem to be involving younger individuals, not infrequently those in their fourth and fifth decades. Curiously, particularly among women with *Mycobacterium avium* complex (MAC) or rapid-growing mycobacterial infections, certain body features are commonly seen: slender/asthenic habitus, mild thoracic scoliosis, narrowed anteroposterior chest (AP) dimensions with or without pectus excavatum, and mitral valve prolapse; these are found in variable combination in many such patients. In other cases, the NTM appear to secondarily invade regions of bronchiectasis caused by other disorders. Specific causes of preexisting bronchiectasis include prior histoplasmosis, cystic fibrosis, and alpha₁ antitrypsin deficiency. However, in many instances, the NTM actually are the primary causes of the bronchiectasis and nodular disease. Figures 1 and 2 represent typical examples of these varieties of NTM disease.

Two major clinical issues are apparent regarding the NTM. First, when should clinicians obtain mycobacterial cultures for patients with lung disease? And second, when does a positive mycobacterial culture indicate disease versus benign "colonization"?

Regarding the former, mycobacterial smears and cultures should be obtained whenever typical radiographic, clinical, and epidemiological findings suggest the probability of either TB or NTM disease (see above). Also, such specimens should be sent whenever patients are manifesting cryptogenic pulmonary disease—e.g., cough, sputum, and/or radiographic abnormalities—that has evaded "routine" diagnostic efforts. The NTM have been reported in causal association with a wide array of lung disorders ranging from

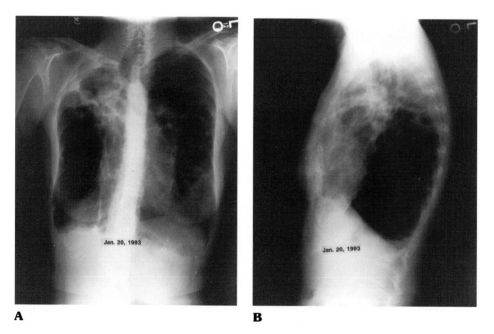

A   **B**

Figure 1 A and B. This 60-year-old woman with cigarette-induced COPD had intensely destructive cavitary disease mainly involving the right upper lobe; it was associated with volume loss and a rightward shift of the trachea. Scattered nodular disease is seen on the left. Increased AP diameter, reduced lung markings, and low, flat diaphragms are manifestations of COPD.

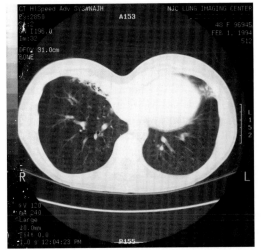
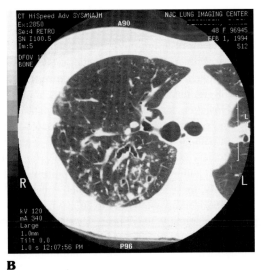

A

B

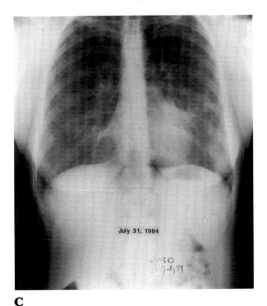

C

Figure 2 A. A thoracic computed tomographic scan of a 48-year-old woman with MAC lung disease. Notable are dense areas of saccular bronchiectasis and atelectasis involving the medial segment of the right middle lobe and the inferior segment of the lingula. Also visible is the pectus excavatum with the deep depression of the sternum displacing the heart into the left thorax. Related to this anomaly, the patient also had mitral valve prolapse, straight-back syndrome, and slender habitus; scoliosis was *not* present. B. A computed tomographic scan of a 40-year-old woman with MAC lung disease. Classical varicoid bronchiectasis is noted in the superior segment of the right lower lobe; multiple nodular shadows are also seen in this segment. This pattern is typical of NTM disease, particularly in women; in our experience, both MAC and RGM are associated with these features. C. A posteroanterior chest radiograph of a 60-year-old woman with MAC lung disease. The findings in plain chest x-rays are typically nondescript and unimpressive. The right heart border is partially effaced and there is a vague shadow in the lower zone of the right lung; the left heart border is also obscured with stellate shadowing extending into the lung. Computed tomographic scans confirmed bronchiectasis and atelectasis of the right middle lobe and lingula.

necrotizing pneumonias to bronchiectasis to hypersensitivity pneumonitis or bronchiolitis obliterans with/without organizing pneumonia; hence, clinicians should have a low threshold for ordering these tests. The debate over whether NTM recovered reflect true ''disease'' or merely ''saprophytic'' states has been sustained for decades. Because the NTM (unlike TB) are organisms found in the environment, including common water sources, an argument can be made that their presence in respiratory specimens is coincidental. However, for the more commonly pathogenic species—such as MAC and *M. kansasii* or the rapid growers, such as *M. abscessus*, *M. chelonae*, or *M. fortuitum*—the likelihood of pathogenicity is quite high in the settings described above. A 1990 American Thoracic Society guideline paper described criteria for disease that were arguably inappropriately strict and limited. By requiring multiple isolations in substantial numbers and smear positivity, these conditions excluded substantial numbers of patients with early, minimal disease, leading potentially to delayed and missed diagnoses and dilatory or missed treatment. More suitably, the revised 1997 American Thoracic Society guidelines recognize that *most* patients with symptoms and radiographic signs such as those noted above *are* infected with the NTM. The issues, which may be subtle, are *which* of these patients needs chemotherapy and *when*.

For those with rapidly progressive or debilitating manifestations, the decision is easy. However, for patients with minimal findings or those without spontaneously volunteered symptoms or signs—whose evaluation may have been prompted by incidental findings—the question of therapy is problematic. Possible strategies might include serial observations for progression or a therapeutic trial in which the patient and clinician collaborate to determine whether a 2- or 3-month course of multidrug treatment results in clinical and radiographic improvements sufficient to justify the side effects of therapy. If the former strategy—observation—is employed, it is vital to realize that NTM disease may advance very slowly and that absence of change over even 3–6 months may not signify the absence of invasive disease. Since some of the NTM cases experience intermittent or stuttering activity spaced out over the course of years, optimal practice might entail interval observations supplemented by admonitions to seek attention promptly in the presence of any extended symptoms.

DIAGNOSIS OF PULMONARY NTM INFECTION

The NTM all share the feature common to mycobacteria: ''acid-fast'' staining. Because of their lipid-rich cell walls, they typically reject Gram's stain reagents, appearing as neutral or ''ghost'' forms. If stained by Gram's reagents, they are positive. In many laboratories, microscopic screening for mycobacteria is performed with the fluorochrome system, a faster, more sensitive technique. If positive organisms are seen, they are confirmed with the older method, either Ziehl-Neelsen or Kenyoun. Mycobacteria cannot be speciated by morphology under the microscope.

Mycobacteria, again probably owing to their complex, lipid-rich walls, grow significantly more slowly than usual bacterial pathogens and generally require specialized media to support their growth. Most pathogenic mycobacteria require 2.5–6 weeks to form grossly visible colonies on solid media. The rapid growers, Runyon's group IV, replicate roughly on order of magnitude more quickly, 3–5 days to form colonies; in some cases, the rapid-growing mycobacteria (RGM) will grow on conventional media. Of note, when recovered from sputum or inflamed tissues, the RGM may not grow well for several weeks.

However, on subculture in the laboratory, their rapid growth is manifest. Currently the preferred method to isolate pathogenic mycobacteria from sputum, tissue, or body fluids is a liquid medium such as Middlebrook 7H-12 broth. Such media appear more sensitive than solid media and offer more rapid species identification. However, solid medium is typically employed to back up the liquid medium.

Various molecular biological techniques are employed to reduce the time required for species identification. Employing the liquid medium radiometric system (Bactec), evidence of mycobacterial growth may appear within 3–10 days of inoculation. When log-phase growth is seen, aliquots may be probed to identify the species. Current kits allow early identification of *M. tuberculosis* complex, *M. avium* complex, *M. intracellulare*, *M. avium*, *M. kansasii*, and *M. gordonae*. If the organisms are from another species, slower conventional techniques must be employed. Direct probes to identify NTM species in sputum or other tissues are not available.

Serological or skin tests are not currently available to help identify persons infected with the NTM. While it is statistically true that persons with NTM infections tend to have low level or indeterminate reactions to PPD-T, the *M. tuberculosis* antigen, this test is so lacking in sensitivity and specificity as to make it virtually worthless for individual patients in this setting.

Most community and regional laboratories are capable of doing routine microscopy and primary isolation of mycobacteria. However, better and more timely results are generally obtained when specimens are sent to specialized laboratories such as those at the National Jewish Medical and Research Center in Denver, those in the Texas State Research Facility in Tyler, Texas, the Mayo Clinic in Rochester, or large national commercial laboratories.

In vitro susceptibility testing is a contentious issue for the NTM. For *M. kansasii*, there is a fairly well-established relationship between in vitro susceptibility and response to treatment. For MAC, such a relationship is less easily discerned but appears to be the most intelligent means available to guide therapy. And for the RGM in vitro susceptibility is a generally satisfactory means of choosing antibiotics, although discordant results between different laboratories are often seen.

PRINCIPLES OF TREATMENT

In vitro susceptibility testing is an integral part of selecting drug agents for these infections. Although the relationship between in vitro susceptibility and response to therapy is not as straightforward as it is in TB, the limited evidence available as well as recent experience indicate that careful, quantitative in vitro susceptibility testing is an appropriate guideline in choosing drugs.

The basic pharmacological principles of antimicrobial therapy should, intuitively, be applicable in NTM disease. At the simplest level, this means that the maximum achievable serum level of any drug should substantially exceed the minimal inhibitory concentration established in vitro. This relationship does not necessarily mean that the drug will be effective, but the converse—failure to achieve inhibition or killing at achievable serum concentration—is quite likely to predict lack of efficacy. In addition, dosing intervals should be established in relation to growth rates of bacilli. Thus, dosing schedules less frequent than commonly employed for conventional pathogenic bacteria appear to be appropriate.

Table 1 Suggested Medical Regimens for Common NTM Pulmonary Disease

	Regimen	Alternative Agents	Comments
Group I *M. kansasii*	Rifampin (RIF) Ethambutol (EMB) Isoniazid (INH) [Amikacin][a] (AK)	Clarithromycin (CLARI) Ciprofloxacin (CIP) Trimethoprim/sulfamethoxazole (TMP/SMX)	Usual duration: 12–18 months. AK may be used initial 2–4 months for more extensive disease.
Group III *M. avium* complex (MAC)	Clarithromycin (CLARI) Ethambutol (EMB) Amikacin (AK) Clofazimine (CFZ)	Azithromycin (AZI) Rifabutin (RBT)[b] Rifampin (RIF)[b] Ciprofloxacin (CIP) Cycloserine (CSN)	Usual duration: 18–24 months.[b] The rifamycins lower the bioavailability of CLARI, RIF more so than RBT. May omit them or adjust dose of CLARI upward.
Group IV *M. abscessus*	Cefoxitin (CEF) Amikacin (AK)	Clarithromycin (CLARI) Minocycline (MINO) Imipenem (IMI)	Usual duration: 6–12 weeks, palliative course. Most strains are resistant to oral meds; Rx is rarely curative.
M. chelonae	Clarithromycin (CLARI) Amikacin (AK) [Cefoxitin][b] (CEF)	Tobramycin (TOB) Imipenem (IMI) Doxycycline (DOXY) Ciprofloxacin (CIP)	Usual duration: 6–12 weeks for palliation. The use of cefoxitin for *M. chelonae* infections is debated.[b]
M. fortuitum	Amikacin (AK) Ciprofloxacin (CIP) Clarithromycin (CLARI)	Sulfamethoxasole (SMX) Imipenem (IMI) Doxycycline (DOXY)	Usual duration: 4–6 months, attempting cure.

[a] The use of AK or other injectable agents is not necessary in most *M. kansasii* cases.
[b] Wallace's laboratory in Texas regards resistance to CEF as a distinguishing feature of *M. chelonae*; but at National Jewish, the great majority of strains we identify as *M. chelonae* are susceptible.

Combination therapy to prevent acquired drug resistance is an essential component of the treatment of TB and should almost certainly be applied to the NTM as well. Single drugs, no matter how efficacious, are subject to selection of drug-resistant variants, leading to clinical resistance to the individual agent. The principle that drug A kills bacilli resistant to drug B and drug B kills bacilli resistant to drug A mandates that in virtually all cases, multiple drugs be used for active disease. Suggested regimens (Table 1) and individual agents employed for groups I, II, and III (Table 2) and group IV (Table 3) are delineated in tabular form.

As in the case of TB, treatment must generally be extended well beyond the time of initial bacteriological and clinical improvement. This is necessary to prevent recurrence by eliminating persistent slow-growing or semidormant bacilli, which may reactivate if chemotherapy is prematurely terminated.

ADJUNCTIVE THERAPY

Surgical treatment for the NTM disease may be useful, including resection of localized and refractory pulmonary disease associated with irreversible damage to the airways or lung parenchyma.

Immunological interventions may be appropriate in selected instances. In some cases where NTM disease has evolved due to immunosuppressive therapy given for other disorders, it is desirable to stop or minimize the predisposing immunosuppressive treatments. Despite aggressive drug therapy, cures are seldom achieved if the host's immune system is substantially inhibited.

On the other side of the coin, we may consider positive immunotherapy using selective agents to enhance the host's immune response, particularly in cases where there is either an underlying or acquired defect of cellular immune capacity. Recent studies have documented the efficacy of interferon-γ in selected patients with disseminated NTM disease, many of whom had non-HIV-related abnormalities of T-cell and/or macrophage function; studies are currently under way to determine whether interferon-γ may also be helpful for patients without discernible defects of cellular immunity but refractory pulmonary disease due to NTMs.

COMMON PATHOGENS

Photochromogenic organisms (group I) are bacteria which, when grown in the dark, have cream- or buff-colored colonial pigment; however, after exposure to light, they rapidly become yellow or orange—photochromogenicity. *M. kansasii* is the most common pathogen in this group and is most commonly distributed in the central and south central United States. *M. simiae* is reported in small but apparently increasing numbers, particularly in the southern and southwestern United States.

Scotochromogenic organisms (group II) are bacilli which, whether grown in the light or dark, produce yellow- or orange-pigmented colonies. *M. scrofulaceum* is the prototype of this group and formerly was a common cause of lymphadenitis in children and pulmonary disease in adults. However, for reasons unclear, it has receded as a human pathogen in the United States and now is reported only episodically. *M. gordonae* is a common contaminant of laboratory specimens. However, there have been occasional re-

Table 2 Medications Commonly Employed for Groups I, II, and III Mycobacterial Infections

Medication	Adult Dose Ranges	Common Toxicity or Side Effects[a]	Comments
Rifampin (RIF) Rifabutin (RBT)	600 mg qd (450 if < 50 kg). 300 mg qd (150 if < 50 kg).	Hepatitis, rash, neutropenia, thrombopenia, discolored urine and tears, numerous drug interactions.[a]	Similar spectrum of activities. RIF more potent stimulator of cytochrome P450 enzyme system. RIF > RBT results in lessened levels of clarithromycin. Neutropenia and thrombopenia more common with RBT, but frank thrombopenic purpura reported more with RIF.
Clarithromycin (CLA)	500 mg bid initial; then 500–750 qd in continuation phase	Dysgeusia, anorexia, nausea (occasionally, vomiting), hepatitis, drug interactions.[a]	CLA more active in vitro vs. most NTMs than AZI; issue of whether ↑ level in macrophages and longer half-life results in enhanced activity of AZI is not resolved.
Azithromycin (AZI)	250–500 mg qd initial; then 250 mg qd in continuation.		CLA ≫ AZI inhibits P450, resulting in slowed catabolism of numerous drugs including the rifamycins, theophylline (and warfarin?) and others.[a]
Ethambutol (EMB)	25 mg/kg body weight qd initial; then 15 mg/kg qd	Must reduce dose with renal insufficiency; optic neuritis, peripheral neuritis, rash.	Rifamycins and EMB often act synergistically vs. MAC strains; macrolides and EMB behave in additive fashion.
Ciprofloxacin (CIP)	500 mg PO bid initially; then 500–750 qd continuation.	Gastrointestinal distress, agitation, insomnia, arthralgias, hepatitis.	CIP is more active in vitro vs. NTM than ofloxacin (vice versa with *M. tuberculosis*); role of later fluoroquinolones such as levo-ofloxacin or sparfloxacin not determined.

Amikacin (AK)	12–15 mg/kg ideal body weight IV twice weekly.	High-frequency hearing loss, tinnitus, vestibular dysfunction, renal impairment, rash.	May give IV or IM; peripherally inserted central catheter (PICC) line very useful for prolonged IV access. High-frequency hearing loss usually precedes vestibular dysfunction with AK; measure audiograms. Reduce dose with preexisting or acquired renal impairment. (May administer via nebulization in rare cases.)
Clofazimine (CFZ)	100–200 mg PO qd initially; then reduce to 50 mg qd when pigmentation appears.	Skin-bronzing a predictable side effect; gastrointestinal distress, eosinophilia. (Note tissue half-life is 70–90 days.)	CFZ has not performed well in therapy of disseminated MAC in AIDS patients but appears well tolerated and efficacious in pulmonary MAC. Long half-life makes detection of intolerance difficult—symptoms may persist weeks after drug is held.
Isoniazid (INH)	300–450 mg PO qd initially; then 300 qd	Hepatitis; peripheral neuritis; lupus syndrome; rash.	INH is rarely very active versus NTMs but it may be efficacious in some cases with *M. kansasii, M. Szulgai,* or others.

[a] See the *Physicians' Desk Reference* for comprehensive listing of toxicities/side effects.

Table 3 Medications Commonly Employed for Group IV (RGM) Infections

Medication	Adult Dose Ranges	Common Toxicity or Side Effects	Comments
Amikacin (AK)	12–15 mg/kg ideal body weight IV qd.	High-frequency hearing loss, tinnitus, vestibular dysfunction, renal impairment, rash.	Prefer to give IV; PICC line very useful for access; high-frequency hearing loss usually precedes vestibular dysfunction with AK; measure audiograms. Reduce dose with preexisting or acquired renal dysfunction. (May administer via nebulization in rare cases.)
Cefoxitin (CEFOX)	2 g IV q8–12h.	Rash, diarrhea including *C difficile* colitis, thrombopenia.	Cefoxitin nearly unique for activity vs. RGMs; only cefmetazole shares activity.
Clarithromycin (CLA)	500 mg PO bid.	Dysgeusia, anorexia, nausea, occasionally vomiting, hepatitis, drug interactions.[a] Give with food to ↓ gastrointestinal effects.	Wallace's lab in Texas reports higher probability of in vitro susceptibility to CLA than does Heifets's in Denver; unsure of true utility of this agent in RGM disease.
Doxycycline (DOX) Minocycline (MINO)	100 mg PO bid. 200 mg PO loading dose; then 100 mg PO bid.	GI distress with anorexia, nausea, vomiting, glossitis, and enterocolitis; rash, photosensitization, hypersensitivity reactions, (minocycline given for extended periods may produce gray/slate skin hues).	May be given IV if oral access is problematic. Mino ≫ DOX has vestibular effects. Absorption impaired by antacids or other divalent or trivalent cations.
Imipenem (IMIP) (Primaxin = imipenem and cilastin)	IM = 500–750 mg q12h. IV = 500–1000 mg q8–12h.	Pain with IM injection; therefore give with lidocaine. May cross-react with prior beta-lactam hypersensitivity; CNS effects including confusion, myoclonus or seizures; nausea with IV infusion—try slowing rate.	Limited clinical experience with RGMs; usually not a first-line choice.
Trimethoprim/sulfamethoxazole (TMP/SMX)	1000 mg PO bid; i or ii double-strength bid.	Hypersensitivity including rash, fever, major dermatopathies; bone marrow suppression; hepatitis; gastrointestinal distress.	Most likely to be active vs. *M. fortuitum* or *M. smegmatis*.

[a] See the *Physicians' Desk Reference* for comprehensive listing of toxicities/side effects.

ports of pulmonary disease associated with this microbe. *M. szulgai* is an infrequent pathogen in this group.

Nonchromogenic mycobacteria (group III) are the most significant cluster of NTM producing human disease. Two closely related species, *M. avium* and *M. intracellulare*, have been lumped together taxonomically as *M. avium* complex (MAC). These organisms historically were associated with disease mainly in the southeastern United States. However, over the past quarter-century, MAC cases have been seen in apparently increasing numbers from all of the continental states, Alaska, and Hawaii. Less frequent pathogens of this group include *M. xenopi* and *M. malmoense*.

Currently, MAC is most notorious for producing bacteremic, diffuse, reticuloendothelial system infection in AIDS patients. However, totally independent of this phenomenon, pulmonary disease associated with MAC appears to be increasing in prevalence. Historically it has been most common among males with cigarette-induced COPD, pneumoconioses, or prior inflammatory lung disease including TB. However, more recently the disease has shifted to involve women, often younger, many without overt preexisting lung conditions. In male patients, the disease tends to resemble typical tuberculosis with extensive upper lung zone fibronodular and cavitary disease (see Fig. 1 above). However, among the females, it produces a more subtle clinical and radiographic picture with scattered, lower-lung-zone subpleural nodulation; computed tomography scans typically demonstrate both cylindrical and saccular bronchiectasis, most prominently involving the right middle lobe and lingula but commonly involving other lung zones as well (see Fig. 2 above). Among women patients we have recognized the association of the nodular bronchiectatic disease with an unusual phenotype that variably involves features of pectus excavatum, mitral valve prolapse, subtle thoracic scoliosis, and a slender or asthenic habitus. Other subtle risk factors for pulmonary MAC disease include prior histoplasmosis, cystic fibrosis and alpha$_1$ antitrypsin deficiency status. Of note, HIV infection is not a risk factor for MAC pulmonary disease in either males or females and HIV screening is not indicated unless independent risk factors are identified.

Rapid-growing mycobacteria (group IV) are emerging as a relatively more common form of NTM disease, following MAC and *M. kansasii* in prevalence. *M. abscessus*, formerly designated as a subspecies of *M. chelonae*, is now the commonest rapid-growing mycobacterium (RGM). Other RGMs such as *M. chelonae* and *M. fortuitum* may produce pulmonary infections, but significantly less often than *M. abscessus*. The RGMs have predispositions similar to those of MAC (see above); in addition, RGMs appear to be associated with achalasia in some cases.

The RGMs most frequently are associated with the diffuse, bronchiectasis-nodular form of disease seen with MAC (see above). Occasionally, tuberculosis-like cavitary lung disease is seen with RGMs.

RECOMMENDED MANAGEMENT

Recommended regimens for the common NTM diseases are outlined in Table 1. It should be emphasized that these represent generally uncontrolled experience with use of individual agents or regimens. In most cases, treating individuals with deep, invasive disease entails aggressive long-term management and probably should be conducted by specialists. Resectional surgery may be considered for younger patients with localized cavitary or intensely destructive disease. However, surgery does not replace chemotherapy. Patients must be treated preoperatively to reduce the mycobacterial burden and postoperatively to reduce the likelihood of disruption of the bronchial closure or recrudescence elsewhere in the lungs.

SUGGESTED READING

1. American Thoracic Society. Diagnosis and treatment of disease caused by nontuberculous mycobacteria. Am Rev Respir Dis 1990; 142:940–953.
2. American Thoracic Society. Diagnosis and treatment of disease caused by nontuberculous mycobacteria. Am J Respir Crit Care Med 1997; 156:S1–S25.
3. Brown BA, Wallace RJ Jr, Onyi GO. Activities of clarithromycin against eight slowly growing species of nontuberculous mycobacteria, determined by using a broth microdilution MIC system. Antimicrob Agents Chemother 1992; 36:1987–1990.
4. Falkinham JO. Epidemiology of infection by nontuberculous mycobacteria. Clin Microbiol Rev 1996; 9:177–215.
5. Griffith D, Girard W, Wallace RJ Jr. Clinical features of pulmonary disease caused by rapidly growing mycobacteria: an analysis of 154 patients. Am Rev Respir Dis 1993; 147:1271–1278.
6. Holland S, Eisenstein E, Kuhns D, Turner ML, Fleisher TA, Strober W, Gallin JI. Treatment of refractory disseminated nontuberculous mycobacterial infection with interferon gamma. N Engl J Med 1994; 330:1348–1355.
7. Iseman M. Nontuberculous mycobacterial infections. In: Gorbach S, Bartlett J, Blacklow N, eds. Infectious Diseases, 2d ed. Philadelphia: Saunders, 1992:1246–1256.
8. Iseman M, Buschman D, Ackerson L. Pectus excavatum and scoliosis: thoracic anomalies associated with pulmonary disease due to M. avium complex. Am Rev Respir Dis 1991; 144: 914–916.
9. Lynch D, Simone P, Fox M, Bucher B, Heinig M. CT features of pulmonary Mycobacterium avium complex infection. J Comput Assist Tomogr 1995; 19:353–360.
10. Wallace RJ Jr. Treatment of infections caused by rapidly growing mycobacteria in the era of newer macrolides. Res Microbiol 1996; 147:30–35.
11. Wallace RJ Jr, Brown BA, Griffith DE, Girard W, Tanaka K. Reduced serum levels of clarithromycin in patients treated with multidrug regimens including rifampin or rifabutin for Mycobacterium avium-Mycobacterium intracellulare infection. J Infect Dis 1995; 171:747–750.
12. Wallace RJ, Glassroth J, Griffith DE, Olivier KN, Cook JL, Gordin F. Diagnosis and treatment of disease caused by nontuberculous mycobacteria. Am J Respir Crit Care Med 1997; 156: S1–S25.

37

Chronic Fungal Pulmonary Infections

Scott F. Davies

University of Minnesota Medical School
Hennepin County Medical Center
Minneapolis, Minnesota

INTRODUCTION

Fungal pathogens are rare but important causes of pneumonia. Acute infections can mimic typical and atypical pneumonias caused by other pathogens. Chronic forms of infection can mimic tuberculosis and lung cancer. Involvement of hilar and mediastinal nodes can cause special problems. Consideration of a fungal etiology for a specific illness depends either on specific clinical features of the illness, factors relating to the host, or a progressive course of illness that drives aggressive diagnostic testing. Sometimes a diagnostic test such as a lung biopsy confirms a fungal diagnosis even when it was not the prime consideration. The main focus here is on symptoms and signs that suggest a fungal pulmonary disease, diagnostic approaches likely to be helpful, and basic principles of treatment. Only histoplasmosis, blastomycosis, coccidiodomycosis, and aspergillosis are covered in any detail.

There are two main groups of fungal pneumonias. The first are caused by T-cell opportunists, including the endemic mycoses and cryptococcosis. The infecting particles are respirable spores, either geographically restricted (the endemic mycoses) or, for cryptococcosis, worldwide in distribution. Nonimmune phagocytes (macrophages and neutrophils) cannot kill these spores and normal hosts who inhale them often develop a primary pneumonia. Normal hosts also usually recover uneventfully when specific immunity develops. Patients with T-cell defects, including patients treated with corticosteroids and especially patients with AIDS, are vulnerable to severe and progressive infections. Patients with normal immunity sometimes suffer more from granulomatous response to the infection than from unchecked spread of the fungus. The second group of illnesses is caused by phagocyte opportunists, of which *Aspergillus* species are by far the most common. The infecting particles are respirable spores that are ubiquitous in the environment. Nonimmune phagocytes can kill these spores and normal hosts can inhale them without fear of pulmonary infection. These infections occur in specific settings. When the lung is abnormal structurally [old cavities or even upper lobe changes of chronic obstructive pulmonary disease (COPD)], the fungus can smolder in the poorly defended spaces, causing local problems. When the host is neutropenic or receiving high-dose corticosteroids, the fungus

639

can become invasive in the lung, often in an angioinvasive manner, and can even spread through the blood to distant organs. Distant spread is more common with profound neutropenia than with corticosteroid therapy.

HISTOPLASMOSIS

Primary Histoplasmosis

The endemic area includes much of the central United States, especially the Ohio and Mississippi River valleys, as well as the Champlain and St. Lawrence River valley in the northeast. Primary infections are very common and usually are not diagnosed but rather buried in the vast numbers of nonspecific respiratory tract infections. Many patients are asymptomatic. Most symptomatic patients have a fever and nonproductive cough, sometimes with body aches and headache. Symptoms resolve in a few days and most patient never see a physician or get a chest x-ray. Occasional patients have severe arthragias and/ or erythema nodosum. With these features or with unusually severe respiratory symptoms, the patient is more likely to see a physician and perhaps have a chest radiograph. A focal infiltrate with prominent hilar adenopathy suggests histoplasmosis more than a viral or mycoplasmal infection. A follow-up radiograph showing hardening of the infiltrate into a discrete residual nodule also favors histoplasmosis over competing diagnoses. Some patients with severe respiratory symptoms have a diffuse micronodular infiltrate on the chest radiograph. This results from a high density of inhaled organisms, and these patients, unlike those with focal infiltrates, often describe a specific high-risk exposure approximately 2 weeks before onset of symptoms (the incubation period is quite uniform), including such activities as cleaning or demolishing an attic, barn, or chicken coop; exploring a cellar or a cave; or cutting dead firewood with a chain saw.

Primary histoplasmosis is diagnosed serologically. Unfortunately, the serologies do not turn positive for 2–4 weeks after onset of the illness. By then the patient has usually recovered, lessening the diagnostic imperative. A positive complement fixation (CF) titer of 1:32 or higher or a positive M band by immunodiffusion is diagnostic. Lower CF titers (1:8 or 1:16) also have considerable positive predictive power if the clinical features suggest a strong pretest likelihood of histoplasmosis (e.g., atypical pneumonia with arthralgias or erythema nodosum, patchy infiltrate with hilar adenopathy, or diffuse micronodular infiltrates with appropriate exposure history). Sputum cultures are not very helpful. Rarely, a patient with progressive focal or diffuse infiltrates or with a nonresolving pneumonia will require invasive diagnosis, with the usual escalation of tests, including bronchoscopic lavage and biopsy, fine-needle aspiration for culture and morphology, and even thoracoscopic or traditional open-lung biopsy.

Primary histoplasmosis rarely needs treatment. Rare patients with diffuse infiltrates can have severe hypoxemia—it is prudent ot treat these patients with amphotericin B. Occasional patient with prolonged subacute symptoms (fever, cough, malaise beyond 2–3 weeks) can be treated with itraconazole (200 mg PO for 6 months) but this is seldom necessary.

One possible sequela of pulmonary histoplasmosis (silent or symptomatic) is a pulmonary nodule. The initial infiltrate does not resolve but contracts and hardens into a focal nodule, which is often discovered on a routine chest radiograph years after the primary infection. Although histoplasmal nodules (histoplasmomas) rarely cause problems, they must be distinguished from early cancers. If the nodule has become densely calcified, it can be assumed to be a granuloma and ignored. If by chance there is a radiograph showing size stability for 2 years, the nodule can be followed. If the nodule is noncalcified and of unknown duration, it must be evaluated as a possible malignancy. The interested reader is referred to the discussion regarding this evaluation in Chap. 20.

Chronic Cavitary Histoplasmosis

Chronic cavitary histoplasmosis usually occurs in patients with underlying destructive bullous or cavitary disease, most often severe COPD. The disease mimics tuberculosis. Patients have subacute illness with low-grade fever, chronic, usually productive cough, malaise, weakness, and sometimes weight loss. Fibrocavitary infiltrates usually involve the upper lobes, because that is where the emphysema is most severe. The infection smolders in the abnormal lung and may spread to adjacent areas of lung and even to the pleura. Distant spread is very unusual.

Diagnosis is usually easy once tuberculosis has been excluded and the differential has been expanded to other chronic infections. Serological tests are positive in up to 80% of patients and sputum cultures (of little benefit in acute histoplasmosis) are also positive in the majority of patients. Only rare patients require more invasive tests, including bronchoscopic lavage and biopsy, fine-needle aspiration for culture and morphology, and even thoracoscopic or traditional open-lung biopsy.

Most cases of chronic cavitary histoplasmosis can be treated with itraconazole 200–400 mg day PO for 6 months. Occasional patients need a longer duration of therapy and rare patients who are severely ill or who are intolerant or poorly responsive to itraconazole can be treated with amphotericin B, usually a total cumulative dose of 2 g.

Mediastinal Histoplasmosis

Histoplasmosis often prominently involves draining lymph nodes in the hilum and mediastinum, which become infected and develop granulomatous inflammation as cell-mediated immunity is engaged. The nodes enlarge and often develop necrosis and subsequent calcification. A variety of complications can develop, which are mostly grouped under the diagnoses of mediastinal granuloma and mediastinal fibrosis. In general, mediastinal granuloma involves a large, discrete nodal mass that causes symptoms by compressing adjacent structures, including the trachea or a proximal bronchus (cough), the esophagus (dysphagia), or the superior vena cava (SVC syndrome). A discrete node can erode into an airway, presenting as a broncholith with cough, hemoptysis, or lithoptysis. Mediastinal fibrosis involves a more diffuse scarring process, often comprising but not confined to discrete nodes, that can entrap and obstruct peripheral bronchi, pulmonary arteries, and pulmonary veins. Symptoms include dyspnea, chest pain, and hemoptysis. Patients with isolated pulmonary veno-occlusion sometimes present with patchy infiltratesand hemoptysis. In some cases the hemoptysis occurs with exercise. If mediastinal fibrosis is bilateral, it can progress to pulmonary hypertension, cor pulmonale, and early death.

Mediastinal granuloma and fibrosis are often diagnosed presumptively. A patient in the endemic area who has calcified hilar and mediastinal nodes with a negative tuberculin skin test likely has histoplasmosis. Serologies are often normal or positive in nonspecific low titer. Even tissue biopsies are often negative by culture and have nonspecific histopathology. Computed tomographic scans of the chest usually include the spleen. The presence of focal calcifications in the spleen offers strong evidence that the process in the chest is histoplasmosis and not tuberculosis or other granulomatous process. Other tests besides computed tomography (CT) that are helpful in defining the extent of disease include ventilation/perfusion lung scans and transthoracic and especially transesophageal echocardiograms. Pulmonary angiograms are helpful in some cases.

Treatment is difficult. In general mediastinal granuloma can be removed surgically, but there is little need to do so, since the clinical syndromes are usually self-limiting. Broncholiths can be treated surgically if they cause major symptoms or proximal obstruction with distal collapse or infection. The surgical approach should be planned and executed by a highly experienced surgeon. Mediastinal fibrosis is seldom a surgical illness. Resection of fibrotic mediastinal tissue is seldom possible, rarely helpful, and can lead to complications including death. Proximal vascular obstructions are sometimes bypassed. Hemoptysis due to localized pulmonary venous obstruction can sometimes be cured by resecting the involved lobe or lung. More commonly, hemoptysis is due to abnormal inflammatory vessels supplied by the bronchial arteries. Bronchial artery embolization can control hemoptysis in many cases, but sometimes there are extensive collaterals from intercostal arteries or even the chest wall vessels feeding into the areas of chronic inflammation. In general, the prognosis of mediastinal fibrosis is reasonably good if the disease is on one side and does not involve the subcarinal area. Bilateral disease leading to pulmonary hypertension has a more guarded prognosis.

There is no direct proof of benefit from antifungal therapy or corticosteroids. Empirical therapy with these agents is sometimes given with the thought that treatment of any active infection may reduce the antigen available to trigger immune response. At the same time, contemporaneous therapy with corticosteroids may reduce inflammation and thereby reduce later scarring. No direct evidence supports these therapies. If there is a decision to treat, one reasonable regimen might be itraconazole 200–400 PO/day for 6 months, prednisone 20–30 mg/day for 3–6 weeks, and then a slow taper off over an additional 3–6 weeks.

Histoplasmosis in AIDS

Most patients have systemic febrile illness. The chest radiograph can be normal or diffusely abnormal, mimicking *Pneumocystis carinii* pneumonia (PCP). In this setting, pancytopenia, abnormal liver function tests, and splenomegaly can be clues to the diagnosis of histoplasmosis, but these clinical features are neither sensitive nor specific. Diagnosis is usually easy. Most patients (70 of 72 in one series) have a positive histoplasmal polysaccharide antigen (HPA) in the urine. The high density of organisms ensures that blood cultures, buffy-coat smears of peripheral blood, and bronchoalveolar lavage (BAL) fluid direct stains and cultures are usually positive. Serological testing for antibodies plays no important role. Treatment requires induction and lifetime maintenance to prevent relapse. Amphotericin B should be used for initial therapy if the patient is critically ill, followed by itraconazole 200 mg twice daily for life. More stable patients can be treated with itraconazole from the onset.

BLASTOMYCOSIS

Acute Pulmonary Blastomycosis

Blastomycosis is coendemic with histoplasmosis over most of the central United States, but disease activity extends further northward across northern Wisconsin and northern

Minnesota and into adjacent provinces of Canada. Blastomycosis elicits a mixed pyogenic and granulomatous inflammatory response. Unlike those with histoplasmosis, most patients with acute pneumonia cough up pus, and the illness resembles bacterial pneumonia more than atypical pneumonia.

Some patients with acute blastomycosis have no symptoms or only minimal symptoms of mild cough and low-grade fever. These patients are usually identified only if they acquire the illness as part of a point-source outbreak of illness. Other patients are more toxic, with high fevers, purulent sputum, and chest pain. The chest radiograph shows dense alveolar or even lobar infiltrates, mimicking pneumococcal pneumonia. Pleural effusions are seen in a minority of cases; intrathoracic adenopathy is uncommon. In some cases the infiltrate is multifocal with some nodular areas, a picture unusual for bacterial pneumonia. With or without antibacterial therapy, the patient can remain ill for several weeks, often with systemic features including malaise and weight loss. The severity and chronicity of the process and the lack of response to antibacterial therapy leads to a broader differential diagnosis and an escalation of diagnostic tests. Some patients start to disseminate and develop skin lesions and/or bony lesions in the context of a pyogenic bacterial process; this raises suspicion of blastomycosis. Some patients with acute blastomycosis present with a picture of infectious acute respiratory distress syndrome (ARDS) with diffuse infiltrates and severe hypoxemia. Others present with lobar or multilobar pneumonia but progress to diffuse infiltrates. Patients with edematous lobar pneumonia with bulging fissures may be especially toxic and at higher risk of progression to diffuse infiltrates and respiratory failure.

In this condition, as opposed to histoplasmosis, serological tests are relatively unimportant. Diagnosis of blastomycosis is usually made by examining secretions or biopsy material directly (either after KOH digestion or after staining with special stains including Papanicolaou and Giemsa stains for cytological material and PAS and silver stains for histopathological material) or by culturing the fungus from these biological materials. Direct methods are important because the process is pyogenic (the patient can usually produce a specimen) and because there is a characteristic morphology that is diagnostic if it is observed—a large 8- to 20-μm yeast with a large single bud with a broad neck of attachment to the parent cell. If sputum smears are not diagnostic, the patient will require more invasive tests, including bronchoscopic lavage and biopsy, fine-needle aspiration for culture and morphology, or even thoracoscopic or traditional open-lung biopsy, as determined by the clinical and radiographic features of the individual case. There is an immunodiffusion test for blastomycosis. It is usually negative in cases of acute pneumonia, so that a negative test has no weight. However, a positive test has reasonable specificity and should never be ignored in any patient with a consistent clinical syndrome. Rather it should prompt a more directed diagnostic progression.

Treatment options include intravenous amphotericin B and oral itraconazole. Patients with severe infections that threaten life should always be treated with amphotericin B. This includes all patients with diffuse infiltrates, severe hypoxemia, edematous lobar pneumonia, and all who are extremely toxic. However, most patients do not meet these criteria. Itraconazole is suitable and highly effective for most patient with acute blastomycosis, even to the point of moderately severe disease with considerable fever and toxicity. Obviously the boundary between the two treatments is difficult and needs to be individualized. Amphotericin B is given daily in doses of 40–50 mg until there is a good clinical response with decrease in fever and overall improvement. Then it is continued at 40–50 mg every Monday, Wednesday, and Friday to a total cumulative dose of 2 g. Itraconazole is given at 200 to 400 mg PO daily for 6 months. Hybrid therapy can be used with amphotericin B to clinical improvement and a 500- or 1000-mg total dose. Then a switch is made to itraconazole, usually 200 mg for 6 months.

Chronic Pulmonary Blastomycosis

Many patients with blastomycosis present with chronic pulmonary illness. Fever, if any, is low-grade. Some but not all patients have chronic productive cough. Some have malaise, weakness, and weight loss. Sometimes an abnormal chest radiograph is the only clinical abnormality. About 50% of patients with chronic pulmonary blastomycosis have skin and/or bone lesions. If present, these distant sites of infection can be both a clue to the diagnosis and a source of diagnostic material. The chest radiograph can show one or multiple nodules or focal or multifocal infiltrates. Fibrocavitary disease is also seen. Sometimes there is a dominant mass, mimicking carcinoma. Commonly that mass is located in the superior segment of the lower lobe, projecting over the hilum on the PA radiograph of the chest.

Direct examination of sputum and other specimens and culture of the same material provides the diagnosis in most cases. Diagnostic testing starts with sputum smear and culture and escalates as needed to bronchoscopic lavage and biopsy, fine-needle aspiration for culture and morphology, or even thoracoscopic or traditional open-lung biopsy. Many times the bronchoscopy is done with suspicion of cancer, but there is no endobronchial tumor and the brushings and/or lavage reveal blastomycosis either directly or by culture. (Fortunately, the fungus stains well with the standard Papanicolaou stain used for cytology.) In fact, a mass-like presentation similar to carcinoma is common enough that blastomycosis is the most common fungal diagnosis made at thoracotomy for presumed but not yet proven carcinoma. Patients with skin or bone disease are often diagnosed by tissue biopsies of those sites. Serological testing is probably better than for acute pneumonia but still lacks adequate sensitivity to become a very important diagnostic tool. If serology is negative, it never rules out blastomycosis. If positive, it has considerable diagnostic weight and should drive further testing to confirm the diagnosis.

A large majority of patients with chronic pulmonary blastomycosis can be treated with a 6-month course of oral itraconazole, 200–400 mg/day. Amphotericin B can be used in selected cases but is rarely needed.

COCCIDIODOMYCOSIS

Acute Pulmonary Coccidiodomycosis

Coccidiodomycosis is endemic in the desert areas of the southwestern United States, particularly in the central desert of Arizona, which includes the Phoenix area and the San Joachim Valley of southern California, including Bakersfield. Disease activity extends eastward as far as San Antonio, Texas, where the endemic area touches but barely overlaps the endemic area for histoplasmosis. There are also endemic regions in Mexico and South America.

Acute pulmonary coccidiodomycosis is somewhat similar to histoplasmosis. Many patients are asymptomatic; others have fever and a dry, nonproductive cough, similar to the symptoms of other nonspecific respiratory infections. Many symptomatic patients have headaches and a minority have sore throats. A syndrome of prolonged cough and fever in the endemic area is sometimes referred to as valley fever. One quantitative difference from acute histoplasmosis is a higher incidence of diffuse arthralgias and erythema multiforme, which occur in up to 10% of patients with acute pulmonary coccidiodomycosis. Within the endemic area, these clinical features are referred to as "desert rheumatism" and "the bumps." Chest radiographs may show a focal patchy or rounded infiltrate, sometimes with enlargement of draining hilar lymph nodes. Some patients have bilateral and extensive infiltrates. Symptoms can persist for several days to several weeks. Fever beyond 6 weeks suggests persistent pulmonary coccidiodomycosis.

One possible sequela of acute pulmonary coccidiodomycosis (silent or symptomatic) is a pulmonary nodule. The initial infiltrate does not resolve but contracts and hardens into a focal nodule. When such a nodule is discovered, there is no ready way to be sure it is a granuloma. It is often discovered on a routine chest radiograph years after the primary infection. It must be distinguished from an early cancer, using the approach as outlined above for histoplasmomas.

About 1% of patients with pulmonary coccidiodomycosis present with diffuse macronodular infiltrates. This pattern likely represents hematogenous dissemination to the entire lung. These patients can have severe hypoxemia and can progress to respiratory failure. Patients with this form of coccidiodomycosis are considered to have disseminated disease and are treated aggressively with amphotericin B.

Serodiagnosis is more advanced for coccidiodomycosis than for other fungal infection. Immunodiffusion for IgG and IgM antibodies is available with good sensitivity (within a week or two of onset) and good specificity. For coccidiodomycosis, there is some evidence that serological tests are not only diagnostic but have some prognostic import. A CF titer of 1:32 or higher correlates with an increased risk of progressive dissemination. The research was done in one reference laboratory, however, and it is somewhat of a stretch to extrapolate the result to different labs and methodology.

Cell-mediated immunity is highly effective against coccidiodomycosis, in the same range as for histoplasmosis. Only one-quarter of 1% of patients with primary coccidiodomycosis develop progressive disease. Differences from histoplasmosis include a higher chance of meningitis if the fungus disseminates and lesser efficacy of antifungal therapy, including both oral azoles and amphotericin B when needed for those with serious disease. Partly for fear of dissemination, many patients in the endemic area with severe or prolonged symptoms are often treated with fluconazole for varying periods, ranging from weeks to months. This may shorten the symptomatic period, and there is the hope (not yet proven) that such treatment may perhaps decrease the already low likelihood of dissemination even further.

Persistent Pulmonary Coccidiodomycosis

This term is often used to describe patients with prolonged illness and those with active nodules. Infiltrates and fevers lasting more than 6 weeks are obviously quite persistent, raise worry of dissemination, and are generally treated with fluconazole. Many patients with persistent infiltrates have fever and cough, which accounts for the serial chest radiographs.

Nodules from coccidiodomycosis often follow a different course than nodules from histoplasmosis. The nodule necroses and the contents are expectorated, leaving a characteristic thin-walled cavity the same size as the previous nodule. There is usually some active infection around the cavity. Also, cavities can be secondarily infected with bacteria. Hemoptysis is common and may be recurrent but is seldom massive. Some patients have a productive cough either due to active coccidiodomycosis or a superinfection. Most patients with persistent pulmonary coccidiodomycosis have positive serological tests, and sputum cultures are positive in a sizable minority.

Cavities that are large, subpleural, and increasing in size may rupture into the pleura and present with a pyopneumothorax. Surgical resection of cavities with this feature is likely appropriate, but they represent only a tiny minority of thin-walled coccidiodomycosis cavities. In fact, the majority of coccidiodomycosis cavities close within 2 years. Small cavities (less than 2 cm) are especially likely to close. Most patients with chronic persistent coccidiodomycosis are given a prolonged course of oral fluconazole.

Chronic Fibrocavitary Coccidiodomycosis

Like chronic cavitary histoplasmosis, chronic fibrocavitary coccidiodomycosis usually occurs in patients with underlying lung disease, most often severe COPD from long-term cigarette smoking. The disease mimics tuberculosis. Patients have subacute illness with low-grade fever and chronic, usually productive cough, malaise, weakness, and sometimes weight loss. Fibrocavitary infiltrates usually involve the upper lobes, because that is where the emphysema is most severe. Dissemination is unusual. This form of coccidiodomycosis is much less common than is chronic cavitary histoplasmosis.

Diagnosis is usually easy once tuberculosis has been excluded and the differential has been expanded to other chronic infections. Serological tests are positive in more than 90% of patients and sputum cultures are also positive in the majority. Only rare patients require more invasive tests, including bronchoscopic lavage and biopsy, fine-needle aspiration for culture and morphology, and even thoracoscopic or traditional open-lung biopsy.

Most cases of chronic cavitary coccidiodomycosis are treated with fluconazole 200–400 mg/day PO for 6–12 months or even longer. Occasional patients need very prolonged therapy, and rare patients who are severely ill or who respond poorly to fluconazole must be treated with amphotericin B, usually to a total cumulative dose of 3 g or more.

Coccidiodomycosis in AIDS

Coccidiodomycosis often explodes in patients with AIDS, especially if they have advanced T-cell immunodeficiency. This is a progressive respiratory illness over days to weeks. Patients have fever, cough, and sputum production. Weight loss is common. About one-third have meningitis, with a range of symptoms including headache, nausea, and vomiting, and decreased level of consciousness. Some 50% of patients have diffuse macronodular infiltrates. Hilar and mediastinal adenopathy is common. Patients with milder degrees of immunosuppression can present with focal infiltrates, nodules, and thin-walled cavities similar to the presentation in normal hosts.

Serodiagnostic tests are positive in up to 75% of patients. The density of organisms is high and coughed up sputum usually shows spherules on direct smear and is positive by culture. BAL fluid is usually positive by direct smear and by culture. Bronchoscopy often shows large, even dime-sized, ulcers. Biopsy shows inflammation and usually spherules in the tissue.

Treatment in AIDS is very difficult. Average survival is just a few months in those who present with aggressive disease, including those with diffuse macronodular infiltrates. Amphotericin B should be used for initial therapy. If the patient stabilizes with 1000–1500 mg total dose of amphotericin B, then fluconazole (at least 400 mg/day) can be used for disease suppression for the rest of the patient's life. Patients with less immunosuppression often have milder disease and can be treated successfully with fluconazole for years.

CRYPTOCOCCOSIS

Cryptococcal Pneumonia

The inflammatory reaction in the lung is not very impressive. Many patients have minimal and nonspecific symptoms. Cough is the most common symptom, but sputum production is minimal. Very few patinets are hightly febrile or otherwise toxic. Symptoms are chronic or subacute. Radiographs sometimes show large round masses. Many other patterns are possible but very nonspecific, including focal, single nodules and multiple nodules. Some patients have pleural effusions. About half of the patients are immunosuppressed; conversely, about half have normal immune status.

Most patients are given antibacterial therapy, do not improve, and then undergo workup for a nonresolving pneumonia or a mass. Cryptococcal antigen in the serum is usually negative. Sputum cultures may be positive, but many patients cannot produce sputum. Other patients require more invasive tests, including bronchoscopic lavage and biopsy, fine-needle aspiration for culture and morphology, or even thorascopic or traditional open-lung biopsy.

When amphotericin B was the only antifungal therapy, the standard approach was treatment for the immunosuppressed patients because they were likely to progress to meningitis and observation for the normal hosts because they were likely to recover without difficulty. The availability of fluconazole has changed the risk-versus-benefit equation. Since this is a rare diagnosis and adequate studies of treatment versus no treatment cannot be done, I favor treatment with fluconazole for all proven cases because the risk of meningitis in normal hosts, while small, is not zero.

Cryptococcal Pneumonia in AIDS

Cryptococcal infection is AIDS is a systemic disease. Some 80% of patients have fever. Meningitis is almost universally present and usually symptomatic, with headache as the primary symptom. Half of the patients have respiratory symptoms, including cough, dyspnea, and chest pain. Chest radiography frequently shows diffuse infiltrates similar to those seen in PCP. Other patterns include localized infiltrates, single or multiple nodules, and small pleural effusions. There is nothing specific about the radiographic presentation.

In patients with AIDS, cryptococcal antigen in the cerebrospinal fluid (CSF) is always positive. Of interest (and unlike the case in other patient groups), cryptococcal antigen is always positive in the serum as well, with titers higher than the CSF titer. A negative serum cryptococcal antigen in an AIDS patient with fever, cough, and diffuse pulmonary infiltrates rules out cryptococcal disease as the cause of that syndrome. The high density of organisms ensures that blood cultures, buffy-coat smears of peripheral blood, and BAL fluid direct stains and cultures are usually positive.

Treatment requires induction to reduce symptoms. Inravenous or high-dose oral fluconazole is usually adequate unless there is meningitis with a depressed level of consciousness. In that case, amphotericin B is used alone or with flucytosine. Flucytosine is particularly toxic in AIDS patients and therefore is used in reduced doses, if at all. Successful induction therapy must be followed by lifetime suppressive therapy with fluconazole to prevent relapse.

ASPERGILLOSIS

Invasive Aspergillosis

Aspergillus species are ubiquitous fungi that are important in the breakdown of dead vegetation. Decaying leaves and compost materials have very high concentrations. Spores are present everywhere and will settle on a piece of bread left on a kitchen shelf. All humans regularly inhale these spores without ill effect. They are cleared by nonspecific lung defenses and can be killed by nonimmune phagocytes. They have virtually no ability to invade normal tissue defended by normal phagocytes.

The clinical setting is the major clue to invasive aspergillosis, which virtually never occurs in normal hosts (the only exception is a massive inhalation of spores that overwhelms host defense). If the total neutrophil count is less than 500/dL, the risk of invasive fungal infection is about 1%/day. It increases to about 4%/day after 3 weeks of severe neutropenia. High-dose corticosteroid therapy, usually for at least several weeks, is the other major risk factor. Organ-transplant recipients receive corticosteroids in combination with other immunosuppressive agents and also are prone to cytomegalovirus infection, which has additional immunosuppressive effects.

In an appropriate setting, several clinical features serve as clues to diagnosis. These include pleuritic chest pain and hemoptysis, either with a normal x-ray or with a focal infiltrate corresponding to the location of the pain. Single or multiple wedge-shaped peripheral infiltrates, single or multiple nodules, and cavitary nodules are all radiographic findings that suggest invasive aspergillosis in the narrow clinical settings with highest risk. Any dense focal infiltrate that progresses despite aggressive antibacterial antibiotics also raises suspicion of invasive aspergillosis. Sometimes a diagnostic bronchoscopy done mainly to obtain a lavage sample reveals endobronchial ulcers. This is an uncommon finding but is more common with fungal, mycobacterial, and viral (usually herpes) infections than with bacterial pneumonias. Biopsy of these ulcers has a high diagnostic yield.

Invasive *Aspergillus* can also spread through the blood to any distant organ. Such spread is more common in patients with profound neutropenia than in glucocorticoid-treated patients, including organ-transplant recipients. Distant spread of the fungus provides clinical combinations of findings that can be helpful in differential diagnosis. A focal or multifocal infiltrate and any of the following findings suggests invasive aspergillosis with pyemic spread: (1) a focal neurological defect and/or one or more focal lesions on CT scan or on magnetic resonance imaging (MRI) of the brain, (2) episodes of left-upper-quadrant pain and/or focal lesions in the spleen on CT scan of the abdomen, (3) episodes of flank pain and/or one or more focal kidney lesions on CT scan of the abdomen, and (4) peripheral skin lesions ranging from red nodules to round areas of cutaneous hemorrhage.

Positive sputum cultures have high specificity in extremely high-risk settings, especially prolonged neutropenia. Fiberoptic bronchoscopy with bronchoalveolar lavage is useful for sampling areas of dense infiltrates. Curiously, some studies have shown higher return from bronchial washings than from lavage samples. Endobronchial biopsies should be done in the rare cases with endobronchial ulcers or nodules. Transthoracic fine-needle aspiration is useful to sample peripheral nodules and cavitites in selected patients. Peripheral skin lesions can easily be biopsied. Blood cultures are usually negative, even in patients with widespread multiorgan disease. Positive urine cultures always imply pyemic spread to the kidneys and never result from genitourinary tract colonization. More invasive tests—including video-assisted thoracoscopic or traditional open-lung biopsy—are sometimes needed; in other cases the risk of such procedures is too high and empirical therapy is initiated based on compatible clinical setting and findings. Serological tests measuring antibodies against aspergillosis are neither useful nor promising. Ultrasensitive assays for *Aspergillus* antigens are more promising (performed on serum and also BAL and body fluids) but are not commercially available.

Amphotericin B is preferred treatment for neutropenic patients. Liposomal formulations are more expensive but minimize renal insult. Most successfully treated patients have been treated with amphotericin B and have had full bone marrow recovery coinciding with their recovery. Residual nodules may activate during subsequent neutropenic episodes (for diseases treated with multiple cycles of chemotherapy). Management includes presumptive treatment with amphotericin B during all subsequent cycles and also (in selected cases) resection of one or several residual pulmonary nodules prior to further chemotherapy. Invasive aspergillosis is seldom curable when there has been extensive distant spread (especially to the brain) and when the underlying disease is not controllable and neutrophil function does not recover. Itraconazole is an alternative therapy for invasive aspergillosis, especially for isolated pulmonary disease in organ-transplant recipients and in other nonneutropenic settings.

Aspergilloma

Aspergillus organisms can colonize any cavitary space in the lung, creating a rounded intracavitary fungus ball. In countries where tuberculosis is common, negative open tuberculous cavities (residual after treatment) are the most common sites for aspergillomas, but any destructive lung disease that leaves a space with poor blood supply and no phagocytic defense can be complicated by an aspergilloma. Stage four sarcoidosis, incompletely resolved lung abscesses, and cystic and bullous areas of emphysema are all settings where aspergillomas occur. The chest radiograph shows a round lesion within a cavity, often surrounded by a crescent of air. Hemoptysis is usually the only symptom directly due to the aspergilloma. It is usually modest but can be persistent, recurrent, and even massive and life-threatening. Any other pulmonary symptoms (especially cough and dyspnea) are usually related to the destructive underlying lung disease that provided the site for the fungus to grow.

Diagnosis is usually based on a typical radiographic presentation. Fine-needle aspiration has the highest diagnostic yield. Suptum cultures and cultures of bronchoscopic specimens may be positive for the fungus. Anitbodies against *Aspergillus* are often positive (precipitins) but lack specificity.

Aspergillomas do not need treatment if the patient does not have hemoptysis. If there is troublesome hemoptysis, surgical resection of the lesion is one good option. Unfortunately, many patients have such severe underlying lung disease that the surgical risk is prohibitive. Medical treatment is less satisfactory but can be successful in many cases. Options include bronchial artery embolization of vessels feeding the area and local intracavitary instillation of potassium iodide or amphotericin B via a small catheter usually placed percutaneously. Systemic therapy with amphotericin B or with itraconazole is unlikely to work, probably because effective levels of drug cannot be achieved within the cavitary space.

Chronic Necrotizing Aspergillosis

Chronic necrotizing aspergillosis (or semi-invasive aspergillosis) is more similar clinically to tuberculosis or chronic cavitary histoplasmosis than it is to invasive aspergillosis. The usual setting is underlying destructive bullous or cavitary disease, most often severe COPD from long-term cigarette smoking. If there is a typical fungus ball localized in a space within an area of destroyed lung and the patient has cough, productive cough, fever, night sweats, or other symptoms suggestive chronic or subacute infection, chronic cavitary aspergillosis is a more likely diagnosis than simple aspergilloma, which is usually asymptomatic unless complicated by episodic hemoptysis. The problem is that many of these same symptoms may result from the underlying disease, thus confounding the diagnostic process. Other patients have no fungus balls but simply extensive fibrocavitary infiltrates.

Chronic cavitary aspergillosis is diagnosed when cultures are negative for tuberculosis and escalation of diagnostic efforts reveals *Aspergillus* (on direct smears or by culture) in coughed sputum or in samples obtained bronchosopically, by needle biopsy, or by thoracoscopic or traditional open-lung biopsy. Positive sputum cultures in patients with advanced COPD lack specificity because patients are often colonized with *Aspergillus* species. Reliable diagnosis usually requires histopathology or cultures from BAL fluid or fine-needle aspiration. Tuberculosis, atypical mycobacterial infections, chronic cavitary histoplasmosis, sporotrichosis, and coccidiodomycosis can all produce the same syndrome with upper lobe fibrocavitary disease, especially in patients with underlying COPD. Fibrocavitary infiltrates that slowly develop extensive pleural thickening over the area of involved lung are also very typical for chronic cavitary aspergillosis, though not specific.

Patients with chronic necrotizing aspergillosis usually have severe underlying lung disease. Surgical resection of localized disease can be curative but is usually prohibited by the lack of pulmonary reserve. Amphotericin B can suppress symptoms, but patients often relapse when it is stopped. Itraconazole is also effective and can be continued for a prolonged time. One strategy in sick patients is to give a 1-g course of amphotericin B (a week of daily therapy followed by 40–50 mg every Monday, Wednesday, and Friday for an additional 6–8 weeks) and then switch to itraconazole 200–400 mg PO daily for a year or more, sometimes indefinitely. Antibiotic therapy tends to be suppressive rather than curative. In general, resectional surgery is helpful for selected patients with reasonable pulmonary reserve and the highest chance of cure; surgery is almost never helpful for patients with the worst disease and the least reserve who fail medical therapy.

Pulmonary Aspergillosis in AIDS

Patients with advanced HIV infection have profound T-cell defects that predispose to severe infection with cryptococcosis and the endemic mycoses. Because the immune system is integrated, humoral and phagocyte defects are also present, although less severe. Neutropenia can result from advanced HIV infection by itself. More commonly, neutropenia results from antiretroviral therapy, from other infections complicating HIV infection (e.g., cytomegalovirus infections, histoplasmosis, *Mycobacterium avium-intracellulare* infections, and others), or from therapy required for opportunistic infection (e.g., ganciclovir, trimethoprim/sulfamethoxazole, pentamidine, and others). HIV-related cancers and the agents used for treating them (immunosuppressive chemotherapy and high-dose corticosteroids) also predispose to phagocyte defects.

Only about 0.1–0.5% of HIV-infected patients ever develop invasive aspergillosis. Infection is most common in patients with advanced disease (CD4 cell count usually less than 50/dL). Half of these patients have classical risk factors including neutropenia and/ or previous high-dose corticosteroid therapy. Some patients have heavy exposure to *Aspergillus* spores, sometimes from smoking marijuana. Other cases likely reflect the complex integration of the immune system and the eventual negative effect of advanced HIV infection on all of its components.

Most cases involve only the lung. The clinical spectrum of pulmonary illness is broad and includes several unusual patterns of disease. Nondescript focal infiltrates resembling bacterial pneumonia occur in one-quarter of the patients. They can be surprisingly indolent over weeks or months and can slowly enlarge or spread to other areas of the lung.

Cavitary infiltrates are common. The cavities can be large (up to 10 cm in size), and often there is little surrounding infiltrate (different than the picture in chronic necrotizing aspergillosis in normal hosts with abnormal lungs). Complications of large *Aspergillus* cavities include serious and sometimes fatal hemoptysis and rupture into the pleural space with presentation as a pneumothorax or pyopneumothorax. Obstructing bronchial aspergillosis occurs fairly commonly in patients with AIDS but is uncommon in other immunosuppressed patients. Bronchial casts laden with *Aspergillus* organisms are sometimes coughed up as visible plugs. The disease progresses to bronchial ulceration, pseudomembranes, and plaque-like lesions, all of which can obstruct distal airways. Cough and hemoptysis are common symptoms. The chest x-ray may be clear or may show patchy bilateral infiltrates due to obstructed airways with distal atelectasis and infection. Finally, diffuse interstitial or alveolar infiltrates are another presentation, mimicking *Pneumocystis carinii* infection and other opportunistic pulmonary infections. Prognosis here is poor, with spread of infection to distant organs in many cases.

Positive sputum cultures have less specificity, intermediate between prolonged neutropenia (very high) and advanced COPD with chronic cough (very low). Fiberoptic bronchoscopy is the best test to diagnose obstructing endobronchial aspergillosis. Diagnosis of parenchymal disease is more difficult, partly because of the high risk of invasive procedures. Bronchoalveolar lavage, transbronchial biopsies, and fine-needle aspiration biopsies are all useful in selected patients. Thoracoscopic and traditional open-lung biopsies have a high diagnostic yield but are done rarely for diagnosis and should be considered only if appropriate in the overall context of the patient's illness.

Overall results of treatment are poor. Localized lung disease can be indolent and can be suppressed with amphotericin B or itraconazole. There are also some treatment responses in patients with obstructing endobronchial aspergillosis. Most patients with diffuse pulmonary disease do not respond to treatment and die quickly.

Management options for hemoptysis include surgical resection of a single cavity in highly selected patients with good overall clinical status. Bronchial artery embolization can be tried in patients who are not good surgical candidates. Treatment of pneumothorax from a ruptured *Aspergillus* cavity is also difficult. If the cavity can be resected, it is sometimes possible to control the pleural leak and eventually remove all chest tubes. Otherwise many patients are fated to long-term chest-tube drainage with a chronically infected pleural space and sometimes a poorly expanded lung.

SUGGESTED READING

1. Binder RE, Faling LJ, Pugatch RD, Mahasaen C, Snider GL. Chronic necrotizing pulmonary aspergillosis: a discrete clinical entity. Medicine 1982; 61:109–124.
2. Davies SF. Fungal pneumonia. Med Clin North Am 1994; 78:5:1049–1065.
3. Davies SF, Sarosi GA. Pulmonary complications of HIV infection: fungal pulmonary complications. Clin Chest Med 1996; 17:4:725–743.
4. Davies SF, Sarosi GA. Epidemiological and clinical features of pulmonary blastomycosis. Semin Respir Infect 1997; 12:206–218.
5. Drutz DJ, Catanzaro A. Coccidiodomycosis: state of the art, part 1. Am Rev Respir Dis 1979; 120:911–938.
6. Goodwin RA Jr, DesPrez RM. Histoplasmosis: state of the art. Am Rev Respir Dis 1978; 117: 929–956.
7. Lorholary O, Meyohas MC, DuPont B, et al. Invasive aspergillosis in patients with acquired immunodeficiency syndrome: report of 33 cases. Am J Med 1993; 95:177–187.
8. Sarosi GA, Davies SF. Blastomycosis: state of the art. Am Rev Respir Dis 1979; 120:911–938.
9. Sarosi GA, Davies SF. Concise review for primary-care physicians: therapy for fungal infections. Mayo Clin Proc 1994; 69:1111–1117.
10. Sarosi GA, Davies SF. Fungal Diseases of the Lung. 2d ed. New York: Raven Press, 1993.
11. Schaffner A, Davis CE, Schaffner T, et al. In vitro susceptibility of fungi to killing by neutrophil granulocytes discriminates between primary pathogenicity and opportunism. J Clin Invest 1986; 78:511–524.
12. Strimlan CV, Dines DE, Payne WS. Mediastinal granuloma. Mayo Clin Proc 1975; 50:702.

38

Occupational and Environmental Airway Disease

Joel N. Kline and David A. Schwartz
University of Iowa
Iowa City, Iowa

INTRODUCTION

Occupational and environmentally induced airways diseases are a common problem for the primary care practitioner as well as the pulmonologist. These disorders may often be unrecognized or misdiagnosed, sometimes with serious consequences. For example, the patient with toluene diisocyanate (TDI)-induced asthma who returns to work in an automobile body shop may develop steroid-dependent asthma, fixed airways obstruction, and serious disability. This chapter outlines the approach to patients with airways disorders associated with environmental or occupational exposures. Some pulmonary airway disorders that are affected by environmental exposures are not included in this chapter. For example, any of the obstructive lung diseases discussed elsewhere will be adversely affected by inhalation of cigarette smoke and common air pollutants. Rather, we focus on those disorders whose exposure is more commonly occupational or accidental rather than routine.

Many substances previously thought to be benign may sensitize susceptible individuals and lead to the development of asthma. Other individuals, with previously known or unrecognized asthma, may develop exacerbations or worsening of the disease subsequent to certain occupational exposures. Acute exposure to irritants at high concentrations may lead to a persistent asthma-like condition (reactive airways dysfunction syndrome, or RADS) in previously healthy patients, just as massive inhalation of organic dusts may lead to a self-limited febrile disorder with significant constitutional symptoms (organic dust toxic syndrome, or ODTS). A note of caution: any category of disease with the term *syndrome* prominent in its discussion is clearly incompletely understood. Knowledge of these conditions has greatly increased in the past two decades and is likely to improve further in the future.

OCCUPATIONAL HISTORY

Diagnosis of a patient's occupational lung disease is predicated on an understanding of his or her occupation and exposures. Although some patients with occupationally induced airways disease present with a complaint of dyspnea, cough, or chest tightness that clearly develops only while they are at work, others are less aware of the connection with their employment. It is the practitioner's responsibility to identify potential job-related exposures and to connect these exposures with the patient's complaints. Often a detailed history taken by the physician is sufficient; sometimes an investigation by an industrial hygienist is necessary to identify the occupational risk factors.

The occupational history must start with identification of the patient's current (and often multiple previous) employment. Although a job title is an important first step, the practitioner must seek an understanding of the patient's specific daily and exceptional duties. In industrial and agricultural workplaces, it is also relevant to note what other exposures may be in the patient's immediate work environment, though not his or her responsibility. This may lead to surprising discoveries, such as finding that a secretary's office is next to the grain elevator entrance, or that an accountant regularly audits an auto body shop. In large companies, material safety data sheets (MSDS) are often available for all known compounds to which workers are exposed; although mandated by law, these may be out of date or inaccurate and are more useful for irritant than sensitizing exposures. When there is doubt, on-site review by an industrial hygienist is critical.

In addition to evaluating exposures, it is also important to inquire about safety measures in the workplace. These may include fixed or portable ventilation systems, personal respirators or masks, and protective clothing. Symptoms and diagnoses of coworkers can also provide clues to the etiology of worker's complaints. Depending on the presenting complaint, exposure to specific compounds—such as organic dusts, isocyanate-containing compounds, irritants, and solvents relevant to the patient's occupation—may also be directly sought out.

Although an exhaustive occupational history often provides clues to patients' disorders, this is not always achieved. The best care requires the cooperation of the patient as well as his employer. Either party may have reasons to provide inaccurate or incomplete information. The employer may be reluctant to supply proprietary information because of security concerns, ignorance of the potential outcome for the worker, concern regarding possible litigation or compensation, or sheer disinterest. The worker, as well, may be reluctant to reveal the possibility of an association with his occupation for fear of losing his or her job or some other adverse consequence. In addition, malingering and compensation seeking must be considered when symptoms and exposures are not consistent.

Although obtaining an accurate occupational history is fraught with challenges, a detailed occupational history is vital to the accurate diagnosis of work-related conditions (Table 1). The essential features of an occupational history include a job history, listing of known toxic exposures, semiquantitative assessment of exposures, use of protective equipment to minimize exposures, ascertainment of the temporal relationship between exposures and symptoms, and identification of the existence of similar problems in coworkers. Questions about the patient's job should focus on specific duties at the work site and include an exhaustive list of all recognized exposures, length of exposure in work-years, and the number of hours of exposure in a typical day. Many workers have part-time or summer employment, have been enlisted in the military, or participate in hobbies

Table 1 Essential Components of the Occupational
and Environmental History

A job history including previous work exposures
Duties at specific worksites
Assessment of similar symptoms in coworkers
Hobbies or summer jobs
Identification of known toxic exposures
Duration, intensity, frequency, and peak exposures to
    specific agent
Length of exposure in work-years
Use of protective equipment to minimize exposures

---

that may account for additional exposure risks. Other risk factors such as cigarette smoking
should be sought and characterized.

OCCUPATIONAL ASTHMA

Occupational asthma is the most common and most costly occupation-associated pulmonary disorder. It is defined as recurrent episodes of airflow obstruction induced or exacerbated by exposures in the workplace. Occupational exposures are responsible for 5–15%
of adult asthma, and these cases can be therapy-resistant. The true incidence of occupational asthma is probably underestimated, as self-selection often causes workers who develop asthma to leave occupations that would cause continued respiratory problems. A
wide range of occupations poses risks for the development of asthma; relevant inhalation
exposures may include dusts, gases, vapors, and fumes. This section concentrates on
asthma induced by occupational exposures. Reactive airways dysfunction syndrome
(RADS), which is an asthma-like condition resulting from inhalation of irritants at high
concentrations, is discussed subsequently in a separate section. Underlying asthma (nonoccupational) can also be exacerbated by exposures in the workplace to irritants (such as
those which cause RADS), allergens, and dusts.

Etiology

A great number of inhaled irritants have been associated with the development of occupational asthma. While each of these has not been fully characterized or tested in a controlled
clinical laboratory setting, these agents can be generally grouped by mechanism of action
into immunological and nonimmunological causes. Immunological causes include most
high-molecular-weight compounds and some low-molecular weight compounds that cause
occupational asthma. High-molecular-weight compounds include proteins and complex
polysaccharides, such as cereal grain dusts, seafood, enzymes, and animal proteins. These
are generally associated with the development of a specific IgE antibody against the offending agent. Low-molecular-weight compounds can also induce the development of IgE
antibody responses by acting as haptens that associate with circulating proteins. Examples
of these agents include acid anhydrides and platinum salts. Other low-molecular-weight
compounds may cause direct activation of T lymphocytes; these include agents such as

Table 2 Common Agents and Occupations in Occupational Asthma

Exposure	Antigen or Source	Occupation
High-molecular-weight agents		
Laboratory animals	Dander and urine	Laboratory workers
Livestock	Dander	Agricultural workers
Grain	Grain mites, grain dust	Grain workers
Flour	Wheat, fungal amylase	Bakers
Crab	Unknown	Snow crab processors
Low-molecular-weight agents		
Polyurethane	Diisocyanates	Paint, plastics industry
Epoxy	Trimellitic anhydride	Chemical, industrial
Western red cedar	Plicatic acid	Cedar workers
Welding flux	Zinc chloride	Welding
Chromium	Chromium	Metal plating
Laxatives	Psyllium	Pharmaceutical
Formaldehyde	Formaldehyde	Laboratory, industrial
Latex gloves	Latex	Laboratory, health care

nickel and toluene diisocyanate. Nonimmunological causes of asthma most likely cause direct airway epithelial damage and are considered subsequently in the discussion of RADS.

Preexisting asthma exacerbated by working conditions may be due to inhalation of irritants or allergens. Asthmatic airways are hyperresponsive to many inhaled irritants and pollutants, such as NO_x, SO_2, and particulate suspensions encountered in many occupational settings. Other irritants include a broad array of solvents, acids, and other toxins that can cause bronchospasm in an individual with bronchial hyperreactivity. Allergens may also be encountered by the asthmatic that are not specifically related to occupational exposure, as among veterinary or laboratory workers with preexisting sensitization to dog or cat dander who are subsequently exposed to the animals in the course of employment.

High-molecular-weight agents associated with occupational asthma include animal proteins, insects, plants, enzymes, and gums. Low-molecular-weight compounds include diisocyanates, acid anhydrides, amines, wood dusts, metals, drugs, and multiple chemicals. Table 2 lists some agents reported to cause occupational asthma and the associated occupations. Although a few agents have been carefully characterized and studied and the mechanism through which they may cause asthma has been defined (such as plicatic acid in western red cedar), other agents have merely been associated with airway obstruction in surveys or case reports. Careful clinical exposure studies need to be carried out before any agent can be proved to be a causative factor in occupational asthma.

Pathogenesis

As with all other forms of asthma, the pathogenesis of occupational asthma is multifactorial; no single mechanism of injury can explain all cases. IgE-dependent occupational asthma (including asthma caused by most high-molecular-weight compounds and some low-molecular-weight compounds) is similar to nonoccupational atopic asthma. IgE antibodies formed against inhaled antigens (or endogenous antigen-hapten conjugates) trigger mast-cell degranulation and a series of inflammatory responses that lead to eosinophil and mast-cell chemotaxis, activation and degranulation, and the release of mediators (including prostaglandins, leukotrienes, histamine, and cytokines), causing airway epithelial damage and bronchospasm. Other forms of asthma may be modulated through direct induction of T-lymphocyte responses. T-lymphocytes may activate eosinophils and other effector cells through elaboration of cytokines in the Th2 family, including interleukin-4 (IL-4) and IL-5. Some low-molecular-weight agents that cause occupational asthma, such as cobalt and isocyanates, cause peripheral lymphocytes to proliferate in vitro, leading to speculation that this activation may be a clue to their mechanisms of injury. However, occupational asthma is often mediated by nonallergic mechanisms, with the airway epithelia and the alveolar macrophages initiating the recruitment of inflammatory cells. Moreover, local production and release of inflammatory mediators may contribute to the chronic remodeling of the airway observed in patients with persistent occupational asthma.

Clinical Features

Diagnostic criteria for occupational asthma rely on both a firm diagnosis of asthma and the determination of a relationship between asthma and work (see algorithm, Fig. 1). In occupational asthma, the presence of airway hyperreactivity and bronchospasm can be demonstrated by serial spirometry examinations, a methacholine challenge, or demonstration of a bronchodilator effect of inhaled beta-agonists. Since symptoms tend to develop several hours after starting work and then improve following several days away from exposures, the use of a peak flowmeter throughout the workday (for at least 2 weeks) and then through a prolonged absence from work can be very useful in documenting the

Initial Complaint: A High Index of Suspicion of Asthma
⇓
Occupational History:
       Job History, Tasks, Exposures, Co-workers' Illnesses
⇓
Documentation of Asthma
       History, Peak Flows, Spirometry, Methacholine or ß-Agonist Response
⇓
Treatment of Asthma
⇓
Documentation of Association With Workplace:
       Work-related airflow obstruction (Peak Flows, Spirometry, Specific
       Airway Challenge), Symptom Diary
⇓
Workplace Measures
       Ventilation, Move Worksite, Personal Respirator
⇓
If inadequate response, perform worksite evaluation by industrial hygienist
⇓
Possible Legal Recourse
       ⇒ Report OSHA
       ⇒ Impairment and Disability

Figure 1 Algorithm for evaluation of suspected occupational asthma.

association between airflow obstruction and employment. In general, there is a period of latency between initial exposure and the development of symptoms, which also contributes to patients' doubts about the work-related nature of their condition. This latent period is longer for asthma associated with the IgE than in cases where IgE does not appear to be pathogenic, as would be anticipated for the development of IgE formation to inhaled allergens. Subsequent exposures may lead to a typical dual responses in IgE-mediated asthma, with initial bronchospasm within minutes to an hour following exposure and a late response that is generally more severe and longer-lasting at 4–6 h after exposure. IgE-independent cases of asthma may present with a single phase of symptoms intermediate between the early and late responses.

Clinical signs and symptoms range from chest tightness and cough to wheezing, diminished airflow, severe dyspnea, and even respiratory failure. No physical diagnostic feature reliably distinguishes occupational from nonoccupational asthma except the association of specific work exposures and the development of airflow obstruction. Physiological testing—either by spirometry, peak flow measurements, or periodic nonspecific broncho-provocative challenges—can and should be used to evaluate the temporal relation between occupational exposures or environmental agents and the development of airflow obstruction. For instance, demonstration of consistent decreases in peak flows of at least 20% when the patient is exposed to a specific agent in the workplace not only helps establish a diagnosis of occupational asthma but may also help to identify the agent. Although specific airway challenges are the most definitive method for making the diagnosis, these tests are not entirely accurate, and very few centers are equipped to perform these potentially hazardous studies of exposure response. Chest radiographs are generally normal but may reveal hyperinflation. Nor does invasive assessment, including bronchoalveolar lavage and lung biopsy, help with this differentiation. Those measures reveal airway inflammation (often eosinophilic but possibly neutrophilic), hypersecretion of mucus, epithelial desquamation with thickened basement membrane, and (chronically) the development of subepithelial fibrosis. Laboratory studies can be useful in some cases; many of the IgE-associated causes of asthma can be evaluated using skin testing, specific IgE measurement, or RAST examination. Specific IgG may be found in patients with non-IgE-associated causes of asthma; this is less helpful because there is no clear connection between the antibody response and pathogenesis of asthma, so the antibodies serve only as markers of exposure. In vitro lymphocyte proliferation assays have been developed for diisocyanates, cobalt, and platinum, but the clinical utility of these tests remains unproven.

The "gold standard" to demonstrate an asthmatic response to occupational exposures is a graded airway challenge in a controlled setting. Unfortunately, clinical exposure testing is not standardized and is currently available in only a few research centers. Thus, indirect measures such as peak-flow and symptom diaries and cross-shift spirometry remain the most useful clinical tools for diagnosing occupational asthma.

Management and Outcome

Once occupational asthma has been identified, the most important management issue is to minimize exposure to the offending agent. The likelihood of complete recovery to normal lung function is inversely related to the total duration of occupational exposure. In some circumstances, avoidance of further exposure may be accomplished through alteration of job requirements, increased ventilation, relocation of the patient within the workplace, or substitution of a nonallergenic material for an allergenic material. Industrial hygienists can be helpful in evaluating specific job needs and in recommending solutions to exposure problems. Mask filtration units are almost never adequate for avoidance of allergen inhalation. Personal respirators—which are expensive, heavy, and uncomfortable—are likewise a poor solution and are only rarely appropriate for long-term usage. If no remediation is possible, the patient should be urged to avoid the workplace. This will usually lead to workmen's compensation and permanent disability actions, which require careful documentation before eligible workers can obtain benefits.

Although continued exposure to allergens may lead to airway remodeling and fixed airway disease, the converse is not always true; avoidance of subsequent allergen exposure does not necessarily lead to resolution of airway inflammation and nonspecific hyperreactivity. Some unfortunate patients develop persistent symptomatology and require vigorous anti-inflammatory therapy. Systemic corticosteroids may be required intermittently or persistently, perhaps lifelong. These patients should be treated as described previously for severe persistent asthma, as recommended by the NIH Expert Panel Report, with efforts made to reduce their usage of steroids as much as possible.

CHRONIC AIRWAY DISEASE—CHRONIC OBSTRUCTIVE PULMONARY DISEASE, INDUSTRIAL BRONCHITIS, AND BYSSINOSIS

Etiology

Although cigarette smoke is the major cause of COPD, COPD may occur following chronic exposure to mineral dusts, fumes, and mixtures of organic and inorganic dust. Epidemiological evidence suggests that combinations of dust and either gas or fumes may be more potent than the dust alone in causing COPD. In addition to the cumulative burden of dust, younger age at exposure, peak exposures, and the combination of dust plus irritant gas or fumes appear to be important at predicting the development of COPD.

Industrial bronchitis, a disorder characterized by dyspnea and a cough productive of sputum at least 3 months each year, is associated with occupational exposure to high concentrations of airborne dust, such as cement dust, or particles encountered in the mining or textile industries. Workers exposed to dust from cotton, flax, hemp, or jute used in the textile industry may experience chest discomfort, cough, or dyspnea. Characteristically, patients complain of ''Monday morning fever,'' referring to the onset of symptoms immediately following reexposure after a period of time away from the work environment. This suggests that at least one component of the disorder may lead to the development of tolerance, as can be seen with chronic exposure to endotoxin. Unlike organic dust toxic syndrome (see below), the response in chronic bronchitis and byssinosis may lead to airway remodeling. Organic dust contains live microorganisms, endotoxin, mycotoxins, and tannins, all of which are capable of initiating an inflammatory response in the airway and causing the development of byssinosis (in the case of cotton workers) or chronic bronchitis.

Pathogenesis

Epidemiological studies have shown that the acute airway response to a variety of occupational agents is predictive of the chronic airway response. Thus, the acute decline in airflow during a work shift is independently associated with accelerated longitudinal declines in lung function among grain handlers, cotton workers, and agricultural workers. These findings suggest that the acute physiological and biological response to specific agents in the workplace may place individuals at risk for developing progressive airway disease. The chronic airway remodeling seen in COPD may be directly related to the acute recurrent inflammatory episodes following exposure to a variety of workplace agents. Chronic histological changes include epithelial metaplasia and desquamation; thickening of the basement membrane, lamina propria, and smooth muscles of the airway; and inflammatory cell infiltration. Abnormal deposition of types III and V collagen results in thickening of the subepithelial basement membrane. However, the relationship between acute inflammation and chronic airway remodeling remains elusive and continues to be a particularly important area of investigation.

Clinical Features

Industrial bronchitis is a disorder characterized by dyspnea and a cough productive of sputum for at least 3 months each year. Individuals may present with airflow obstruction due to hypersecretion of mucus in the proximal airways. As with other forms of chronic bronchitis, nonspecific airway hyperreactivity may be present, as demonstrated by positive methacholine inhalation challenge tests. This is not necessary to make the diagnosis, however; similarly, specific exposure challenges add to neither the sensitivity nor the specificity of diagnosis and are not recommended in this setting.

Characteristically, patients with byssinosis complain of ''Monday morning fever,'' referring to the onset of symptoms immediately on exposure after some time away from the work environment. The majority of patients with these symptoms experience a decrease in their FEV$_1$ over the course of a work shift; at least initially, they develop symptoms to exposures only after having been away from the inciting agent. As the disease progresses, the symptoms of dyspnea, wheezing, and cough persist and are exacerbated throughout the work week.

The diagnosis of COPD is made using standard diagnostic criteria which include symptoms of dyspnea, cough, sputum production, and persistent declines in airflow. Findings on physical examination are notable for a prolonged expiratory phase, and radiographic findings include hyperinflation.

Management and Outcome

These individuals are at high risk for progressive airflow obstruction, and exposure to the specific agent (inorganic dust, organic dust, or fumes/gas) should be completely eliminated. This may require leaving the workplace; however, in many cases, modifications can be made in the work environment to eliminate the exposure. Medical treatment should be initiated in all individuals with airflow obstruction and should include inhaled corticosteroids and possibly bronchodilators. In addition, antibiotics should be used in individuals with industrial bronchitis.

TOXIC FUMES

Many fumes, gases, vapors, dusts, and inhaled substances have potentially toxic effects manifest by pulmonary and extrapulmonary injury. Exposure by inhalation occurs in industrial settings as well as in the home, in public places, and in other environments. The acute and long-term effects of many of these inhaled agents are predominantly mediated through irritant mechanisms.

Etiology

Inhaled toxins exist in many forms and may be categorized according to their physical properties. General categories include gases, vapors, fumes, aerosols, and smoke. Table 3 summarizes the physical properties of these inhalants. The initial pathogenic responses to a harmful inhaled agent depend on a number of factors, including the concentration of the substance in the ambient air, the pH of the inhaled substance, the presence and size of particles, the relative water-solubility of the inhaled agent, the duration of exposure, and whether the exposure occurs in an enclosed space or in an area with adequate ventilation and free circulation of fresh air. In addition, an undetermined number of host factors—including age, smoking status, the presence of preexisting pulmonary or extrapulmonary disease, and the use of respirators or protective breathing apparatus—all affect a person's response to the inhalation of a toxic substance.

Pathogenesis

Inhaled gases with potential irritant effects manifest their actions at different anatomic locations in the respiratory system. In general, substances that are highly water-soluble—such as ammonia, sulfur dioxide, and hydrogen chloride—can cause immediate irritant injury to the upper airway. The acute effects of highly water-soluble irritants on the upper airway, exposed skin, and other mucous membranes often produce such unpleasant symptoms that exposed persons quickly leave the area of exposure and avoid continued inhalation of the harmful toxins. In contrast, inhaled toxins that have low water-solubility—such as phosgene, ozone, and oxides of nitrogen—often have little or no acute effect on the upper airway and instead produce irritant effects at the level of the bronchiole and alveolus. Because agents of low water-solubility do not produce immediate, noticeable upper airway irritation (except in episodes of massive acute exposure), exposed persons may inadvertently remain in the area of exposure and increase their duration of exposure to harmful agents. Agents that exhibit intermediate water-solubility, such as chlorine, can have pathological effects throughout the respiratory system. However, extreme exposure

Table 3 Types of Irritant Gases and Mechanisms of Injury

Irritant Gas	Water Solubility	Mechanisms of Injury
Ammonia (NH_3)	High	Alkali burns
Chlorine (Cl_2)	Intermediate	Acid burns
		Free radical formation
Hydrogen chloride (HCl)	High	Acid burns
Oxides of nitrogen	Low	Acid burns
(NO, NO_2, N_2O_4)		Free radical formation
Ozone (O_3)	Low	Free radical formation
Phosgene ($COCl_2$)	Low	Acid burns
Sulfur dioxide (SO_2)	High	Acid burns

to any one of these irritants may result in involvement of the upper and lower respiratory tract. Absorption of any one of these irritants onto particulate matter may also alter the area of involvement.

Irritants enter cells directly through nonimmunologically mediated mechanisms of injury and inflammation. Cell injury involves the deposition or formation of an acid (chlorine, hydrogen chloride, oxides of nitrogen, phosgene, and sulfur dioxide), alkali (ammonia), or reactive oxygen species (oxygen, oxides of nitrogen, and possibly chlorine). A primary injury is localized in airway epithelial tissues, but excessive damage may also occur in subepithelial and alveolar regions. Acid injury results in coagulation of the underlying tissue, while acute injury due to alkali results in liquefication of the mucosa and deep penetrating lesions in the airway. Reactive oxygen species include oxygen-derived metabolites (such as hydrogen peroxide and hydrochloric acid) and oxygen-derived free radicals (such as superoxide anions and hydroxyl radicals). These reactive oxygen species may injure tissues and cells through lipid peroxidation, which can directly injure cells and lead to elaboration of inflammatory mediators; these can perpetuate the initial damage. Regardless of the initial mechanism of irritant injury, inflammatory mechanisms that involve networks of proinflammatory cytokines may be subsequently initiated. The resulting inflammation may be important with regard to perpetuation of the acute injury as well as long-term sequelae. In addition, disruption and eventual repair of the airway epithelia may decrease the host's ability to defend against inhaled infectious or irritant substances inhaled at a future time.

Clinical Features

Inhalation of irritant gases may cause airway hyperresponsiveness by initiating a localized inflammatory response resulting in the development of airway disease. Inhaled irritants may enhance epithelial permeability, exposing subepithelial irritant receptors, which are subsequently at risk of being stimulated by a variety of agents, including cold air, changes in humidity and temperature (exercise), and cigarette smoke. The chronic inflammatory response in the subepithelial region can result in remodeling of the underlying airway architecture. Striking inflammatory changes—such as extensive collagen deposition beneath the epithelial basement membrane, eosinophilic infiltration, and mass cell degranulation—are seen in transbronchial biopsy specimens obtained from individuals previously exposed to toxic fumes.

Course and Management

Spirometry findings may initially be normal, but in some cases progressive airflow obstruction develops; thus, a case can be argued for obtaining baseline airflow indices and following the exposed subject with spirometry over the 24–48 h after exposure. For persons without significant decrements in airflow but with symptomatic chest tightness or wheezing, inhaled steroids are essential and bronchodilators may be useful. In cases that demonstrate airflow obstruction (FEV_1 of 80% or less than predicted or 10% less than the patient's initial baseline), a short course of systemic corticosteroids may be beneficial in addition to the use of inhaled steroids and bronchodilators. However, there is no definitive evidence that treatment with parenteral corticosteroids substantially relieves the acute airflow obstruction or prevents the onset of either reactive airways dysfunction syndrome (see below) or bronchiolitis obliterans.

Bronchiolitis obliterans may be a late or delayed consequence of the inhalation of toxic fumes. The clinical presentation is characterized by a persistent, nonproductive cough, fever, sore throat, and malaise. The lung exam typically reveals late inspiratory crackles but no wheezes; many patients may have no abnormalities on physical examination. Characteristic chest radiographic features include bilateral patchy, ground-glass densities that begin as focal lesions but may coalesce with time. Obstructive physiology is often seen with bronchiolitis obliterans; however, individuals with bronchiolitis obliterans organizing pneumonia (BOOP) may present restrictive ventilatory patterns. Treatment of bronchiolitis obliterans with corticosteroids may result in a dramatic improvement. However, many patients with bronchiolitis obliterans do not respond to medical intervention.

REACTIVE AIRWAYS DYSFUNCTION SYNDROME (RADS)

Etiology

RADS was first described in 1985 as an asthma-like syndrome with bronchial hyperreactivity that developed after inhalation of a high dose of irritant fumes, gases, or smoke. It is defined (see Table 4) as a single exposure to high concentrations of irritant gas, smoke, fumes, or vapors that results, in an individual with no prior respiratory problems, in cough, wheeze, dyspnea, airflow obstruction, and nonspecific bronchial hyperreactivity. These symptoms must develop within 24 h of exposure and persist for at least 3 months.

Exposures that have been reported to cause RADS include, among others, ammonia, chlorine, sulfur dioxide, formic acid, sulfuric acid, hydrochloric acid, smoke, and swine-confinement gases. In most cases, the injuring exposure has been brief but at a high concentration.

It is unclear whether RADS and "irritant asthma" are the same or different entities. It is possible that in the future, the term *RADS* will describe the result of high-level irritant inhalations leading to airway injury and bronchial hyperreactivity in all exposed subjects, whereas *irritant asthma* will refer to the development of nonspecific bronchial hyperreactivity and bronchospasm following lower levels of inhaled irritants in susceptible individuals.

Table 4 Diagnostic Criteria for Reactive Airways Dysfunction Syndrome (RADS)

Absent prior pulmonary disorder or symptoms
A single documented exposure leading to onset
of symptoms
Exposure to high concentrations of irritant gas, smoke,
fumes, or aerosol
Onset of symptoms within 24 h of exposure and
lasting at least 3 months
Symptoms resembling asthma; may include wheezing,
coughing, dyspnea
Spirometry may demonstrate obstructive indices
Methacholine challenge test is positive
No other pulmonary disorder can be diagnosed

Pathogenesis

The pathogenesis of RADS is uncertain but most likely involves generation of a localized inflammatory response in the airways following epithelial and subepithelial mucosal injury. The epithelial damage leads to increased epithelial permeability and exposes subepithelial irritant receptors to inhaled and environmental influences, including cold air, smoke, pollutants, and nonspecific irritants. Stimulation of the subepithelial receptors can cause nonspecific bronchial hyperreactivity and bronchospasm.

Clinical Features

RADS is characterized by the development of bronchospasm and nonspecific bronchial hyperreactivity for at least 3 months following the inciting exposure. Patients have a positive bronchospastic response to inhaled methacholine and generally respond to inhaled beta agonists with significant bronchodilation. Clinically, they may be indistinguishable from asthmatic patients. Chest radiography is usually normal, but patients may present with chemical pneumonitis acutely.

Bronchial biopsies have been obtained on a number of patients with RADS, although this is generally not clinically indicated. These biopsies demonstrated a chronic inflammatory response characterized by lymphocytic and monocytic infiltrates and some epithelial desquamation. Eosinophilia is not characteristic of RADS. Sensitization to allergens does not play a role in the development of RADS, and immunological testing is not helpful.

Management and Outcome

Management of patients with RADS is supportive and based on symptoms. Most patients require treatment of their airway obstruction, and use of inhaled bronchodilators is common. For persistent and serious cases of airway inflammation, inhaled steroids are helpful; some patients require systemic steroids at least initially. All patients should be urged to stop smoking and to avoid subsequent inhalation of irritants. Unfortunately, symptoms of RADS can persist for years after the initial injury.

ORGANIC DUST TOXIC SYNDROME (ODTS)

Etiology

Organic dust toxic syndrome (ODTS) is an acute systemic inflammatory response induced by inhalation of high concentrations of organic dust, as may be generated in the storage or handling of grain, cotton, animal bedding, compost, or other sources. ODTS was first reported in 1986, but the danger of inhaling concentrated agricultural dust suspensions had long been recognized. Other terms for ODTS include *pulmonary mycotoxicosis, silo unloader's syndrome, grain fever syndrome*, and *inhalation fever*. Although moldy dusts have frequently been implicated in this disorder, the presence of mold or fungi is not mandatory. Table 5 summarizes exposures and settings reported to be associated with the development of ODTS. ODTS must be distinguished from hypersensitivity pneumonitis (HSP, or "farmer's lung") since HSP, unlike ODTS, may lead to chronic progressive pulmonary dysfunction. Unlike the case in HSP, antibody-mediated responses do not play a role in the development of ODTS, nor is previous exposure to the inhaled agent required.

Table 5 Specific Exposures and Settings Associated with Organic Dust Toxic Syndrome

Grain dust
Moldy silage
Compost
Wood chips
Animal bedding
Silo unloading
Cleaning of swine confinement buildings
Cleaning of poultry confinement buildings

Exposure to high levels of dust is required to diagnose ODTS but not HSP. ODTS also is clearly distinct from reactive airways dysfunction syndrome (RADS), since the latter requires inhalation of high levels of irritants and leads to persistent bronchial hyperreactivity, whereas ODTS resolves without adverse sequelae. This also distinguishes ODTS from chronic bronchitis or byssinosis, which may lead to persistent changes in airway structure and function.

Pathogenesis

ODTS results from the acute inflammatory response to inhaled toxins. These toxins include endotoxins (from gram-negative bacteria) and components of molds, fungal spores, and thermophilic bacteria. As with all such nonspecific responses, multiple aspects of the lung's defenses are activated.

The alveolar macrophages and neutrophils appear to be the primary cells responding to the inhaled organic dust. Endotoxin and fungal spores activate macrophages to release a number of inflammatory mediators, including cytokines and metabolites of arachidonic acid, which act in a cascade to attract and subsequently activate other inflammatory cells, such as neutrophils. Products of these cells, especially the proinflammatory cytokines IL-1β and tumor necrosis factor-α, can cause a systemic inflammatory response.

Clinical Features

The syndrome has been characterized as a flu-like illness that develops within 6 h of exposure to high concentrations of organic dusts. The patient can almost always provide a compatible history, which generally involves manipulating or moving dusty agricultural products in an enclosed environment. Interestingly, ODTS develops in only 10–30% of individuals with similar exposures, suggesting a range of susceptibility to this process. In recurrent cases, tachyphylaxis is common, with symptoms most common early in the work week but subsiding after 1 day back on the job, leading to the coining of the phrase "Monday morning fever." Complaints often include fever, myalgias, headache, weakness and malaise. Shaking chills, nausea, and vomiting have been reported but are uncommon. Although cough and dyspnea are often present, the physical examination is relatively normal. Patients are frequently tachypneic and tachycardic, but abnormal breath sounds, such as crackles or wheezes, are rare; chest x-ray is almost always normal. Although mild obstructive indices may be seen on spirometry, these are transient; lung volumes and diffusion capacity are normal. Arterial blood gas may demonstrate a widened alveolar-arterial oxygen gradient with an acute respiratory alkalosis. Examination of peripheral blood may demonstrate leukocytosis (with or without a left shift); laboratory test results are otherwise unremarkable. Precipitating antibodies to antigens commonly associated with hypersensitivity pneumonitis are not associated with ODTS.

MANAGEMENT AND OUTCOME

Since ODTS is almost always self-limited, its management centers on recognition, distinguishing it from other illnesses, and education on how to prevent recurrences. Patients are markedly improved within 24 h and generally have no sequelae from their illness. Supportive care includes the careful use of nonsteroidal anti-inflammatory drugs to improve the constitutional symptoms as well as rest. We have previously mentioned the importance of distinguishing ODTS from HSP, as HSP can lead to irreversible pulmonary fibrosis if not recognized and treated. In general, ODTS is a preventable disorder. Individuals of risk should be alert for signs of heavy dust levels in the workplace and use appropriate ventilation measures or personal respirators as appropriate. If ODTS recurs in the workplace, consultation with an industrial hygienist experienced in dust-control measures is recommended.

SUGGESTED READING

1. Chan-Yeung M, Malo JL. Aetiological agents in occupational asthma (review; see comments). Eur Respir J 1994; 7:346–371.
2. Chan-Yeung M, Malo JL. Occupational asthma (review). N Engl J Med 1995; 333:107–112.
3. Chan-Yeung M. Assessment of asthma in the workplace. Chest 1995; 108:1084–1117.
4. Brooks SM, Weiss MA, Bernstein IL. Reactive airways dysfunction syndrome (RADS): persistent asthma syndrome after high level irritant exposures. Chest 1985; 88:376–384.
5. Von Essen S, Robbins RA, Thompson AB, Rennard SI. Organic dust toxic syndrome: an acute febrile reaction distinct from hypersensitivity pneumonitis. Clin Toxicol 1990; 28:389–420.
6. Cartier A. Definition and diagnosis of occupational asthma. Eur Respir J 1994; 7:153–160.
7. Goldman RH, Peters JM. The occupational and environmental health history. JAMA 1981; 246: 2831–2836.
8. Schwartz DA. Acute inhalational injury. Occup Ref 1987; 2:297–318.

39

Occupational and Environmental Lung Diseases Caused by Inhaled Particles and Fibers

Gerald S. Davis

University of Vermont College of Medicine
Fletcher Allen Health Care
Burlington, Vermont

Inhalation of mineral dusts can cause chronic diffuse parenchymal lung diseases associated with fibrosis (the pneumoconioses), chronic airway irritation (industrial bronchitis), and increased risk for neoplasms; occasionally it can initiate hypersensitivity reactions as well. The many various particles and fibers of occupational and environmental origin carry different risks for causing lung disease; some are relatively inert despite intense exposure, while others carry substantial risk with slight contact. This chapter presents concepts that are common to most diseases caused by inorganic particles and fibers and then offers specific information about individual agents and diseases.

Occupational lung disease is a changing field. Many of the "classic" pneumoconioses, such as silicosis and asbestosis, have been nearly eradicated in most industrialized nations by measures to reduce ambient dust levels. These diseases remain widespread in many developing countries, however, and may actually be increasing as hand processes are replaced by power tools with the capability for generating dense aerosols. New diseases caused by exposures to new processes involving hard metals, synthetic mineral fibers, petrochemicals, and many other substances are of growing concern. At the same time that severe chronic parenchymal fibrosis resulting from occupational exposure has decreased among workers, less obvious diseases—such as chronic bronchitis and cancer in the elderly—have been unmasked. An understanding of the principles that underlie exposure, deposition, and disease caused by inhaled particles and fibers should help to manage these new diseases as well as to prevent the more traditional ones.

DIAGNOSIS OF OCCUPATIONAL PARENCHYMAL LUNG DISEASES

The diagnosis of an occupational lung disease due to inhaled fibers or particles can be established in most instances by a compatible work history linked with characteristic abnormalities on chest radiography and the exclusion of other diseases that might present these features. Appropriate signs and symptoms help support other evidence but are rarely specific. In some instances, a lung biopsy or other more detailed diagnostic studies may be needed to confirm the diagnosis.

Patients with occupational parenchymal lung disease present in two broad patterns. One group presents with known exposure and apparent symptoms, where confirmation of the diagnosis (and exclusion of other diseases) is required in order to qualify for disability or compensation. Many of these workers will have bona fide pneumoconiosis and impairment, while others will have limited exposure and no disease or an unrelated disease such as chronic obstructive pulmonary disease (COPD) caused by tobacco smoking. A second group presents with diffuse interstitial lung disease of unknown etiology, and the clinician must determine a specific diagnosis. Within this group, a detailed history may reveal unexpected past exposure to inhaled fibers or particles, or a lung biopsy may reveal characteristic pathology and minerals. The evaluation of patients in the second group is dealt with primarily in Chap. 29. The first group is considered below.

The Workplace, the History, and the Physical Examination

A detailed occupational history is essential for the diagnosis of pneumoconiosis or other mineral-induced lung diseases. The approach to this history is discussed in detail in Chap. 6; the determination of impairment and disability is presented in Chap. 41. It is essential to record all past work and hobbies that might include relevant exposures as well as current work exposure. The actual tasks performed ("I swept up asbestos waste from the floor") as well as the job title ("I was a custodian") must be recorded. The tobacco-smoking history is essential in order to weigh the possibility of COPD as an alternate diagnosis. Current symptoms, limitations on work performance, and changes over time are important in estimating impairment.

The cardinal symptoms of diffuse interstitial lung disease of occupational origin are gradually progressive shortness of breath with exertion and cough. Sputum production is usually modest unless industrial bronchitis or chronic smoker's bronchitis is also present. More acute complications may develop, such as pleural effusion in asbestosis or tuberculosis with silicosis, and should be sought if symptoms change rapidly. The symptoms of occupational interstitial disease are very nonspecific and do not by themselves permit diagnosis.

The physical examination is rarely of great assistance in evaluating the patient with occupational lung disease. Radiographic disease and physiological abnormalities are often far greater than would be expected from physical findings. Crackles at the lung bases are common with asbestosis and are sometimes found in silicosis and other conditions. Silicosis and coal worker's pneumoconiosis may present with virtually normal chest examinations despite significant physiological disturbances. In these diseases, prolonged expiration and even wheezing may sometimes occur as a result of scarring around airways. Digital clubbing is found in many patients with asbestosis (pulmonary fibrosis associated with asbestos), but the extent of abnormality does not match the degree of lung scarring. Clubbing is only very rarely found in other pneumoconioses.

The history and physical examination are useful for excluding other diseases that may cause lung dysfunction or confound a diagnosis of primary disease due to inhaled particles or fibers. Signs and symptoms of asthma, COPD, or other lung diseases should be evaluated further. Systemic diseases or limited involvement of other organ systems should suggest alternative diagnoses, because the pneumoconioses involve only the lungs. In particular, collagen vascular diseases that can be associated with diffuse parenchymal lung disease should be excluded.

Radiology

Radiographic features of occupational lung diseases are often unique or highly suggestive. When coupled with an appropriate exposure history, distinctive chest radiographic abnormalities may be sufficient to establish a diagnosis of pneumoconiosis and even to confer disability and workmen's compensation. The chest x-ray also serves as a powerful tool for epidemiological studies of industries or worker groups and as a means of following the progress of individual subjects over time. The radiological features of specific pneumoconioses are described along with each of the individual diseases discussed below. A standardized scoring method, the ILO U/C Classification System, has been developed for the description and grading of chest radiographs in the pneumoconioses.

High-resolution computed tomography (HRCT) provides thin 1 to 2-mm slice thickness (collimation) and high spatial reconstruction algorithms to produce a detailed image of the fine structure of lung parenchyma. The techniques and applications of CT are presented in detail in Chap. 11. HRCT has become a powerful tool in the diagnosis of pneumoconiosis, offering both sensitive and specific images. The HRCT patterns of silicosis, asbestosis, and other diseases caused by inhaled particles and fibers are distinctive but not unique and must be coupled with an appropriate occupational history and other compatible features. HRCT is highly sensitive in detecting subtle abnormalities that may not be appreciated by plain film, such as early pleural disease, mild alveolitis or fibrosis, and small nodules. This technique may also reveal centrilobular emphysema indicative of smoking-induced lung disease in association with pneumoconiosis. Studies with groups of asbestos workers have shown superior sensitivity with HRCT as opposed to conventional chest radiography in detecting early disease and in correlation with physiological impairment. Not every worker needs an HRCT. In many instances, a compatible exposure history and a plain chest radiograph will be sufficient to establish a diagnosis or to follow the progression of abnormalities. When the diagnosis is in doubt or when impairment may be due in part to other confounding lung diseases, HRCT can be extremely valuable for the diagnosis of occupational lung disease.

Pulmonary Function Testing

Measurements of pulmonary function quantitate the severity of pneumoconiosis but do not provide a specific diagnosis. These diffuse parenchymal lung diseases are traditionally viewed as causing a "restrictive" pattern of abnormality, but mild to moderate airflow limitation is commonly present as well. Scarring and/or nodule formation around small and medium-sized airways may explain the airflow reduction. Typically, the vital capacity and the total lung capacity with its relevant subdivisions will be reduced. The single-breath diffusing capacity will be decreased. Oxygenation and ventilation will usually be normal at rest or show mild hypoxemia. Incremental exercise will often reveal desaturation, and therapeutic oxygen may be needed with walking but not at rest.

All patients with suspected or confirmed pneumoconiosis should have at least simple measurements of pulmonary function: forced expiratory spirometry and digital oxygen saturation. These tests will help determine the degree of impairment and the assignment of disability. Some patients will require more extensive testing and evaluation under exercise conditions in order to assess their ability to perform work-related tasks. All of these tests may be confounded by COPD due to smoking, but they will at least provide an estimate of the total impairment experienced by the patient.

Lung Biopsy, Bronchoalveolar Lavage, and Detection of Minerals

Examination of lung tissue reveals distinctive patterns of response to each of the mineral fibers and particles that cause occupational parenchymal lung disease and usually permits a specific diagnosis. The demonstration of the causative particles or fibers in the lung strengthens the diagnosis. Transbronchial biopsy may sometimes be adequate to establish a diagnosis, but in most instances it provides too small a piece of tissue to observe the distinctive pathology or to estimate the dust burden. Because the minerals are sometimes aggregated in local concentrations of particles, a very small sample may miss the mineral by chance. Video-assisted thoracoscopic biopsy or limited open lung biopsy (minithoracotomy) is usually preferable for definitive diagnosis of occupational parenchymal disease.

Most patients do not require lung biopsy to establish a diagnosis of pneumoconiosis. If an appropriate exposure history is present and the chest radiograph or HRCT scan are compatible, then biopsy is not needed. In some patients a biopsy will have been performed to diagnose an unknown disease, and particles, fibers, and/or a distinctive histopathological pattern will be found. When the exposure history is slight or confused, then lung biopsy may be very helpful in establishing or rejecting the diagnosis of pneumoconiosis.

Bronchoalveolar lavage (BAL) cell profiles may be abnormal in pneumoconiosis but are neither specific nor sensitive and thus are not useful clinically. The exception is chronic beryllium disease, where lung lymphocytes recovered by BAL may provide immunological confirmation of the diagnosis. BAL may be helpful in documenting exposure to specific minerals by recovering them from the lung. A reasonable relationship has been established between the number of fibers per milliliter of BAL fluid and the likelihood of asbestos-related lung disease. With other minerals, it is vital to recognize that recovery of the particulates documents exposure; it does not document lung disease. At present, Vermont granite workers have exposure to silica that is low enough that virtually none develop radiographic or physiological abnormalities, but more than 20% of the macrophages recovered by BAL from these healthy granite workers contain silicates. BAL might be a useful and relatively noninvasive method of confirming pulmonary exposure to a mineral if the exposure were in doubt.

DOSE, TIME, EXPOSURE, AND BIOLOGICAL RESPONSE

Work activities that produce dust create aerosols of particulates suspended in air. In general, in order to be a significant respiratory health hazard, the particles must be small enough to reach the lower respiratory tract. Coarse particles that are too large to reach the lower respiratory tract cause little problem; thus relatively dense clouds of sand on a dusty road or in a desert sandstorm create little hazard. Respirable aerosols can be created as rock, ore, or metal are drilled, crushed, ground, chipped, or polished. Many materials create hazards for the miner who first extracts them from the earth, the worker who mills or processes them to extract metal or create a useful product, and the worker who utilizes or installs that product. Once in place, these products are usually inert and pose no further risks. Asbestos is an exception, because this hazardous aerosol can be generated from installed products during its removal as well as during its manufacturing processes.

Factors That Influence Disease

The extent of lung disease that results from exposure to respirable particulates in the workplace is determined by the interactions of many factors, including the characteristics of the particle or fiber, the concentration of the dust in the air, the duration of exposure, environmental factors that alter the intensity of exposure, and the personal characteristics of the worker. These factors are summarized in Table 1. For most of the pneumoconioses, the extent of disease follows a dose-effect relationship in which higher ambient doses and longer exposure leads to more disease. The lung diseases caused by inhaled particles and fibers follow a sigmoid dose-response curve: at low levels of dust exposure, no workers demonstrate disease; at intermediate levels of exposure, the most susceptible workers show abnormalities; while at very high levels, all become ill.

The characteristics of airborne particles govern their behavior in an aerosol and their deposition in the lung. Particles that remain suspended in air are generally 0.01–100 μm in diameter; larger particles settle out rapidly by gravity. Particles between 0.2 and 10 μm are effectively deposited in the lower respiratory tract and may be retained there; thus

Table 1 Factors That Influence Lung Disease
Caused by Particles and Fibers

Characteristics of the particle or fiber
   Biological activity of the material
   Aerodynamic size
   Aerodynamic shape
Airborne dust concentration
   Average dust level in the air
   Intermittent peak dust levels
Timing of exposure
   Duration of work exposure (years)
   Frequency of exposure at work (hours)
Environmental factors
   Ventilation in the workplace
   Direct dust extraction (stone cutting)
   Water spray on cutting surface
   Isolation of machinery from workers
   High-temperature operations (metals)
Personal characteristics
   Comorbid disease
   Tobacco smoking
   Work and safety habits
   Genetic susceptibility

they are of most concern for human disease. The ambient concentrations of different particles and fibers that are considered safe for long-term human exposure are usually expressed in terms of "threshhold limit values" (TLV) or "permissible exposure levels" (PEL). The current U.S. PELs recommended by the Occupational Safety and Health Administration for some particles and fibers of interest are presented in Table 2.

For most of the diseases caused by inhaled particles and fibers, the reaction in the lung continues long after the inhalation exposure ends. Therefore patients may have no evidence of disease while they are working in an industry but develop clinical symptoms and signs decades after leaving the industry. This phenomenon highlights the importance of a complete work history in the evaluation of a patient with diffuse parenchymal lung disease.

In contrast to the pneumoconioses, some industrial lung diseases strike only a small fraction of the exposed workforce despite a wide range of doses. These individuals are unusually sensitive to the offending agent or develop immune reactivity to it while most workers do not. Very small doses are all that is required to provoke disease in susceptible individuals. Hypersensitivity pneumonitis, "hard metal disease" due to cobalt, and berylliosis are examples of this unusual reactivity. The occurrence of disease resembles an all-or-none phenomenon in these circumstances, and neither the prevalence nor the severity of illness follows a simple dose-response relationship.

Pathogenetic Mechanisms

A chain of complex events leads from the inhalation of harmful dusts to chronic lung injury, inflammation, and fibrosis with respiratory dysfunction. There are very great differences between the extent and patterns of disease caused by various materials, as detailed in the sections that follow. Asbestos fibers, silica particles, and cement dust would not produce identical reactions in the lung even if the doses were similar. Nonetheless, there are also many common features to these diseases, and there appear to be common pathways by which the lung reacts to inhaled particulates. A detailed presentation of the biological processes that occur in the lung in response to particles and fibers is beyond the scope of this chapter.

Table 2 Regulated Exposure Levels for Selected Particles and Fibers

Material	Permissible exposure level (PEL)[a]	Comment
Asbestos	0.2 fibers per cubic centimeter of air	
Beryllium	0.002 parts per million (ppm)	
Cobalt—metal	0.05 mg/m^3 air	Dust or fumes
Cobalt—carbonyl	0.10 mg/m^3 air	Carbonyl or hydrocarbonyl
Coal	2.00 mg/m^3 air	Silica less than 5%[b]
Silica—quartz	0.10 mg/m^3 air	Respirable fraction
Silica—cristobalite	0.05 mg/m^3 air	Respirable fraction
Silica—tridymite	0.05 mg/m^3 air	Respirable fraction

[a] Standards established by the U.S. Occupational Safety and Health Administration. The PEL is expressed as the time-weighted average for an 8-h workday assuming a 40-h work week.
[b] For silica fraction greater than 5%, the limit is 10 mg/m^3 air divided by the percentage of silica.

Particles and fibers appear to injure structural lung cells directly through physico-chemical interactions between reactive moieties on the crystal surface and cell membranes as well as through the generation of high-energy oxygen radicals. Most particulates are ingested rapidly by macrophages, activating these phagocytes and leading to the elaboration of cytokines that recruit additional inflammatory cells, promote fibroblast proliferation, and lead to excessive connective tissue matrix deposition. The time course of events in silicosis, asbestosis, and other dust diseases represents a paradox between the very prolonged course of disease observed clinically and the very rapid sequence of individual events inferred by the cytokine and oxygen radical pathways outlined from laboratory research. The diseases stretch over years or decades, while the cell interactions take place in hours or days. It is assumed that the slow progression of pulmonary fibrosis and dysfunction is the aggregate result of many brief focal events occurring at different times throughout the lung.

LUNG DISEASES CAUSED BY INHALED PARTICLES

Silica

Silicosis is a chronic fibronodular lung disease caused by the long-term inhalation of dust containing crystalline free silica. Silicosis can result from exposure to airborne silica in a wide variety of trades and industries in which stones are drilled, quarried, crushed, shaped, or utilized as abrasives.

Mineralogy

The term *silica* implies a compound with the chemical formula SiO_2. The crystalline forms, such as quartz, are fibrogenic and inflammatory, while the noncrystalline forms, such as glass, are generally not fibrogenic. The most common by far is α-quartz; cristobalite and tridymite are much less abundant but are somewhat more biologically active. Silica makes up about 25% of the earth's crust and may occur in pure form, such as sand or sandstone, or as a component of mixed conglomerate rocks such as granite or basalt.

Occupational Exposure

Numerous industries pose risks for exposure to silica. These can be grouped broadly into trades where rock is drilled or removed from the earth, trades where silica-containing stone is worked to produce other products, jobs that use silica as abrasives for cleaning or shaping other materials, or occupations that use powdered silica as an additive in manufacturing. Dust generated from drilling rock in the confined tunnel of a mine provides an obvious exposure. Airborne silica can result from the use of grinding wheels containing silica, such as the sandstone wheels used for sharpening knives, abrasives used for cleaning castings in a foundry, or sand powder used as a blasting material. Silica exposure can also occur when a stone containing silica is the target of a nonsilica abrasive, as in the manufacture of granite monuments or sandblasting of buildings made of stone. Silica powder, or ''silica flour,'' is divided into very small particles and thus is easily aerosolized in handling; it is used widely for its absorptive and bulking properties in the manufacture of plastics, ceramics, paint, and other products. Table 3 lists some of the occupations with exposure to silica.

Silicosis demonstrates dose-effect relationships in producing lung disease, as evidenced by longitudinal and cross-sectional studies of workers in several industries. Work-

Table 3   Occupations with Exposure
to Silica

Rock drilling
  Hard rock mining
  Tunnel drilling
Stone working
  Stone quarrying
  Stone crushing
  Masonry
  Monument manufacture
  Sculpting
Abrasives
  Foundry casting
  Tool grinding
  Knife sharpening
  Sandblasting
Silica powder
  Silica flour production
  Diatomaceous earth production
  Glass manufacture
  Ceramic production
  Plastics and paint manufacture

---

ers with jobs creating the highest levels of dust in the air and those with the longest employment develop the most severe disease. In most circumstances, silicosis requires decades of exposure to become evident as clinical disease. Personal work habits, smoking, genetic susceptibility, and comorbid diseases will also affect the extent of silicosis, but to a lesser degree than the intensity and duration of exposure.

Industrial hygiene measures to reduce silicosis have been highly effective in most industries. These measures include strategies such as substituting other materials for silica (e.g., iron carbide in sandblasting applications), replacing human workers with machines at dusty locations (drilling machines that work at the tunnel faces of mines), spraying water on grinding surfaces (tool manufacture), extracting air at high volume from the grinding surface (stone polishing), or providing respiratory protection and an independent air source for workers (sandblast engraving). Most of these measures require technology and a substantial investment and thus are used most widely in the industrialized nations.

Silicosis was once a common disease in the United States and throughout the world. It is also an ancient disease, having been recognized for both its cause and consequences in ancient Greece and Rome. The application of modern industrial hygiene measures during the middle years of the twentieth century have led to a dramatic decrease in the incidence of silicosis among workers in the industrialized countries of the world. Tunnel drillers, sandblasters, foundrymen, and granite cutters develop new silicosis only rarely in most developed countries. Elderly workers, now retired from trades they began in the 1930s, may still present with significant silicosis. This disease is still a major public health problem in those developing nations where mining, ore extraction, the crafting of building stone, and other trades depend heavily on human labor, with few machines and little attempt to control dust. Thus the prevalence of silicosis is rising in China, while it is falling abruptly in North America and Europe.

The practitioner in an industrialized nation must remain alert for silicosis under several circumstances. Obviously, it must be considered if a worker, particularly an elderly one, reports an occupation with recognized exposure risks. Workers in small industries, owner-worker shops, and miscellaneous trades may not be aware of the risks, knowledgeable about dust-control measures, or willing to spend money on them. These small businesses may not come under government scrutiny and thus may not be regulated with regard to industrial hygiene measures. New applications of finely divided silica as an additive in paints, plastics, and other materials may subject particular workers to high exposure levels during the manufacturing process.

Clinical Features of Silicosis

The responses to inhaled silica occur in three patterns: (1) as chronic nodular silicosis (simple or progressive massive fibrosis), (2) as accelerated silicosis, or (3) as acute silicosis. Simple nodular silicosis develops slowly over decades. Individuals affected with mild disease, evident by x-ray only, are generally asymptomatic unless there is associated chronic bronchitis or COPD. As the disease progresses, dyspnea is common, and cough and sputum due to coincident bronchitis are frequent as well. If progressive massive fibrosis supervenes, shortness of breath may become disabling. Specific physical findings are often lacking; digital clubbing and rales are rare. The course of the disease is often insidious, and progression occurs in the absence of continued exposure to silica. Cor pulmonale is occasionally an end-stage feature but is not common. The diagnosis of silicosis is made on the basis of a work history with silica exposure of substantial length and intensity linked with compatible chest radiograph abnormalities.

The clinical and radiographic features of silicosis are caused by the development of numerous sites of tissue reaction to deposits of mineral dust within the lung. Although the dust is spread throughout the lung initially, it is translocated to peribronchial, subpleural, and interstitial sites, where groups of particles are found clustered together. At these sites the lesions of silicosis, referred to as "silicotic nodules," develop. The typical silicotic nodule occurs near the respiratory bronchiole and is composed of whorled collagen and reticulin centrally, with surrounding macrophages, fibroblasts, and lymphocytes, as shown in Fig. 1. As the disease progresses in time and extent, the center of the nodule becomes fibrotic and acellular, fibrosis extends outward in bands, and ultimately multiple nodules become fused into larger complex masses of granulomatous inflammation and scar.

The chest radiograph in *chronic nodular silicosis* demonstrates several characteristic features. Simple silicosis is manifest as diffuse rounded opacities with a modest upper lobe predominance (see Fig. 2). Calcification of the lung lesions of simple nodular silicosis or "eggshell" calcification of the hilar nodes may occur infrequently. With advanced disease, the discrete rounded opacities may coalesce and fuse to form large, irregular-shaped masses, as shown in Fig. 3—a stage referred to as *progressive massive fibrosis*. The degree of pulmonary function impairment is generally related to the severity of the radiographic abnormalities.

HRCT offers a distinctive picture of silicosis, as illustrated in Fig. 4. A profusion of small, rounded opacities throughout the lung parenchyma is seen with mild disease; the coalescent larger opacities occur with more advanced silicosis. Calcifications within

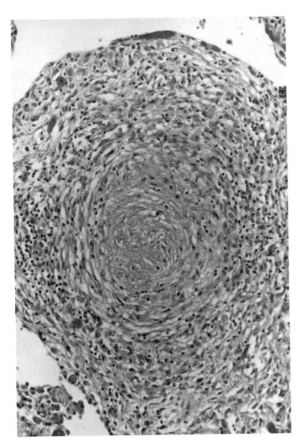

Figure 1 Silicosis. A lesion of silicosis (silicotic nodule) shows a whorled connective tissue center with concentric layers surrounded by mononuclear cells and fibroblasts. (From Davis GS, Calhoun WJ. Occupational and environmental causes of interstitial lung disease. In: Schwarz MI, King TE, Jr, eds. Interstitial Lung Disease, 2nd ed. St. Louis, MO: Mosby Year Book, 1993: 179–229.)

enlarged hilar nodes and lung opacities can often be seen by HRCT while not evident by plain chest radiograph. Multiple subpleural nodules with calcification are characteristic of silicosis.

Accelerated silicosis is relatively rare but can develop in 2–5 years if exposure to free silica is intense. Cases have been reported from sandblasting, tunnel drilling, and other industries. Dyspnea is apparent early and soon becomes disabling. The radiographic picture is of diffuse, small, irregular opacities or reticulonodular opacities rather than the upper-lobe nodular opacities typical of simple silicosis. Accelerated silicosis appears to be uniformly fatal within several years after the appearance of clinical signs.

Acute silicosis is a rare consequence of exposure to free silica at very high levels, usually related to tunneling through hard rock, sandblasting, or the use of finely divided silica powder. Acute silicosis presents as rapidly progressive dyspnea and respiratory insufficiency. Radiographically, the appearance is that of a diffuse perihilar alveolar filling process with ground-glass opacities. Upon pathological examination, the alveolar spaces are filled with a lipoid and proteinaceous exudate and cellular debris; damage to the epithe-

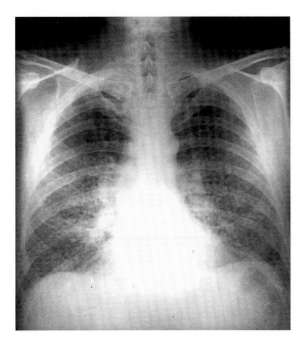

Figure 2 Silicosis. Chest radiograph from a granite worker with 25 years of exposure shows simple nodular silicosis with diffuse small, rounded opacities (ILO U/C classification system = type p and q opacities). The hilar lymph nodes are enlarged. (From Davis GS, Calhoun WJ. Occupational and environmental causes of interstitial lung disease. In: Schwarz MI, King TE, Jr, eds. Interstitial Lung Disease, 2nd ed. St. Louis, MO: Mosby Year Book, 1993: 179–229.)

lium is extensive. Thus, acute silicosis more closely mimics pulmonary alveolar proteinosis than it does interstitial fibrosis; it is sometimes referred to as silicoproteinosis. Acute silicosis appears to be a uniformly fatal disease.

Associated Conditions

Mycobacterial infection can be exceedingly difficult to differentiate from the progression of underlying silicosis. Thus, in patients with silicosis, such evidence as radiographic or clinical progression of pulmonary parenchymal disease or the development of constitutional symptoms should prompt a search for *Mycobacterium tuberculosis* infection. Infections with nontuberculous mycobacteria (see Chap. 36) occur with higher frequency among silicotics than among those without such exposure; thus identity by culture of the mycobacterial species must guide therapy. The means by which silicosis may predispose an individual to tuberculosis are uncertain but are probably related to a reduced capacity for intracellular killing of *Mycobacteria* by silica-laden macrophages and sequestration of viable microorganisms within silicotic lesions. Treatment of tuberculosis associated with silicosis follows usual guidelines, but complete eradication may be difficult. Some experts advise very prolonged or even "lifetime" therapy with a single agent, usually isoniazide, after conventional treatment is complete.

Cough, sputum, and mild airflow obstruction associated with occupational exposure to dusts or fumes has been termed *industrial bronchitis* and is discussed in detail in Chap. 38, on occupational airways diseases. Exposures to mixed dusts or pure silica can

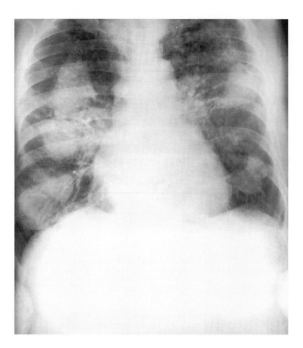

Figure 3   Silicosis. An elderly granite worker shows advanced silicosis by chest radiograph, with coarse, rounded opacities (ILO U/C classification = q, r) and large, conglomerate lesions of progressive massive fibrosis. (From Davis GS, Calhoun WJ. Occupational and environmental causes of interstitial lung disease. In: Schwarz MI, King TE, Jr, eds. Interstitial Lung Disease, 2nd ed. St. Louis, MO: Mosby Year Book, 1993: 179–229.)

cause this form of chronic bronchitis along with true silicosis; thus patients may evidence symptoms or signs of both conditions.

Epidemiological studies from around the world reveal an increased risk for lung cancer among workers exposed to silica, although the effect is nowhere as great as for asbestos. The statistics suggest a clear increase in risk for workers who have overt silicosis and smoke tobacco, with an adjusted odds ratio for death (standardized mortality ratio) of two- to sevenfold. There is compelling evidence for increased risk among workers with silicosis who never smoked. Some data suggest slightly increased risk for workers who are nonsmokers with exposure to silica but without clinical silicosis. Thus silica appears to function as a cocarcinogen with tobacco smoke and possibly as an independent agent as well.

Therapy

No specific therapy is available for silicosis; the emphasis must rest on prevention through industrial hygiene and healthy work practices rather than on treatment after the disease develops. Small case series have reported clinical improvement during corticosteroid therapy in patients with rapidly progressive (probably accelerated) silicosis, but the long-term benefit has not been assessed. For most patients with silicosis, clinical impairment develops late in life and is disabling but not fatal. Many have been smokers and suffer from coincident COPD. Removal of the worker from a hazardous environment and smoking cessation are essential if not already accomplished. Supportive measures such as therapeu-

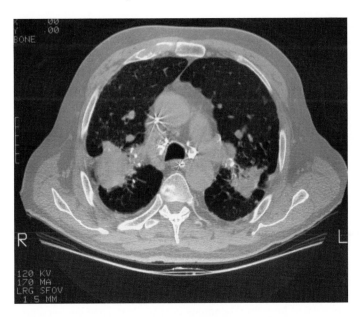

Figure 4 Silicosis. High-resolution computed tomography demonstrates small, rounded opacities in low profusion, large bilateral conglomerate lesions with calcifications, surrounding emphysema, and hilar lymph node enlargement with calcifications.

tic oxygen, physical rehabilitation, bronchodilator therapy if indicated, and early treatment of complicating infection are helpful. For patients with advanced disease at a younger age, lung transplantation offers a solution, with no expectation of disease recurring in the transplanted lung.

Coal

Exposure to coal dust in mines and in processing applications results in several forms of lung disease that often overlap: coal worker's pneumoconiosis (CWP), progressive massive fibrosis (PMF), and chronic airflow obstruction. Defined by radiographic findings, pulmonary dysfunction, or pathology, the prevalence of each of these abnormalities is related to the amount of airborne dust, the duration of exposure, the type of coal, and to a lesser degree the amount of crystalline free silica mixed with the coal. Successful reduction of dust exposure through industrial hygiene measures in the industrialized nations has led to demonstrable improvement in the prevalence and severity of lung disease among coal workers.

The Mineral and the Workplace

Coal is formed by the decomposition and compression of organic matter and is composed primarily of carbon with hydrogen and oxygen, trace quantities of sulfur, and many other elements. Up to 40% of coal may be noncarbonaceous minerals, including 5–10% silica. Coal type is described by "rank," an expression of hardness. The hardest or highest-rank coal is anthracite, followed by medium-hard/medium-rank bituminous and subbituminous coal, soft/low-rank lignite, and ultimately peat. The prevalence of lung disease is incrementally greater with harder grades of coal at comparable ambient dust levels.

Coal is used primarily as fuel for electrical power generation in the industrialized nations, but it is still a major source for home and building heat and for industrial furnace applications in developing countries. Increasing amounts of coal are being processed for conversion to gas (gasification), oil, and gasoline. Most of the 1 billion tons of coal mined annually in the United States is bituminous or subbituminous, as it is no longer cost-effective to mine anthracite. Traditional underground coal mines now provide about 40% of the coal mined in the United States and may produce substantial exposure to coal dust as well as inhaled silica and silicosis. Approximately 60% of coal is extracted from surface mines where the "overburden" of soil is stripped away with huge earth-moving machines, the coal seams exposed, and the coal broken and transported for further processing. Strip mining offers less ambient dust hazard to workers than tunnel mining, but drilling and selected other tasks can cause significant exposure. Workers employed in crushing coal, handling it for transport or fueling, or processing it for gasification extraction can also receive hazardous exposures to coal dust.

Governmental surveillance and regulations in many countries have improved conditions for most coal workers, including the United States Coal Mine Health and Safety Act of 1969 (the "black lung" law). These measures have resulted in a substantial reduction in mine air dust concentrations and closer monitoring of worksites for safety compliance. Prevalence rates for industry-related lung disease among coal workers have declined progressively since the early 1970s.

Clinical Features

The pathological processes caused by coal dust appear first as *simple coal worker's pneumoconiosis* (CWP), "macules" of black dust–laden macrophages with little or no scarring near respiratory bronchioles. With progression, these macules coalesce to form hard black nodules up to 10 mm in diameter, with scarring. The alveoli surrounding these sites become overdistended and alveolar walls may be destroyed, creating adjacent emphysema. Further aggregation of the CWP nodules into larger masses with more advanced adjacent lung distortion is described as *complicated coal worker's pneumoconiosis*. Conglomerate lesions greater than 2 cm in size define *progressive massive fibrosis* in coal workers. This process can occur with exposure to pure coal or even pure carbon (graphite) and does not require silica. If the coal has a substantial silica content, silica nodules (see above) may also form, and silicosis can complicate CWP.

The symptoms of CWP are nonspecific except for the expectoration of black or gray sputum. Dyspnea with exertion, cough, and progressive impairment become evident as the disease advances. A small number of workers develop severe pulmonary dysfunction, cor pulmonale, and ultimately die of respiratory insufficiency.

The typical chest radiographic findings in simple CWP are small, rounded opacities, and/or less abundant irregular shadows with somewhat of an upper-lobe predominance. A chest radiograph from a coal worker with simple CWP is shown in Fig. 5. When these phenomena are present in low profusion, the workers usually have no respiratory symptoms and normal pulmonary function. As profusion increases and the opacities become larger, symptoms develop and a picture of a restrictive pulmonary function deficit appears, often with airflow obstruction. Advanced PMF with multiple large, sometimes calcified bilateral opacities and surrounding emphysema identifies severe disease. Among workers who began employment after the imposition of stricter dust controls in 1970, an abnormal chest x-ray has been found in approximately 5%, and less than 1% of these workers evidenced PMF.

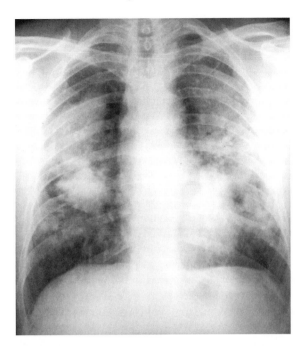

Figure 5 Coal workers' pneumoconiosis. Chest radiograph from an anthracite coal miner shows coarse, round opacities in high profusion and multiple coalescent masses typical of progressive massive fibrosis. (From Davis GS, Calhoun WJ. Occupational and environmental causes of interstitial lung disease. In: Schwarz MI, King TE, Jr, eds. Interstitial Lung Disease, 2nd ed. St. Louis, MO: Mosby Year Book, 1993: 179–229.)

Cough, sputum production, and chronic airflow limitation complicate lung disease in coal workers in several ways. First, substantial symptoms of bronchitis may be present before or without CWP, and workers may evidence spirometric airflow reduction with a normal chest radiograph. Second, emphysema is part of the pathological process of CWP and becomes widespread with advanced PMF; thus airflow limitation may be substantial. Last, tobacco smoking is common among miners (although prohibited at the coal face!), and conventional COPD may complicate the picture of lung disease in coal workers. Epidemiologically, the adverse effects of coal dust and smoking on lung function appear to be additive, not synergistic.

No specific treatments are known for the lung diseases caused by coal. As described for silica, supportive measures may be helpful. Prevention through reduction of inhaled coal dust must be the basis for control of these diseases.

Silicates, Clays, and Other Particles

Particles from a wide variety of stones, metals, and inorganic materials can be aerosolized during the course of working with them. Workers who inhale these dusts may develop respiratory symptoms, abnormal chest radiographs, and occasionally severe chronic lung disease if the exposure is sufficiently intense. These materials do not cause lung disease that is as prevalent or as severe as that due to silica or coal; many are considered to be "nuisance dusts" rather than specific respiratory toxicants. Exposure to these materials

Table 4 Activities That Produce Exposure to Nuisance Dusts

Activity or process	Industrial example
Mining to remove ore from the earth	Tin mining
Quarrying to remove stone from the earth	Slate quarry
Crafting stone into a final product	Cutting and polishing marble
Crushing or smelting ore to extract a metal	Iron smelter
Crushing stone to produce a powder product	Talc manufacturing
Adding a powder to a product mixture	Cement mixing
Utilizing a powder for an industrial process	Kaolin in porcelain china

takes place in many occupations but occurs through a few common types of activities, as summarized in Table 4.

Most of the materials considered in this section can be cleared successfully from the respiratory tract without causing a significant inflammatory response or structural damage as long as the dose is moderate. The materials considered to be nuisance dusts are believed to be nonfibrogenic and thus safe for human exposure at relatively high levels. Very high levels of dust exposure to virtually any material will cause cough, chest tightness, and a sense of dyspnea.

The mining and manufacturing processes involved with these less toxic materials often create exposures to silica, asbestiform fibers, chemical fumes, oxides of nitrogen, and other substances that can cause lung disease. For example, underground iron miners may need to drill through silica-bearing "hard rock" in order to access seams of iron ore. Asbestos minerals often contaminate industrial-grade talc. It may be very difficult to separate out the effects of individual components with this type of mixed exposure. A few of these materials are discussed below because they can cause recognizable pneumoconiosis or because exposure to them is very common.

Talc is a hydrated magnesium silicate, $Mg_3Si_4O_{10}(OH)_2$, with variable amounts of aluminum, iron, and calcium. The mineral occurs as a soft rock (soapstone), which fragments into small plates when crushed. Talc powder is used in a wide variety of applications that take advantage of its properties as a dry lubricant, an absorbent, and a bulk filler. Workers may be exposed to talc aerosols during the primary mining and milling of the mineral or during its secondary use for industrial processes. Talcosis develops slowly in heavily exposed individuals; this may be due to pure talc alone and also to contamination of talc with amphibole asbestos fibers and other minerals.

Pure talc, used for cosmetic purposes as face and body powder, is white in color and contains virtually no contaminants. Low-grade "fibrous" talc is widely used for industrial purposes; is tan, reddish, or gray in color; and contains up to 50% tremolite or anthophyllite asbestos with varying amounts of quartz and other crystalline silicates. Talc is used in the rubber industry to line molds, coat products, and keep sticky surfaces from adhering to one another. Talc is added as a filler or a smoothing agent in paints, plastics, and ceramics.

Talc can produce nodular lung lesions that may coalesce, diffuse interstitial fibrosis, and foreign-body granulomatous reactions. These patterns frequently coexist in a single patient, although they may appear independently. The chest radiograph shows small, rounded opacities with a middle-lung-zone predominance. These nodular infiltrates may coalesce with advanced disease and produce compensatory overinflation and distortion of adjacent upper and lower lung zones. Diffuse interstitial fibrosis can be seen in workers who have exposure to low-grade industrial talc, which contains tremolite and anthophyllite asbestos. The clinical course and features of the disease resemble those of asbestosis (see below) and are believed to be due to the contaminating fibers. The pathology of talcosis demonstrates ill-defined nodules composed of collagen, connective tissue matrix, and occasional cells. Talc particle plates can be seen within these lesions by polarized light microscopy.

Exposures to kaolin (china clay), diatomaceous earth, mica, and a variety of other silicates can cause moderately severe lung disease if the exposure is adequately intense and prolonged. These agents may be a problem for small numbers of workers in a particular industry, but they are not common causes of occupational lung disease. *Kaolin* is used to make porcelain china and also extensively in the manufacture of paper products and ceramics and as a filler in paint, rubber, and plastics. Heavily exposed workers develop small, irregular opacities on chest x-ray and also rounded opacities if silica is intermingled. Amorphous (noncrystalline) SiO_2 forms the skeleton of unicellular marine diatomes, settles to the sea floor when they die, and is compacted into *diatomaceous earth*. This easily powdered stone is used for lining molds, for its absorptive properties in filters, and as an additive in explosives. For some applications, the diatomaceous earth is heated intensely or "calcined," and some of it converts to crystalline cristobalite silica. Diffuse lung disease caused by diatomaceous earth resembles silicosis and is probably attributable to the silica component. *Mica* refers to a family of aluminum silicates with varying amounts of iron and magnesium that form dense, thin plates. The mica rock can be split or crushed to produce thin plates with useful thermal and electrical properties; it is used extensively for insulation, boiler liners, as a nonabsorptive bulk additive, and as a dry lubricant. Heavy exposure to mica dust can cause reticulonodular infiltrates of the lower lung zone and fine interstitial fibrosis.

Exposure to *cement* dust is often suggested as possibly causing lung disease, but it does so rarely. Portland cement is made from a mixture of stone and mineral powders. Clay, sand, oxides of aluminum, iron and magnesium, calcium silicate and calcium carbonate, gypsum, and other materials are mixed, ground together, and then heated to drive off impurities. The dry powders combine chemically when water is added to form a fused conglomerate mass. Cement is used widely throughout the world, and many thousands of workers are exposed to this material in a powdered form. Fortunately, most of the powder is composed of large particles, exposure is often out of doors, and the material is not highly fibrogenic. Workers involved in cement manufacture with high levels of exposure may show abnormal chest radiographs with small rounded and irregular opacities, and some studies have detected mild reductions in airflow rates. Clinically significant pneumoconiosis is rare.

Iron metal is extracted from iron oxide and carbonate ores by smelting at high heat. Respirable dust can be generated as the ore is mined from the earth in open pits or, more rarely, in underground tunnels. Iron in metallic form may also be aerosolized as it is formed into products and alloys, cut, ground, and abraded. Inhalation of iron and iron ore in pure form can result in densities on the chest radiograph, but it probably does not cause significant pulmonary dysfunction. The iron is so radioopaque that small amounts of it create quite abnormal x-rays. Many of the processes involved in iron mining, extraction, and fabrication involve coincident exposure to silica dust, chemical fumes, and other metals. It is probably these other materials that cause a decrement in pulmonary function in some iron workers.

LUNG DISEASES CAUSED BY INHALED FIBERS

Asbestos

Asbestos mineral fibers produce four major categories of human disease: pulmonary fibrosis (asbestosis), benign asbestos-related pleural responses, bronchogenic carcinoma, and mesothelioma. The likelihood of developing each of these conditions is generally related to the cumulative dose of asbestos received. True asbestosis (pulmonary fibrosis) is limited to individuals who receive high doses of exposure and requires many decades to develop fully, while pleural plaques can develop with much lower exposure, and mesothelioma is sometimes attributed to quite brief asbestos exposure.

The fibers of asbestos have wide application for insulation, friction-bearing surfaces, and composite materials to strengthen them. Asbestos-related diseases appear in workers involved in the primary extraction of asbestos from rock deposits, the fabrication and installation of products containing asbestos, the use of these products in a wide variety of unrelated trades, and their repair and removal. The common denominator of all these instances is occupational or environmental exposure to airborne asbestos fibers.

Mineralogy

Asbestos minerals occur in almost pure form in natural deposits in many parts of the world. These fibrous magnesium silicates have industrial value because of their physical properties and their great resistance to alteration by either chemical or physical means. The loose packing properties and heat-resistance of asbestos make it an excellent material for insulation of all sorts. The long, tough fibers can be woven into cloth with remarkable heat resistance. Asbestos added to resins or cement confers added strength to these composites.

Asbestos falls into two major mineral groups. *Chrysotile* (serpentine) asbestos appears physically as long, curly fibers. The *amphibole* asbestos types appear as needle-like crystals. The amphibole group of crocidolite, amosite, and others are important for their special properties, but their use has been progressively curtailed because of the excessive health risks that may be associated with them. Chrysotile accounts for more than 70% of the estimated annual world production of asbestos and for virtually all of the asbestos used in the United States. It is recovered from open-pit mines in Quebec, Russia, and elsewhere. Crocidolite, amosite, and anthophyllite are less important commercial sources of fiber. During the first two-thirds of the twentieth century, asbestos was used extensively for industrial products and for building or pipe insulation. Usage has decreased tremendously over the past 30 years since the health hazards have become widely known, and asbestos is now used primarily in applications where no safer substitute is available.

Occupational Exposure

Asbestos is removed from the earth in large blocks of virtually pure fibrous mineral. The crude rock is crushed and processed in mills, usually near the mine, in order to separate the fibrous material from contaminating bed rock. The fibers may then be carded like wool to align them for later weaving. Milling, carding, and packaging can aerosolize large numbers of small fibers and can present major health hazards unless dust levels are strictly controlled.

Asbestos is mixed with asphalt tar to produce roofing tiles and with other binders and resins to make brake linings, clutch pads, flooring and wall materials, insulation for electrical circuits, and many other products. Loose asbestos was used extensively for insulation in former times, particularly in ships' boilers and steam fittings, and insulation workers in all industries received exposure. Asbestos insulation, or lagging, was sprayed with a binder onto pipes, walls, ceilings, and other surfaces. About 75% of the current U.S. asbestos utilization is in the construction trades, where insulation, tiles, wallboards, cement foundations, and other materials may contain asbestos. The fibers are tightly bound in resins or composites as these products come from the factory, but fibers may be aerosolized as they are cut, drilled, ground, or shaped during installation.

There is great public concern over health risks from asbestos in schools, homes, and office buildings, where it may be present in floor tiles, ceiling tiles, acoustic ceiling coverings, wall insulation, and pipe coverings. Asbestos may slowly flake off or be eroded into the air of the building from these sources. The amount of asbestos in these environments is too little to cause pulmonary fibrosis. The increased risk of mesothelioma or lung cancer due to these exposures has not been precisely defined but is probably slight. Properly installed, intact building materials that contain asbestos probably represent a very minimal health risk for those who live and work around them. Quite a different risk may be present when installed asbestos materials are cut, renovated, removed, or decay with age. Removal or maintenance may generate aerosols with significant asbestos fiber counts, and these environments may become health risks for individuals who spend considerable time in them. Maintenance personnel are at particularly great risk of asbestos exposure, since they may spend a working lifetime disturbing or removing asbestos materials from different sites within the same institution or workplace.

Asbestosis

The symptoms and signs of asbestosis are not distinguishable from idiopathic pulmonary fibrosis (IPF) (see Chap. 29) except for the history of substantial asbestos exposure. The insidious onset of shortness of breath with exertion is usually the first sign of asbestosis but does not appear until many years after asbestos exposure began and may occur only decades after exposure ceased. Thus asbestosis (like IPF) is almost always a disease of persons over the age of 50 or 60 years. Cough is frequent and is usually paroxysmal and nonproductive. Scant mucoid sputum may accompany cough in later stages of disease. Dyspnea at rest, edema associated with cor pulmonale, and ultimately respiratory failure may appear in the final stages of severe asbestosis.

The physical findings of asbestosis are typical of IPF as well. Fine end-inspiratory high-pitched crackles (rales, crepitations) are heard initially over the lung bases and become more extensive as disease progresses. Digital clubbing is common but does not correlate with the extent of pulmonary dysfunction. Symptomatic hypertrophic pulmonary osteoarthropathy is rare and should provoke a search for a bronchogenic carcinoma. Edema, jugular venous distention, a right ventricular heave, and gallop rhythm appear as late signs of cor pulmonale.

The pathology of asbestosis is that of diffuse interstitial fibrosis with the added presence of asbestos fibers and "asbestos bodies." Advanced asbestosis demonstrates small, firm lungs, often with thickened pleura and associated pleural plaques (see below). Seen by microscope, the earliest lesions of asbestosis appear in the respiratory bronchioles. As disease progresses, second- and third-order bronchioles and alveolar ducts become diseased and the process encompasses increasing numbers of lobules. Fibrosis affects the septal planes and appears to radiate out from the central unit. Finally, extensive fibrosis engulfs and distorts the normal structures to create a honeycomb pattern with dense bands of collagen bordering cyst-like empty spaces. Asbestos fibers that have become coated with a bead-like deposit of protein and iron are called asbestos bodies (AB) or ferruginous

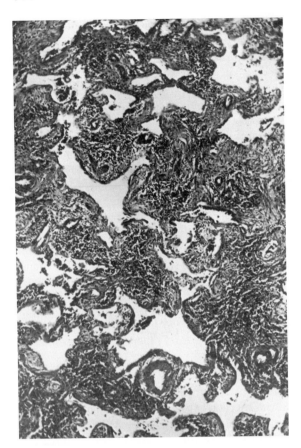

Figure 6   Asbestosis. Lung tissue histopathology demonstrates moderately advanced pulmonary asbestosis with diffuse interstitial disease and marked distortion of lung architecture. (From Davis GS, Calhoun WJ. Occupational and environmental causes of interstitial lung disease. In: Schwarz MI, King TE, Jr, eds. Interstitial Lung Disease, 2nd ed. St. Louis, MO: Mosby Year Book, 1993: 179–229.)

bodies and are found in the lung tissue, BAL fluid, and sometimes sputum of workers with substantial asbestos exposure. Crocidolite and other amphiboles appear to generate AB much more readily than serpentine chrysotile. The abundance of AB or uncoated fibers in tissue sections, ashed tissue samples, and BAL fluid correlates reasonably well with both the magnitude of exposure and the extent of disease. Fig. 6 illustrates the pathology of asbestosis.

Asbestosis provides a characteristic pattern of small irregular shadows with a lower-lung-zone predominance. This is not unique for asbestosis, and asbestosis cannot be distinguished from IPF on these grounds alone. Associated pleural changes of asbestos-related disease (see below) may increase confidence in a purely radiological diagnosis, but an appropriate asbestos exposure history is required to establish the cause of disease. Computed tomography enhances both the specificity and sensitivity of detecting diffuse interstitial lung disease due to asbestos. Figures 7 and 8 illustrate the radiographic features of asbestosis.

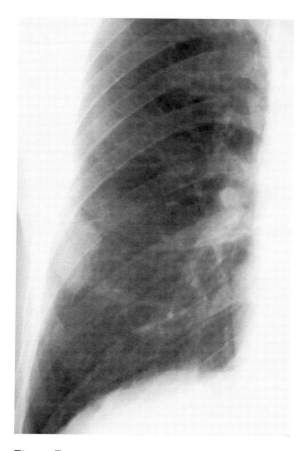

Figure 7   Asbestosis. Chest radiograph from a shipyard worker shows small, irregular shadows in low to moderate profusion and a pleural plaque in the right middle lung zone. (From Davis GS, Calhoun WJ. Occupational and environmental causes of interstitial lung disease. In: Schwarz MI, King TE, Jr, eds. Interstitial Lung Disease, 2nd ed. St. Louis, MO: Mosby Year Book, 1993: 179–229.)

Pulmonary function tests in asbestosis reflect small, stiff lungs with abnormal gas transfer. The vital capacity is reduced. Airflow rates are usually normal unless chronic airways disease of other cause is present as well. The total lung capacity and its subdivisions are reduced proportionately. Carbon monoxide gas transfer (single-breath DL_{CO}) is typically reduced. Arterial hypoxemia is initially detected only with exercise and then becomes abnormal at rest as well as with advancing disease. Hypercarbia is found only in the terminal stages of severe asbestosis. In contrast to silicosis or coal worker's pneumoconiosis, substantial physiological abnormality and disability may be present in asbestosis with only relatively mild changes on the chest radiograph.

The clinical course of asbestosis is usually protracted, and progression is very gradual. A worker with 10 years of moderate exposure during his twenties and thirties might not evidence symptoms or radiographic changes until his late forties or fifties, might retire early with disability in his late fifties or sixties, and might die prematurely of respiratory insufficiency in his sixties or seventies. There is no specific treatment for asbestosis; prevention is the only means of controlling this disease. The anti-inflammatory/cytotoxic drug treatments offered for IPF have not been tested rigorously in asbestosis, but clinical experience suggests no benefit from these agents. Lung transplantation offers hope for younger, otherwise healthy patients with advanced asbestosis.

Benign Asbestos-Related Pleural Disease

Pleural plaques appear as patches of fibrous thickening on the parietal pleura in response to asbestos. These lesions are distinctive on chest radiographs but cause little or no significant symptoms or disability. Plaques are a marker of substantial asbestos exposure rather than a cause of substantial disease. Pleural plaques are illustrated in Fig. 8. The prevalence of pleural plaques in groups of asbestos workers increases with age and the intensity of exposure. Families of asbestos workers and people living near asbestos manufacturing sites may also have asbestos-related plaques. The pleural plaques are dense, raised lesions found almost exclusively on the parietal surface, with normal or nearly normal visceral pleura apposed to them. Central plates of dystrophic calcification often form within the plaques.

Pleural plaques appear on the chest radiograph as multiple round or irregularly shaped flat lesions several centimeters or more in diameter and several millimeters in thickness. They occur most frequently against the inner surface of the ribs, particularly in a posterior and lateral position, and over the central tendinous portion of the diaphragm. Distribution is bilateral, and the appearance of a single lesion alone should prompt consideration of diagnoses other than asbestos-related disease. Calcified plaques appear to have a dense white line within them when viewed in profile. The presence of bilateral linear diaphragmatic or midlung pleural calcifications is strongly supportive of a diagnosis of

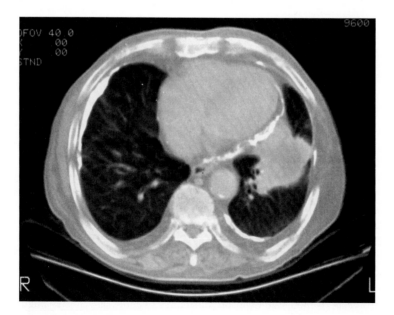

Figure 8 Asbestos-related disease. Computed tomography of the lower thorax in a 71-year-old asbestos worker reveals a mass of trapped left lung; this proved to be rounded atelectasis. Peripheral irregular opacities in the lung parenchyma, as well as extensive pleural calcification along the right anterolateral and left posterior chest wall and the pericardium, are also evident.

significant asbestos exposure and asbestos-related disease. Computed tomography demonstrates these pleural abnormalities beautifully.

Pleural plaques are associated with mild pulmonary physiological abnormalities. Although pleural plaques without other disease were originally believed to be of no clinical significance, more recent studies indicate that these lesions are associated with decreased vital capacity and FEV_1. Plaques with an otherwise normal plain chest roentgenogram may be associated with diffuse interstitial lung disease detectable by HRCT scan.

Benign pleural effusions sometimes occur in patients with asbestos exposure, asbestosis, or pleural plaques. The effusions are exudates but may be serous or serosanguinous. They are more common early in the course of asbestos-related disease, usually small in volume, and generally asymptomatic. Substantially compromised lung function is unusual; the effusions can, however, be associated with chronic chest pain. They may be quite chronic or may recur intermittently in one or both lungs. The main problem with asbestos pleural effusion is the diagnostic concern that it may represent a malignant effusion associated with mesothelioma or bronchogenic carcinoma in patients who are at greatly increased risk for these diseases. Unfortunately, no definitive features other than negative test results and the passage of time can rule out malignancy in these cases.

Lung Cancer

Bronchogenic carcinoma is linked to asbestos exposure in tobacco smokers. The mineral appears to act as a cocarcinogen and primarily as a ''promoter'' under circumstances where tobacco smoke substances are ''inducers'' of neoplasia. The cancer risk appears to be dose-related with both asbestos exposure and smoking intensity and increases cancer incidence rates up to 50-fold. Nonsmokers who are exposed to asbestos have slight or no increased risk of bronchogenic carcinoma. Enhanced cancer risk encompasses all commercial types of asbestos and all major cell types of bronchogenic carcinoma. Lung cancer is a substantial risk for smokers even at levels of asbestos exposure that are below those expected to produce pulmonary fibrosis. The presentation, diagnosis, and management is the same as for lung cancers in the general population. Individuals with exposure to asbestos must be encouraged most strongly to stop smoking, and smokers with asbestos exposure must be watched with unusual vigilance for the appearance of bronchogenic carcinoma. Surveillance programs involving annual or semiannual chest radiographs and sputum cytology examinations may be justified in this high-risk group.

Mesothelioma

Malignant mesothelioma is an aggressive mesenchymal tumor that can arise in the peritoneal or pleural space. It develops in a small proportion of individuals many years after asbestos exposure and very rarely in those with no known exposure to this fiber. Mesothelioma presents with dyspnea due to effusion and loss of lung volume as well as with chest wall pain. This tumor may occur after relatively slight asbestos exposure, and environmental fiber pollution levels which are quite safe regarding pulmonary fibrosis may not be safe regarding mesothelioma. It is a major source for the concern surrounding asbestos insulation and building products in schools and homes. Unfortunately, no effective treatment for mesothelioma has been found; aggressive surgery, radiotherapy, or chemotherapy must be viewed with little enthusiasm, and care is largely supportive.

Wollastonite

Wollastonite is a calcium silicate mineral fiber quarried from surface mines at several locations. The crushed stone yields relatively short, thick, straight fibers with a low length-to-width ratio. Wollastonite is used as a strengthening agent in plastics and ceramics and as an asbestos substitute in other industrial applications. Reports from Finland have indicated an excess prevalence of pleural plaques and one possible case of mesothelioma among wollastonite workers, but it is unclear whether contaminating asbestos or other minerals could have complicated the exposure. Cross-sectional surveys of mine and mill workers exposed to wollastonite at a New York State site have not shown excess respiratory disease.

Glass and Ceramic Fibers

Synthetic glass and ceramic fibers are used widely, and exposure to them is often considered as a possible cause of lung disease. They deserve discussion for this reason, although they rarely cause significant illness. Synthetic vitreous fibers include what is commonly called fiberglass or glass wool as well as long glass fibers and ceramic fibers. These materials have experienced intense industrial development and wide use as substitutes for asbestos in providing insulation and durability. All of these products are manufactured by heating minerals to a molten state and then using centrifugal force to spin the pliable material into long, thin fibers. Rapid cooling leaves the compound in an amorphous noncrystalline state. The fibers are all similar in appearance: straight or slightly curved with blunt angulated ends and a high length-to-width ratio.

Glass wool is used extensively for heat and sound insulation in homes and businesses, where it may be installed as a loose blown wool fiber or preformed into batts, panels, tapes, or tiles. It has completely replaced asbestos in these applications. Workers may be exposed to airborne respirable fibers in the plant where the glass wool is produced, in secondary manufacturing facilities where panels or tiles are made, and during installation or removal from building sites. The health effects of glass wool have been studied extensively in animal models and in cohorts of human workers; virtually no adverse effects have been observed. Irritation of the skin and mucous membranes is common with extensive contact and is attributed to larger fibers. Prolonged inhalation studies in rodents showed no pulmonary fibrosis and only a minimal cellular inflammatory response. Human surveys have not shown excess respiratory symptoms, radiographic opacities, or pulmonary function deficits in manufacturing plant or product installation workers.

Refractory ceramic fibers are made from kaolin or other aluminum silicates and are used in special applications where highly heat-resistant, chemically inert insulating materials are needed. Insulation for furnaces and kilns, papers, and textiles used under highly adverse conditions; high-temperature gaskets; and similar products are made from ceramic fibers. The health effects of refractory ceramic fibers may be less benign than those of glass wool. Studies in rodents have revealed variable pulmonary fibrosis and occasional examples of mesothelioma and lung cancer. Surveys in human workers suggest an increased prevalence of pleural changes but not pulmonary fibrosis.

LUNG DISEASES CAUSED BY COBALT

Cobalt causes three patterns of lung disease: (1) a chronic diffuse interstitial lung disease that leads to pulmonary fibrosis (cobalt pneumoconiosis), (2) a relatively acute interstitial disease with features of hypersensitivity pneumonitis, and (3) an obstructive airways disease that resembles occupational asthma. The same industrial exposure can cause each of these patterns in different workers. Even more confusing, features of more than one pattern may be seen in the same patient.

Mineralogy

Elemental cobalt is used widely as a hardener and binder in metal alloys of tungsten, aluminum, chrome, molybdenum, beryllium, and others. It is employed also to bind microdiamond dust to surfaces for use as abrasives. Tungsten carbide, the "hard metal" that originally gave cobalt pneumoconiosis its name, is made by mixing very small particles of tungsten, carbon, and up to 25% cobalt and then sintering the mixture at high heat to produce an extremely hard and heat-stable alloy. The particles of the original mixture of powdered metals are very fine, with most in the 1- to 2-μm range; thus they are easily inhaled and deposited deep in the lung. Small particles liberated from the abrasive wheel or cutting tool may also be inhaled, carrying cobalt with them into the lung. Cobalt is relatively soluble and may form salts under biological conditions. Although often detectable in the lung with electron probe analysis or other special techniques, the cobalt may also be leached out of the tissue, leaving only the inert carrier particles.

Workplace Exposure

Tools made of tungsten carbide are used extensively for drilling, cutting, or milling where heat resistance or longevity are important features. Particles of tungsten carbide are bound or glued to the surfaces of plates or wheels to produce durable grinding implements for shaping and polishing other materials. Metal foundry workers have exposure to the original powdered mixture of cobalt and other metals and may inhale this dust during the manufacture of alloy ingots or the fabrication of the alloy into secondary products. Tool makers may be exposed to sizable aerosols of particles as they grind, bore, and shape hard metal blanks into tools and parts. Coolants and cutting oils are used to cool and lubricate the cutting point as tools are fabricated, and may be aerosolized with small particles as they are sprayed onto the cutting surface of the rapidly moving parts. Cobalt is soluble in certain coolants and may accumulate in the liquid as cobalt-alloy metals are cut. Workers using abrasives that contain tungsten carbide chips or cobalt binders may receive exposure as their grinding wheels decay and liberate aerosols from the rapidly turning surfaces. Dental technicians who work in close proximity to the crowns and prostheses they are grinding can develop cobalt pneumoconiosis. Thus lung disease due to cobalt may occur among those who make tools or parts from hard metal or sintered diamond dust abrasives, and also among those who grind or polish a variety of other materials with abrasives.

Cobalt Pneumoconiosis (Hard Metal Disease)

A distinctive chronic interstitial lung disease occurs in workers exposed chronically to cobalt: it is referred to as cobalt pneumoconiosis, cobalt-tungsten-carbide pneumoconiosis, or hard metal disease. The association with cobalt rather than the other hard metal components was confirmed when typical features of the disease were found in diamond polishers with no exposure to tungsten carbide but who used abrasives composed of diamond dust bound with cobalt.

Dyspnea with exertion and nonproductive cough are early symptoms of cobalt pneumoconiosis and worsen as exposure continues and disease progresses. Physical examina-

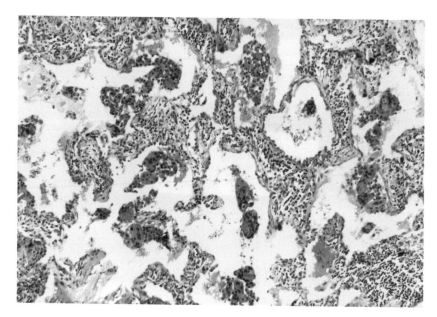

Figure 9   Cobalt pneumoconiosis. A lung biopsy specimen from a tungsten-carbide worker demonstrates interstitial pneumonitis with occasional very large, bizarre multinucleated giant cells—a pattern consistent with giant-cell interstitial pneumonitis. (From Davis GS, Calhoun WJ. Occupational and environmental causes of interstitial lung disease. In: Schwarz MI, King TE, Jr, eds. Interstitial Lung Disease, 2nd ed. St. Louis, MO: Mosby Year Book, 1993: 179–229.)

tion demonstrates fine basilar crackles that become more coarse with progression of disease. Digital clubbing is common. Pulmonary function abnormalities include a reduction in all lung volumes, lowered carbon monoxide gas transfer (DL_{CO}), and hypoxemia at rest that worsens with exercise. Airflow reduction is variable but usually not prominent. Cobalt pneumoconiosis usually develops in workers only after prolonged exposure, often 10 or more years in the industry.

"Giant-cell interstitial pneumonitis," as described by Liebow before the cause was known, is the distinctive pathological change associated with cobalt pneumoconiosis. The giant cells have a different appearance than is usually seen with either foreign-body reactions or sarcoidosis and assume bizarre forms. The alveolar spaces are packed with macrophages and type II pneumocytes, suggesting desquamative interstitial pneumonitis. Alveolar walls show proliferation of type II epithelium (cuboidalization). Bronchiolitis obliterans may be seen, but vasculitis is not. The particulates related to abrasives and sometimes elemental cobalt may be found by scanning electron microscopy and electron probe analysis but are usually too small and nonrefractile to be found by polarized light microscopy. Cobalt pneumoconiosis in the lung tissue of a tungsten carbide worker is illustrated in Fig. 9.

The chest radiograph shows small, irregular opacities predominantly in the lower lung zones, although coarser patterns and more widespread infiltrates can also be seen and honeycombing may develop in late disease. A pattern of perihilar ground-glass infiltrates is sometimes seen in more acute disease. Symptoms and pulmonary functional impairment often precede radiographic changes. Thus, the chest radiograph may appear normal despite significant complaints, definite physiological impairment, and pathological changes on lung biopsy. One should not await x-ray changes before pursuing hard-metal disease in appropriately exposed workers.

The clinical course of cobalt pneumoconiosis is variable. Most workers have prolonged exposure before the disease becomes apparent, and the onset of symptoms is insidious. Many improve after ceasing exposure to the offending agent; with time, cobalt should be leached from their lung tissues. Some patients experience persistent symptoms and progression of disease after exposure stops. The most important aspect of treatment is removal of the cobalt-alloy aerosol from the work environment. In some instances this can be achieved by industrial hygiene measures that extract air and dust from the cutting or grinding surface. In other cases it may be necessary for the sensitized worker to change jobs or leave the industry. Corticosteroid therapy has resulted in improvement in several reported cases; steroids are more likely to be helpful if the disease is relatively acute and in its early stages. A trial of steroid therapy is probably warranted in most cases of proven cobalt pneumoconiosis.

Cobalt Hypersensitivity Pneumonitis

Features that suggest hypersensitivity pneumonitis (see Chap. 40) have been found in several cases of cobalt exposure and may represent one clinical form of cobalt pneumoconiosis. Symptoms developed rather abruptly, were persistent, or appeared to follow exposure immediately, and the disease improved with removal of exposure to the offending agent. Increased numbers of lymphocytes with a predominance of CD8+(suppressor-cytolytic) cells and eosinophils were found in BAL specimens. It is not clear whether hypersensitivity pneumonitis due to cobalt is a separate disease from the more common chronic progressive form of hard metal disease or whether they represent two clinical extremes of the same spectrum.

Cobalt Asthma

Cobalt sintered in hard metal and other abrasives can cause occupational asthma (see Chap. 26), highlighting the variety of pulmonary immunological responses to cobalt in provoking lung disease. In contrast to the pneumoconioses, occupational asthma due to cobalt may develop soon after work exposure begins and presents with a different symptom complex. Patients with acute airflow limitation occurring upon exposure to the work environment or to bronchial provocation challenge with cobalt were included in several case series of apparent cobalt pneumoconiosis. The symptoms and airflow obstruction in these patients occurred promptly upon exposure and persisted for hours or days after challenge. These responses occurred in workers who did not appear to have diffuse interstitial lung disease. Rhinitis, conjunctival irritation, and contact dermatitis have also been attributed to cobalt sensitivity. These reports suggest that cobalt shares with platinum, nickel, and other metals the ability to sensitize exposed workers and to provoke a variety of hypersensitivity reactions; cross-reactivity among these metals can sometimes be found in sensitive patients. It is not clear whether the responses are directed to the metal as an antigen or, more likely, whether it denatures autologous proteins to form unique haptens or neoantigens.

LUNG DISEASES CAUSED BY BERYLLIUM

Exposure to the metal beryllium produces chronic beryllium disease, or berylliosis, a lung disease that is clinically identical to sarcoidosis. The disease is caused by sensitization resulting in a cell-mediated immune response, with chronic granulomatous inflammation and fibrosis. Although relatively few individuals receive exposures to beryllium that cause lung disease, it is an important model for genetics, immune responses, and pathogenetic processes in lung diseases where the causative agent is not known.

The Metal and the Workplace

Beryllium (element Be) is a light metal with applications in specialized industries. It occurs in beryl (beryllium aluminum silicate), euclase, bertanite, and other ores, from which it is extracted by smelting. The metal is used in pure form or alloyed with aluminum, copper, or nickel to craft nuclear reactor components, nuclear weapons parts, tools and dies of special purpose, aircraft parts, and electronic components. Internalization and sensitization to beryllium takes place primarily by aerosol inhalation and can occur from exposure to ore, purified metal, or even alloys with less than 5% beryllium.

Workers may be exposed to aerosolized beryllium during ore processing, secondary metal manufacture, or tooling and fabrication of final products. People living in the vicinity of beryllium processing plants and family members of beryllium workers may develop berylliosis. The exposure required to cause sensitization varies greatly, from a few months to more than four decades, but the risk is related to the intensity of exposure. With stringent industrial hygiene measures that provide low ambient levels and current limitation of the use of beryllium to a few selected industrial applications, the prevalence of the disease has decreased greatly in recent decades.

Clinical Features

The symptoms, signs, radiographic abnormalities, and histopathology of chronic beryllium disease are essentially those of sarcoidosis, as described in detail in Chap. 28. The insidious onset of dyspnea and nonproductive cough are typical symptoms. Some patients may also develop fever, central chest pain, and arthalgias. Although involvement of the skin, liver, heart, and other organs can occur, most patients demonstrate only thoracic disease. Physical examination is nonspecific and often unrevealing unless extrathoracic disease is present. The radiographic features include diffuse parenchymal nodules and opacities, particularly along the course of bronchovascular bundles and at subpleural locations. Hilar adenopathy is common. Calcification within lymph nodes and lung nodules may occur over time. Large, conglomerate masses with adjacent traction emphysema may form in advanced disease. The pathology of involved tissue is noncaseating granulomas with fibrosis. Beryllium may or may not be detectable within affected tissue; special techniques are required to identify this low-molecular-weight element. The diagnosis of chronic beryllium disease is established—and distinguished from sarcoidosis—by compatible granulomas or mononuclear cell infiltrates in tissue, a history of beryllium exposure, and demonstration of an immunospecific cell-mediated response to beryllium.

If the disease is not recognized and exposure continues, progressive lung dysfunction can proceed rapidly. Slower progression can occur long after exposure ceases, presumably due to persistent beryllium in lung tissue as an antigen. Specific therapy is similar to that for sarcoidosis. Corticosteroids usually suppress symptoms and slow or stop organ dysfunction. Prolonged treatment, the use of alternative cytotoxic agents, and ultimately lung transplantation may be needed for some patients.

Intense high-dose exposure to aerosolized beryllium can cause an acute chemical pneumonitis, a problem largely seen before the imposition of strict environmental control measures. A high proportion (15–30%) of workers who experienced the acute beryllium pneumonitis went on to develop chronic beryllium disease. Exposure to beryllium carries a slightly increased risk for lung cancer, after adjustment for smoking and other factors, with a standard mortality ratio (SMR) of approximately 1.5 in several studies.

Immune Mechanisms and Genetics

Patients with chronic beryllium disease demonstrate T-lymphocyte activation and proliferation upon exposure to beryllium compounds. This cell-mediated immune response forms the basis for an in vitro laboratory test available at a few national centers that allows identification of sensitized individuals, the *beryllium lymphocyte proliferation test*. The peripheral blood lymphocytes from most patients with chronic beryllium disease demonstrate a positive proliferation response, while in other patients only lung lymphocytes recovered by BAL show a positive test. A proportion of beryllium workers demonstrate positive in vitro tests without symptoms or signs of disease. A greater than expected fraction of these sensitized individuals will progress to overt disease if exposure continues.

CONCLUSIONS

Occupational lung disease occurs at the interface between industry and medicine. The diseases cannot be understood without a clear picture of the materials and work environments responsible for them. The workplaces cannot be modified and made safe without an understanding of the diseases that develop in them. This process is constantly changing as new materials, new industries, and changing economic forces create new diseases or a different environment in which old ones develop. Within this dynamic process there is always the potential for tension between the health concerns to create as safe a workplace as possible and the economic motives to operate an industry as efficiently as possible. It is the challenge of health care providers to identify and treat occupational lung diseases when they occur and to help guide safe, economically sound work practices that prevent them from occurring.

SUGGESTED READING

Silica

1. American Thoracic Society Committee of the Scientific Assembly on Environmental and Occupational Health. Adverse effects of crystalline silica exposure. Am J Respir Crit Care Med 1997; 155:761–768.
2. Craighead JE, Kleinerman J, Abraham JL, Gibbs AR, Green FHY, Harley RA, Ruettner JR, Vallyathan NV, Juliano EB. Diseases associated with exposure to silica and nonfibrous silicate minerals. Silicosis and Silicate Disease Committee. Arch Pathol Lab Med 1988; 112:673–720.
3. Davis GS. Pathogenesis of silicosis: current concepts and hypotheses. Lung 1986; 164:139–154.

4. Weill H, McDonald JC. Exposure to crystalline silica and risk of lung cancer: the epidemiological evidence. Thorax 1996; 51:97–102.

Coal

1. Remy-Jardin M, Remy J, Farre I, Marquette CH. Computed tomographic evaluation of silicosis and coal workers' pneumoconiosis. Radiol Clin N Am 1992; 30:1155–1176.
2. Weeks JL. From explosions to black lung: a history of efforts to control coal mine dust. Occup Med 1993; 8:1–18.

Silicates, Clays, and Other Particles

1. Abrams HK. Diatomaceous earth silicosis. Am J Ind Med 1990; 18:591–597.
2. Short SR, Petsonk EL. Respiratory health risks among nonmetal miners. Occup Med 1993; 8:57–70.
3. Wergeland E, Andersen A, Baerheim A. Morbidity and mortality in talc-exposed workers. Am J Ind Med 1990; 17:505–513.

Asbestos

1. Craighead JE, Abraham JL, Churg A, Green FHY, Kleinerman J, Pratt PC, Seemayer TA, Vallyathan V, Weill H. The pathology of asbestos-associated diseases of the lungs and pleural cavities: diagnostic criteria and proposed grading schema. Arch Pathol Lab Med 1982; 106:540–597.
2. Kamp DW, Weitzman SA. Asbestosis: clinical spectrum and pathogenic mechanisms. Proc Soc Exp Biol Med 1997; 214:12–26.
3. Mossman BT, Bignon J, Corn M, Seaton A, Gee JBL. Asbestos: scientific developments and implications for public policy. Science 1990; 247:294–301.

Glass and Ceramic Fibers

1. Bignon J, Brochard P, Brown R, Davis JM, Vu V, Gibbs G, Greim M, Oberdorster G, Sebastian P. Assessment of the toxicity of man-made fibres: a final report of a workshop held in Paris, France 3–4 February 1994. Ann Occup Hyg 1995; 39:89–106.
2. Glass LR, Brown RC, Hoskins JA. Health effects of refractory ceramic fibres: scientific issues and policy considerations. Occup Environ Med 1995; 52:433–440.

Cobalt

1. Cugell DW, Morgan WK, Perkins DG, Rubin A. The respiratory effects of cobalt. Arch Intern Med 1990; 150:177–183.

Beryllium

1. Kreiss K, Miller F, Newman LS, Ojo-Amaize EA, Rossman MD, Saltini C. Chronic beryllium disease—from the workplace to cellular immunology, molecular immunogenetics, and back. Clin Immunol Immunopathol 1994; 71:123–129.
2. Newman LS, Lloyd J, Daniloff E. The natural history of beryllium sensitization and chronic beryllium disease. Environ Health Perspect 1996; 104(suppl 5):937–943.

40

Hypersensitivity Pneumonitis

Gerald S. Davis

University of Vermont College of Medicine
Fletcher Allen Health Care
Burlington, Vermont

Hypersensitivity pneumonitis (HP) is a diffuse parenchymal lung disease produced by the immunological response to an inhaled antigenic agent, usually as a result of intense and sometimes prolonged exposure in the workplace, through a hobby, or in the home. In the United Kingdom the condition is referred to as extrinsic allergic alveolitis (EAA). Although the list of agents and exposures that may cause the disease is long and growing, the pathogenetic mechanisms and clinical features are the same in all instances. The common features appear to be (1) an intense and/or repeated exposure to an inhaled, usually particulate antigen small enough to reach the distal lung; (2) a susceptible individual; (3) a T lymphocyte–driven cell-mediated pulmonary immune response that results in transient or persistent lung parenchymal inflammation; and (4) possible fibrosis if the disease persists. The clinical features are often highly suggestive but may be nonspecific and confused with other diseases. Treatment rests on recognition and avoidance of the offending antigen.

CLINICAL FEATURES

HP can present in an acute form characterized by distinct episodes of brief illness or in a chronic form with gradually progressive symptoms. Both patterns respond favorably to antigen removal. In a minority of patients, the chronic form can manifest diffuse interstitial scarring and resemble idiopathic pulmonary fibrosis (IPF). Some authors refer to the chronic progressive pattern as "subacute" and identify only the end-stage fibrotic disease as "chronic." The pattern that develops in a particular patient will depend on the antigen, the nature of the exposure, and possibly on the immune response characteristics of the individual.

Acute Hypersensitivity Pneumonitis

Patients with the acute form of HP develop shortness of breath, cough with little or no sputum production, pulmonary infiltrates, fever, muscle aches, and generalized malaise 2

697

to 9 h following exposure to an antigen to which they are sensitized. The peak of symptoms occurs typically about 6 h after exposure. Physical examination of the chest may be normal, or it may demonstrate scattered rhonchi or reveal bilateral crackles. Leukocytosis with neutrophilia (but without eosinophilia), hypoxemia at rest that worsens with exertion, and a reduced vital capacity may be found on diagnostic testing. The symptoms and signs improve spontaneously within 24–72 h of their onset, although subtle abnormalities may persist for weeks after an episode of exposure. As described below, the type of exposure that leads to episodes of acute HP usually involves periodic, intense contact with the antigen rather than continuous daily exposure.

For the patient, the illness develops many hours after the exposure; thus the link between cause and effect may not be obvious. For the clinician, the signs and symptoms are identical to those of an acute respiratory tract infection. The chest radiograph (Fig. 1) may be normal, demonstrate subtle diffuse abnormalities, or show patchy or lobar consolidation. For these reasons most initial or infrequent episodes of acute HP are diagnosed as influenza, viral bronchitis, or community-acquired pneumonia. It is only after repeated episodes occur too frequently to be written off as "the flu" or when signs and symptoms become chronic that many patients undergo the evaluation needed to produce a definitive diagnosis.

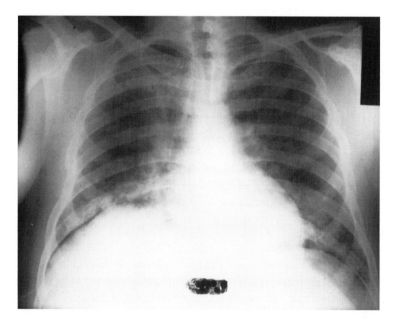

Figure 1 Acute hypersensitivity pneumonitis. A 34-year-old Vermont dairy farmer worked in a 100-year-old barn feeding baled hay and milking tied cows at stations. He developed repeated episodes of cough, dyspnea, and low-grade fever through November and December, and made several physician visits where antibiotics were prescribed. By January he had also noted exercise limitation and weight loss. A seaside vacation relieved all symptoms, but he became acutely ill on the first day of milking after his return. Evaluation revealed scattered crackles on examination, leukocytosis, and restrictive pulmonary physiology. The chest radiograph (above) showed patchy bilateral infiltrates. His serum contained precipitating antibodies against *Faeni rectivirgula*. He left the barn work temporarily and all symptoms cleared. He was able to return to work after the farm was modernized with a free-stall barn and a milking parlor and was converted to chopped silage for feed.

Chronic Hypersensitivity Pneumonitis

The chronic form of hypersensitivity pneumonitis (HP) presents as a progressive diffuse parenchymal lung disease. Dyspnea with exertion that is relatively constant from day to day, chronic cough with little sputum, and mild malaise or anorexia bring the patient to medical attention. Some patients may present with symptoms resembling chronic bronchitis and relatively little dyspnea. Physical examination typically reveals bi-basilar or diffuse crackles in the chest, or it may be normal. Wheezing is uncommon. Digital clubbing is generally not seen in HP, although it may be a feature of very late fibrotic disease. Routine laboratory studies are generally unrevealing and nonspecific. The radiograph usually demonstrates small irregular or rounded opacities in a diffuse pattern (see Fig. 2).

Patients with chronic HP may not be able to date the onset of their symptoms precisely, may or may not be aware of variation in symptoms at different times, but usually describe gradual worsening of their condition. If exposure ceases, they will almost always improve spontaneously within days or weeks.

Radiology

The features of HP on conventional posteroanterior and lateral chest radiographs are highly variable. With the acute form of HP, ground-glass opacities are often present; they may be patchy or may be localized in one or more sites resembling a community-acquired pneumonia. Pleural abnormalities or calcifications are very rare. Slight hilar adenopathy may be seen occasionally, but it is never prominent. A pattern of ill-defined small, rounded opacities and/or small, irregular shadows is common in both the acute and chronic forms of HP and probably corresponds to the typical abnormality found on high-resolution computed tomography (HRCT). A normal chest radiograph can be found in many patients with the acute form of HP, particularly between episodes. A pattern of peripheral fibrosis and ''honeycombing'' occurs in patients with advanced, chronic HP and may be indistinguishable from IPF on plain films.

The pattern of HP revealed by HRCT scanning is quite distinctive and may be virtually diagnostic if the clinical setting is appropriate. Small nodules with a surrounding rim of ground-glass opacity found at the center of each lobule represent the typical (possibly almost pathognomonic) HRCT pattern of HP. This abnormality is illustrated in Fig. 2 of this chapter and in Fig. 11 in Chap. 11. The centrilobular nodules are usually most abundant in the mid- and lower lung zones, sparing the apices, and are distributed uniformly from central to peripheral tissue. Mild enlargement of hilar and mediastinal lymph nodes may be seen. The pleura and airways are usually normal. These abnormalities appear to be entirely reversible with an end to exposure. A pattern of fibrosis resembling IPF, sometimes with zones of hyperinflation and emphysema, may be found in advanced chronic disease.

The radiographic patterns of HP may resemble those of other diffuse lung diseases. Sarcoidosis usually demonstrates nodules adjacent to larger airways and vessels (axillary pattern) and at subpleural locations. IPF is typically more patchy and more peripheral within the involved lobes; it shows early bands of fibrosis and a reticular pattern. Bronchiolitis obliterans organizing pneumonia (BOOP) can resemble acute HP, with patchy ground-glass opacities but usually can be distinguished radiographically from the picture of chronic HP.

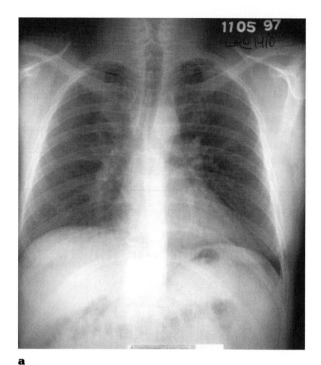

a

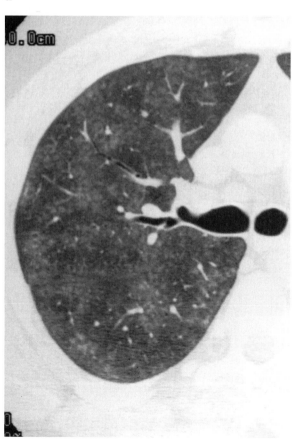

b

Pulmonary Function Testing

Pulmonary function testing typically demonstrates a "restrictive" pattern, a reduced vital capacity and a proportionately decreased FEV_1, and a reduced total lung capacity with its subdivisions. Airflow rates (FEV_1/FVC ratio, peak flow, $FEF_{25-75\%}$) are usually normal. Measures of gas exchange (P_{O_2}, O_2 saturation, DL_{CO}) are typically decreased at rest but may be normal. Oxygen desaturation with exertion may be striking and may appear to be out of proportion to the degree of other physiological or radiographic abnormalities. For this reason, it is very useful to routinely test oxygen saturation with walking in patients with suspected or confirmed HP.

Nonspecific airway hyperreactivity (manifest by increased sensitivity to methacholine inhalation challenge) is common in HP, although wheezing is not heard on physical examination, airflow rates are normal, and the primary pathophysiologic site of antigen-immune cell interaction appears to be the alveolus. This observation, and the presentation of some patients with primarily bronchitis symptoms, suggests that airway inflammation as well as alveolitis is an important part of HP. As noted elsewhere in this book, many agents can cause either HP or asthma in different subjects and occasionally even in the same person. *Aspergillus* species fungi, cobalt metal, and the diisocyanate chemicals are examples of this variation in responses.

AGENTS AND ENVIRONMENTAL EXPOSURES

The agents that cause HP share the common features that they are respirable, they are antigenic, and they can trigger a cell-mediated immune response in susceptible individuals. Most of these agents are inhaled as particles, although some may be fumes or chemical materials that are adsorbed to particle surfaces. In almost all instances the inhaled materials are very small (0.5–5.0 μm diameter) and are deposited at an alveolar level; some larger particulate antigens may be deposited within the airways and then solubilized, such as the spores of *Alternaria* fungi.

Most of the materials that cause HP are complex organic particles, not single pure antigens. Fungal spores, bacterial debris, or bird droppings and feathers all contain many proteins and glycoproteins that may be antigenic to differing degrees or may trigger responses of different intensity in different individuals. The complex nature of this material

---

Figure 2 Chronic hypersensitivity pneumonitis. A 36-year-old computer company engineer sought medical evaluation for 6 weeks of gradually worsening malaise, cough without sputum, and dyspnea with exertion. No clues to diagnosis were elicited at the initial evaluation. Spirometry showed mild reduction in volume without airflow obstruction; arterial blood gases at rest were normal but with a slightly widened alveolar–arterial oxygen gradient of 30 torr, and oxygen desaturation to 80% was observed with walking. A chest radiograph showed diffuse small, irregular opacities (panel A); high-resolution computed tomography demonstrated centrilobular nodules with surrounding ground-glass opacities (panel B). Further questioning revealed that he owned two cockateel birds that had been in his home for 5 years. He took a scheduled 1-week vacation, the birds were removed, and the home cleaned thoroughly. After 1 week his symptoms had improved but pulmonary function remained abnormal; after 6 weeks, he had complete resolution of symptoms and all tests were normal.

Table 1   Agents and Exposures Associated with Hypersensitivity Pneumonitis

Agent	Source	Disease
Microbiological agents		
Faeni rectivirgula	Moldy hay	Farmer's lung disease
Thermoactinomyces vulgaris	Mushroom compost	Mushroom worker's disease
Aspergillus species	Moldy beer malt	Malt worker's disease
Cryptostroma corticale	Decaying maple bark	Maple bark stripper's disease
Penicillium casei	Cheese mold	Cheese worker's lung
Penicillium frequentans	Moldy cork	Suberosis
Pullularia species	Moldy redwood	Sequoiosis
Aureobasidium species	Sauna, hot-tub water	Sauna taker's disease
Trichosporon cutaneum	House dust	Japanese summerhouse disease
Bacillus subtilus	Detergent enzymes	Detergent worker's disease
Animal proteins		
Pigeon proteins	Serum, feathers, droppings	Pigeon breeder's disease
Parakeet proteins	Serum, feathers, droppings	Budgie fancier's disease
Turkey proteins	Turkey materials	Turkey handler's lung
Rat proteins	Rat urinary proteins	Laboratory worker's lung
Chemicals		
Toluene diisocyanate	Epoxy polymers, plastics industry	Hypersensitivity pneumonitis
Phthalic anhydride		

is probably important in causing the features of HP as it is clinically recognized, but the mechanisms are not known.

People encounter respirable particulate antigens in a vast variety of environments, but the dose and duration of exposure are not usually sufficient to induce complete sensitization. As noted below, many individuals with appropriate exposure will evidence a humoral immune response (serum antibody), and some may even demonstrate cell-mediated immune responses (lymphocyte transformation) with no clinical features of disease. Most of the occupations, hobbies, or living environments that produce HP create exposures to distinctive antigenic materials that involve repeated high-dose inhalation and/or prolonged contact. The agents that cause HP can be grouped broadly into three categories: microbiological agents, proteins, or chemicals. Many of these occur in distinctive work environments, and HP in those settings has been labeled with the name of the job. Table 1 lists a selection of these conditions.

Farmer's Lung Disease

HP was described for the first time in farmers handling moldy hay and was dubbed Farmer's lung disease (FLD). It has become the prototype for HP, and is described in detail to illustrate several features of both the environmental circumstances and the clinical consequences associated with this condition. FLD is due in most instances to the growth of heat-loving bacteria that participate in the decomposition of organic material. If wet hay is baled in the field or packed tightly into a hay mow, the hay begins to ferment and decompose. Wet climates such as those of Britain, New England, and the northern Midwest favor this circumstance, as frequent rains prevent complete drying of the hay before bailing. The initial stages of decomposition are dominated by molds and bacteria that function at ambient temperatures, but fermentation produces heat. Chopped silage ferments more rapidly, creates acid conditions, and does not heat as much as baled hay. As the temperature within the hay bale or mow rises to 56°–60°C, the conditions become disadvantageous for most microorganisms but ideal for the thermophilic actinomycetes and related bacteria. *Faeni rectivirgula* (formerly *Micropolyspora faeni*) and *Thermoactinomyces vulgaris* are the most common agents, with *T. candidus*, *T. viridis*, and others also found. These organisms proliferate and secrete degradative enzymes as long as the temperature remains high and water is plentiful. The heat drives off water through evaporation, and fermentation consumes water. As the hay dries out and begins to cool, the thermophilic organisms stop proliferating and undergo sporulation. The spores of *F. rectivirgula* are extremely small (1–2 μm), and very lightweight; thus they are easily aerosolized when the hay is disturbed.

Farmers break open bales of hay to feed cows and other livestock. When a bale of "moldy hay" contaminated by thermophiles is opened, a puff of white, smoke-like dust rises from the bale. This puff of dust is distinctive and looks quite different from the heavier, tan, less easily distributed field soil dust that is present in most bales. Virtually all farmers will recognize this feature. Most bales of hay will not have this appearance, but occasional bales will be readily identified as moldy. As the farmer breaks open a moldy bale by hand, his face will be immediately next to the bale and will be surrounded by a cloud of respirable spores.

In the conventional "tie-stall" or "station" dairy barn, cows are immobilized by their necks at their stations; the dairyman breaks open a bale of hay and spreads slabs of hay in front of the cows. He then returns to place and later removes mechanical milkers while they eat. Finally, the scattered or uneaten hay will be swept up and removed, along with manure and bedding. The exposure to moldy hay in the barn is most intense during the winter and early spring months. The hay harvested in the fall has had time to ferment, the cows are dependent on stored feed, and the barn is closed up to preserve heat. In this workplace the farmer has close contact with hay throughout the work cycle, but particularly during the morning and afternoon milking times.

If most of the hay is clean, and only the rare bale is moldy, the dairyman may have only occasional intense exposure to thermophilic antigens, and may likely develop the acute form of HP. Exposure to a bale of moldy hay might occur at 4 P.M., but peak symptoms of acute HP would not be apparent until about 10 P.M. If many bales are moldy or moldy hay remains scattered in the barn, chronic HP may be more likely. Chronic HP could develop in this setting because most dairymen work in the barn all day, even when new feed is not being placed before the cows. The symptoms would become gradually more apparent as the winter progressed.

The economics of dairy farming have changed the workplace and made FLD less common. Few farmers today can earn a living working with a small dairy herd feeding baled hay and milking at stations in a tie barn. Larger-scale mechanized farming allows more cows to be managed by fewer farmhands and has replaced the labor-intensive traditional approach of the family farm. Large "free-stall" barns, open on three or four sides to a surrounding paddock, allow cows to move about at will. Hay and corn are chopped for silage in the field, stored in large silos or bunkers, and fed into troughs at the center of the free-stall barns. The fodder is never moved by hand but is harvested and distributed by power machinery. The cows move periodically into a milking parlor, where they receive grain and where 4–20 cows can be milked simultaneously by one person in a central pit.

These newer methods reduce thermophilic bacterial growth because the hay is not baled, improve ventilation because the barn is open, and decrease human contact with the feed material because it is handled by machinery and located away from the milking activities.

Microbiological Agents

Numerous microbial agents can cause HP. The thermophilic actinomycetes implicated in FLD grow in decaying vegetable matter in many other environments and cause diseases such as mushroom worker's lung among those composting the substrate for commercial food mushrooms. Common molds are ubiquitous but can grow to high concentrations in wet environments or where commercial materials decay. Diseases such as maple bark stripper's disease (*C. corticale* growing beneath the bark), malt worker's lung (*Aspergillus* species growing on the malt), cheese worker's lung (*Penicillium caseii*), or suberosis (*P. frequentans* growing on moldy cork) are examples of fungi that cause HP. Roof thatching, wine grape pressing, brewing soy sauce, and numerous other occupations that involve exposure to organic materials that may become moldy have been linked with colorful names for HP. Bacteria can also produce HP, and notable outbreaks have been associated with *Bacillus subtilis* enzymes used in laundry detergent and with *Pseudomonas* growing in cooling fluid for tool machining.

Domestic as well as commercial environments can produce HP due to microbial contamination. A form of HP known as Japanese summerhouse disease is due to *Trichosporon cutaneum* growing in moist wood and floor mats; it is common among those who spend substantial time in their houses in wet parts of Japan during the summer months. The thermophilic actinomycetes can grow in the water pans of humidifiers that are in the ducts of home heating systems using forced hot air furnaces and also in the condensate of air conditioning units, causing humidifier lung or air conditioner lung. Molds growing around hot tubs, saunas, and spas can be domestic or resort sources of disease.

Proteins

Avian proteins are a common cause of HP; proteins in serum, droppings, and feathers are implicated. Pet parakeets (budgerigars, or budgies in Britain) are a frequent source of continuous exposure to avian antigens and often cause the chronic form of HP. Virtually all varieties of domestic pet birds have been associated with HP, including parrots, cockateels, canaries, and love birds. Although exposure is maximum when the bird's cage is being cleaned, the antigens may linger in the home for many months after the birds are removed.

Pigeon breeders have been studied extensively with regard to HP, because the disease is common among them. These hobbyists raise flocks of homing pigeons for racing, transport the birds to remote locations, and then time their return to the home roost. The fancier's pigeon coop or dove cote typically is located on the roof of a city building or in a rural outbuilding. Exposure to the avian antigens may occur intermittently when the birds are fed or cleaned and is often intense. Family members occasionally may develop HP from contact with contaminated clothing even if they have no direct contact with the birds. Pillows and quilts stuffed with feathers can cause HP, but it is rare. Typical disease has been found among workers who raise geese, ducks, turkeys, and other birds for commercial purposes. Although chickens are abundant, these birds seem to be an uncommon cause of HP.

Mammalian proteins cause HP only very rarely. A similar disease has been described among furriers, possibly due to skin and hair antigens. Research laboratory workers may occasionally develop HP from rodent antigens in urine, but occupational asthma is much more common in this setting. Insect proteins can cause HP, as with *Sitophilus granarius* grain weevils causing miller's lung or silkworm larvae proteins causing disease in silk workers. Even molluscan proteins can be antigenic, as with oyster shells causing HP in workers crafting mother-of-pearl.

Chemicals

Chemicals can trigger the immune responses that produce HP. The responsible materials are believed to act as haptens and/or to denature host proteins to create neoantigens that are recognized as foreign. The same materials that commonly cause occupational asthma through this mechanism occasionally produce HP (see Chap. 38). Toluene diisocyanate and other isocyanates used in two-part paints and varnishes, phthalic anhydride and related compounds used in the plastics industry, pyrethrum insecticide, and other chemicals have been implicated in isolated cases. These materials do not appear to be as important a cause of HP as organic particulates.

PATHOGENESIS

The mechanisms of disease leading to the clinical expression of HP appear to rest on a cell-mediated immune response to the offending antigen and on a consequent cascade of events resulting in tissue inflammation, injury, and eventually altered connective tissue matrix with fibrosis. Although this general sequence of events can be invoked for many or acute and chronic lung diseases, there are unique and distinguishing features in HP.

The tissue pathology is believed to reflect the mechanisms of disease. Lung biopsies are usually obtained in patients with chronic HP or frequent and prolonged episodes of acute HP; thus the pathology of early acute HP is usually not captured. Lung biopsy tissue from a patient with HP shows interstitial mononuclear cell infiltrates, a cellular bronchiolitis, and loosely formed non-necrotizing granulomas. The infiltrate is very bronchocentric, surrounding small airways with mononuclear cells and filling adjacent alveoli with lymphocytes, macrophages, and cellular debris. This is probably a parallel to the pattern seen on HRCT radiographs. Neutrophils usually are few in number and eosinophils are uncommon. Vasculitis is not seen. Many specimens demonstrate areas of bronchiolitis with organizing pneumonia (BOOP), but a mononuclear infiltrate and loose granulomas are also seen in these specimens. Sites of emphysema and areas of interstitial fibrosis may be found, particularly in more advanced disease. The pathological pattern of HP is usually distinct enough to allow a specific diagnosis, particularly in an appropriate clinical setting. This pattern could suggest sarcoidosis or idiopathic BOOP; it could also suggest fungal or mycobacterial infection, and these should be ruled out by appropriate stains and culture. If the disease is very patchy, relatively indolent, or only a small specimen is available, a specific diagnosis may not be possible. Transbronchial biopsy may be sufficient to establish a diagnosis of HP in some instances but offers only 50% specificity; a more generous thoracoscopic or open lung biopsy may be needed in many cases.

Immunological Features in Humans

Characterization of the immune responses has been limited by the availability of suitable antigens. Avian serum proteins can serve as a source of antigens that are free of contaminating toxins, can be quantified in dose, and can be purified into single proteins; thus the immunology of HP has been elucidated using pigeon serum for antigen and breeders as sources of responding cells. Extracts of fungal or thermophilic antigens are problematic because they frequently include exotoxins or other materials that may stimulate or poison test cells nonspecifically.

The key feature of the immune response in HP appears to be a sensitized population of T lymphocytes that is responsive to the offending antigen. In humans, these cells can sometimes be detected in peripheral blood and almost always in bronchoalveolar lavage (BAL) cell populations by exposing lymphocytes in culture to the cognate antigen and observing blast transformation or other indices of a cellular response.

The BAL fluid of patients with HP is believed to offer a reflection of the disease process. The percentage of lymphocytes is greatly increased, exceeding 40% of all cells in most cases and approaching 80% in many instances. In contrast, normal subjects have approximately 10% lymphocytes, and patients with active sarcoidosis will usually demonstrate 20–40% lymphocytes. The BAL lymphocyte population in HP is dominated by CD8+ rather than CD4+ T cells, with ratio of a CD4+ to CD8+ of less than 1.0 and often less than 0.5. By comparison, normal subjects exhibit a ratio of CD4+ to CD8+ of about 1.5; active sarcoidosis shows a strong CD4+ predominance with ratios in excess of 2.0. These patterns may be useful clinically in establishing a diagnosis of HP.

The CD8+ suppressor/cytolytic T-cells in the lungs of HP patients appear to participate in a chronic granulomatous inflammatory response that is associated with elaboration of the cytokine interferon-γ and follows a pattern characterized as a T response of the Th1 type. This might be expected in a granulomatous disease. In this paradigm, lymphocytes of the Th2 type would be scarce and interleukin-4 (IL-4) and IL-5 would not be produced in abundance; thus eosinophils would not be attracted or activated at sites of disease. This concept highlights an essential difference in mechanisms between HP and asthma (a Th2-type, IL-4 and IL-5–abundant, eosinophil- and IgE-mediated disease). It is clinically relevant in explaining the absence of eosinophils from the blood, lung biopsy, and BAL fluid of patients with HP.

A BAL fluid sample with increased lymphocytes and a CD8+ predominance can be found in exposed workers who do not have clinical HP. Although this result does not appear to predict future disease, its implications are not fully understood. An essential difference between subjects without overt lung disease may be the function of CD8+ cells as suppressor cells, rather than those with disease, in whom these cells may function as amplifiers of the inflammatory response.

Humoral immune responses can be detected routinely in patients with HP, but they appear to be secondary or incidental rather than a direct cause of lung disease. Antibodies directed against multiple antigens from the offending agent can be detected in the serum of patients with HP. When patient serum is placed in a well cut in agar on a glass slide, an extract of the offending agent is placed in a second well nearby, and the materials allowed to diffuse toward one another through the agar, one or several lines of antigen-antibody precipitate will form between the wells. This "double-diffusion Ouchterlony" test is the basis of clinical tests for "precipitins" or "precipitating antibodies" against suspected antigens. It is used to screen patients for possible HP. These antibodies are of the IgG class. Notably, IgE antibodies are not found in HP, patients are usually not atopic, and thus HP is not an "allergic" disease.

Unfortunately, humoral antibodies against the environmental agents that trigger HP are entirely nonspecific. These precipitating antibodies are an indication of substantial exposure but not of clinical disease. Precipitating antibodies are very common among appropriately exposed individuals, and relevant precipitins can be found in up to 50% of pigeon breeders or dairy farmers who have no clinical evidence of lung disease. Testing an individual patient for precipitins may be helpful in confirming a suspected exposure or searching for a possible antigen when none is known, but a positive precipitin test does not in any way establish the diagnosis of HP.

Animal Models of Disease

Models of HP in rodents provide insight into which immune responses are important and clinically relevant. As shown by Schuyler and associates, the disease can be created by sensitizing animals through repeated respiratory exposure to appropriate antigens. Populations of lymphocytes from sensitized mice can be expanded in culture in vitro with antigen, transfused into naive animals, and produce lung disease upon initial inhalation challenge. Although CD8+ lymphocytes are numerous in vivo, successful adoptive transfer depends on naive and memory-type activated CD4+ lymphocytes from the sensitized animal. Cell-free serum from sensitized mice contains antibodies but cannot transfer experimental HP to naive animals. These observations highlight the importance of cell-mediated immunity in the pathogenesis of HP.

PREVALENCE

A small fraction of people exposed to respirable antigens develop HP. The exposure must be intense and must be repeated on multiple occasions or involve relatively continuous contact. As many as 50% of dairy farmers, pigeon breeders, or mushroom workers with appropriate exposure may demonstrate precipitating antibodies in their serum, but only a minority will evidence clinical disease. Population studies based largely on symptom questionnaires have detected HP in as few as 0.5% or as many as 20% of exposed individuals. On average, about 5–8% of people with suitable exposure may be expected to develop clinical symptoms and signs of HP. These observations suggest that the genetics of immune responsiveness must coincide with exposure to produce disease. No specific associations between the prevalence of histocompatibility locus markers (HLA-A, -B, -C, -DR) and HP has been detected despite attempts in several surveys.

There is an unexpectedly low incidence of HP among tobacco smokers. While about 30% of the adult population are smokers, only 5–20% of HP patient groups are smokers. The prevalence of serum antibody is skewed similarly away from smokers in exposed populations. It is postulated that the immune suppressant effects of tobacco smoke decrease sensitization and/or the intensity of the immune response. These statistics do not exclude the possibility of HP as a cause of an unknown lung disease in a smoker, but they do make it less likely.

DIAGNOSIS

Establishing a diagnosis of HP requires key elements of history coupled with objective findings. Although the diagnosis may be obvious in some cases, it is often obscure and difficult to pin down in others. The diagnostic studies that may be useful in establishing a diagnosis of HP are summarized in Table 2. A secure diagnosis requires an appropriate exposure to a candidate antigen (sometimes confirmed by serum antibody), compatible clinical symptoms and signs, distinctive findings on chest CT, lung biopsy, or BAL fluid analysis, and the exclusion of other diseases that might be mistaken for HP. Combinations of these concepts have been proposed by Terho as major and minor criteria for the diagnosis of FLD. An additional criterion might include clinical improvement following removal from antigen exposure, and this is essential for a favorable outcome. In some instances, clinical improvement upon withdrawal from the suspected antigen and worsening with reexposure to the antigen may serve as adequate proof for diagnosis, and invasive studies may not be required.

A detailed environmental and occupational exposure history by an interviewer who is knowledgeable about HP is an essential component of this evaluation. Work type, chemicals and materials used, hobbies and crafts, pets, contact with large animals and their feed or bedding, home heating and air-conditioning systems, and known exposure to moldy environments must be explored in detail. Physical examination should seek chest crackles as confirmatory findings or wheezes as evidence against the diagnosis. A plain chest x-ray may be useful, but an HRCT scan will offer much more detailed and specific information. Pulmonary function testing can offer compatible abnormalities but is quite nonspecific; it may be more useful in establishing the severity of the disease than its cause. Serum precipitin testing may be useful to document exposure if it is in doubt, but it is not essential and a positive test is not proof of disease. Skin testing for either immediate or delayed-type hypersensitivity is not useful. Transbronchial or thoracoscopic lung biopsy can be used to confirm the diagnosis of HP if necessary; in other cases it is the histology that suggests the diagnosis before the offending antigen exposure is known. These test results may strongly suggest a diagnosis of HP and a likely agent that is causing it. Reproduction of the disease upon reexposure and/or disappearance of the disease when exposure stops are required in many cases to confirm the diagnosis of HP.

Exposure of sensitized patients with HP to the offending antigen can be dramatic and even hazardous. Direct bronchial provocation or laboratory exposure to purified antigens is rarely wise, practical, or necessary except for research protocols. There are few if any purified HP antigens suitable for human inhalation exposure, and extracts of microbial

Table 2   Diagnostic Tests for Hypersensitivity Pneumonitis

Detailed occupational, hobby, and environmental history
Chest examination with crackles
Chest radiograph with patchy or diffuse infiltrates
High-resolution computed tomography scan with centrilobular densities
Pulmonary function testing with
    A restrictive pattern
    Exercise hypoxemia
    A reduced diffusing capacity (DL_{CO})
Serum antibodies against potential offending agents
Lung biopsy with granulomatous alveolar and bronchiolar infiltrates
Bronchoalveolar lavage fluid with high lymphocyte fraction
Bronchoalveolar lavage fluid with CD8+ lymphocyte predominance
Compatible symptoms and signs upon natural exposure to the antigen
Clinical improvement following antigen removal

agents may contain toxins that produce nonspecific responses. Doses are not standardized, and may be too low to produce the desired responses or dangerously high and produce excessive disease. Although laboratory bronchial provocation testing is rarely indicated, monitoring the response to a natural exposure that may have caused the disease in the first place is often a useful clinical tool. Similarly, stopping exposure and documenting improvement provides valuable information as well as treatment. A brief vacation for the patient provides an excellent opportunity to test both aspects of exposure; interviews and pulmonary function testing before the holiday, immediately upon return but before reexposure, and then after exposure may document both improvement and acute deterioration. Similar testing before and several hours after a work shift can provide useful information. Complete spirometry (vital capacity) is usually needed because a ''restrictive'' test pattern is typical, and home peak flow monitoring by patients may not be sensitive.

PROGNOSIS

The prognosis for patients with HP is generally excellent if a diagnosis is made early in the course of disease and exposure to the offending antigen ceases. Pulmonary function and chest radiograph findings return to normal in most patients if exposure stops. Resolution can be expected in several weeks or less in the acute form of the disease, while the chronic form may require a longer time for symptoms and pulmonary tests to normalize. Continuing exposure will lead to repeated episodes of acute illness or progressive loss of lung function. Among dairy farmers, long-term pulmonary function abnormalities are uncommon even if occasional exposure occurs, although some groups have shown more substantial deterioration. Pigeon breeders in the United States and Europe have a good prognosis. Significant morbidity and mortality have been observed in other countries, possibly because the birds are customarily kept in the home rather than in a separate dovecote. Among pigeon breeders, the severity of abnormalities at presentation did not predict their long-term outcome, but a shorter duration of exposure to the hobby and a younger age at presentation were favorable predictive factors. Patients with the chronic pattern of disease who present with more advanced abnormalities and honeycomb changes on HRCT scan may not recover full function, and some degree of disease progression may occur.

THERAPY

The treatment of HP rests primarily on separating the patient from the antigen responsible for the disease. This treatment requires correct identification of the specific agent (e.g., *F. rectivirgula*), or at least the environment in which it is located (the barn). For most patients, this identification may have great financial or emotional implications, since they may need to give up their occupation, their hobby, or a favorite pet. Separating the patient from these activities may be far more difficult than making the diagnosis. Because of the importance of these changes in the life of the patient, it is essential that a secure diagnosis be established and that the clinician's advice be based on sound evidence and not speculation. The most definitive treatment will be for the dairy farmer to stop farming and move away from the farm, for the pigeon racer to give up both birds and hobby, or for the parakeet owner to sell the bird and clean the house intensively. This ideal solution may not be possible or acceptable for some patients.

Respiratory protection devices offer a limited solution to decreasing antigen exposure for some workers. Once sensitized, HP patients need only a very small exposure to antigen in order to trigger a significant response. Respiratory protection strategies usually reduce exposure but do not eliminate it entirely; thus they may not provide adequate treatment for many patients. Simple paper dust masks are virtually useless because they do not filter out small particles effectively, and substantial air flows around the mask and into the respiratory tract. Fitted rubber face masks with dual filter units offer better protection but may still allow some entry of antigen. A full hood respirator with an independent positive-pressure air source does offer a clean breathing environment. All of these devices have substantial shortcomings, however. The independent air source units are expensive, heavy, and cumbersome to move about; they require a hose to an isolated compressor or an independent portable tank. Both air hoods and fitted rubber masks may be hot, confining, and very difficult to use for heavy work that requires a high minute ventilation. These devices are practical for short-term intermittent use, particularly at low-intensity tasks. They are not a practical solution for a lifetime of day-long use in the workplace. The clothes worn by workers are contaminated with antigen particles and may provide secondary exposure after the mask is removed.

Modification of the environment to reduce or prevent antigen exposure appears to be an adequate solution for some patients with HP. It may be possible for pigeon breeders to contact their birds for short periods of time out of the roost if someone else cleans and cares for them in the roost. Modernization of a dairy farm may reduce the abundance of antigen by shifting away from baled hay and may reduce exposure by building new barns. If a worker contacts antigen only during selected, infrequent activities, it may be possible to shift that worker to other tasks or to use respiratory protection during that activity.

Corticosteroid therapy is effective in the short term for relieving symptoms and accelerating the resolution of disease. It is not a substitute for ending antigen exposure and is not needed for most patients. If corticosteroids are to be used, doses of prednisone (or equivalent) in the range of 30–60 mg per day for 5–10 days, then tapering to complete therapy in 2–4 weeks would be appropriate. Occasional patients experience intense exposure and intense acute reactions that require hospitalization and immediate steroid therapy, but this is rare. Supplemental oxygen may be required for patients during acute episodes or during recovery, particularly with exertion, and should be prescribed using the usual guidelines (see Chap. 22).

HP is a fascinating disease involving complex cell-mediated immune responses, substantial individual differences in susceptibility, and a wide variety of colorful occupations that provide exposure to suitable antigens. HP offers a great diagnostic challenge in many instances, and successful treatment often involves major lifestyle changes. Fortunately, for the great majority of patients with HP, the prognosis is very good if the correct diagnosis is made and appropriate changes in exposure can be achieved.

SUGGESTED READING

1. Ando M, Suga M, Nishiura Y, Miyajima M. Summer-type hypersensitivity pneumonitis. Intern Med 1995; 34:707–712.
2. Baur X. Hypersensitivity pneumonitis (extrinsic allergic alveolitis) induced by isocyanates. J Allergy Clin Immunol 1995; 95:1004–1010.
3. Daroowalla F, Raghu G. Hypersensitivity pneumonitis. Comp Ther 1997; 23:244–248.

4. Lacasse Y, Fraser RS, Fournier M, Cormier Y. Diagnostic accuracy of transbronchial biopsy in acute farmer's lung disease. Chest 1997; 112:1459–1465.
5. Lynch DA, Newell JD, Logan PM, King TEJ, Muller NL. Can CT distinguish hypersensitivity pneumonitis from idiopathic pulmonary fibrosis? AJR 1995; 165:807–811.
6. Reynolds HY, Fulmer JD, Kazmierowski JA, Roberts WC. Analysis of cellular and protein content of bronchoalveolar lavage fluid from patients with idiopathic pulmonary fibrosis and chronic hypersensitivity pneumonitis. J Clin Invest 1977; 59:165–175.
7. Richerson HB, Bernstein IL, Fink JN, Hunninghake GW, Novey HS, Reed CE, Salvaggio JE, Schuyler MR, Schwartz HJ, Stechschulte DJ. Guidelines for the clinical evaluation of hypersensitivity pneumonitis: Report of the Subcommittee on Hypersensitivity Pneumonitis. J Allergy Clin Immunol 1989; 84:839–844.
8. Rose C, King TEJ. Controversies in hypersensitivity pneumonitis. Am Rev Respir Dis 1992; 145:1–2.
9. Schuyler M, Gott K, Cherne A, Edwards B. Th1 CD4+ cells adoptively transfer experimental hypersensitivity pneumonitis. Cell Immunol 1997; 1997; 177:169–175.
10. Schuyler M, Cormier Y. The diagnosis of hypersensitivity pneumonitis. Chest 1997; 111:534–536.
11. Sharma OP. Hypersensitivity pneumonitis. Disease-a-Month 1991; 37:409–471.
12. Terho EO. Diagnostic criteria for farmer's lung disease. Am J Ind Med 1986; 10:329–334.

41

Evaluation of Respiratory Impairment and Disability

Akshay Sood and Carrie A. Redlich
Yale University School of Medicine
Yale–New Haven Hospital
New Haven, Connecticut

INTRODUCTION

Health care providers are frequently asked to determine whether individuals have any respiratory impairment and/or disability. To evaluate respiratory impairment and disability, the physician must assess both the patient's clinical condition and the job requirements. Two important questions should be addressed: Are there objective impairments in lung function? Will these impairments in lung function limit the patient's ability to work?

Impairment and disability evaluations are frequently performed in the context of an evaluation for benefits or compensation, such as social security disability or workmen's compensation. It is important that the physician understand the system of evaluation and his or her specific role in the process.

BASIC DEFINITIONS

Practitioners need to understand some basic terms used in disability evaluation.

Impairment means loss of physical or physiological function. *Disability* refers to the impact of the impairment on the person's life. An impairment or disability may be characterized in terms of expected duration and severity. A permanent impairment or disability is not expected to substantially improve with time and/or further treatment. A temporary impairment or disability can be expected to improve to a higher level of function with time and/or further treatment. An impairment or disability may also be characterized as partial or total. Impairment is usually characterized and "rated" from mild to severe or by more specific categories using specific guidelines, as noted below. *Total disability* usually implies that an individual is unable to perform gainful employment. *Partial disability* refers to a lesser degree of disability than total, usually implying that the individual can do certain types of work.

Impairment may occur without any disability. For example, a person with moderate emphysema whose work entails word processing at a desk may have measurable impairment but little resultant disability. Similarly, disability may occur without a measurable impairment. For example, a painter at an auto body shop with isocyanate asthma may be 100% disabled from working in the shop but may have no measurable impairment if removed from work early on in the disease process. Two people with the same degree of impairment may have quite different resultant disabilities, based upon occupational, psychosocial, and educational factors.

GUIDELINES FOR DISABILITY EVALUATION

Patients may seek disability benefits under a number of different entitlement programs that frequently have different eligibility criteria. The physician's role is not to determine whether the patient is entitled to certain benefits but to determine, objectively, the presence and extent of any respiratory problem and—in the case of workmen's compensation— whether the problem is work-related.

The U.S. Social Security Administration, Department of Veterans' Affairs, American Medical Association (AMA) (*Guides to the Evaluation of Permanent Impairment*), and the American Thoracic Society (ATS) official statements are the most commonly used guides for evaluating pulmonary disability. For pulmonary disability arising from occupational disorders, criteria from the various state workmen's compensation boards are also used. Many states use the AMA guidelines for determining workmen's compensation.

CLINICAL APPROACH TO EVALUATING PULMONARY DISABILITY

Impairment evaluations are based on the subject's history, general physical examination, pulmonary function tests, and chest radiograph.

The relevant features to elicit in the history include dyspnea, cough, sputum production, wheezing, environmental exposures, tobacco use, and a careful occupational history. The occupational history should focus on a description of relevant current and past employment including exposures, the relationship between exposures and symptoms, and the use of personal protective equipment. Patients should be encouraged to obtain Material Safety Data Sheets (MSDS) from their employers to better identify exposures.

Physical examination should include a description of breathing pattern, cyanosis, clubbing, adventitious lung sounds, and evidence of cor pulmonale.

Pulmonary Function Tests (PFTs)

The tests most commonly used for impairment evaluation are spirometry and diffusing capacity for carbon monoxide (DL_{CO}). It is important to make sure that the patient understands the test and gives a good reproducible effort according to the ATS guidelines.

The spirometric test results are expressed as percentage predicted based on the individual's height, age, and sex. The prediction equations commonly used are those of Crapo et al. from nonsmoking, asymptomatic individuals. Adjustments for predicted normal values have been recommended for race by some authors. The single-breath (DL_{CO}) is a test which can be prone to substantial inter- and intralaboratory variations and thus must be performed carefully according to the ATS performance criteria.

Table 1 American Medical Association Classification of Respiratory Impairment[a]

American Medical Association	Class 1 (0%, no impairment of the whole person)	Class 2 (10–25%, mild impairment of the whole person)	Class 3 (26–50%, moderate impairment of the whole person)	Class 4 (51–100%, severe impairment of the whole person)
FVC	≥80%	60–79%	51–59%	≤50%
FEV$_1$	≥80%	60–79%	41–59%	≤40%
DL$_{CO}$	≥70%	60–69%	41–59%	≤40%
ABG				Resting hypoxia[b]

Key: FVC, forced vital capacity; FEV$_1$, forced expiratory volume in the first second; DL$_{CO}$, diffusing capacity of carbon monoxide; ABG, arterial blood gases.

[a] Predicted values are based on height, age and sex of white Americans, from Crapo et al. The FEV$_1$, FVC, and DL$_{CO}$ numbers are expressed as percentages of the predicted value.

[b] Resting hypoxia is defined as Pa$_{O_2}$ of 50 mmHg on room air or less than 60 mmHg on room air in presence of pulmonary hypertension, cor pulmonale, or erythrocytosis documented on two occasions at least 4 weeks apart.

Source: Adapted from American Medical Association. Guides to the Evaluation of Permanent Impairment, 4th ed. Chicago: American Medical Association, 1993:153.

Table 1 outlines the frequently used AMA classification of respiratory impairment, which is quite similar to the ATS classification. At least one of the measures of ventilatory function should be abnormal to the degree described if the impairment is to be rated in that class.

Chest Roentgenograms

Chest roentgenograms are helpful in establishing a pulmonary diagnosis but generally are not useful in determining the level of impairment.

Arterial Blood Gas Determination

Resting arterial Pa$_{O_2}$ frequently does not correlate well with exercise capacity or symptoms of breathlessness. Arterial blood-gas determination may be useful if hypoxemia is suspected. According to the AMA guidelines, resting hypoxia is defined as Pa$_{O_2}$ of 50 mmHg on room air, or a Pa$_{O_2}$ of less than 60 mmHg on room air in the presence of pulmonary hypertension, cor pulmonale, worsening hypoxemia during exercise, or erythrocytosis. Hypoxemia should be documented on two occasions at least 4 weeks apart; if present, it indicates severe impairment by itself, as per the AMA guidelines.

Cardiopulmonary Exercise Testing

Cardiopulmonary exercise testing is not routinely recommended for assessing disability as it can be difficult to perform, is expensive, and may not be readily available. Cardiopulmonary exercise testing can be useful in cases where subjective dyspnea is disproportionate to the pulmonary function test results or when the latter are difficult to interpret because of submaximal performance. This test may be useful in measuring a subject's aerobic capacity and determining whether the individual can perform a job with a known energy requirement. Under the ATS guidelines, a worker should be able to perform comfortably at 40% of his or her $\dot{V}_{O_2max}$ (maximal oxygen consumption).

EVALUATION OF COMMON DISEASES

Obstructive Pulmonary Disorders

Chronic Obstructive Pulmonary Disease

The impairment rating for patients with chronic obstructive pulmonary disease is usually based upon pulmonary function test (PFT) results. Concomitant disorders like cor pulmonale may compound the degree of impairment. Disability assessments must take into account the impact of the patient's lung disease on the ability to work and function. For example, patients with chronic bronchitis may have relatively modest impairment based upon their PFTs yet may be unable to wear respirators because of heavy phlegm production, affecting the ability to perform certain jobs.

Example   A 62-year-old chronic smoker with emphysema presents for disability evaluation. He works as a bookkeeper and has chronic dyspnea progressing over 10 years. The dyspnea has become so severe that he is unable to perform routine daily activities such as walking on level ground. Lung examination reveals poor air movement bilaterally. Chest x-ray shows overinflated lungs. His PFT results are as follows:

Study	Observed	Predicted	% Predicted
FVC (L)	2.94	4.82	61
FEV$_1$ (L)	1.16	3.75	31
FEV$_1$/FVC	39%		

This patient has severe emphysema. Using the AMA guidelines (Table 1), the impairment is rated as severe or class 4 based upon the PFT results.

Asthma

The episodic and reversible nature of asthma makes impairment assessments difficult. The different entitlement systems have different eligibility criteria for asthmatics. The commonly used ATS guidelines for asthma attempt to rate impairment by using a composite clinical score based on medication use, spirometry, and reversibility of airflow obstruction (Table 2).

Occupational Asthma

It has been estimated that about 10–15% of cases of adult-onset asthma may be due to occupational exposures, and all patients should be evaluated for possible occupational or environmental triggers. Physiological tests may be normal and symptoms may be absent in the absence of exposure to the specific agent. Impairment is assessed as in any patient with asthma. However, depending on the causative agent and the patient's work, patients with occupational asthma may be disabled from certain types of work despite limited impairment.

Example   A 40-year-old automobile spray painter has had new-onset asthma over the past year requiring several emergency department visits and intermittent use of oral prednisone. His other medications include inhaled bronchodilators and steroids. His symp-

Table 2 Asthma Impairment Rating Using American Thoracic Society Guidelines

A. Postbronchodilator FEV_1

Score	FEV_1 (% Predicted)
0	>lower limit of normal
1	70–lower limit of normal
2	60–69
3	50–59
4	<50

B. Reversibility of FEV_1 or Degree of Airway Hyperresponsiveness

Score	% FEV_1 Change
0	<10
1	10–19
2	20–29
3	≥30

C. Minimum Medication Needs

Score	Medication
0	No medication
1	Occasional bronchodilator or cromolyn, not daily
2	Daily bronchodilator and/or cromolyn and/or inhaled low-dose inhaled steroid
3	Bronchodilator on demand and daily high-dose inhaled steroid (>800 μg beclomethasone or equivalent) or occasional course (1–3/years) of systemic steroid
4	Bronchodilator on demand and daily systemic steroid

D. Summary of Impairment Rating Classes[a]

Impairment rating	Score
0	0
I	1–3
II	4–6
III	7–9
IV	10–11
V	Asthma not controlled despite maximal treatment

[a] The impairment rating is calculated as the sum of the patient's scores from parts A, B, and C of this table.
Source: Adapted from American Thoracic Society: Guidelines for the evaluation of impairment/disability in patients with asthma. Am Rev Respir Dis 1993; 147:1056–1061.

toms occur after spray painting at work and improve away from the workplace. His lung examination reveals expiratory wheezes. His PFTs demonstrate the following:

Study	Prealbuterol	Postalbuterol	% Change
FVC	3.00 (75%)[a]	3.68 (92%)	23%
FEV_1	2.12 (62%)	3.01 (88%)	42%

[a] The numbers in parentheses represent the percent predicted values, based on reference equations generated by Crapo et al., 1981.

Further occupational history reveals that the patient has a history of work-related exposure to isocyanates, a common cause of occupational asthma. Charting of peak expiratory flow confirms reduced peak expiratory flow rates temporally associated with spray painting and improvements away from work. A diagnosis of occupational asthma is made. Despite attempts to reduce exposures in his workplace, his symptoms persist—a common problem with sensitizing agents such as isocyanates. Complete removal from further exposure to isocyanates is recommended. Given the work-related nature of his asthma, he is eligible for workmen's compensation. Under the ATS guidelines, he is considered 100% disabled from his current work, irrespective of the severity of the measured impairment, which is determined using the same scaling systems as for nonoccupational asthma (Table 2). He should undergo vocational training and rehabilitation for another job while receiving compensation for the loss of his employment.

Restrictive Lung Disorders

Most compensation systems base the impairment ratings for restrictive lung diseases on the PFT results. As in the case of asthma, disability assessments must also take into account the patient's workplace exposures and ability to continue current employment.

Example   A 45-year-old carpenter with a diagnosis of idiopathic pulmonary fibrosis was discharged from the hospital on steroids. He gets short of breath walking 50 m and is unable to carry out his prior job. Six months later, he shows no improvement of symptoms. Physical examination shows no clubbing; fine midinspiratory crackles are heard in all zones of the lung. His spirometric results are as follows:

Study	Observed	Predicted[a]	% Predicted
FVC	2.3	5.5	42%
FEV$_1$	1.9	4.8	40%
FEV$_1$/FVC	83%	—	—

[a] The predicted spirometric values are based on reference equations generated by Crapo et al., 1981.

Comments   The patient has chronic interstitial lung disease. His occupational history reveals no history of exposure to asbestos or other exposures of concern. He is severely limited by his disease and will probably apply for social security disability. Since there has been no improvement over 6 months with maximal medical intervention, this is a permanent disability rating. Using the relevant social security disability rating scheme for restrictive lung disorders, he qualifies as "impaired."

Lung Cancer

Evaluation of patients with lung cancer depends both on the presence of tumor and the degree of physiological impairment. Although cigarette smoking accounts for the great majority of lung cancer cases, it is important to identify other possible causes, such as asbestos. According to the AMA guidelines, lung cancers are a cause of severe impairment at the time of diagnosis. If, at reevaluation a year later, no evidence of tumor is found, respiratory impairment is recalculated on the basis of the degree of physiological impairment present at that time. If there is evidence of tumor, the patient remains severely impaired.

Example   A 65-year-old office secretary with a 60-pack-per-year smoking history is diagnosed with squamous cell cancer of the right lung. It is staged as a T2N1 lesion and undergoes right upper lobectomy. No chemotherapy or radiation therapy is given postoperatively. She continues to work at her job but has noticed dyspnea on climbing a flight of stairs. Her examination and radiological studies a year later confirm that she is tumor-free, and her PFTs are as follows:

Study	Observed	Predicted	% Predicted
FVC	1.5	2.15	70
FEV$_1$	1.1	1.73	71
FEV$_1$/FVC (%)	73		
D$_{CO}$ (mL/min mmHg)	15.5	19.7	78

At this point, a year after surgical resection, she is tumor-free. According to the AMA classification of respiratory impairment, she has mild impairment. Since she can continue her job as a secretary at this time, she has no resultant disability.

Three years later, she is noted to have a recurrence of her previous primary tumor. Based on the presence of tumor, she is rated as severely impaired under the AMA system and also rated as "impaired" under the social security system.

WORKMEN'S COMPENSATION

Patients with work-related lung diseases can seek disability benefits under the workmen's compensation system. This is a "no-fault" system of medical care and disability insurance in which private insurers or self-insured employers pay benefits to an employee who sustains an injury or illness due to a workplace exposure. In return, the workers cannot sue their employers for the work-related injury or illness. Workmen's compensation laws frequently vary from state to state. In the United States, some states require the physician to report all occupational injuries and illnesses.

The level of certainty required in determining causation for workmen's compensation is different from the usual standard of 95% certainty used in medical research. The commonly accepted standard of certainty is that the illness was substantially caused or exacerbated by an occupational exposure on a "more probable than not" basis, or a level of certainty greater than 50%. This decision is made by the attending physician.

When there may be more than one contributing factor to a patient's disease, apportionment describes the relative contribution of multiple factors to the total impairment or disability. For example, both asbestos exposure and cigarette smoking can be contributory factors to lung cancer. Often it is difficult or impossible to quantitate the relative roles of different factors in disease causation. The usual standard is whether the occupational exposure has been a "substantial contributing factor" in causing or increasing the impairment.

REPORTING DISABILITY AND COMPENSATION EVALUATIONS

It is important that a disability report be accurate and clear, answering all the specific questions asked. The practitioner does not make the determination as to whether a patient is entitled to benefits. This task is usually entrusted to an administrative agency that reviews the report and makes a decision regarding the benefits a patient is entitled to receive. The disability report should be tailored to the compensation program the patient is applying for, since requirements vary. Most reports contain the following key components: a summary of the patient's relevant symptoms, physical findings, and medical problem(s); the ''objective data,'' such as results of pulmonary function testing; and an assessment of the patient's impairment and/or disability (in response to what is specifically requested). It is best to provide the specific findings and criteria used, such as the AMA *Guides to the Evaluation of Permanent Impairment*. Workmen's compensation evaluations must address whether the patient's problem is caused or aggravated by the workplace. Reports should always address the specific questions being asked. It should be remembered that the person reviewing the report is frequently a nonphysician; the report should be written so that it can be understood by a nonmedical professional.

SUGGESTED READING

1.   American Medical Association. Respiratory system. In: Guides to the Evaluation of Permanent Impairment, 4th ed. Chicago: American Medical Association, 1993:153.
2.   American Thoracic Society. Evaluation of Impairment/Disability Secondary to Respiratory Disorders. Am Rev Respir Dis 1986; 133:1205–1209.
3.   American Thoracic Society. Standardization of Spirometry, 1994 Update. Am Rev Respir Dis 1995; 152:1107–1136.
4.   American Thoracic Society. Guidelines for the evaluation of impairment/disability in patients with asthma. Am Rev Respir Dis 1993; 147:1056–1061.
5.   Barnhart S, Balmes JR. Respiratory impairment and disability. In: Harber P, Schenker MB, Balmes JR, eds. Occupational and Environmental Respiratory Diseases. St. Louis: Mosby–Year Book, 1996:868–882.
6.   Crapo RO, Morris AH, Gardner RM. Reference spirometric values using techniques and equipment that meets ATS recommendations. Am Rev Respir Dis 1981; 123:659–664.
7.   Epstein P. Impairment and disability evaluation in lung disease. In: Elias JA, Fishman AP, Grippi MA, eds: Pulmonary Diseases and Disorders, 3rd ed. New York, Mc Graw-Hill, 1998: 631–641.
8.   Sood A, Beckett WS. Determination of disability for patients with advanced lung disease. Clin Chest Med 1997; 18:471–482.
9.   Sue DY. Exercise testing in the evaluation of impairment and disability. Clin Chest Med 1994; 15:369–387.
10. U.S. Department of Health and Human Services, Social Security Administration. *Disability Evaluation under Social Security*. HHS-SSA Publication No. 64-039. Baltimore: USDHHS-SSA, 1992.
11. Veterans Administration. *Physician's Guide for Disability Evaluation Examination of Pulmonary Diseases*. IB 11-56. Washington, D.C.: U.S. Government Printing Office, 1985:5-1–5-7.

42
Altitude and Illness

William G.B. Graham
University of Vermont College of Medicine
Fletcher Allen Health Care
Burlington, Vermont

INTRODUCTION

An immutable but usually benign feature of our earthly existence is that the oxygen supply available to us varies depending on the altitude. Oxygen is most plentiful at the highest barometric pressures. Usually this means at sea level, where the barometric pressure is 760 torr.* At locations below sea level, such as the Dead Sea or Death Valley, or in deep mines, oxygen is even more plentiful. As one ascends to higher terrain, artificially levitates oneself in balloons or aircraft, or simulates altitude by sitting in an airlocked decompression chamber, the barometric pressure drops, becoming 47 torr at 63,000 ft, at which point no gases are present in alveolar air, only drops of moisture. The reduced barometric pressure in densely populated areas of the world, such as Denver (altitude 5280 feet, barometric pressure of 622 torr, normal arterial P_{O_2}, 65 torr), hardly stress normally functioning mechanisms, which provide oxygen for aerobic metabolism. However, when patients living at these same moderate altitudes have disease-limited adaptive mechanisms brought on by a wide range of medical conditions, the coping responses may be sluggish or ineffective, producing, at least, uncomfortable symptoms and in some cases more severe clinical illness. An illustrative epidemiological example concerns chronic obstructive pulmonary disease (COPD). A large multihospital Veterans Administration (VA) study of the prognosis of COPD included two participating hospitals located at moderate altitude (Salt Lake City, at 4300 ft, and Albuquerque at 5400 ft). Patients at those altitudes compared with similar patients at sea level had a significantly higher mortality, the precocious development of cor pulmonale, and lower oxygen saturations.

Adaptive mechanisms to lower barometric pressure are often stressed in normal healthy individuals when they find themselves at higher altitudes, even those between 8000 and 10,000 ft. From 25–50% of healthy recreational skiers staying at resorts located at these levels have symptoms of altitude illness; in one study, those with the most severe

---

* Torr is an equivalent term for millimeters of mercury. The term derives from Evangelisto Torricelli (1608–1647), who invented the barometer.

symptoms of headache and dyspnea had small but significant decreases in spirometric volumes. High-altitude pulmonary edema (HAPE) has been observed at a ski resort located at 9600 ft. The popularity of mountain climbing and trekking is increasing yearly, in many cases involving trips at altitudes over 14,000 ft. Unless they are fully acclimatized, many people engaging in and hoping to enjoy these recreational activities will at least be uncomfortable or at worst jeopardize their lives.

Patients with underlying illness—such as symptomatic obstructive lung disease, angina, congestive heart failure and other cardiovascular diseases, or obstructive sleep apnea—undergo a more complex interaction on ascending to altitude. Such exposures involve the variables of the severity and category of underlying illness, the actual altitudes to which patients go, and the duration of time spent there. Few clinical studies have addressed these issues; there are only sparse or nonexistent epidemiological data supplemented by a certain amount of unsubstantiated speculation. Aircraft flight is undoubtedly the commonest setting where altitude interacts with human disease. The plane's cabin pressure may be equivalent to altitudes as high as 8000 ft, and the duration of flight, which is probably important as a clinical variable in inducing illness, may vary from short exposures of less than an hour to those lasting up to 15 h.

Two other common settings for the interaction of preexisting or developing disease and altitude involve prolonged exposure to areas of lower barometric pressure when traveling or because of long-term residence at higher altitude. Individuals living permanently at high altitudes develop the same spectrum of diseases as those living at sea level, but the clinical presentation of many illnesses, particularly pulmonary and cardiovascular disease, may be altered by an adverse reaction to the altitude. An example already mentioned is the different mortality of patients with COPD at moderate altitude.

GENERAL ADAPTIVE MECHANISMS IN NORMALS

Ascending from sea level to various altitudes—the ultimate earth-based elevation being 29,000 feet on Mt. Everest—involves exposing oneself to decreasing barometric pressure, with attendant decreases in ambient, tracheal, and alveolar oxygen tension. Regardless of the altitude, the percentage of oxygen in the air remains at approximately 20.93%.

As an example of how reduced barometric pressure influences oxygen tensions, the barometric pressure at the summit of Mt. Washington, New Hampshire (6288 ft) is 608 torr. Barometric pressure at sea level is approximately 760 torr. Mt. Washington is an instructive altitude to examine because the barometric pressure is in the general range of many aircraft flights, and it approximates the altitudes of many large population centers such as Denver, Albuquerque, or Mexico City. The pressure of water vapor at body temperature is 47 torr independent of barometric pressure and must be subtracted from total barometric pressure: $608 - 47 = 561$ torr. Multiplying 561 by the percentage of oxygen (20.93%) gives a tracheal oxygen tension of 117 torr, compared with a value of 150 at sea level. When tracheal air is taken down to the alveoli, the air is diluted by carbon dioxide; a correction has to be made for the respiratory exchange ratio ($\dot{V}_{O_2}/\dot{V}_{CO_2}$), based on the fact that more carbon dioxide is manufactured than oxygen is taken up. The corrected alveolar carbon dioxide pressure is 45 torr; this value is then subtracted from the tracheal air pressure for oxygen (117 in our example) to give an alveolar oxygen pressure of 72 torr. The penalty for going from sea level barometric pressures to the altitude of 6300 ft is to lower the alveolar oxygen tension from 102 torr—a drop of 39 torr.

This reduction in alveolar oxygen tension in a normal, healthy individual will reduce the arterial oxygen tension to approximately 65 torr at Mt. Washington's altitude unless there is some compensatory hyperventilation. At a value of 65 torr, there will be little drop in the oxygen saturation because of the shape of the oxygen dissociation curve: a drop in the oxygen tension from 72 to 65 torr will result in no more than a 1 to 2% change in oxyhemoglobin saturation. Oxygen transport carried to tissues will not be affected and requires only minor compensatory adjustments.

As barometric pressure decreases with increasingly higher altitude, alveolar gas tensions for both carbon dioxide and oxygen undergo complex changes, as illustrated in Fig. 1. As oxygen tension drops in alveolar air, with consequent reductions in arterial oxygen tensions, the carotid and aortic chemoreceptors drive the respiratory centers to increase alveolar ventilation and reduce alveolar and arterial carbon dioxide tensions. According to our illustration, the drop in Pa_{CO_2} initially is slight, up to about 10,000 ft, but it then becomes steeper with increasing altitude, finally dropping below 20 torr over altitudes of 20,000 ft. This extreme alveolar hyperventilation is the main respiratory compensation in the adaptation to altitude because it enables the alveolar and arterial oxygen tensions to remain far higher than would otherwise be the case. The hyperventilation has another effect, however, and that is a respiratory alkalosis that occurs as carbon dioxide is blown off. This change in pH is gradually compensated by renal excretion of bicarbonate, which tends to normalize to pH 7.4, though the compensation is rarely complete. Losing bicarbonate reduces the buffering capacity of the blood, which means that changes in pH will be more severe with a given change in alveolar ventilation.

Despite the progressive changes in alveolar and arterial P_{O_2} and P_{CO_2} that occur as barometric pressure decreases, the changes in oxygen at the tissue level appear to be attenuated. These changes are illustrated in Fig. 2, the oxygen cascade. The alveolar-arterial oxygen tension gradient (A-a DO_2) narrows due to the shape of the oxyhemoglobin

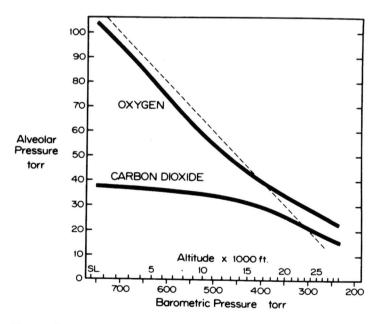

Figure 1   Changes in alveolar oxygen and carbon dioxide tensions with increasing altitude.

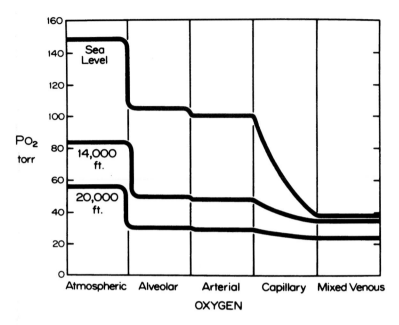

Figure 2 Changes in oxygen tension as oxygen passes through the respiratory and circulatory systems. Note the relative stability of the mixed venous P_{O_2} until very high altitudes are achieved.

dissociation curve. The mixed venous P_{O_2}, which at sea level is about 40 torr, is well maintained at this level up to an altitude of about 14,000 ft, after which it drops progressively into the twenties with increasing altitude. At the level of the mitochondria, it is postulated that oxygen tensions are maintained sufficiently high that anaerobic metabolism does not occur and metabolic acidosis due to anaerobic metabolism is avoided except with extreme exertion.

Other compensations that enable humans to live more energetically and comfortably at altitude come into play. There is an early increase in cardiac output both at rest and during exercise, which helps to maintain oxygen delivery to tissues. This is apparently mediated by hypoxic stress, producing both tachycardia and an increase in stroke volume, but it gradually returns to baseline. Other compensatory mechanisms occur more slowly. If prolonged exposure to altitude occurs, hypoxia leads to an increased production of erythropoietin and an increase in the red cell mass, which again allows increased oxygen delivery for a given cardiac output. Finally, it has been postulated that capillary density increases in muscle, which allows a shortening of the diffusion path of oxygen from the red cell to the metabolizing tissues. A possible compensatory mechanism that is thought to be short-lived is the generation of 2,3 diphosphoglycerate in the red cell, which tends to shift the oxygen dissociation curve to the left, thus facilitating the unloading of oxygen at the capillary level.

ALTITUDE AND ILLNESS

These adaptive responses to a lower barometric pressure, and the attendant drops in arterial oxygen tension, generally occur with relatively minor symptoms at altitudes below 8000 ft, except for a definite sense of dyspnea with exercise in some individuals. Others may experience a feeling of fatigue, headache, and poor sleep. Above the altitude of 8000 ft, however, an increasing proportion of individuals develop more severe symptoms as the altitude increases. These symptoms can be placed within three major categories, although all are related to hypoxia and comprise a continuum that overlap and may coexist.

The categories are: (1) acute mountain sickness (AMS); (2) high-altitude pulmonary edema (HAPE); and (3) high-altitude cerebral edema (HACE). AMS and HACE are due to effects of hypoxia on the central nervous system but are of different severity and prognosis. Another manifestation of hypoxia is the occurrence of retinal hemorrhages, which can be commonly observed at extremely high altitudes. Unless the macular area of the retina is the site of hemorrhage, visual symptoms do not occur.

ACUTE MOUNTAIN SICKNESS

This symptom complex occurs commonly in unacclimatized individuals who travel to altitudes over 8000 ft, especially if they are physically active, skiing or climbing at higher altitudes, and if they sleep over at this critical altitude. The syndrome consists of headache, loss of appetite, insomnia, bad dreams, unusual fatigue, exaggerated shortness of breath either with mild exercise or at rest, and in some cases nausea and vomiting. The symptoms are probably aggravated by drinking alcohol and becoming dehydrated. The incidence appears to increase with the altitude, the quickness of ascent, and a younger age. No gender bias exists, and—unfortunately—exceptional physical fitness is not protective. Estimates of incidence are from 20–50% at altitudes below 10,000 ft. The incidence at much higher altitude depends critically on how well acclimatization has been managed by pace of ascent, regulation of activity, and even the use of medications. The onset of symptoms may begin as quickly as 6–8 h after ascent to within 24 h and they may be worse on the second day. Remaining at the same altitude and avoiding exercise usually results in a decrease in the severity of symptoms over a few days' time.

Symptoms may become severe and be associated with pulmonary complaints such as cough. Examination of the chest may reveal rales. If symptoms become too severe for comfort and immediate relief is a priority—as opposed to waiting for the unpleasantness to subside by gradual adaptive mechanisms—descent is the safest and quickest solution. Descending only 2000 ft may result in a quick amelioration of altitude illness.

Over years of observation, the carbonic anhydrase inhibitor acetazolamide (Diamox) has proved to have both therapeutic effects in ameliorating AMS symptoms in individuals already ill and in preventing or modifying symptoms when taken as a preventive measure. Climbers who had become ill and were diagnosed as having AMS at 4200 m (13,780 ft) on Mt. McKinley were treated with 250 mg of acetazolamide in two doses 8 h apart, and were compared with a group of climbers who received a placebo. In several of these climbers, arterial blood gases were measured. The conclusion of this study was that such treatment not only alleviated symptoms but also improved gas exchange. The alveolar-arterial oxygen tension gradient narrowed in the treatment group but widened in the placebo group. Acetazolamide leads to the excretion of bicarbonate by the kidney, reducing the alkalosis (from hypoxic hyperventilation), which, in turn, blunts the full effect of the increased chemoreceptor drive. The net effect is to actually increase the arterial oxygen tension.

Using acetazolamide as prevention has also proved effective in preventing or reducing symptoms of AMS when the drug is taken before ascent or during ascent before symptoms have developed. The dosage used is generally 125 mg twice a day beginning on the day of ascent or as treatment at altitude after symptoms develop. Doubling of the dose is acceptable, though side effects will occur more commonly. Side effects described include a metallic taste, mild paresthesias, and an unpleasant modification of the taste of beer. In most cases, the symptoms of AMS are not severe enough to recommend therapy unless the individual has had previous severe illness or in those such as rescue workers who must ascend rapidly to altitude without adequate time for acclimatization. Diamox is a sulfa drug and should not be used in individuals sensitive to sulfas.

Other therapies used to treat severe symptoms have included oxygen, which will give temporary relief but is not as effective as descent to lower altitude, and diuretics. These therapies, of course, can be used as well in the more severe forms of altitude illness, HAPE and HACE.

HIGH-ALTITUDE PULMONARY EDEMA (HAPE)

High-altitude pulmonary edema is considerably less common than acute mountain sickness, occurring in perhaps 2% of people traveling to 9000 ft; it probably increases in severity at higher altitude if ascent is rapid and physical activity strenuous. It is definitely more serious than AMS and may end fatally unless recognized early and handled appropriately. It may occur uncommonly in individuals at altitudes of 7000–8000 ft. Individuals with only one pulmonary artery may be unusually susceptible.

For many years, allusions to or descriptions of symptoms at altitude among high-altitude climbers or skiers have included nonproductive cough, extreme breathlessness out of keeping with the level of activity and the altitude, and breathlessness at rest. Eventually, as the disease progresses, foamy and then blood-tinged sputum and severe cyanosis may occur as gas exchange worsens. The patient may die of severe hypoxia and presumably cardiac arrhythmias.

The pathophysiology of this disorder has been extensively studied but has not been convincingly explained. The most important datum is pulmonary hypertension with normal wedge pressures. HAPE is therefore classed as noncardiogenic pulmonary edema. A leading hypothesis regarding the basic mechanism is that the increase in pulmonary capillary permeability is due to hyperreactive pulmonary vessels. When these vascular beds constrict, the resulting pulmonary hypertension directs blood flow to other areas of the pulmonary vasculature and perhaps produces shear forces that disrupt pulmonary capillaries. Other mechanisms include possible pulmonary vein constriction and an inflammatory component that may enhance capillary leakage. Pulmonary hypertension is a key player in this scheme, since nifedipine, which reduces pulmonary hypertension, reverses the syndrome, as does nitric oxide. The latter treatment of HAPE increases arterial oxygen tensions and is believed to improve the distribution of blood flow in the lungs. A supporting clinical observation is that individuals with a single pulmonary artery are at increased risk of HAPE; the entire cardiac output goes to a single vascular bed, with higher pulmonary artery pressures.

Physical examination will show coarse rales, cyanosis, and an extremely rapid respiratory rate. When HAPE occurs, the most important step is to descend as quickly as possible. Often a reduction in altitude of only 1000–2000 ft will improve symptoms. Nifedipine will tend to prevent HAPE in patients known to be susceptible and can also be used as therapy. The dose is 10 mg sublingually, then 30 mg of an extended-release tablet twice a day for up to a week. It should be used with caution and under medical supervision because of side effects of hypotension. Strong diuretic therapy should be used cautiously if at all. Supplemental oxygen should be used to correct hypoxemia. But the most important therapeutic maneuver is descent. Within recent years, body bags (Gamow), which can be inflated with positive pressure by foot pumps, have been used for temporary reversal of symptoms. They provide a small hyperbaric environment. The duration of treatment with such devices is only 1–2 h, which can produce an astonishingly quick reversal of dyspnea and cyanosis; but the improvement is only temporary, providing precious additional time available for descent.

Obviously, the prevention of HAPE is far more important than allowing it to happen. The most important factors are educating the climbing community about the disease and emphasizing the preventive measures. These include a slow ascent in any major climb after 8000 ft, increasing altitude by no more than 1000 ft per day, and taking every fourth day off for rest. This may be too pokey for some climbers but will protect their more susceptible colleagues and avoid problems that could make everyone's life miserable. Sleeping at high altitude rather than descending during the night will increase the likelihood of the disease, as will high levels of activity.

HIGH-ALTITUDE CEREBRAL EDEMA

This syndrome is part of the spectrum of symptoms that occur in relation to altitude hypoxia, and it is certainly related to changes in blood gases (low oxygen, carbon dioxide, and alkalosis). This is the least common of the hypoxic disorders and is probably the most serious. It tends to occur at higher altitudes than either AMS or HAPE. The symptoms are more severe than those of AMS and include intense headache, lassitude, ataxia, loss of judgment, disorientation, hallucinations, and ultimately coma and death. The onset of any of these symptoms should be, to other climbers, a clear indication to evacuate the individual to a lower altitude as quickly as possible.

We have mentioned two medications that can be used in the treatment or prevention of altitude-related illness, acetazolamide (Diamox) for AMS and for HAPE and nifedipine for HAPE. The latter drug is not recommended for AMS. A third drug, dexamethasone, has been shown to relieve the severe headache of AMS and HACE, and it may also be useful in HAPE. However, it does not help the process of acclimatization and, when discontinued, a rebound of symptoms may occur. The usual dosage of this medication is 8 mg as the initial dosage and 4 mg every 6 h until symptoms abate. Some studies suggest that a combination of dexamethasone and Diamox is superior to either medication alone.

Nonsteroidal anti-inflammatory drugs such as ibuprofen may help headache, and prochlorperazine may help with nausea or vomiting. Sedatives and tranquilizers are not generally recommended because of possible interference with respiratory control.

The essence of the above discussion is that prevention of these illnesses is of fundamental importance. Physicians who educate their patients (although healthy young people do not often consult their doctors about risks of this sort) will do an important service, but more important is that the climbing community, ski areas, leaders of trekking parties, and outdoor recreation programs educate themselves and pass this information on to their clientele. Not warning people and exposing them to known risks is an open invitation to liability litigation.

ALTITUDE AND EXISTING LUNG DISEASE

Any disease affecting the lungs will ultimately affect gas exchange, initially by lowering of arterial oxygen tensions and, in more advanced disease, particularly COPD, increasing the carbon dioxide tension. In a broader context, such primary lung disease will adversely affect coexisting illnesses, such as cardiac disease (congestive heart failure, angina), hematological conditions (sickle cell anemia), peripheral vascular disease with claudication, etc. The hypoxemia due to lung disease will reduce oxygen delivery to any organ system compromised by another disease process and either require adjustments or produce a worsening of symptoms.

The complex interaction between distinct diseases at the barometric pressure of sea level is analogous to the interaction between primary lung disease and ascent to altitude. This occurs in several different contexts: (1) residence at moderate or high altitude for a long period of time, during which primary lung disease such as COPD or silicosis may develop, involving a very slow adaptive process measured in months or years; (2) travel to altitude by "sojourners" from sea level or thereabouts who intend to stay at altitude for variable periods of time; and (3) the acute and relatively short-lived exposure to altitude in aircraft flight. The latter exposure occurs because cabin barometric pressure is not maintained at the equivalent of sea level pressure but may be as low as the pressure at 8000 ft. The risks of long-term exposure to moderate altitude and those of short-term exposure undoubtedly differ, but more attention has been paid to aircraft hypoxemia. Many studies have dealt with the effects of simulated or actual flight on blood gases, with speculation as to whether flights are harmful. A number of committees and advisory panels have made recommendations for providing supplemental oxygen. The basis for making these recommendations is not often provided. It has been suggested that Pa_{O_2} values below 50 torr during aircraft flight will lead to serious medical consequences; this may be true, but clinical data are lacking, especially for the usually short exposures on commercial aircraft flights, in fact, the number of incidents causing emergency landings due to hypoxic illness appears to be astonishingly low. In a different context, little attention has been paid to the medical penalties for living at altitude with coexisting disease. The following discussion focuses on lung disease and altitude; the issues regarding other diseases such as cardiac and hematological illnesses (e.g., sickle cell disease) are not addressed.

LUNG DISEASE AND ADAPTATION TO ALTITUDE

There was little documentation of the interaction of long-term exposure to altitude and lung disease until a clinical study of COPD patients in Mexico City (altitude 7080 ft) was done. The results showed a high prevalence of cor pulmonale, extreme levels of arterial hypoxemia (mean resting Pa_{O_2} of 43 torr; range, 15–56 torr) and normal carbon dioxide tensions (mean Pa_{CO_2}, 38 torr). Normal values at this altitude are Pa_{O_2} of 57–71 torr and Pa_{CO_2} of 33–38.5 torr. Five years later, a multicenter study of prognosis in COPD was published by the Veterans Administration. Two of the participating hospitals were located at moderate altitude (Salt Lake City and Albuquerque). Patients studied at these sites compared with those studied at sea level had a mortality rate one-third greater and the earlier development of electrocardiographic changes of cor pulmonale. This study was carried out before the therapeutic advance of supplemental oxygen for severely hypoxemic patients. A later study relating mortality from COPD to the altitude of various counties in Colorado confirmed the initial results. Presumably the lower barometric pressures even at moderate altitudes resulted in lower alveolar oxygen tensions and provoked the well-known hypoxic reflex, which produces elevation of pulmonary artery pressure. This latter effect of ascent to higher altitude was demonstrated in a simulated aircraft flight lasting $2^1/_2$ h where extensive measurements of cardiovascular and ventilatory adjustments were made. The pulmonary artery pressure increased, as did cardiac output, and the patients developed unpleasant symptoms. An additional factor in the multicenter Veterans Administration mortality study was that the patients at altitude had higher hematocrits; the authors speculated that the increase in blood viscosity was partly responsible for the increase in pulmonary artery pressure.

The physiological adjustments that take place as patients with COPD ascend to altitude and lower their arterial oxygen tensions include alveolar hyperventilation, which lowers the arterial carbon dioxide tension, and an increase in minute ventilation, which may be observed only at exercise. The magnitude depends on the altitude and the complex responses of the respiratory control centers to hypoxemia. Other changes include a probable increase in cardiac output and pulmonary artery pressure, though these have not been documented in more than brief exposures. The extent to which these changes occur in a given individual depends on two major factors: the arterial oxygen tension at the lower altitude and the altitude to which the patient ascends. Physiologically, there is a big difference between 4000 ft in Salt Lake City and 7080 ft in Mexico City. As time of residence increases, according to the data in Mexico City and the VA study, hematocrit increases and the elevated pulmonary artery pressures induce right ventricular hypertrophy.

Symptoms that patients may experience on ascent include loss of appetite, headache, insomnia, increased exercise dyspnea, and cough. These symptoms are reminiscent of symptoms occurring in healthy individuals at much higher altitudes and are consistent with the same mechanisms that cause acute mountain sickness. Other patients may develop much more severe illness; the author has observed patients who went into right heart failure with the development of peripheral edema after being transferred to New Mexico from lower altitudes in Texas. The experience of physicians in Santa Fe (7000 ft), NM indicates that some patients who have traveled to this altitude require hospitalization for severe dyspnea and hypoxemia, and require transfer back to lower altitudes or the institution of chronic supplemental oxygen therapy. One patient we observed on Mt. Washington (BP 608, altitude 6288 ft) developed severe hypoxemia due to greatly increased shunting, severe hyperventilation, atrial arrhythmias, and electrocardiographic changes of acute right heart strain with a shift in the QRS axis rightward. These symptoms were reversed within minutes after oxygen therapy was started.

Assessments of the degree of pulmonary impairment are obviously important to patients with symptomatic COPD at or near sea level who plan for long-term residence at moderate altitude or even sojourning for a period of a few days or weeks. Such an assessment requires as the basic datum the measurement of arterial blood gases and an estimate of how low arterial oxygen tensions will fall after ascent. The long-term adjustments will depend most importantly on the altitude of residence, but also important are physiological adjustments such as the degree of alveolar hyperventilation due to increased arterial chemoreceptor drive. So-called ''high-altitude stress tests,'' during which a patient breathes a lower percentage of oxygen (say 15%) for a short period of time and has blood gas determinations done, may provide some information. It is impossible to predict with certainty what the long-term resident will experience in terms of eventual adaptation, particularly the crucial question of elevations of pulmonary artery pressure.

Table 1 Recommendations for Healthy Individuals Traveling at Altitudes Above 8000 Ft

---

Acclimatize at lower elevations; ascend no more than 1000 ft/day above 8000 ft.

Drink fluids and avoid alcohol.

Do not overexert yourself.

Consider use of prophylactic acetazolamide if prior symptoms have appeared at altitude or for those individuals who must ascend rapidly (e.g., rescue workers). Contraindicated in individuals with sulfa allergy.

Make sure travelers are familiar with the symptoms of high-altitude pulmonary edema and high-altitude cerebral edema and that the onset of these symptoms requires rapid descent.

Thus, any individual with underlying COPD who is planning to sojourn or reside at altitudes over 3000–4000 ft should have a careful medical evaluation. If the Pa_{O_2} at sea level is less than 65 torr, it is probable that the patient on arrival at altitude will have symptoms of poor sleep and definitely increased dyspnea, fatigue, and malaise. In our studies, when patients with mean Pa_{O_2} values of 63 torr ascended to 6288 ft, a high percentage had these symptoms, which tended to improve within 48 h. The average Pa_{O_2} at altitude was about 50 torr. No studies have attempted to follow the course of adaptation longer than 72 h.

AIRCRAFT FLIGHT

Among the millions of people who fly in aircraft, some will surely have underlying COPD or other diseases that will lower oxygen tensions at sea level. The question of how far arterial oxygen tensions will fall as aircraft cabin pressures decline has been a concern since aircraft flight became popular. This question has been investigated systematically in both actual short-term flights, where cabin pressure becomes equivalent to as high as 8000 ft, and in decompression chambers. The duration of these experiments is always short. In patients with advanced COPD and sea-level hypoxemia, oxygen tensions fall from resting levels of 60–65 torr to about 48–50 torr, values that would be considered an indication for oxygen supplementation in an acutely ill patient at sea level. It is surprising to find that in these studies, patients have very few symptoms, probably because of relatively short exposure and lack of physical exertion. At least one study has observed asymptomatic ectopic heart beats. Nomograms have been developed that will predict in a general way the fall of arterial oxygen tensions, depending on the cabin pressure and the preexisting arterial oxygen tension in the individuals.

Tables 1, 2, and 3 contain recommendations for healthy travelers going to altitude,

Table 2 Recommendations for Patients with Chronic Lung Diseases Traveling to Altitudes Above 4000 Ft

---

These patients should have a careful medical evaluation prior to travel, including measurement of arterial blood gases.

Consider supplemental oxygen at altitude for patients with Pa_{O_2} below 65 torr ($\leq 92\%$ saturation) at sea level, depending on altitude of travel location and duration of stay.

Patients should know to seek medical attention if they experience onset of increased dyspnea or signs of right heart failure (peripheral edema).

Avoid sedative medications.

Table 3   Recommendations for Patients with Chronic Lung Disease Who Plan Aircraft Travel

Patients should be evaluated prior to travel with measurement of arterial blood gases or oxygen saturation.

Patients with Pa_{O_2} less than 55 torr at sea level should have in-flight supplemental oxygen at 2 LPM by nasal cannula or 28% Ventimask.

Patients with hypercapnia, CHF, or angina should have inflight supplemental oxygen if $Pa_{O_2} \leq$ 60 or oxygen saturation $\leq$ 91% on room air at sea level.

Patients already on supplemental oxygen may require an increase in flow rates during the flight and will require their home care supplier to make arrangements for oxygen at their travel destination.

Prescriptions for in-flight oxygen must be arranged at least 2 weeks in advance with the airline.

and for patients with chronic lung diseases. The recommendations are drawn as a consensus from the Suggested Readings and other sources. Recommendations have also been published for in-flight oxygen supplementation, with oxygen provided either by nasal cannula or ventimask. The consensus is that patients whose resting sea- or low-level altitude arterial oxygen tensions are 50–55 torr or less should have in-flight supplemental oxygen. For patients who have carbon dioxide elevation and are therefore in mild respiratory failure, oxygen is probably even more important because carbon dioxide retention implies problems in respiratory control (that is, inability to respond appropriately to lower arterial oxygen tensions) and a higher pulmonary artery pressure.

Nonetheless, little information exists regarding medical emergencies in patients with COPD in aircraft flight, although a compilation of data from four air carriers suggested that COPD was a factor in approximately 10% of in-flight emergencies. There was little indication of what caused the flight crews to judge that the passengers' symptoms merited an emergency landing.

The indications for oxygen therapy during aircraft flight in patients with lung disease have been outlined by a number of committees, but it appears that the most reliable and useful measurement is an arterial blood-gas determination, made shortly before the scheduled flight. Tests such as spirometry, diffusing capacity, maximum voluntary ventilation, etc., are not useful. One certain indication for providing in-flight oxygen is that the patient at sea level requires ambulatory or nocturnal oxygen. In this case the dose of oxygen will have to be increased during flight. For patients recognized as having a severe degree of airflow limitation at sea level, a resting arterial oxygen tension below 50 to 55 torr would be considered an indication, and a provision of 2 L of oxygen by nasal cannula or a 28% Ventimask would provide levels of arterial oxygen tension similar to sea level values if the aircraft cabin altitude were equivalent to 8000 ft. The Federal Aeronautical Agency's guidelines mandate oxygen for everyone, including crew members, when cabin altitude is over 10,000 ft. From anecdotes, it is probably true that very long flights at lower cabin pressures are much more likely to produce adverse symptoms, such as 15-h flights from Chicago to Japan. Short flights lasting 3–4 h or less are intuitively less likely to cause symptoms.

Another firm recommendation for in-flight oxygen therapy exists when the patient is in respiratory failure, with elevation of the carbon dioxide pressure. With such advanced lung disease and problems with gas exchange, it would be likely that pulmonary artery pressure would be chronically raised and exposure to lower alveolar oxygen tensions might provoke the development of tachycardia and arrhythmias.

Certain practical points should be mentioned in the planning of in-flight oxygen therapy. Commercial aircraft do not allow patients to bring their own oxygen equipment on the plane unless the tanks are emptied. Provision for oxygen therapy requires a doctor's prescription for dose and duration of therapy. This should be done at least 2 weeks before scheduled departure. If the patient is going to require oxygen during long layovers at sea level, arrangements should be made with an oxygen supply company at that location. Finally, if oxygen is going to be prescribed at the final destination, similar arrangements should be made (see also Chap. 22).

In a patient with chronic lung disease going to altitude, the only measure needed to prevent possible adverse symptoms is the provision of properly calibrated supplemental oxygen therapy. Other medications that the patient is taking are maintained at their same dose.

SUGGESTED READING

1. AMA Commission on emergency medical services: medical aspects of transportation aboard commercial aircraft. JAMA 1982; 247:1007–1010.
2. Berg BW, Dillard TA, Rajagopal KR, Mehm WJ. Oxygen supplementation during air travel in patients with chronic obstructive lung disease. Chest 1992; 101:638–641.
3. Goetz AE, Kuebler WM, Peter K. High-altitude pulmonary edema (letter). 1996; 335: 206.
4. Gong H, Tashkin DP, Lee EY, Simmons MS. Hypoxia-altitude simulation test. Am Rev Respir Dis 1984; 130:980–986.
5. Gong H. Air travel and oxygen therapy in cardiopulmonary patients. Chest 1992; 101:1104–1113.
6. Graham WGB, Houston CS. Short-term adaptation to moderate altitude: patients with chronic obstructive pulmonary disease. JAMA 1978; 240:1491–1494.
7. Grissom CK, Roach RC, Sarnquist FH, Hackett PH. Acetazolamide in the treatment of acute mountain sickness: clinical efficacy and effect on gas exchange. Ann Intern Med 1992; 116: 461–465.
8. Honigman B, Read M, Lezotte D, Roach RC. Sea-level physical activity and acute mountain sickness at moderate altitude. West J Med 1995; 163:117–121.
9. Honigman B, Theis MK, Koziol-McLain J, Roach R, Yip R, Houston C, Moore LG. Acute mountain sickness in a general tourist population at moderate altitudes. Ann Intern Med 1993; 118:587–592.
10. Hultgren HN, Honigman B, Theis K, Nicholas D. High-altitude pulmonary edema at a ski resort. West J Med 1996; 164:222–227.
11. Jerome EH, Severinghaus JW. High altitude pulmonary edema (editorial). N Engl J Med 1996; 334:662–663.
12. Kaminsky DA, Jones K, Schoene RB, Voelkel NF. Urinary leukotriene E4 levels in high altitude pulmonary edema. Chest 1996; 110:939–945.
13. Renzetti AD, McClement JH, Litt BD. The Veterans Administration cooperative study of pulmonary function. Am J Med 1966; 41:115–129.
14. Scherrer U, Vollenweider L, Delabays A, Savcic M, Eichen Berger U, Kleger G, Fikrle A, Ballmer PE, Nicod P, Bartsch P. Inhaled nitric oxide for high-altitude pulmonary edema. N Engl J Med 1996; 334:624–629.
15. Schwartz JS, Bencowitz HZ, Moser KM. Air travel hypoxemia with chronic obstructive pulmonary disease. Ann Intern Med 1984; 100:473–477.

16. Simonneau G, Escourrou P, Duroux P, Lockhart A. Inhibition of hypoxic pulmonary vasconstriction by nifedipine. N Engl J Med 1980; 304:1582–1585.
17. Soto G, Marquez C. Some features of pulmonary insufficiency at high altitudes. Am Rev Respir Dis 1961; 85:25–29.
18. Tso E. High altitude illness. Emerg Med Clin North Am 1992; 10:231–247.

43
Obesity

Dudley F. Rochester
University of Virginia School of Medicine
Charlottesville, Virginia

INTRODUCTION

The term *morbid obesity* refers to obesity that is severe enough to produce symptoms and complications. Patients with the obesity-hyperventilation syndrome (OHS) have all of the features of morbid obesity with comparable degrees of excess body weight, but OHS patients also have ventilatory failure that is frequently complicated by pulmonary hypertension and right ventricular failure. The diagnosis of OHS is established by demonstrating elevation of the partial pressure of carbon dioxide in arterial blood (Pa_{CO_2}) in the absence of other causes of CO_2 retention, such as coexistent chronic obstructive pulmonary disease (COPD). Morbidity and mortality are higher in OHS than in simple obesity. Both simple obesity and OHS are characterized by significant abnormalities of pulmonary gas exchange, respiratory mechanics and pulmonary function, dyspnea on exertion and decreased exercise capacity, and a predilection for obstructive sleep apnea (OSA). Morbidly obese patients are also at risk for developing postoperative complications such as pneumonia, hypoxemia, and atelectasis.

This chapter covers aspects of respiratory physiology consequent to obesity, indicates the differences between simple obesity and OHS, and delineates relationships between obesity, OHS, and OSA. It also reviews approaches to the differential diagnosis of the respiratory manifestations of obesity and the added complications associated with OHS. Finally, the chapter presents therapeutic approaches to weight loss, which is the mainstay of therapy for all obese patients with and without OHS and OSA; it also outlines additional treatments that are specific for OHS and OSA. Table 1 lists in alphabetical order the abbreviations used in the text and tables.

QUANTIFICATION AND DISTRIBUTION OF OBESITY

Quantification

The severity of obesity is defined by the extent to which the observed body weight surpasses the normal range predicted from height and sex. Obesity is generally considered

Table 1 Glossary of Abbreviations

Abbreviation	Definition
$P_{(A\text{-}a)_{O_2}}$	Alveolar to arterial oxygen pressure gradient
BMI	Body-mass index (body weight/height^2)
BW	Body weight
COPD	Chronic obstructive pulmonary disease
CPAP	Continuous positive airway pressure
DL_{CO}	Diffusing capacity for carbon monoxide
ERV	Expiratory reserve volume
FEV_1	Forced expiratory volume in 1 s
FVC	Forced vital capacity
FRC	Functional residual capacity
HCO_3^-	Bicarbonate
MVV	Maximal voluntary ventilation
NPPV	Noninvasive positive-pressure ventilation
OHS	Obesity-hypoventilation syndrome
OSA	Obstructive sleep apnea
Pa_{CO_2}	Partial pressure of carbon dioxide in arterial blood
Pa_{O_2}	Partial pressure of oxygen in arterial blood
PE_{max}, PI_{max}	Maximal expiratory and inspiratory pressures generated by voluntary effort against a closed airway (reflect respiratory muscle strength)
$P_{0.1}$	Inspiratory mouth occlusion pressure, measured 0.1 s after occlusion (reflects neural drive to breathe)
Sa_{O_2}	Arterial blood oxyhemoglobin saturation
TLC	Total lung capacity
VC	Vital capacity
V_D/V_T	Ratio of dead space to tidal volume
$\dot{V}_E$	Minute ventilation
$\dot{V}_{O_2}$	Oxygen consumption
WHR	Waist/hip ratio

to be mild when body weight (BW) lies between 125 and 150% of ideal and severe when body weight exceeds 170% of ideal. The severity of obesity can also be quantified using the ratio of body weight to height (BW/Ht) or the body-mass index (BMI). BMI is the ratio body weight/height squared. The upper limits of normal for BW/Ht and BMI are 0.50 kg/cm and 28 kg/m^2, respectively; values in excess of 0.70 kg/cm and 40 kg/m^2 correspond to severe obesity.

Distribution of Body Fat

Body fat makes up approximately 15–20% of body mass in healthy men versus 25–30% in healthy women. In obesity, body fat typically makes up 40–45% of body mass but can be as much as 60%. The distribution of fat can be assessed morphometrically by measuring skin-fold thickness in different parts of the body and by calculating the ratio of waist to hip circumference (waist/hip ratio, WHR). In normal-weight men and women, typical values for WHR are 0.90 and 0.83, respectively; WHR increases with obesity in both sexes. The amount of visceral fat in the abdomen can be assessed using ultrasonography, computed tomography, or magnetic resonance imaging. The ratio of visceral fat to subcutaneous fat in normal-weight subjects is 0.80 in men versus 0.35 in women; these values do not change much in obesity.

Fat-Free Mass

The fat-free mass (lean body mass) also increases in obesity, by approximately 0.3 kg per kg increase in body weight. For example, if a male's weight increases from 70 to 105 kg, 63% of the weight gain is fat and 37% is fat-free mass. The ratio of resting energy expenditure to fat-free mass is the same in obesity as it is in normal-weight subjects. Thus oxygen consumption ($\dot{V}_{O_2}$) increases in obesity in proportion to the increase in fat-free mass.

GAS EXCHANGE AND PULMONARY FUNCTION

Gas Exchange

Severely obese patients are usually hypoxemic, with a widened alveolar-arterial oxygen tension gradient [$P(A-a)_{O_2}$]. The partial pressure of oxygen in arterial blood (Pa_{O_2}) may be normal when obese subjects are sitting or standing, but Pa_{O_2} falls when they are supine. Hypoxemia in obesity results from underventilation of the dependent parts of the lung, which continue to be well perfused. In some patients, alveoli in dependent regions are not ventilated at all except after a deep breath or sigh, so most of the time there is a right-to-left shunt through the dependent lung regions. Such patients respond poorly to supplemental oxygen. Hypoxemia is most pronounced in obese subjects with small lung volumes. The single-breath diffusing capacity (DL_{CO}) is normal in simple obesity and slightly reduced in OHS. The physiological dead space (VD), the ratio of dead space to tidal volume (VD/VT), and intrapulmonary gas mixing are normal.

The majority of patients with severe obesity have a normal Pa_{CO_2}, even though obesity increases the demand upon the ventilatory system. Patients with OHS are not only hypercapnic but also have a lower Pa_{O_2} than patients with simple obesity. The $P(A-a)_{O_2}$ is somewhat larger in OHS, but most of the reduction of Pa_{O_2} results from the increase in Pa_{CO_2}.

Spirometry and Lung Volumes

Simple obesity generally exerts only mild effects on pulmonary function (Table 2). The expiratory reserve volume (ERV) is reduced because the obese abdomen displaces the diaphragm into the thorax, and the degree of reduction in ERV is proportional to the severity of obesity. The vital capacity (VC), functional residual capacity (FRC), total lung capacity (TLC), and maximal voluntary ventilation (MVV) are within the normal range in most subjects with simple obesity, but VC falls somewhat in very severe obesity. Men whose obesity is more centrally distributed have lower values of FVC, FEV_1, and TLC than those with more peripheral obesity. For a given BMI, the pulmonary function deficits are more severe in OHS (Table 2).

Table 2 Pulmonary Function in Simple Obesity
(OB) and Obesity Hypoventilation Syndrome (OHS)

Variable	Units	OB	OHS
VC	(% predicted)	95	65
FEV_1/FVC	(%)	80	80
ERV	(% predicted)	60	35
FRC	(% predicted)	85	80
TLC	(% predicted)	95	85

Key: VC, vital capacity; FVC, forced vital capacity; FEV_1,
forced expiratory volume in 1 s; ERV, expiratory reserve volume; RV, residual volume; FRC, functional residual capacity;
TLC, total lung capacity.

RESPIRATORY SYSTEM COMPLIANCE AND RESISTANCE

Compliance

Compliance of the respiratory system is approximately half of normal in both simple obesity and OHS. Part of the decrement in compliance results from a fall in lung compliance and part from a reduction in compliance of the chest wall. With appropriate techniques, it can be shown that the excess weight presents an added inspiratory load of the threshold type, that is, a weight that must be lifted to inspire.

Resistance

The total flow resistance of the respiratory system is increased in obesity, especially in severely obese patients. Resistance is approximately four times normal in simple obesity and eight times normal in OHS. In the absence of underlying lung disease, the FEV_1/FVC ratio is normal in both simple obesity and OHS, indicating that the source of the increased resistance lies in lung tissue and small airways.

Work and Energy Cost of Breathing

As a result of the increased resistance and decreased compliance, the work of breathing is increased by approximately 60% in simple obesity vs. 250% in OHS. The oxygen cost of breathing represents the oxygen consumed by the respiratory muscles per liter of ventilation and is an index of the energy required to breathe. The oxygen cost of breathing is four times normal in simple obesity and almost ten times normal in OHS.

CONTROL OF BREATHING

Pattern of Breathing

The respiratory rate of eucapnic morbidly obese subjects is approximately 40% higher than that of normal subjects during quiet breathing. The tidal volume is normal or slightly reduced, both at rest and at exercise. Patients with OHS have a 25% higher respiratory rate and a 25% smaller tidal volume than subjects with simple obesity. The lower tidal volume and higher respiratory rate of OHS contribute to increased dead-space ventilation and retention of CO_2. Patients with OHS uncomplicated by obstructive airways disease can attain a normal level of Pa_{CO_2} by voluntary hyperventilation, but it requires considerable effort. Thus it is likely that the patient with OHS chooses a more comfortable pattern of breathing through a modification in ventilatory control.

Ventilatory Drive

The ventilatory response to inhalation of CO_2 is often reduced in simple obesity, mostly due to the increase in mechanical load. In OHS, the ventilatory response to CO_2 is usually reduced to an even greater extent. Some patients with OHS have normal responses to CO_2 but markedly reduced ventilatory responses to inhaled hypoxic gas mixtures. The mouth occlusion pressure during quiet breathing ($P_{0.1}$) is about twice normal in obesity and in obese patients who have recovered from OHS. The increase in $P_{0.1}$ represents a compensatory mechanism to preserve ventilation in the face of the increased ventilatory load. Values for $P_{0.1}$ during quiet breathing in OHS patients with hypercapnia are not available. The $P_{0.1}$ and diaphragmatic electrical activity on electromyography (EMG) in response to CO_2 inhalation are twice normal in simple obesity and obstructive sleep apnea, but they are only normal in OHS. In other words, patients with OHS ought to have an increased ventilatory drive to help overcome the added ventilatory load, but they do not.

RESPIRATORY MUSCLE AND EXERCISE PERFORMANCE

Respiratory Muscles

Maximal inspiratory and expiratory pressures (PI_{max}, PE_{max}) are normal in simple obesity, but PI_{max} is 40% below normal in OHS (Table 3). In severely obese subjects, the diaphragm may be overstretched and at a mechanical disadvantage, at least in the supine position. The maximal voluntary ventilation (MVV), an index of ventilatory endurance, is approximately 80% of normal in uncomplicated obesity and 55% of normal in OHS; maximal exercise ventilation is approximately 60% of MVV (Table 3)—i.e., a level that can be sustained for 15 min or more.

Table 3 Ventilatory and Exercise Capacity in Normal Subjects (NLS), Simple Obesity (OB), and Obesity Hypoventilation Syndrome (OHS)

Variable	Units	NLS	OB	OHS
PI_{max}	cmH_2O	100	95	60
PE_{max}	cmH_2O	150	125	—
MVV	L/min	160	130	90
VE_{max}	L/min	90	80	—
$\dot{V}_{O_2max}$	mL/min/kg BW	45	30	—

Key: PI_{max}, maximal inspiratory pressure; PE_{max}, maximal expiratory pressure; MVV, maximal voluntary ventilation; VE_{max}, minute ventilation at maximal exercise; $\dot{V}_{O_2max}$, oxygen consumption at maximal exercise; BW, body weight.

Exercise Capacity

Young adults with uncomplicated obesity have a near normal capacity for physical exercise. At the onset of exercise, obese subjects tend to have transient hypoventilation and arterial blood oxyhemoglobin desaturation. At rest and moderate exercise, they consume approximately 25% more oxygen than nonobese subjects. Much of the excess $\dot{V}_{O_2}$ can be attributed to movement of the leg mass. The maximal cycle ergometer work rate, maximal exercise $\dot{V}_{O_2}$ and maximal exercise VE are approximately 90% of normal in young obese subjects. Maximal $\dot{V}_{O_2}$, expressed as mL/min/kg body weight, is low in obesity (Table 3) but would be near normal if it were expressed as mL/min/kg fat-free mass.

CLINICAL COMPLICATIONS RELATED TO THE RESPIRATORY SYSTEM

Dyspnea

Dyspnea on exertion is one of the most prevalent complications of morbid obesity (Table 4). Moreover, it can be difficult to distinguish dyspnea due to obesity per se from dyspnea associated with congestive heart failure, pulmonary embolic disease, or obstructive disease of the airways. Many obese patients have systemic hypertension and compromised left ventricular function; pulmonary embolism occurs more often in obesity, and some obese patients also have COPD. Thus it is important to evaluate the dyspneic obese patient carefully to rule out heart failure, pulmonary vascular disease, and obstructive lung disease (Table 5).

The medical history is of limited value in differential diagnosis. Dyspnea on exertion is characteristic of obesity, congestive heart failure, pulmonary vascular disease, and obstructive airways disease. However, dyspnea at rest points to pulmonary embolic disease, and paroxysmal nocturnal dyspnea suggests left ventricular failure. Associated symptoms such as angina pectoris in coronary artery disease and cough and sputum production in chronic bronchitis give added diagnostic clues when present.

The physical examination is also not too helpful. Peripheral edema is very common in severe obesity and is not a sensitive indicator of congestive heart failure. Obesity may mask other physical evidence of congestive heart failure, such as venous distension and hepatomegaly, and makes it hard to detect a left or right ventricular gallop rhythm. Severely obese patients may have rales at the lung bases that are hard to distinguish from the rales of pulmonary edema.

The most useful screening laboratory tests are chest x-ray, spirometry, and electrocardiogram. The heart may appear somewhat enlarged in relation to lung size in obesity because of an increase in total blood volume and reduced descent of the diaphragm. The

Table 4 Clinical Complications of Morbid Obesity

Dyspnea and reduced capacity for physical exercise
Ventilatory failure
Obstructive sleep apnea, nocturnal hypopnea, and central apnea
Deep vein thrombosis and pulmonary embolism
Atelectasis, pneumonia
Pulmonary hypertension and right ventricular failure

Table 5 Differential Diagnosis of Dyspnea in Obesity and Diagnostic Approach

Underlying cause	Diagnostic tests
Morbid obesity	Negative test results
Obstructive lung disease	Spirometry
Other lung disease	Chest x-ray, spirometry, lung volumes
Respiratory muscle weakness	PI_{max} and PE_{max}
Congestive heart failure	ECG, echocardiogram
Pulmonary embolism	$\dot{V}/\dot{Q}$ scan, pulmonary angiogram

Key: PI_{max}, maximal inspiratory pressure; PE_{max}, maximal expiratory pressure; ECG, electrocardiogram; $\dot{V}/\dot{Q}$, ventilation/perfusion.

principal value of the chest x-ray is to detect pronounced cardiomegaly and to rule out other processes such as pneumonia, interstitial lung disease, pleural effusion, pneumothorax, masses, and unilateral paralysis of the diaphragm. Bilateral paralysis of the diaphragm is harder to detect radiographically in obesity because the diaphragm is already high, and the sniff test is of limited value.

The spirometric finding of a reduction in FEV_1/FVC indicates obstructive disease of the airways, since FEV_1/FVC is normal in obesity and OHS in the absence of airflow limitation. If the spirogram shows a small VC, then lung volumes should be measured to see if the residual volume (RV) and FRC are large, as in chronic obstructive lung disease, or if the FRC and TLC are small, as in interstitial lung disease. In addition, one should measure PI_{max} and PE_{max} to rule out weakness of the diaphragm or other respiratory muscles as a cause of dyspnea.

The electrocardiogram can document arrhythmias that either reflect heart disease or, like atrial flutter, occur in response to pulmonary vascular or pericardial disease. The electrocardiogram can also provide evidence of left or right ventricular hypertrophy. When the clinician suspects disease of the heart or pulmonary circulation, the next step is to obtain an echocardiogram. Things to look for include evidence of right or left ventricular enlargement, abnormalities of the ventricular wall, dilation of the pulmonary artery, heart valve abnormalities, and intracardiac thrombus. A ventilation/perfusion ($\dot{V}/\dot{Q}$) scan should be obtained to look for evidence of pulmonary embolism. If clinical suspicion is high but the scan is indeterminate, then a pulmonary angiogram should be done. An echocardiogram can screen for primary pulmonary hypertension, but the definitive diagnosis rests on catheterization and measuring pulmonary artery systolic, diastolic, and wedge pressures.

Ventilatory Failure

Hypercapnia in obesity is mainly associated with OHS. To a lesser extent, CO_2 retention in obesity may result from a sleep-related breathing disorder or from associated COPD. Patients with OHS lack the increase in ventilatory drive needed to overcome the increased ventilatory load, the ventilatory load is much higher in OHS than in simple obesity, the inspiratory muscles are weaker and the tidal volume is smaller in OHS, and pulmonary function and gas exchange are correspondingly worse in OHS than in simple obesity. It is still not clear what causes OHS, but it seems likely that a combination of genetic predilection for lower ventilatory drive coupled with a higher work of breathing, weaker inspiratory muscles, and smaller tidal volume are jointly responsible for CO_2 retention in OHS patients.

Sleep-Related Breathing Disorders

Obese patients are at risk for several types of disordered breathing during sleep. These include obstructive apneas, hypopneas, central apneas, and overt hypoventilation. Obese patients with a history of snoring and daytime irritability or somnolence should have a sleep study. At the very least, they should be screened to see how much and how often arterial oxyhemoglobin saturation (Sa_{O_2}) falls during sleep. However, to differentiate central from obstructive apneas, assess the response to nasal CPAP, and rule out other forms of sleep-related breathing disorder, a full polysomnographic sleep study is necessary. All patients with OHS should have a polysomnographic sleep study, since the prevalence of OSA is high in OHS.

The most vulnerable period for hypopneas and obstructive apneas is during rapid-eye-movement (REM) sleep, when the tone of limb, trunk, chest wall, and upper airway muscles is markedly diminished; only the tone of the diaphragm is relatively well preserved. Collapse of the pharynx and chest wall during inspiration may cause nocturnal hypoventilation and even daytime CO_2 retention. A clinical clue to nocturnal hypoventilation is early-morning headache; this results from cerebral vasodilation induced by the acute rise in Pa_{CO_2} overnight.

The prevalence of obstructive sleep apnea (OSA) in simple obesity is approximately 50% in men vs. 10% in women. The higher prevalence of OSA in obese men is associated with more upper-body fat and higher waist/hip ratios, thicker skin folds, and lower $P_{0.1}$ at rest as well as lower $P_{0.1}$ and ventilatory responses to carbon dioxide and hypoxia. The prevalence of sleep apnea in OHS is probably higher, ranging between 40 and 80%. Thus, OSA may not be an essential component of OHS, but it certainly aggravates hypoxemia and hypercapnia. Conversely, hypercapnia is not a feature of uncomplicated obstructive sleep apnea. When patients with OSA retain CO_2, they usually have diffuse airway obstruction or obesity.

The rate at which Sa_{O_2} falls during an apnea and the extent of the decrement in Sa_{O_2} are clinically important. During voluntary breath-holding, alveolar P_{O_2} falls much faster in obese subjects than in normals, and the magnitude of the fall in 15 s is correlated with the severity of obesity and the reduction of FRC. Under anesthesia and after 5 min of 100% oxygen, the time required for Sa_{O_2} to fall to 90% during a deliberately induced apnea was 6 min for normal subjects vs. less than 3 min for obese subjects. Patients with higher degrees of nocturnal desaturation have more organ dysfunction and are at greater risk of developing pulmonary hypertension and right ventricular failure.

Anesthesia and Surgery

Anesthetic management of the obese patient is difficult. Technical problems include transfers from bed to operating table, locating veins and arteries, tracheal intubation, and placement of epidural cannulas. Postoperative positioning and cardiopulmonary monitoring are also difficult. The FRC and Pa_{O_2} often fall further with anesthesia. Atelectasis occurs in up to 30% of patients, especially heavier patients with smaller FRC, but less than 5% develop pneumonia. In patients with OSA, postoperative analgesics may increase upper airway collapse and lead to respiratory arrest and death.

Pulmonary Embolism and Pulmonary Hypertension

The risk of deep vein thrombosis and pulmonary embolism in obesity is twice that in normal subjects. Postoperative pulmonary embolism occurs in up to 5% of patients undergoing weight-reduction surgery. It is difficult to make a definitive diagnosis of pulmonary embolism in the obese patient because the overlying adipose tissue and small lung volume makes it hard to read $\dot{V}/\dot{Q}$ scans. Recurrent or chronic pulmonary embolism is one of the causes of pulmonary hypertension in obesity. A second cause is pulmonary arterial vasoconstriction consequent to alveolar hypoxia in OHS. A third cause of pulmonary hypertension is a drug or drugs taken to suppress appetite. Two of the more effective appetite suppressants, fenfluramine and dexfenfluramine, were withdrawn from the market in 1997 because they appear to cause heart valve lesions as well as persistent and even fatal pulmonary hypertension.

WEIGHT LOSS IN MORBID OBESITY

Diet and Exercise

The optimal treatment of morbid obesity is weight loss, but this is hard to achieve and often transitory. Obese people underestimate their caloric intake to a substantial degree, and weight loss induces a reduction in metabolic rate that offsets the effect of dieting. Use of behavior modification and a diet of 1200 kcal/day can lead to a weight loss of 8.5 kg in 20 weeks, as compared with a 20-kg loss in 12–16 weeks with a medically supervised diet of 400–800 kcal/day. Approximately 60% of the weight loss is maintained for 1 year, but patients return to their original weight in 5 years.

Physical exercise is an important component of the weight-loss regimen because it increases energy expenditure and helps with loss of body fat. Exercise also helps to lower blood pressure and improve the lipid profile. Dieting without exercise leads to loss of fat-free mass, but this can be prevented by combining diet with physical exercise. A typical exercise prescription involves both endurance and strength training. Endurance training consists of walking, cycling, or other aerobic activity to approximately 85% of predicted maximal exercise heart rate, starting at 20 min a day, 3–4 times a week, and gradually increasing the duration of each session to 1 h. Strength training can be accomplished using weight or exercise machines 3–4 days a week with increasing intensity.

Drugs

Several types of pharmacological agents have been used in obesity clinics. Fluoxetine is an antidepressant; in doses of 20–60 mg/day it leads to weight loss of approximately 10 kg in 2–3 months. Higher doses produce side effects such as headache, diarrhea, and overstimulation but have no additional effect on weight loss. Patients tend to become resistant to fluoxetine after the first several months. Phenteramine is an amphetamine-like anorectic drug. Given in a dose of 15–30 mg once a day, it may facilitate mild weight loss, but it too is not effective for long-term weight reduction. Drugs such as Orlistat, which block cleavage and absorption of fat from the gut, have recently received preliminary FDA approval and are beginning to come on the market.

Surgery

If medical treatment fails, patients may be referred for surgery. Current surgical procedures for weight loss include vertical-banded gastroplasty and Roux-en-Y gastric bypass; these effectively make the stomach smaller and produce a malabsorption syndrome. Patients who undergo such surgery lose 50–70% of their excess weight in 2 years, but approximately one-third to one-half of those who lose weight regain much of it after 5–10 years. The magnitude and duration of benefits of gastric surgery are the same for patients with OHS and/or sleep apnea as they are for simple obesity. An alternative surgical approach for certain patients is panniculectomy. This procedure can reduce body weight by 20%, but the long-term results are not known.

In simple obesity, pulmonary function and arterial blood gases improve after weight loss induced by surgery or by low-calorie diets. The most striking change in pulmonary function is a marked increase in ERV. Weight loss in simple obesity is also associated with a small but statistically significant increase in VC, but there is little change in FEV_1/FVC, TLC, or compliance. Some patients develop mild respiratory muscle weakness after stringent dieting or surgery. Weight loss increases Pa_{O_2} in eucapnic obese patients provided that body weight falls to less than 130% of ideal.

The effects of weight loss on pulmonary function are far more striking in OHS. In addition to improvement in ERV, there are substantial increases in FRC, VC, and MVV. Concomitantly, Pa_{CO_2} falls and Pa_{O_2} rises. Indeed, weight loss is the most important component of the short- and long-term management of ventilatory failure. Patients with both OHS and OSA experience fewer and less severe nocturnal desaturations as well as improvement in daytime Pa_{O_2} and Pa_{CO_2}.

TREATMENT OF OSA AND VENTILATORY FAILURE

Obstructive Sleep Apnea

The best treatment for OSA in obesity is weight loss, and the next best for most patients is continuous positive airway pressure (CPAP). Because the level of pressure needed to maintain upper airway patency is quite high in obesity, CPAP alone may be poorly tolerated (Table 6).

Table 6 Treatment of Obstructive Sleep Apnea and Ventilatory Failure

Condition	Treatment
Obstructive apnea	CPAP (single level or bilevel)
	Mandibular advancement device
	Tracheostomy in refractory cases
Hypopnea, central apnea	CPAP
	Mechanical ventilation via mask
Acute hypercapnia	Intubation and mechanical ventilation
	Supplemental oxygen, phlebotomy
	Acetazolamide, potassium chloride, furosemide, spironolactone
Chronic hypercapnia	Mechanical ventilation via mask
	Tracheostomy and mechanical ventilation

Patients with OSA may develop central apneas and hypopneas sufficient to cause nocturnal or daytime CO_2 retention after their obstructive apneas have been relieved by CPAP or a bilevel pressure device. Because it is difficult to obtain a sample of arterial blood for gas analysis without waking the patient, patients must have their Sa_{O_2} monitored with an ear or pulse oximeter. Supplemental oxygen alone is not sufficient to correct the hypoxemia; these patients need to be ventilated mechanically with supplemental oxygen as needed to achieve an Sa_{O_2} of at least 90%. Mechanical ventilation may be accomplished using a nasal mask attached to a volume-cycled ventilator (Table 6). In some cases a bilevel pressure support device that includes a respiratory rate control to deliver tidal volumes periodically may be substituted for the volume-cycled respirator.

Other treatments for OSA include the use of devices and surgery. A mandible advancement appliance pulls the jaw forward and thus helps prevent inspiratory occlusion of the pharynx. This has replaced an earlier device that pulled the tongue forward. The mandibular advancement appliance works well in mild OSA and occasionally in moderate OSA, but experience with it in obese OSA patients is limited. A surgical operation called uvulopharyngopalatoplasty yields modest improvement in about half the people who undergo it. Another surgical operation advances the mandible. Again, there is limited experience with these procedures in OSA associated with obesity. The one definitive surgical approach to OSA is tracheostomy. This completely bypasses the upper airway obstruction, but, like CPAP, it does not correct hypopneas and central apneas. Complications of chronic tracheostomy are fewer with new, smaller endotracheal tubes.

Acute Ventilatory Failure

In the obese patient with acute ventilatory failure, mechanical ventilation should be accomplished using tracheal intubation and a volume-cycled positive-pressure ventilator in the assist-control mode (Table 6). Selected patients who are alert may be tried initially on volume-cycled ventilation delivered via nasal mask. Once the patient has been stabilized, pressure-support ventilation may be more comfortable, and it can also be used as a technique for weaning. In acute ventilatory failure, it is critically important to provide adequate oxygenation—i.e., maintain Sa_{O_2} above 90%. The severe hypoxemia of OHS often responds poorly to supplemental oxygen because of shunting through unventilated alveoli. This problem is alleviated partly but not completely by mechanical ventilation. Systemic complications of ventilatory and right heart failure will not resolve without adequate oxygenation.

Even though patients with OHS have been living with an elevated Pa_{CO_2}, many will readjust to a lower Pa_{CO_2} after treatment for ventilatory failure if given a chance. To that end, one should lower Pa_{CO_2} with mechanical ventilation to below 50 mmHg. At the same time it is necessary to give acetazolamide to promote renal excretion of excess bicarbonate and to give potassium chloride to replace chloride that was lost when bicarbonate rose in response to elevation of Pa_{CO_2}. In order for patients to increase ventilatory drive and maintain a lower Pa_{CO_2} after discontinuing mechanical ventilation, their chloride and bicarbonate have to be normalized along with the Pa_{CO_2} (Table 6).

Additional measures in the treatment of acute ventilatory failure include phlebotomy and diuresis. Phlebotomy is indicated when the hematocrit is greater than 55%, but it should not be undertaken until the patient is adequately oxygenated and ventilated and has a stable blood pressure. The rate of phlebotomy should not exceed 500 mL every other day. Obese patients in acute ventilatory failure will begin to diurese once they are adequately oxygenated and out of respiratory acidosis. Loop diuretics may be given, but caution should be used so as not to increase the hematocrit. In the presence of right ventricular failure, it is helpful to give spironolactone to treat presumed secondary hyperaldosteronism and to provide a slow, steady, sustained diuresis. After appropriate phlebotomy and diuresis, there is often significant further persistent improvement in oxygenation.

Chronic Ventilatory Failure

For management of chronic ventilatory failure, mechanical ventilation may be given on a prolonged intermittent basis—i.e., for 4–8 h during each day or night. Negative-pressure body respirators allow patients to be ventilated and oxygenated without concern about worsening hypercapnia. Unfortunately, negative-pressure ventilation may induce OSA. Oxygen therapy tends to aggravate sleep apnea, but CPAP added to negative-pressure ventilation alleviates apnea.

Noninvasive positive-pressure ventilation (NPPV) may also be provided by a nose mask or a mask that covers both nose and mouth (Table 6). NPPV can be added when regular CPAP or bilevel positive airway pressure alone fails. NPPV is generally driven by conventional ventilators in the assist-control mode or by a bilevel pressure device equipped with the respiratory rate control. When NPPV is used for chronic ventilatory failure, tidal volume and Pa_{CO_2} should be monitored initially to ensure that NPPV is being used correctly. In contrast to negative-pressure ventilation, NPPV improves sleep substantially, and this may be one of its most important benefits.

The complications from nose-mask CPAP or NPPV include erosion of skin, especially over the bridge of the nose, and exacerbation of nasal stuffiness or sinusitis. These can be minimized by using a custom-fitted mask, temporarily switching to nasal pillows, keeping the face and mask clean, and not overtightening the head straps that secure the mask. Alternatively, CPAP or positive-pressure ventilation can be delivered using a lip-seal device; but when used chronically, the lip-seal device may cause problems with dentition.

CASE PRESENTATION

A 64-year-old obese woman was admitted to a hospital with chest tightness and dyspnea at rest. Overweight for many years, she had lost 40 kg a year prior to admission but recently gained it back. In the month prior to admission she had progressive exertional dyspnea with chest and abdominal tightness. She also noticed increasing abdominal girth and swelling of the legs.

Physical examination revealed an obese woman in respiratory distress. Blood pressure was 142/100, heart rate 124, respiratory rate 36, and weight 144 kg (225% ideal). Wheezes and rales were present over the lower chest bilaterally, and she had tachycardia with gallop and jugular venous distension. The abdomen was obese and there was 3+ pitting edema of legs. Initial arterial blood-gas analysis on room air showed that Pa_{O_2} was 43 mmHg, Sa_{O_2}, 78%; pH, 7.29; Pa_{CO_2}, 75 mmHg; HCO_3^- 32 meq/L, and hematocrit 55%. The electrocardiogram showed atrial flutter with 2:1 block. The chest x-ray showed poor inspiration and a $\dot{V}/\dot{Q}$ scan was consistent with high probability for pulmonary embolism.

She was anticoagulated with heparin and given digoxin and procainamide without supplemental oxygen. Her somnolence worsened, and on the third hospital day another room-air blood-gas analysis showed that Pa_{O_2} was 40 mmHg; SaO_2, 75%; pH, 7.22; Pa_{CO_2}, 85 mmHg; and HCO_3^-, 34 meq/L. She was given metoprolol and intravenous diltiazem for the atrial flutter, but she became hypotensive and was transferred to the intensive care unit. There she was intubated, mechanically ventilated, and oxygenated. The Sa_{O_2} was maintained above 90% and Pa_{CO_2} was lowered slowly to <50 torr. After stabilization, she received furosemide for diuresis, acetazolamide to promote HCO_3^- excretion, and later spironolactone. She lost a total of 20 kg, was cardioverted on the fifth hospital day, and was extubated on the eighth hospital day.

At this point she was ventilated with a bilevel pressure-support device and given supplemental oxygen at 2 L/min. She was switched to bilevel pressure support ventilation at night only on the tenth hospital day and was discharged home on the thirteenth hospital day. Medications were digoxin, spironolactone, oxygen at 2 L/min, and nocturnal bilevel CPAP. On discharge, a room-air blood-gas analysis showed that Pa_{O_2} was 47 mmHg; SaO_2, 83%; pH, 7.40; Pa_{CO_2}, 59 mmHg; and HCO_3^-, 35 meq/L. Polysomnography after discharge showed central apneas and hypopneas with desaturation to 65% without CPAP and marked improvement with CPAP. In the subsequent 3 years, she has not been rehospitalized.

This case illustrates several important therapeutic points: (1) It is absolutely necessary to maintain adequate oxygenation. Trying to treat the arrhythmia without oxygenation led to hypotension, which was rapidly reversible with intubation, mechanical ventilation, and oxygenation. (2) Hypoxemia was relatively resistant to therapy, a common problem in OHS. (3) Mechanical ventilatory support coupled with diuretics that promoted bicarbonate excretion and inhibition of aldosterone facilitated weight loss as well as normalization of pH and Pa_{CO_2}. (4) This patient with OHS did not have OSA, but she needed CPAP to relieve hypopneas.

SUMMARY

Morbid obesity without hypoventilation is characterized by marked increases in body weight and body-mass index. Most of the excess weight is fat, but some is increased fat-free mass. Obesity markedly reduces the expiratory reserve volume (ERV) and has a lesser effect on the functional residual capacity (FRC). The vital capacity (VC) and total lung capacity (TLC) are normal except in very severe obesity. Hypoxemia results from overperfusion of dependent lung zones, which are very poorly ventilated or even acting as shunts. With weight loss, the biggest improvements are restoration of the ERV and Pa_{O_2} substantially toward normal.

Obesity triples respiratory resistance and halves respiratory system compliance. Obesity doubles the work of breathing and quadruples the energy cost of breathing. Compensatory mechanisms include doubling of ventilatory drive and shifting to a higher respiratory rate with a smaller tidal volume. Inspiratory muscle strength is well preserved, maximal voluntary ventilation is somewhat reduced, and obese subjects have a relatively normal capacity for physical exercise. However, they have to expend more work during treadmill or bicycle exercise owing to the excess load imposed by the mass of their bodies or their legs, and impaired pulmonary gas exchange limits the available energy supply to a mild degree.

In the obesity hypoventilation syndrome (OHS), body weight is the same as in uncomplicated morbid obesity, but the respiratory abnormalities are more severe. The VC is reduced by one-third, ERV is reduced by two-thirds, and compliance is halved. Respiratory resistance, the work of breathing, and the oxygen cost of breathing are approximately twice as high in OHS as in simple obesity at the same body weight. Furthermore, patients with OHS have moderate inspiratory muscle weakness, their ventilatory drive is not increased to meet the increased work of breathing, the respiratory rate is higher, and the tidal volume is smaller than in uncomplicated obesity.

It is likely that the ventilatory abnormalities of OHS suffice to explain CO_2 retention without having to invoke obstructive sleep apnea (OSA). When present, central apneas, hypopneas, and obstructive sleep apneas only make matters worse. OSA is five times as common in obese men as in obese women, and men with OSA have a more visceral distribution of fat and a lower sensitivity to inhaled CO_2. Many but not all patients with OHS have severe OSA.

Dyspnea in obesity may result from morbid obesity alone, but it is important to rule out other cardiac and pulmonary causes. Many obese patients have coexisting heart or lung disease, so workup with chest x-ray, spirometry, electrocardiogram, echocardiogram, and $\dot{V}/\dot{Q}$ scan is indicated. It is also important to look for evidence of pulmonary hypertension and to determine its underlying cause—i.e., hypoxic vasoconstriction or pulmonary embolism or prior treatment with fenfluramine anorectic drugs.

The best treatment for morbid obesity and its complications is weight loss. The optimal regimen is a combination of low-calorie, high-protein diet and exercise. Anorectic drugs may be useful, but only to help initiate weight loss. Surgery to make the stomach smaller and to minimize intestinal absorption is indicated when medical treatment fails. Weight loss in OHS is associated with increased ERV and VC, decreased FRC, increased Pa_{O_2}, lowering of Pa_{CO_2}, and lessening of sleep-related apneas and hypopneas.

Key elements in the treatment of ventilatory failure are oxygenation, relief of upper airway obstruction when present, and mechanical ventilation to correct hypercapnia. Hypoxia is relatively resistant to treatment if there is severe shunting through nonventilated regions. Treatment generally involves CPAP, mechanical ventilation, and supplemental oxygen, because oxygen alone is not sufficient. Providing CPAP or NPPV by nose mask is often sufficient, but intubation is usually necessary to treat acute ventilatory failure in obesity.

SUGGESTED READING

1. Abenhaim L, Moride Y, Brenot F, Rich S, Benichou J, Kurz X, Higenbottam T, Oakley C, Wouters E, Aubier M, Simonneau G, Begaud B. Appetite suppressant drugs and the risk of primary pulmonary hypertension. N Eng J Med 1996; 335:609–616.
2. Collins LC, Hoberty PD, Walker JF, Fletcher EC, Peiris AN. The effect of body fat distribution on pulmonary function tests. Chest 1995; 107:1298–1302.
3. Donnelly JE, Pronk NP, Jacobsen DJ, Pronk SJ, Jakicic JM. Effects of a very-low-calorie diet and physical-training regimen on body composition and resting metabolic rate in obese females. Am J Clin Nutr 1991; 54:56–61.
4. Hakala K, Mustajoki P, Aittomaki J, Sovijarvi AR. Effect of weight loss and body position on pulmonary function and gas exchange abnormalities in morbid obesity. Int J Obesity 1995; 19:343–346.
5. Hood DD, Dewan DM. Anesthetic and obstetric outcome in morbidly obese patients. Anesthesiology 1993; 79:1210–1218.

6. Leibel RL, Rosenbaum M, Hirsch J. Changes in energy expenditure resulting from altered body weight. N Engl J Med 1995; 332:621–628.
7. Millman RP, Carlisle CC, McGarvey ST, Eveloff SE, Levinson PD. Body fat distribution and sleep apnea severity in women. Chest 1995; 107:362–366.
8. Pelosi P, Croci M, Ravagnan I, Vicardi P, Gattinoni L. Total respiratory system, lung, and chest wall mechanics in sedated-paralyzed postoperative morbidly obese patients. Chest 1996; 109:144–151.
9. Piper AJ, Sullivan CE. Effects of short-term NIPPV in the treatment of patients with severe obstructive sleep apnea and hypercapnia. Chest 1994; 105:434–440.
10. Ramsey-Stewart G. Vertical banded gastroplasty for morbid obesity: weight loss at short and long-term follow up. Aust NZ J Surg 1995; 65:4–7.
11. Rochester DF. Obesity and pulmonary function. In: Alpert MA, ed. Cardiopulmonary Effects of Obesity. Armonk, NY: Futura, 1997, Chap. 5.
12. Rochester DF, Enson Y. Current concepts in the pathogenesis of the obesity-hypoventilation syndrome. Am J Med 1974; 57:402–420.
13. Ross R, Shaw KD, Rissanen J, Martel Y, de Guise J, Avruch L. Sex differences in lean and adipose tissue distribution by magnetic resonance imaging: anthropometric relationships. Am J Clin Nutr 1994; 59:1277–1285.
14. Shenkman Z, Shir Y, Brodsky JB. Perioperative management of the obese patient. Br J Anaesth 1993; 70:349–359.
15. Sugerman HJ, Kellum JM, Engle KM, Wolfe L, Starkey JV, Birkenhauer R, Fletcher P, Sawyer M.-J. Gastric bypass for treating severe obesity. Am J Clin Nutr 1992; 55:560S–566S.
16. Vgontzas AN, Tan TL, Bixler EO, Martin LF, Shubert D, Kales A. Sleep apnea and sleep disruption in obese patients. Arch Intern Med 1994; 154:1705–1711.
17. Zerah F, Harf A, Perlemuter L, Lorino H, Lorino A-M, Atlan G. Effects of obesity on respiratory resistance. Chest 1993; 103:1470–1476.

44

Pregnancy

Jing W. Liu
University of Virginia School of Medicine
Salem Veterans Administration Medical Center
Salem, Virginia

Dudley F. Rochester
University of Virginia School of Medicine
Charlottesville, Virginia

INTRODUCTION

The most common lung diseases in pregnancy are asthma, pulmonary embolism, acute bronchitis, pneumonia, and tuberculosis. This chapter covers pulmonary problems with particular reference to their impact on pregnancy and vice versa. Most of the risk of maternal pulmonary disease to the fetus is related to maternal hypoxemia. We do not cover in depth aspects of pulmonary diseases that are dealt with in other chapters, but we do cover issues in diagnosis and management that are relevant to the pregnant woman.

Fetal radiation exposure consequent to diagnostic imaging is summarized in Table 1. The exposure from a chest x-ray is very small, so a chest x-ray should be obtained whenever there is a good clinical indication. The exposure from most other procedures is also quite low and can often be minimized by using the appropriate technique.

The Food and Drug Administration (FDA) assigns medications into Category A, no known risk; Category B, no evidence of risk in humans; Category C, risk cannot be excluded but benefits may outweigh risks; Category D, risk to fetus established but in some situations benefits may outweigh risks; Category X, contraindicated in pregnancy. FDA ratings for antibiotics are summarized in Table 2. The FDA category of certain medications is indicated in the text using parentheses—for example, tetracycline (D) and streptomycin (X).

RESPIRATORY PHYSIOLOGY IN PREGNANCY

Pulmonary Function

Pregnancy is associated with an increase in the central nervous system's drive to breathe that results from stimulation of the respiratory center by a sixfold increase in circulating progesterone. Ventilatory drive promptly returns to normal after delivery. Ventilation in-

Table 1 Fetal Radiation Exposure from Diagnostic Testing

Procedure	Fetal radiation (Rad)
Chest roentgenogram, PA and lateral	<0.001
Ventilation lung scan	
^{133}Xe	0.004–0.019
^{99m}Tc DTPA	0.007–0.035
^{99m}Tc SC	0.001–0.005
Perfusion lung scan	
3 mCi ^{99m}TcMAA	0.018
1 mCi ^{99m}TcMAA	0.006
Bilateral venography without abdominal shield	0.63
Unilateral	0.31
Limited, abdomen shielded	<0.05
Pulmonary angiography	
Femoral approach	0.41
Brachial approach	<0.05

Key: Xe, xenon; Tc, technetium; DTPA, diethyline triamine pentaacetic acid; S.C., sulfur colloid; MAA, macroaggregates of human albumin.
Source: Adapted from Ginsberg JS, Hirsh J, Rainbow AJ, Coates G. Risks to the fetus of radiologic procedures used in the diagnosis of maternal venous thromboembolic disease. Thromb Haemost 1989; 61:189–196.

Table 2 Risks in Pregnancy of Antibiotics Commonly Used to Treat Pulmonary Infections

Recommended use	FDA rating	Agent
As needed	B	Amphotericin B
	B	Aztreonam
	B	Cephalosporins
	B	Erythromycins except estolate
	B	Penicillins
Only for strong indication	C	Acyclovir
	C	Amantadine
	C	Aminoglycosides
	C	Clindamycin
	C	Imipenem-cilastin
	C	Sulfonamides except at term
	C	Trimethoprim
	C	Trimethoprim/sulfamethoxazole except at term
	C	Vancomycin
	D	Chloramphenicol except at term
Contraindicated	C	Quinolones, ciprofloxacin
	D	Tetracyclines
	X	Streptomycin

creases by about 50%, mainly due to an increase in tidal volume, but oxygen consumption ($\dot{V}_{O_2}$) increases by only 20%. Because hyperventilation is in excess of the increase in metabolic rate, the partial pressure of carbon dioxide in arterial blood (Pa_{CO_2}) falls to around 30 mmHg. However, the compensatory renal excretion of bicarbonate allows arterial blood pH to be normal.

Changes in respiratory mechanics are related to the gravid uterus, which not only distends the abdomen but also causes flaring of the lower rib cage. The diaphragm is displaced headward and the expiratory reserve volume (ERV) decreases markedly. The functional residual capacity (FRC) falls by as much as 20% in late pregnancy, but vital capacity (VC) and total lung capacity (TLC) are usually normal. The compliances of the lung and the chest wall are nearly normal in pregnancy. The large airways are normal, as are expiratory flow rates such as forced expiratory volume in 1 s (FEV_1). The nasal mucosa is hyperemic during the second and third trimesters; this is thought to be a result of the elevated estrogen levels.

Lowering of Pa_{CO_2} with hyperventilation tends to increase the partial pressure of oxygen in arterial blood (Pa_{O_2}). However, owing to reduction in caliber of the small airways, some alveoli may remain poorly ventilated or unventilated during ordinary tidal breathing. As a result, Pa_{O_2} tends to fall, especially on changing from sitting to the supine position. The pulmonary diffusing capacity is essentially normal throughout pregnancy.

Respiratory Muscles and Exercise Capacity

The respiratory muscles most affected by pregnancy are the diaphragm and the abdominal inspiratory muscles. Data concerning the function of the abdominal muscles in pregnancy are lacking, but if the abdominal muscles were overstretched, capacity to cough and to generate the high intraabdominal pressures needed for expulsive maneuvers would be impaired. Diaphragmatic position is shifted headward and diaphragmatic excursion is curtailed, but the other inspiratory muscles help to accomplish the increase in tidal volume. The diaphragm may become fatigued during labor.

The capacity for physical exercise is quite well preserved throughout pregnancy. Peak work capacity and maximal $\dot{V}_{O_2}$ are mildly impaired, but $\dot{V}_{O_2}$ at submaximal work is the same in pregnant and normal women. Pregnant women can usually carry on activities of daily living without difficulty.

Dyspnea

Approximately half of healthy pregnant women experience mild dyspnea by midterm and about three-quarters do so at full term. Dyspnea results from a combination of factors including increased central nervous drive to breathe, hyperventilation, the mechanical changes of the chest and abdomen, weight gain, increased blood volume, and mild anemia. Dyspnea in an otherwise normal pregnancy is usually not severe and tends to level off.

Less than 5% of pregnant women experience dyspnea because they have cardiac or pulmonary disease. Cardiac conditions include cardiomyopathy as well as valvular, congenital, and ischemic heart disease and arrythmias. Dyspnea due to heart disease tends to get much worse as term approaches, is intensified by exertion, and may be accompanied by significant orthopnea or paroxysmal nocturnal dyspnea. There may also be symptoms such as chest pain, palpitation, or syncope. Diagnosis of heart disease during pregnancy is essentially the same as in the absence of pregnancy.

Dyspnea due to pulmonary disease is also intensified by exertion and becomes more severe in later pregnancy. Dyspnea due to asthma may be either intermittent and episodic or chronic, depending on whether asthma is acute or chronic. Dyspnea due to pulmonary infection is usually associated with other evidence of infection, such as cough, production of purulent sputum, and fever. When dyspnea results from interstitial lung disease, pulmonary embolism, or other pulmonary vascular disease, the cause may be harder to discover.

Sleep-Related Breathing Disorders

During the first trimester, pregnant women experience an increase in total sleep time and in daytime sleepiness. In contrast, during the third trimester there is a decrease in sleep time and an increase in number of nocturnal awakenings. Most of the awakenings are due to nonrespiratory factors such as urinary frequency, heartburn, fetal movements, leg cramps, and general discomfort. Polysomnographic sleep studies show that late pregnancy is associated with significantly less rapid-eye-movement (REM) sleep and an increased number of arousals. Pregnant women change position frequently during sleep, and they spend less time in supine and prone positions.

For the most part, women at the end of pregnancy have fewer apneas and hypopneas than nonpregnant women. In addition, they either do not exhibit nocturnal arterial oxyhemoglobin desaturation or they have a small decrease in baseline saturation and a small increase in the number of desaturations during sleep. However, women with obesity or other risk factors for sleep apnea continue to have sleep apnea during pregnancy; indeed, pregnancy may make sleep apnea worse.

Severe maternal arterial oxyhemoglobin desaturation has grave consequences for the fetus. Thus it is necessary to treat sleep apnea during pregnancy, and the principal modalities recommended are nasal continuous positive airway pressure (CPAP), supplemental oxygen, avoidance of the supine position, and attempts to minimize weight gain. Tricyclic antidepressants cause fetal abnormalities and should be avoided.

OBSTRUCTIVE LUNG DISEASES

Smoking

Women who smoke during pregnancy may have mild obstructive disease of the airways, but the fetal complications are the real problem. Smoking increases maternal and fetal carbon monoxide and reduces fetal oxygen carrying capacity by 25%. Moreover, nicotine causes uterine vasoconstriction. Complications associated with maternal smoking include abruptio placenta, placenta praevia, premature rupture of membranes, spontaneous abortion, low birth weight, and fetal death. The prevalence of complications is dose-related. It is extremely important to enroll pregnant women smokers into an effective smoking cessation program.

Asthma

Asthma affects approximately 4% of the population and is equally common in pregnancy. About one-third of pregnant asthmatics experience amelioration of asthma, one-third have no change, and one-third get worse during the course of pregnancy. Pregnant adolescents with asthma do worse, probably because they have more upper respiratory infections and are often poorly compliant with treatment. The risks to the fetus during an asthma attack include uterine vasoconstriction consequent to lowering of maternal Pa_{CO_2}, reduction in placental blood flow owing to reduced maternal cardiac output, and maternal hypoxemia. Fetal problems include growth retardation and low birth weight. Although asthma can cause significant maternal and fetal morbidity and mortality, pregnant asthmatics with proper management have normal pregnancies and give birth to normal children. Asthma tends to return to its prepregnancy status within the first 3 months postpartum. The current classification of asthma severity is summarized in Table 3.

The management of asthma in pregnant women is the same as in those who are not pregnant. It is important for women to know what triggers their asthma attacks and to avoid those triggers. Immunotherapy that is begun before pregnancy may be continued during pregnancy, but immunotherapy should not be started during pregnancy because of the small but finite risk of anaphylaxis.

The pregnant asthmatic should monitor her peak expiratory flow rate (PEFR) using a peak flowmeter twice daily. She should establish her best peak flow range and strive to keep her peak flow above 80% of her personal best PEFR. When PEFR falls below 80% of the personal best, it is time to increase the frequency and/or dose of medication; when PEFR falls below 50% of the personal best, she needs to seek medical attention at once. When asthma is not well controlled, fetal monitoring for heart rate, movement, and intrauterine growth is indicated.

The current recommendations for the treatment of asthma (Table 4) stress the use

Table 3 1997 Recommendations About Classification of Asthma

Severity	Symptoms	Lung function
Mild intermittent	Daytime wheeze, cough, chest tightness occur twice a week or less. Nocturnal symptoms occur less than twice monthly. Often associated with exercise.	PEFR and/or FEV_1 are 80% of normal or better; values vary less than 20%.
Mild persistent	Daytime symptoms occur more than twice a week but less than daily. Nocturnal symptoms occur more than twice a month. Severe attacks may affect activity.	PEFR and/or FEV_1 usually 80% or more of normal, but values vary up to 30%.
Moderate persistent	Bouts of wheeze, cough, and tight chest occur daily and nightime symptoms occur more than once a week. Attacks severe enough to affect activity may occur two or more times a week.	PEFR and/or FEV_1 range between 60 and 80% of normal; values vary up to 30%.
Severe persistent	Continual wheeze, cough, chest tightness day and night. Physical activity is limited by breathing problems. Severe attacks are frequent.	PEFR and/or FEV_1 less than 60% of normal; values vary more than 30%.

Table 4 1997 Recommendations for Treatment of Asthma

Severity	Quick relief	Long-term control
Mild intermittent	Short-acting beta$_2$ agonist such as albuterol.	None, or consider inhaled steroid if quick relief needed more than twice a week.
Mild persistent	Short acting beta$_2$ agonist such as albuterol; may need to take bid–qid for short periods.	Use low dose of inhaled steroid such as budesonide or use cromolyn.
Moderate persistent	Use short-acting beta$_2$ agonist such as albuterol on a daily basis.	Use medium dose of inhaled steroid such as budesonide on daily basis or a low dose plus long-acting drug such as salmeterol or theophylline.
Severe persistent	Use short-acting beta$_2$ agonist such as albuterol on a daily basis.	Daily use of high dose of inhaled steroid plus oral steroid such as prednisone plus salmeterol.

of inhaled steroids for all but the least symptomatic patients. Inhaled short-acting beta$_2$ adrenergic agonist bronchodilators such as albuterol should be used along with inhaled steroids, either as needed to control infrequent symptoms or on a regular schedule if symptoms occur more frequently. When using inhaled medications, it is better to use a spacer with the metered-dose inhaler to reduce oral complications and increase the pulmonary dose of the drug.

When symptoms persist most days or nights, the dose of inhaled steroid should be increased. It may also be necessary to add a long-acting bronchodilator such as salmeterol and also oral steroids, usually prednisone or methylprednisolone. Women whose asthma is not well controlled should always have oral prednisone on hand in case of worsening symptoms and/or falling peak flow; it is better to start the steroid and then seek medical help. Aminophylline (C) in a long acting preparation may be a useful adjunct therapy for poorly controlled asthma.

Treatment of an acute asthma attack involves inhalation of a beta$_2$ agonist such as albuterol or subcutaneous injection of 0.25 mg terbutaline (B) or 0.3 mL of 1:1000 epinephrine (C) solution. Epinephrine may be given every 20 min for a total of three doses. If there is a poor response to the bronchodilators, intravenous hydrocortisone or other corticosteroids should be given. Dehydration should be corrected with caution in pregnancy so as not to precipitate pulmonary edema. Hospitalization for an asthma attack is indicated when the patient has a history of frequent attacks, is already on oral steroids, and has had prior hospitalization for asthma and prior treatment for ventilatory failure.

Approximately 10% of asthmatics will have an attack during labor. Women who have been on oral prednisone should be given hydrocortisone intravenously during labor to prevent adrenal insufficiency. Although beta$_2$ adrenergic agonists might stall the progression of labor, the stress of asthmatic wheezing and coughing has a greater inhibitory effect. Ketamine is the drug of choice for general anesthesia because it has bronchodilating effects; halogenated anesthetics also lead to bronchodilation. Epidural anesthesia is safe in asthma. Fentanyl is the preferred analgesic; drugs such as morphine and demerol that release histamine should be avoided. Oxytocin is the agent of choice for inducing labor and for treating postpartum hemorrhage. Ergotamine and prostaglandin F2-alpha should be avoided because they aggravate asthma.

None of the usual asthma medications is considered to be teratogenic. Beta$_2$ adrenergic agonists such as albuterol (C), metaproterenol (C), and terbutaline (B) may be used. Inhaled ipratropium bromide (B) is also considered to be safe and useful in pregnancy. Cromolyn (B) has few side effects and may be used in pregnancy; there is no experience with nedocromil in pregnancy. Aminophylline (theophylline, C) should be used only when needed to treat asthma that is not well controlled by the agents listed above and by inhaled steroids.

Beclomethasone (C) is the preferred inhaled steroid, but flunisolide (C), fluticasone (C), and triamcinolone (D) may also be used. Oral steroids may be used in tapering doses for short courses. A placental enzyme metabolizes 87% of prednisone before it crosses to the fetus. Steroids may cause a 300- to 400-g decrease in birth weight, and high doses of steroids may induce maternal gestational diabetes.

Cystic Fibrosis

Women with cystic fibrosis have anatomically normal reproductive systems and live long enough to have multiple pregnancies. Women who meet the criteria for good clinical status [Schwachman score > 75, body-mass index (BMI) > 20 kg/m^2, no pancreatic insufficiency, and forced expiratory volume in 1 s (FEV$_1$) > 60% of predicted] tolerate pregnancy well, but women with more severe disease may have problems with congestive heart failure, prematurity, inadequate maternal weight gain, and ventilatory failure. The prepregnancy FEV$_1$ is the best predictor of the outcome of pregnancy in cystic fibrosis; FEV$_1$ values lower than 60% of predicted are associated with higher rates of fetal prematurity and maternal mortality.

Management of the patient with cystic fibrosis requires attention to nutritional status. The woman considering pregnancy should attempt to increase her BMI to above 20 kg/m^2 before pregnancy; during pregnancy, she should gain at least 9 kg. Poor outcome is associated with weight gain of less than 4.5 kg. Pancreatic enzymes, fat-soluble vitamins, and oral nutritional supplements should be given as needed. Some women may need nocturnal feedings by nasogastric tube; to minimize aspiration, continuous rather than bolus feedings should be given and the head of the bed elevated.

Bronchopulmonary infections must be controlled. Oral and inhaled antibiotics may be used in some cases, but severe infections must be treated in hospital with postural drainage, chest physiotherapy, and intravenous antibiotics. Combination beta-lactam/beta-lactamase inhibitor drugs such as anti-*Pseudomonas* or anti-*Staphylococcus* penicillins and the cephalosporins are considered safe during pregnancy. Use of aminoglycosides is discouraged because they cause fetal ototoxicity, but in severe infection the benefit of aminoglycoside therapy may outweight the risk. Quinolones, tetracyclines, and sulfonamides are contraindicated because of fetal toxicity.

Pulmonary hypertension is a leading cause of maternal mortality in pregnancy and labor; one cause of pulmonary hypertension is severe pulmonary disease in cystic fibrosis. Patients with cystic fibrosis who experience a marked sustained decline of lung function during pregnancy, with FEV$_1$ falling below 40% predicted, should be advised to terminate the pregnancy.

RESTRICTIVE DISORDERS OF THE LUNGS AND CHEST WALL

General Characteristics

Almost all restrictive disorders are characterized by small VC, FRC, and TLC. However, the ratio of FEV_1/FVC is normal, indicating that there is no airflow limitation. If there is combined airways obstruction and restriction of the lung or chest wall, then the ratio FEV_1/FVC will be low. Hypoxemia is present, especially in restrictive diseases of the lung, and the DL_{CO} is reduced in restrictive lung diseases.

Interstitial Lung Diseases (ILD)

In interstitial lung disease, the chest x-ray, and computed tomography (CT) show an interstitial pattern, and in later stages there is cystic enlargement of airspaces referred to as honeycombing. The interstitial lung diseases most likely to be encountered during pregnancy are sarcoidosis, hypersensitivity pneumonitis, and idiopathic pulmonary fibrosis. Pulmonary fibrosis also occurs in association with rheumatoid arthritis, polymyositis, and progressive systemic sclerosis.

Lymphangiomyomatosis is a rare disease that occurs in women of childbearing age. There is proliferation of cells that resemble smooth muscle and have receptors for estrogen and progesterone. Clinical manifestations are a mixed interstitial and emphysema-like pattern, plus chylous pleural effusion and pneumothorax. Lymphangiomyomatosis often worsens with pregnancy. Tuberous sclerosis causes nearly identical lung lesions; about 80% of cases are in women, and most of these die of multiple extrapulmonary causes before age 20.

Patients with interstitial lung diseases are often advised against pregnancy, since the lung disease may progress and increase the risks of pregnancy and labor. The highest risk to mother and fetus occurs in women who have progressive systemic sclerosis or tuberous sclerosis with renal disease. When the disease process is limited to the lung, women with interstitial lung disease may complete pregnancy successfully despite having VC and DL_{CO} less than 50% predicted. Successful pregnancy has also occurred after pneumonectomy. Supplemental oxygen for documented hypoxemia is the most important component of treatment.

Restrictive Diseases of the Chest Wall

The diseases of the chest wall that are most likely to have an effect on pregnancy are kyphoscoliosis and flail chest. Idiopathic kyphoscoliosis is somewhat more common in women, and it is not clear whether or not pregnancy causes spinal curvature to worsen. Most women with kyphoscoliosis have normal pregnancies, although they are more apt to be dyspneic. Serious respiratory complications occur only in women who have extreme spinal curvature, and even these can be supported by mechanical ventilation.

Many neuromuscular diseases cause respiratory muscle weakness and predispose to ventilatory failure. Muscle weakness in myotonic dystrophy, myasthenia gravis, and several types of myopathy may worsen during the third trimester of pregnancy and then ameliorate after delivery. Patients with these disorders are more susceptible than normal women to respiratory depression from anesthetics and neuromuscular blocking agents. Most women with stable neuromuscular diseases such as spinal cord injury, old poliomyelitis, or slowly progessive dystrophies and myopathies are able to carry pregnancy through to successful completion.

Pleural Disease

Benign pleural effusion occurs postpartum in approximately 25–50% of normal pregnancies. Pathological pleural effusions are uncommon and are varied in nature. Causes include chylous effusion associated with lymphangiomyomatosis or trauma, hemothorax with choriocarcinoma or neurofibromatosis, urinothorax associated with hydronephrosis, and effusions associated with rupture of the diaphragm, mycoplasmal infection, and antiphospholipase antibodies.

Spontaneous pneumothorax and pneumomediastinum may occur during labor. The clinical presentation is characterized by chest pain, dyspnea, and sometimes cough. Spontaneous pneumomediastinum usually needs no treatment other than supplemental oxygen to facilitate reabsorption. Spontaneous pneumothorax should be treated with chest tube drainage and oxygen to prevent fetal hypoxemia. Labor may be induced with chest tubes in place. Most women can undergo vaginal delivery rather than cesarean section.

INFECTIOUS DISEASES

Influenza and Pneumonia

Influenza and community-acquired pneumonia occur in up to 1% of pregnancies, with a mortality rate of up to 3% maternal and fetal. The principal obstetrical complications of pneumonia are premature labor, abortion, and both fetal and maternal death. The same holds for influenza, but influenza is not associated with maternal death except when complicated by pneumonia. The most common causes of community-acquired pneumonia in women of childbearing age are *Streptococcus pneumoniae*, *Mycoplasma pneumoniae*, respiratory viruses, *Chlamydia pneumoniae*, and *Haemophilus influenzae*. Miscellaneous other causes include *Legionella* species, *Mycobacterium tuberculosis*, endemic fungi, and aerobic gram-negative bacilli.

Poor outcomes are associated with extensive pulmonary involvement seen on chest x-ray, hypoxemia, and history of smoking more than 10 cigarettes per day. Clinical signs that point to severe pneumonia and need for hospitalization are summarized in Table 5.

Table 5 Indicators of Severe Pneumonia

History	Severe dyspnea
Physical examination	Temperature $< 35°$ or $> 40°$ C
	Diastolic blood pressure < 60 mmHg
	Respiratory rate > 30 breaths per minute
	Recruitment of neck inspiratory muscles
	Retractions, cyanosis
Laboratory	$Pa_{O_2} < 60$ mmHg or $Sa_{O_2} < 90\%$
	pH < 7.35
	WBC $< 4000/\mu L$
	BUN < 30 mg/dL
	Na < 130 meq/L

It is important for clinicians to look for a history of preexisting lung disease, a respiratory rate in excess of 30 breaths per minute and hypoxemia with Pa_{O_2} less than 60 mmHg, and arterial oxyhemoglobin saturation (Sa_{O_2}) less than 90%.

The diagnosis of community-acquired pneumonia rests on the clinical presentation, with variable combinations of cough, fever, sputum production, dyspnea and chest pain, and physical signs of rales and/or consolidation. An abrupt onset with chills and fever and yellow or rusty sputum is more consistent with pneumococcal pneumonia, whereas hacking nonproductive cough, malaise, and headache point toward mycoplasmal pneumonia or influenza. Patients without evidence of severe pneumonia should have a chest x-ray but little else in the way of diagnostic testing. Thoracentesis is recommended if pleural effusion is present.

Most cases of community-acquired pneumonia in pregnant women can be treated at home with oral antibiotics prescribed empirically. Typically, a macrolide (i.e., erythromycin, but not erythromycin estolate) or a second-generation cephalosporin would suffice. Pregnant women should not be given tetracycline or trimethoprim/sulfamethoxazole unless there is a very strong clinical indication.

Patients who meet clinical criteria for severe pneumonia should be hospitalized, and they need more diagnostic testing to judge severity and to look for specific etiological agents and for organisms resistant to antibiotics. Sputum Gram stain, sputum and blood cultures, thoracentesis, bronchoscopy, and serological tests are the usual tools for further investigation. Treatment of the hospitalized patient usually includes a second- or third-generation cephalosporin or a combination beta-lactam/beta-lactamase inhibitor as well as a macrolide. In very severe cases, coverage for *Pseudomonas* species should be added and patients should receive several antibiotics intravenously, including, for example, a third-generation cephalosporin, an aminoglycoside, and erythromycin.

Some forms of pneumonia are especially hazardous. Influenza may be associated with fetal damage. Women who are at risk to contract influenza should be given amantidine prophylactically, as it can prevent 50–70% of infections. Women who are suspected to have influenza should get amantadine, since it reduces fever as well as the duration of symptoms by about 50%. Women of childbearing age probably should have influenza vaccination; the Centers for Disease Control recommend that pregnant women should be vaccinated after the first trimester. In an influenza epidemic, even women in the first trimester should be vaccinated.

Varicella pneumonia is much more common in pregnant than in nonpregnant women and may go on to adult respiratory distress syndrome (ARDS). The treatment is acyclovir (C), which has no known adverse fetal effects. Hantavirus also produces severe ARDS; treatment is supportive. Coccidioidomycosis is 100 times more likely to disseminate in pregnancy, with high risk to the mother. The treatment is amphotericin B (B). Women with HIV infection may contract *Pneumocystis carinii* pneumonia; because of the high maternal risk they need to be treated with trimethoprim/sulfamethoxazole despite its potential for fetal damage.

Tuberculosis

Tuberculosis is most prevalent in areas of poverty where there are indigent and homeless people and among populations of immigrants from areas with a very high prevalence of tuberculosis. Tuberculosis also occurs in intravenous drug abusers and in women who are close contacts of someone with active pulmonary tuberculosis. The prevalence of tuberculosis in pregnancy ranges from 0.3–1.9%. Tuberculosis may get worse during pregnancy and may increase the risk of miscarriage. Pregnant women with tuberculosis are often asymptomatic and are apt to present with unilateral, noncavitary, smear-negative disease. Thus it is important to apply the tuberculin skin test to all pregnant women. At 48 h, induration of 5 mm diameter is considered to be a positive reaction for women who are contacts, who have HIV infection, or who have clinical evidence of tuberculosis. Induration of 10 mm is considered to be a positive reaction for women in high-risk groups, and a 15-mm-diameter induration is considered positive for women at low risk.

Positive reactors should have a chest x-ray, and sputum cultures should be obtained if any infiltrate or suspicious lesion is seen. It may be necessary to collect pooled early-morning specimens, to induce sputum using a saline aerosol, or to obtain specimens of gastric juice for culture. Prophylaxis with isoniazid is indicated for women who have documented recent conversion of their skin test; prophylaxis should be delayed until after the first trimester. Pregnant women who are taking isoniazid should also take a pyridoxine supplement, because pregnancy increases the vitamin B_6 requirement.

If the chest x-ray shows lesions consistent with tuberculosis, treatment should be initiated with isoniazid, rifampin (C), and pyridoxine and continued for 9 months. In patients with extensive cavitary tuberculosis, ethambutol may also be given for the first 2 months. If multiple drug resistance is suspected, pyrazinamide (C) may also be given. The dose schedule of these drugs is shown in Table 6. Standard treatment may be given daily at a lower dose or twice weekly using a higher dose; the latter regimen is indicated for patients whose treatment must be directly supervised by a health care worker. Treatment of multiple-drug-resistant tuberculosis is beyond the scope of this chapter. Streptomycin and ethionamide are contraindicated in pregnancy.

Congenital tuberculosis is rare; it results from hematogenous spread from an infected placenta. Fetal sites of involvement are mainly the liver and lung. Diagnosis is difficult, so newborns of women with active tuberculosis should receive isoniazid for 3 months or until maternal sputum cultures are negative. Rifampin prophylaxis may be indicated if the mother has multiple-drug-resistant disease. Treatment of congenital tuberculosis is similar to treatment in adults, with isoniazid, rifampin, pyrazinamide, and ethambutol or streptomycin if a fourth drug is indicated.

Table 6 Typical Doses for Drugs Used to Treat Tuberculosis in Pregnant Women

Drug	Dose	Toxicity
Isoniazid	300 mg daily 900 mg twice a week[a]	GI distress, hepatitis, seizure, neuritis
Rifampin	600 mg daily 600 mg twice a week[a]	GI distress, hepatitis, headache, fever
Ethambutol	15 mg/kg/day 25 mg/kg twice a week[a]	Decreased visual acuity, optic neuritis
Pyrazinamide	25 mg/kg/day 50 mg/kg twice a week[a]	Hepatitis, hyperuricemia, and gout
Pyridoxine	50 mg daily	

[a] The twice weekly regimens are for patients whose therapy is directly observed by a health care worker.

ACUTE RESPIRATORY FAILURE

Acute respiratory failure is a leading cause of maternal morbidity and mortality. Hypoxic respiratory failure is more dangerous than hypercapnic respiratory failure (ventilatory failure). Hypoxic respiratory failure results from cardiogenic pulmonary edema; severe infectious or aspiration pneumonia; embolism with air, fat, thrombi, or amniotic fluid; and adult respiratory distress syndrome (ARDS).

Permeability Pulmonary Edema

ARDS is characterized by severe injury to the alveolar-capillary membranes, with leakage of protein-rich fluid into alveoli. Even small increases in pulmonary capillary pressure intensify the leakage and worsen the pulmonary edema. Mortality from ARDS still ranges from 30–70%. Leading causes of ARDS is pregnancy are summarized in Table 7. The risk of aspiration during labor and delivery is high because of delay in gastric emptying and atony of the gastroesophageal sphincter. Aspiration can be prevented by using regional anesthesia, not giving patients anything by mouth, and applying cricoid pressure if endotracheal intubation is performed. Amniotic fluid embolism is a very rare but highly lethal event. It can occur any time during pregnancy and up to 48 h postpartum. Maternal mortality approaches 90%, with half of these women dying in the first hour. Diagnosis rests on finding material of fetal origin in blood aspirated from the pulmonary artery. Venous air embolism can occur during the peripartum period; risk factors include central venous access, abortion, and placenta previa as well as labor and delivery.

The clinical presentation of ARDS includes dyspnea, tachycardia and tachypnea, bibasilar rales, and often cyanosis. Chest x-ray shows widespread pulmonary infiltrate, usually bilateral, that ranges from a barely perceptible interstitial pattern initially to a florid alveolar pattern later on. The ratio of Pa_{O_2} to $F_{I_{O_2}}$ is less than 200 (normal is greater than 400). Pulmonary capillary wedge pressure is normal.

Treatment includes intubation, mechanical ventilation with supplemental oxygen and positive end-expiratory pressure (PEEP), fluid restriction, and treatment of the under-

Table 7 Causes of Acute Hypoxic
Respiratory Failure in Pregnancy

Adult respiratory distress syndrome (ARDS)
Obstetrical: Chorioamnionitis
Amniotic fluid embolus
Trophoblastic embolus
Eclampsia
Nonobstetrical: Pneumonia
Sepsis
Aspiration of gastric contents
Pulmonary edema
Cardiogenic
Associated with tocolytic therapy
Preeclampsia
Pulmonary thromboembolism
Pneumothorax

lying cause when one can be identified. However, in catastrophic situations such as amniotic fluid embolism that are associated with hypotension and low cardiac output, it may be necessary at the onset to provide fluid resuscitation as well as oxygenation and mechanical ventilation. The fetus should be delivered promptly and neonatal resuscitation may be needed.

The most important aspects of treatment are to maintain blood perfusion and oxygenation to heart, brain, and fetus. The reader should consult Chap. 25 for details of treatment to minimize barotrauma and maintain adequate oxygenation during mechanical ventilation.

Hydrostatic Pressure Pulmonary Edema

Cardiogenic and fluid overload pulmonary edema results from an increase in pulmonary capillary pressure, and this is abetted by the low serum protein concentration of late pregnancy. Pulmonary edema sometimes occurs in preeclampsia, mainly from volume overload. Cardiogenic pulmonary edema in pregnancy may result from cardiomyopathy, rheumatic heart disease, atrial septal defect, and endocarditis. Unlike the edema fluid of ARDS, cardiogenic edema fluid has very little protein, so it can be reabsorbed into the circulation quite promptly when the capillary pressure falls. Mechanical ventilation often unloads the left ventricle and assists in the resolution of edema.

Tocolysis is the use of beta$_2$ adrenergic agents to inhibit preterm labor. An occasional adverse side effect of tocolysis is a form of cardiogenic pulmonary edema that usually occurs 24–48 h after initiation of tocolytic therapy. The clinical presentation includes dyspnea, tachypnea, tachycardia, bibasilar rales, and a chest x-ray consistent with fluid overload. The key components of treatment are to stop the tocolytic agent and provide supportive care, including a loop diuretic. Resolution usually occurs within 24 h, and mechanical ventilation is usually not necessary.

Ventilatory Failure

Ventilatory failure occurs in obstructive diseases of the airways, morbid obesity, neuromuscular diseases and other forms of severe muscle weakness, and restrictive diseases of the chest wall. Ventilatory failure is rare in pregnancy, because even women in the third trimester have a high ventilatory reserve. Causes of ventilatory failure in pregnancy are listed in Table 8; the most likely are severe asthma (status asthmaticus), myasthenia gravis and Guillain-Barré syndrome. Ventilatory failure sometimes occurs in very slowly progressive conditions such as muscular dystrophy, myopathy, and kyphoscoliosis, but only when there is severe muscle weakness or chest wall deformity.

Physical findings that indicate respiratory distress and a probable need for mechanical ventilation include increasing dyspnea and tachypnea, progressive recruitment of neck inspiratory muscles, and chest-abdomen asynchrony. When ventilatory failure is suspected, it is also necessary to obtain an arterial blood gas analysis. The Sa_{O2} measured by oximeter is too insensitive; it falls only very late in the course of ventilatory failure. One should also measure VC and maximal respiratory pressures made by voluntary effort against a closed airway (PI_{max} and PE_{max} or MIP and MEP). Laboratory markers for ventilatory failure include Pa_{CO_2} greater than 50 mmHg, VC less than 15 mL/kg, and MIP less than 35 cmH$_2$O, but a rising Pa_{CO_2} and falling VC or MIP are reason to consider initiation

Table 8 Causes of Ventilatory Failure in Pregnancy

Airways disease	
Asthma (status asthmaticus)	
Cystic fibrosis	
Neuromuscular diseases	
Rapidly progressive:	Myasthenia gravis
	Guillain-Barré syndrome
Slowly progressive:	Old poliomyelitis
	Muscular dystrophy
	Congenital myopathies
	Acquired myopathy (steroid, polymyositis)
Chest wall disease	
Obesity hypoventilation syndrome	
Kyphoscoliosis	
Flail chest	

of mechanical ventilation even if these variables have not yet reached these limits (see Chap. 25).

When patients with status asthmaticus need mechanical ventilation, it should be provided using positive-pressure ventilation via an endotracheal tube. In contrast, patients with CO_2 retention consequent to neuromuscular or chest wall disease may be ventilated with a negative-pressure device or receive positive-pressure ventilation via a nose mask.

DEEP VENOUS THROMBOSIS AND PULMONARY EMBOLISM

Prevalence and Risk Factors

Pregnancy is associated with some increase in the risk of deep venous thrombosis (DVT) owing to increase in plasma concentrations of coagulation factors and fibrinolytic inhibitors as well as the mechanical factors of venous compression and stasis. The incidence in previously healthy women is 0.5–7 per 1000 deliveries, and pulmonary thromboembolism (PE) is a leading cause of maternal mortality, accounting for up to 17% of maternal deaths. In approximately 95% of patients, PE comes from DVT in the legs. Risk factors for DVT and PE during pregnancy include prior history of DVT or PE during pregnancy or while on contraceptives, prolonged bed rest, cesarean section, complicated vaginal delivery, and thrombophilic states such as deficiencies of antithrombin III, protein C or protein S, and antiphospholipid antibody syndromes.

Diagnosis of DVT and PE

Clinical diagnostic criteria are unreliable because leg pain and swelling are common in pregnancy. Diagnosis often depends on techniques that involve some form of ionizing radiation. It is estimated that with fetal exposure to less than 5 rads, there is a slight increase in childhood cancer but no increase in congenital malformations. With care, the exposure needed to diagnose DVT and/or PE can be kept below 0.5 rads (Table 1).

Tests for DVT include impedance plethysmography (IPG); Doppler and duplex ultrasonography; radioactive iodinated fibrinogen uptake scan, which is contraindicated in pregnancy; and contrast venography. Limited contrast venography with an abdominal shield reduces fetal radiation to <0.05 rads but does not allow visualization of the iliac veins.

IPG is sensitive and specific for DVT in nonpregnant patients. In pregnancy, especially in the third trimester, IPG can yield a false-positive result owing to compression of the iliac vein by the gravid uterus. IPG is insensitive to DVT in the calf, so serial testing over 7–14 days may be necessary to exclude DVT extending proximally from the calf.

Doppler and duplex ultrasound are also sensitive and specific for proximal DVT. Duplex ultrasound combines real-time B-mode and Doppler ultrasound imaging. Limitations include subjectivity of interpretation, dependence on the skill of the examiner, and inability to detect isolated iliac vein thrombosis, which may occur in pregnancy.

A practical diagnostic approach for clinically suspected DVT and/or PE in the pregnant woman is shown in Table 9. Before the third trimester, begin with ultrasound, since an abnormal test will confirm the diagnosis of DVT. If ultrasound is normal, obtain IPG; and if IPG is normal, repeat serially over 7–14 days to exclude propagation from the calf. Anticoagulation can be withheld until DVT is detected proximally. In the third trimester—or earlier if ultrasound and IPG are not available—perform limited contrast venography to differentiate between proximal DVT and venous compression by the uterus. If limited venography is normal and DVT is suspected strongly, then perform complete contrast venography to look for isolated iliac vein thrombosis.

The lung perfusion scan is the most useful test for PE in pregnancy. A normal perfusion scan rules out PE and a high-probability scan indicates the presence of PE in most cases. The dose of radioisotope for the perfusion scan can be reduced from 3 mCI to 1–2 mCi, and the ventilation part of the scan is omitted to minimize fetal radiation exposure. When the perfusion scan is of intermediate or indeterminate probability, then the options depend on the clinical probability of PE. If the clinical and perfusion scan probabilities are low or moderate, then look for DVT in the legs using serial ultrasonography; if results over 2 weeks are negative, PE is essentially excluded. If the clinical proba-

Table 9 Diagnostic Approach to DVT and/or PE in Pregnancy

Suspect DVT and US or IPG is available	
Normal IPG or US:	Follow with serial IPG or US
Abnormal IPG or US in first and second trimester:	Treat
Abnormal IPG or US in third trimester:	Limited venography to confirm, treat if positive
Suspect DVT; if neither US nor IPG is available, perform limited venography	
Limited venography is normal: Perform complete venography, treat if positive	
Limited venography is abnormal: Treat	
Suspect PE, low to moderate clinical probability	
Perfusion lung scan is of low probability, IPG and US are normal: serial IPG or US	
Suspect PE, high clinical probability	
Perfusion lung scan is not of high probability and IPG or US are normal: pulmonary angiogram	

Key: DVT, deep venous thrombosis; US, Doppler ultrasound; IPG, impedance plethysmography.

bility is high and the perfusion scan result is not of high probability, then perform a pulmonary angiogram. Fetal radiation exposure can be reduced by almost 90% by using a brachial rather than a femoral venous approach plus an abdominal shield (Table 1).

Treatment of DVT and PE

Anticoagulation is the preferred treatment for documented DVT or PE during pregnancy and the puerperium. Unfractionated heparin does not cross the placenta and does not harm the fetus. Treatment consists of unfractionated heparin intravenously for 5 days followed by subcutaneous heparin q12 h until delivery. The partial thromboplastin time (PTT) drawn 6 h after heparin dose should be adjusted to approximately 1.5–2.5 times control. The PTT should be monitored every week, as the heparin requirement may vary over the course of the pregnancy. Supplemental calcium should be given to avoid heparin-induced osteoporosis, and platelets should be monitored to look for heparin-induced thrombocytopenia, typically 7–10 days after starting heparin.

Low-molecular-weight heparins (LMWH) do not cross the placenta, and they appear to be suitable substitutes for unfractionated heparin, although data in pregnancy are limited. LMWH cause no more bleeding than regular heparin and their longer half-life permits once-a-day dosing. The anticoagulant responses to LMWH are more predictable, so the need for monitoring PTT is reduced. LMWH are less apt to cause osteoporosis or thrombopenia.

Warfarin crosses the placenta and can cause severe embryopathy, central nervous system (CNS) deformities, and fetal bleeding. Therefore warfarin is contraindicated during pregnancy. However, warfarin is safe for nursing infants and may be given after delivery to complete a course of anticoagulation.

Inferior vena cava filters have been used in pregnancy with no significant maternal or fetal mortality. The indications are recurrent thromboembolism despite adequate anticoagulant therapy or contraindication to anticoagulation such as bleeding or heparin-induced thrombocytopenia.

Thrombolytic therapy is relatively contraindicated in pregnancy and in the first days after delivery. Thrombolytics cross the placenta and may cause fetal bleeding, and they cause excessive postpartum blood loss.

Anticoagulation at Delivery

High doses of heparin can exert an anticoagulant effect for more than 24 h. Elevation of PTT increases the risk of bleeding at delivery and also increases the hazard of epidural anesthesia. Thus one may wish to induce labor electively close to term and stop subcutaneous heparin 24 h prior to induction. If a woman receiving adjusted-dose subcutaneous heparin enters labor spontaneously, heparin should be stopped immediately. If the PTT is greater than 1.5 times control, one may give protamine sulfate. For women who receive 5000 U of heparin subcutaneously every 12 h, stopping heparin at the onset of true labor will suffice. For women at high risk of thromboembolism, intravenous heparin should be started after subcutaneous heparin has been stopped, then intravenous heparin is stopped 6 h before the anticipated time of delivery.

Since the risk of thromboembolism is greatest immediately postpartum, heparin should be restarted as soon as adequate hemostasis has been achieved, and warfarin should be started the same day. Heparin should be continued until warfarin has increased pro-

Table 10 Prophylaxis Recommendations for Pregnant Women with Prior DVT or PE

Group	When given	Heparin dose
ACP	First, second, third trimester	5000 U SC q12h
BSH	First, second, third trimester	10,000 U SC q12h
	or	or
	First, second trimester	5000 U SC q12h;
	and third trimester	adjust dose to obtain PTT 1.5 times control
HTTF	Up to 36 weeks gestation and postnatally	5000 U SC q12h
	36 weeks gestation to term	10,000 U SC q12h

Key: ACP, American College of Physicians; BSH, British Society of Haematology; HTTF, Haemostasis Thrombosis Task Force, Maternal and Neonatal Working Party.

thrombin time to an International Normalized Ratio (INR) of 2–3. Warfarin should be continued for 4–6 weeks postpartum or for 3 months in women who have had venous thromboembolism late in pregnancy.

Prophylaxis

Anticoagulation is also recommended for prophylaxis against venous thromboembolism in women at risk because of prior history of thromboembolism or those who have thrombophilic states such as deficiency of antithrombin III, protein C, or protein S. Recommendations as to heparin dose vary from 5000 to 10,000 units subcutaneously every 12 h, depending on frequency of monitoring APTT or antifactor Xa activity (Table 10). Women at risk who cannot or will not use heparin should have clinical surveillance and periodic IPG or ultrasonography. Heparin should be started 4–6 weeks before the time in pregnancy that a previous thromboembolic episode occurred, or delayed until post partum if the previous episode occcured postnatally. If a woman had previous thromboembolism not associated with pregnancy, she should be anticoagulated in the third trimester and puerperium if the prior event was not severe, and throughout pregnancy if the prior event was severe. Low-molecular-weight heparins are now being used in other conditions as the treatment of choice for prophylaxis against DVT and PE, and it is likely that they will become the preferred mode of prophylaxis in pregnancy as well.

SUGGESTED READING

1. Carter EJ, Mates S. Tuberculosis during pregnancy: the Rhode Island experience, 1987–1991. Chest 1994; 106:1466–1470.
2. Garcia-Rio F, Pino JM, Gomez L, Alvarez-Sala R, Villasante C, Villamor J. Regulation of breathing and perception of dyspnea in healthy pregnant women. Chest 1996; 110:446–453.
3. Ginsberg JS, Hirsh J, Rainbow AJ, Coates G. Risks to the fetus of radiologic procedures used in the diagnosis of maternal venous thromboembolic disease. Thromb Haemost 1989; 61:189–196.
4. Miller JM Jr, ed. Pulmonary diseases in pregnancy. Clin Obstet Gynecol 1996; 39(1):1–52.
5. Niederman MS, ed. Pulmonary disease in pregnancy. Clin Chest Med 1992; 13(4):555–740.
6. Rizk NW, Kalassian KG, Gilligan T, Druzin MI, Daniel DL. Obstetric complications in pulmonary and critical care medicine. Chest 1996; 110:791–809.

7. Rochester DF. Obesity and abdominal distension. In: Roussos C, ed. The Thorax Part C: Disease. New York: Marcel Dekker, 1995:1951–1973.
8. Stenius-Aarniala BS, Hedman J, Teramo KA. Acute asthma during pregnancy. Thorax 1996; 51:411–414.
9. Toglia MR, Weg JG. Venous thromboembolism during pregnancy. N Engl J Med 1996; 335: 108–114.

45

Preoperative Evaluation and Management of the Respiratory Disease Patient

Simon D. Spivack
Albany Medical College
Albany Medical Center
New York State Department of Health

Joseph L. Saraceno
Albany Medical Center
Albany, New York

The prevention of a serious postoperative complication is the most compelling reason to perform a preoperative evaluation on a patient. The most common causes of postoperative morbidity are respiratory in nature. This chapter is aimed at helping the clinician identify the surgical candidate at risk for respiratory complications, quantify that risk if possible, and identify those techniques that have proven useful in minimizing that risk. This chapter is structured to first review the pathophysiological changes inherent in anesthesia and then identify the high-risk surgical procedures from a respiratory standpoint. The convergence of a high-risk procedure with a high-risk patient will be highlighted.

THE SURGICAL PROCEDURE AS A CHALLENGE TO THE RESPIRATORY DISEASE PATIENT

Surgery and the associated anaesthesia present specific challenges to the physiology of the respiratory system. Induction of general anesthesia inhibits central ventilatory and hypoxic drive, alters mechanics of the chest wall and diaphragm, and induces lung parenchymal changes. These combine to present a substantial challenge to the patient with preexisting respiratory disease. The manipulations inherent in surgical procedures are additional insults to the respiratory system and vary widely according to site and nature of the surgery. The anesthesia and surgical aspects to the procedure are briefly reviewed.

ANESTHESIA

General Anesthesia

As the respiratory effects of general anesthesia differ from those of regional anesthesia, these are discussed separately.

Deranged control of breathing and depression of ventilatory drive is common to most general anesthetic agents. Inhalational agents such as isoflurane and enflurane are quite potent in this regard, and their effects linger in proportion to the duration of the operation. These agents go largely unmetabolized and are distributed throughout tissues such as fat and muscle, ultimately to be eliminated by the lungs. Nitrous oxide (N_2O) has the least ventilatory depressant effects of the inhaled agents and is often used to lower the required concentrations of the other agents. Those volatile agents with the shortest biologic half-lives such as desflurane and sevoflurane allow this effect to be transient, with ventilatory drive normalized within 30 min postoperatively. Patients recovering from the use of any of the inhalation agents often have a rapid respiratory rate but a depressed tidal volume, predisposing them to atelectasis. Virtually all the inhaled agents markedly impair the ventilatory response to hypoxia, even at low concentrations. Intravenous narcotics, barbiturates, propofol, and other agents are also potent inhibitors of ventilation, both to hypercarbia and hypoxia. However, the use of ultra-short-acting opiates such as remifentanil, a mu-receptor agonist, may minimize this effect to a few minutes postinfusion.

Patients with chronic obstructive pulmonary disease (COPD) are more sensitive to the ventilatory depressant effects of both inhalation and intravenous anesthetics. The anesthetic-induced impairment of ventilatory response to hypoxia extends into the recovery period when traditional inhaled agents are used, particularly for long-lasting operations and extended anesthesia times. The reduced clearance of the anesthetic in these patients is a result of the impaired ventilatory response to hypoxia as well as the increased dead space and decreased ventilatory drive inherent to their disease. Thus, COPD poses a risk for impaired ventilation following general anesthesia. The degree to which that risk is prohibitive is discussed in a later section.

Lung Mechanical Effects

General anesthesia reduces the inflation status of the lung independent of subsequent surgical manipulation. Generally, the functional residual capacity (FRC) is reduced by approximately 500 mL. This reduction may persist up to 1–2 weeks. The factors leading to this reduction include diaphragmatic relaxation and elevation and chest wall relaxation. More shallow breathing and infrequent sighs contribute to the tendency for atelectasis. Within minutes of induction, atelectasis occurs in roughly 5% of the dependent portions of normal human lungs regardless of potentially confounding factors of type of anesthesia, mode of ventilation (spontaneous or mechanical), or F_{IO_2}. Persistence of atelectasis 24 h into the postoperative period has been reported to occur in 50% of healthy patients. The decrease in the clearance of mucus and increased bacterial colonization in these atelectatic areas predisposes toward infection. The application of modest amounts of positive end-expiratory pressure may be of some value. The use of intravenous "local" anesthetics such as lidocaine has been attempted in other settings to abolish reflexes that subserve the neural component of the postabdominal surgery ileus reflex, but it has not been reported in the context of postsurgical diaphragmatic dysfunction.

Gas Exchange Effects

Hypoxia is a concomitant of atelectasis because of the mechanical forces that predispose to low ventilation/perfusion ($\dot{V}/\dot{Q}$) matching. The absence of nitrogen in the patient breathing an $F_{I_{O_2}}$ of 100% does not appear to be a major contributor to atelectasis. Those most susceptible to hypoxia are the aged, the obese, and those with preexisting lung disease whose propensity for airway closure and low $\dot{V}/\dot{Q}$ areas predate the additional insults of anesthesia.

For the bronchial tree, clearance of mucus has been noted to be depressed for 2–6 days following general anesthesia. The mechanism is unclear but appears to depend on mucus and ciliary properties, not on an impairment in coughing. Additionally, airway smooth muscle tone may be decreased by some inhaled anesthetics agents (e.g., enflurane) and some intravenous agents (e.g., ketamine); therefore, these drugs have been used therapeutically in the operating suite in those with refractory and life-threatening bronchospasm.

Regional Anesthesia

There are considerable theoretical and physiological reasons why the use of regional or spinal-epidural anesthesia might hasten postoperative recovery for the respiratory-impaired patient. Epidural anesthesia using local anesthetics causes less respiratory depression than general anesthesia. In some series, this approach has translated into fewer postoperative episodes of pneumonia and respiratory failure; in hip surgery in patients with substantial medical comorbidities, it has improved mortality. However, there are older studies demonstrating no benefit to the use of combined intraoperative epidural agents over that of general anesthesia.

The postoperative use of regional anesthesia has been reported to be advantageous over that of systemic opioid analgesics with regard to postoperative oxygen desaturation, recovery of vital capacity, and pain control. There are studies on both sides of the issue as to whether clinical bronchitic or pneumonia episodes or chest radiographic abnormalities are less frequent occurrences with the use of postoperative epidural versus systemic analgesia.

The use of regional anesthesia is precluded in laparosopic procedures because of gas insufflation–related discomfort and in thoracotomy, where control of ventilation and lung motion is essential. Complications related to epidural anesthesia, such as hypotension and catheter site infection, are unusual.

In summary, it remains the task of the anesthesiologist to weigh the planned operative approach, the patient's underlying comorbidities, and the regional or spinal versus general anesthesia approaches in a calculus that individualizes the technical approach to anesthesia.

SITE-SPECIFIC RISKS FOR SURGERY

The most important risk factor for respiratory complications is the site of surgery. A well-worn adage is "The more proximate to the diaphragm, the higher the rate of respiratory complications."

Cardiac Surgery

Coronary artery bypass surgery is the most common cardiac surgical procedure in the United States. The invasion of the chest would, at first glance, seem to be a profoundly compromising factor for rapid postoperative recovery, particularly for those with preexisting lung disease. Vital capacity and functional residual capacity have been reported as depressed 4 months after surgery, presumptively due to altered chest mechanics. However, the anesthetic, median sternotomy, graft harvesting, and graft implantation aspects of the procedure have been sufficiently refined to yield overall mortality rates of 1–4%. Patient subgroups with higher overall mortality include those of advanced age, pulmonary disease, and other comorbidities.

Respiratory morbidity may include atelectasis, hypoxia, pneumonia, pulmonary thromboembolism, prolonged mechanical ventilation, and other adverse outcomes. For example, the incidence of postoperative pneumonia has been reported to occur in up to 23% of patients, depending on the study definition of pneumonia and the subgroup examined. Another well-studied outcome is the requirement for prolonged mechanical ventilation. Ventilation for more then 48 h was required by about 8% of patients in a large series. It should be noted that a variety of pulmonary, cardiac, and other insults may lead to the requirement for prolonged mechanical ventilation. By multivariate analysis, the presence of COPD by diagnosis or by surrogate clinical or lung function parameters was not predictive of prolonged mechanical ventilation (>48 h). Left ventricular dysfunction and to a lesser extent other nonpulmonary comorbidities were the only consistent risk factors for this endpoint.

In contrast, an earlier study by Cohen et al. that relied on simple univariate analysis had suggested that COPD carried some prognostic value. Longer ventilation times, more frequent pneumonias, prolonged intensive care, and extended hospital stays were all associated with the diagnosis of COPD. The differences in analytical techniques—multivariate versus univariate—is critical; confounders were controlled quantitatively only in the multivariate analysis. The integration of risk factors for morbidity into a multivariate index has been reported in other studies, and the presence of COPD is not consistently cited as a strong adverse factor.

Therefore, integrating an incomplete body of literature with clinical experience, moderate to severe COPD is considered a risk factor but not an absolute contraindication to surgical intervention for coronary artery or valve surgery. COPD patients with FEV_1 less than 1 L and hypercarbia have been successfully operated. It is apparent that pulmonary complication rates are higher in those with severe COPD than in those matched subjects without this disorder. No clinical parameters clearly predict with certainty a poor respiratory outcome; therefore, the establishment of ''inoperability'' due to respiratory insufficiency remains a matter of judgment of the medical and surgical teams. The acceptance of a higher perioperative respiratory complication risk must be the subject of an open discussion between physician, surgeon, and patient prior to surgery.

The literature does not adequately address the risks of interstitial disease or sleep-disordered breathing for this type of chest surgery. Progressive interstitial disease should be factored in heavily as a life-limiting condition before coronary surgery is undertaken. Sleep-disordered breathing and attendant hypoxia are often confounding factors in the attempt to control coronary ischemia. Clearly, this treatable set of conditions should be well-controlled, with the use of CPAP or BiPAP or with supplemental oxygen, before and during the perioperative period. The presence of sleep-disordered breathing should not preclude coronary artery surgery in and of itself, but associated conditions such as morbid obesity and airway management do add complexity to the procedure.

Thoracic Surgery

An estimated 170,000 patients are diagnosed with lung cancer annually in the United States. For those patients who present with localized non-small-cell carcinoma, thoracic resection is the primary curative option. Even for those who are fortunate enough to be diagnosed with early-stage disease, smoking-related comorbidities such as COPD and coronary artery disease complicate surgical referral. In addition, recent revisions of lung cancer staging and a renewed interest in the potential benefits of lung cancer screening may lead to even more frequent surgical evaluations for smaller, radiographically suspicious, or cytologically defined lesions that are amenable to diagnosis by excision and potential ''cure.''

Assessing who can tolerate surgical resection from a respiratory standpoint is straightforward in the extreme cases; those with no preexisting pulmonary impairment can and those with profound preexisting debility cannot undergo this surgery. The process of risk evaluation is more complex between these extremes. Spirometry, quantitative ventilation perfusion scanning, and arterial blood-gas analysis (ABG) are commonly used evaluations to help stratify potential surgical candidates based upon the premise that each modality has a threshold value below which the perioperative risk is prohibitive.

Thoracic resection adversely affects the respiratory system by a number of pathways. Ventilatory patterns become less effective because of increased respiratory rates, lower tidal volumes, and an increased ratio of dead space to tidal volume. Lung volumes are diminished, with associated atelectasis leading to gas-exchange abnormalities. Pulmonary defense mechanisms are diminished secondary to anesthesia and subsequent instrumentation. Coughing is blunted by both pain and the medications used as sedatives and analgesics. As these abnormalities are seen in the normal individual undergoing surgery, there is particular concern for the patient with preoperative ventilatory impairment. The importance of developing a strategy whereby patients in whom these physiological insults would lead to a significant degree of morbidity and mortality is apparent. Once identified, preoperative preparation or therapeutic alternatives to surgical resection of functional lung tissue could be instituted. The capacity of each test to identify a population at high respiratory risk as well as its predictive value are reviewed briefly.

Since 1955, it has been reported that preoperative spirometry could identify a high-risk population for thoracotomy. Although prediction of morbidity or mortality for an individual patient was not possible, it was concluded that an FEV_1 below 70% of that predicted or a maximum voluntary ventilation (MVV) less than 50% of that predicted was associated with a 40% postoperative mortality in patients undergoing thoracic resection for pulmonary tuberculosis. Reports on lung cancer patients over the next two decades reported similar ''high-risk'' groups based upon simple spirometric and demographic risk factors. In the 1970s, the use of a radionuclide perfusion scan to predict a postoperative FEV_1 and tolerance for thoracic surgery was reported. Patients were able to tolerate resection if the predicted postoperative FEV_1 (using radionuclide perfusion scanning) exceeded 800 mL and there was no associated pulmonary hypertension or severe hypoxemia with exercise. At that time, perioperative mortality rates for pneumonectomy and lobectomy were 17.6 and 7.7%, respectively. These outcomes were considered acceptable given the poor outcome of metastatic bronchogenic carcinoma. Other, more recent studies suggest that the spirometric threshold be a percentage of the predicted factor scaled to factors known to affect spirometry: age, sex, race, and height. An FEV_1 greater than 40% of predicted has been confirmed as a useful threshold for this purpose.

Measurement of gas exchange has been studied as a risk factor for respiratory morbidity. At the present time hypoxemia from COPD cannot be considered an absolute contraindication to lung resectional surgery. Hypercapnia associated with COPD may prove to be more of a barrier, but even that has been broached in recent clinical reports. Other measures of gas exchange, such as carbon monoxide diffusion, have been examined as well. A recent report suggests that a composite index of the percent predicted postoperative FEV_1 and the percent predicted postoperative DL_{CO} may have some predictive capacity, but this remains speculative. At a clinical level, many pulmonologists find diffusion capacity, with its wide standard error of normal values, of little incremental value over and above other available testing and bedside assessments in defining operative candidacy.

Cardiopulmonary exercise testing with expired gas analysis is used in cases where borderline spirometric values are of concern. Exercise is an integrated, dynamic study of both the cardiovascular and respiratory systems; it represents a relatively new addition to the traditional preoperative evaluation. In the lung, exercise requires an increase in minute ventilation, oxygen transfer, carbon dioxide removal, blood flow, and ventilation perfusion matching that is also seen postoperatively in thoracic resection. Although different performance criteria have been used, a maximal oxygen consumption ($\dot{V}_{O_2max}$) of greater than 20 mL/kg/min has been associated with minimal complications and no fatalities in three studies. Conversely, a $\dot{V}_{O_2max}$ oxygen consumption under 10 or 15 mL/kg/min has been associated with a significant postoperative morbidity, and values less than 10 mL/kg/min have been associated with mortality rates as high as 27%.

Many surgeons have been trained to have the patient climb "one or two flights of stairs" and declare a stair-tolerant patient to be a surgical candidate. Unfortunately, the few reported evaluations of this approach in the literature are not rigorous. The metabolic cost of a symptom-limited stair climb has been measured, however, indicating that the $\dot{V}_{O_2}$ correlates well with formal bicycle ergometry workloads and suggesting that an inability to climb three to four flights of stairs is compatible with a $\dot{V}_{O_2}$ max below 20 mL/kg/min. Thus it is possible that the inability to climb three flights of steps may, on further evaluation, predict the inability to tolerate lung resectional surgery. This hypothesis requires formal prospective testing.

While the process of defining high-risk patients based upon preoperative evaluations is well established, controversy does exist over our ability to predict definitively a poor outcome for any individual lung resection patient. While the inverse relationship between predicted postoperative FEV_1 and respiratory complications after traditional thoracotomy has been demonstrated, a large fraction of patients in this group have an uneventful hospital course. Hypercarbia (Pa_{CO_2} greater than 45 mmHg), desaturation with exercise (Sa_{O_2} less than 90% on room air), or current smoking status have *not* been associated consistently with significant postoperative complications. Limited resections (single or multiple wedge resections) by standard thoracotomy or by thoracoscopy can be performed in patients with a preoperative FEV_1 less than 1.0 L, but long-term disease-free survival has generally been inferior. Nonpulmonary factors such as poor nutritional status, neoadjuvant chemotherapy, and cardiac disease have also proven to correlate with major postoperative complications.

Newer anesthetic and critical care techniques have now allowed patients with limited pulmonary function to undergo thoracic resection successfully. Thoracoscopic techniques have been a notable advance. Operative mortality in those with moderate to severely depressed spirometric function has been reported as low as 2.4%. Improved outcomes in high-risk patients are possible, and many teams advocate a less rigid approach to surgical selection criteria.

Combining lung volume reduction surgery (LVRS) with traditional lung resectional surgery may further affect preoperative stratification. LVRS is discussed in Chap. 27. One recent report on a small number of otherwise inoperable patients who underwent combined LVRS and resection of stage I non-small-cell lung cancer was favorable. The mean preoperative FEV_1 was 0.654 L, which rose to over 1 L postoperatively. No deaths were reported.

In summary, the preoperative evaluation for thoracic resection remains a complex and multifaceted issue. Improvements in perioperative patient care, newer anesthetic and thoracoscopic surgical technique, the use of limited resections, and uncertainty associated with the predictive ability of our standard preoperative testing need to be considered in evaluating individual patients. Percent of predicted postoperative FEV_1, percent of predicted postoperative diffusion capacity, and the presence of hypercapnia may not be as prohibitive as originally believed but certainly target a higher-risk subset. Exercise testing has also shown promise as an additional operability criterion. A general preoperative evaluation strategy is outlined in Fig. 1 and summarized below.

The standard evaluation of preoperative risk for potential lobectomy or pneumonectomy begins with simple spirometry: (1) if $FEV_1 > 2$ L and MVV $> 50\%$ predicted, the patient is a surgical candidate unless contraindicated by nonpulmonary factors; (2) if

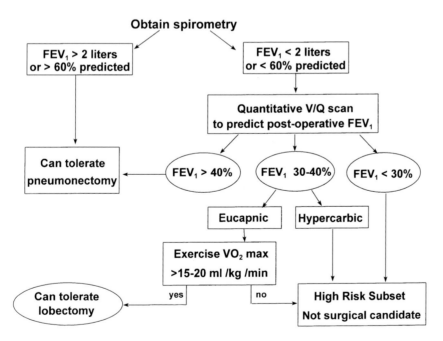

Figure 1 A series of diagnostic studies provides an algorithm for deciding whether or not a patient is likely to tolerate a lobectomy or pneumonectomy. $\dot{V}/\dot{Q}$, ventilation/perfusion radionuclide scan; $\dot{V}_{O_2}$, maximum oxygen consumption during incremental exercise; hypercarbia, $P_{CO_2} > 45$ torr.

$FEV_1 < 2$ L *and* predicted postoperative FEV_1 with quantitative perfusion scans exceeds 1000mL (or 40% predicted) *and* $Pa_{CO_2} < 45$ mmHg, the patient is a surgical candidate unless contraindicated by nonpulmonary factors; (3) if predicted postoperative FEV_1 is less than 800–1000 mL (or 40% predicted) *and* there is baseline hypoxia or hypercapnea, further testing is warranted (cardiopulmonary exercise testing with or without expired gas analysis; see Fig. 1).

Abdominal Surgery

There is ample evidence that abdominal surgery is an insult to the ventilatory function of the lung and exerts its effects by a variety of mechanisms. Anesthesia effects are manifest as decreases in vital capacity, cough, secretion clearance, and lung aeration as well as depressed hypoxic and hypercarbic drive. Surgical manipulation results in direct impairment. Surgical intervention also impairs diaphragmatic function, and this appears to be mediated independently of the presence of pain, as evidenced by afferent nerve blockade studies. Rather, the handling of the viscera appears to result in reflex inhibition of diaphragmatic performance via visceral afferents to central centers and then via phrenic output. This effect persists for hours to days into the postoperative period, depending on the general anesthetic technique. Experimentally, this inhibition can be overcome by volition, phrenic nerve stimulation, and, in part, by aminophylline.

Surgical proximity to the diaphragm therefore has a strong bearing on respiratory outcome postoperatively. There is a substantially increased rate of respiratory complications related to upper abdominal (20–40%) versus lower abdominal (2–5%) surgery by traditional techniques. Duration of surgery, patient age, and morbid obesity also play into the postoperative respiratory complication rate.

Those patients with preexisting lung dysfunction as demonstrated spirometrically are more likely to suffer pulmonary complications from upper abdominal surgery. Pneumonia rates reported in the older literature have ranged as high as 44%, depending on the definition of that complication, severity of underlying lung disease, and additional comorbidities. Current respiratory complication rates are much lower, and further identification of patients at particularly high risk has been attempted.

Preoperative respiratory status has a nonquantitative relationship to postoperative respiratory complications. Indeed, upper abdominal surgery has been successfully performed in COPD patients with FEV_1 less than 1.0 L, though this group has a higher attendant risk. Spirometry does describe the group characteristics of those who will develop postoperative respiratory complications, but it fails in reliably predicting the specific postoperative respiratory outcome for an individual patient. This general position, taken by the American College of Physicians, is discussed in several reviews (see "Suggested Reading" at the end of this chapter).

No definitive lung function threshold has been validated in the literature below which the abdominal surgery candidate is inoperable. Lung mechanical dysfunction in COPD, as assessed spirometrically, down to previously "prohibitive" ranges has been reported. Chronic hypercarbia had been cited as a strong and prohibitive risk factor in several early studies, although this has been challenged recently. Most internists and anesthesiologists would forego *elective* upper abdominal surgery in a patient with active exacerbated airways disease, purulent bronchitis, unresolved pneumonia, or chronic ventilatory failure (hypercarbia) until the situation had been brought under better medical control.

Existing comorbidities such as uncompensated congestive heart failure, unstable angina, renal failure or poorly controlled diabetes mellitus must be considered to confer risk that is synergistic with underlying lung compromise. A discussion of these comorbidities lies outside the scope of this chapter. For *emergent* upper abdominal surgery in those with COPD, the acceptance of risk by the informed patient or surrogate is a prerequisite to essential, lifesaving surgical interventions.

Lower abdominal surgery (such as appendectomy, abdominal hysterectomy, cystectomy, or herniorrhaphy) has generally been associated with very low rates of postoperative respiratory compromise, and further clinical stratification by spirometric or blood-gas parameters is not helpful. The basic principles of postoperative care—adequate postoperative analgesia, early ambulation, and venous thromboembolism prophylaxis—generally prove quite adequate.

The literature reveals a lack of formal study of the pulmonary risk conferred by interstitial, pleural, chest wall, or neuromuscular disease in the context of abdominal surgery. The presence of obstructive sleep apnea may necessitate the use of nasal continuous positive airway pressure through the perioperative period.

Other Surgical Sites

Head-and-neck surgery is often performed in those with cigarette exposure as a risk factor for obstructive lung disease. In the absence of data supporting *routine* spirometric or blood-gas analysis, it again appears prudent to allow clinical warning signs (e.g., active bronchitic symptoms, severe functional limitations due to dyspnea, etc.) to prompt such evaluation. Manipulation of the upper airway during such surgery may predispose to postoperative pneumonia.

Orthopedic and limb surgery is generally considered to confer little risk to the surgical candidate of the sort that is unique to those with preexisting respiratory compromise. However, immobility certainly predisposes to atelectasis, hypoxia, and risk of pneumonia as well as pulmonary thromboembolism. Insofar as underlying comorbidities such as lung disease or cor pulmonale further predispose to these conditions, simple preventive maneuvers such as early ambulation are essential. The specifics of preventing deep venous thrombosis are described further on.

PERIOPERATIVE INTERVENTIONS THAT MINIMIZE RISK

Simple clinical principles guide the perioperative maneuvers that prevent postoperative respiratory complications such as atelectasis, pneumonia, pulmonary embolism, and ventilatory failure. Some have been noted in Tables 1 and 2 with respect to coronary artery bypass grafting (CABG) and abdominal surgery. These measures include early smoking cessation, early but prudent extubation, the aggressive use of lung expansion techniques, liberal bronchodilator use, deep vein thrombosis (DVT) prophylaxis, and adequate pain management permitting a more normal respiratory pattern and early ambulation, as well as vigilance for evolving complications.

Table 1 Preoperative Risk Factors for Post-CABG Respiratory Complications

Preoperative risk factor	Strength of association	Adequacy of literature	Perioperative options[a]
Spirometric obstruction (COPD)	Weak, varies	Inadequate	*Preop*: bronchodilators; avoid elective operation in acute exacerbation, class IV dyspnea from COPD *Postop*: incentive spirometry, ambulation
Spirometric restriction	No data	No data	*Preop*: Chest wall/pleural/parenchymal restriction are unstudied in CABG; severity and progressiveness of disorder important in risk-benefit analysis
Hypercarbia	Weak	Inadequate	*Preop*: Careful risk-benefit analysis of surgery Aggressive bronchodilators, theophylline if tolerant, and pulmonary consultation
Neuromuscular disease	No data	No data	*Preop*: Severity and progressiveness important
Sleep apnea	Unknown	Few data	*Periop*: Continue any applied CPAP/BiPAP or tracheostomy access. Minimize sedatives
Other comorbidities [emergent operation, repeat operation, electrocardiogram, age, cerebrovascular disease, renal disease diabetes]	Strong, in aggregate	Adequate	*Preop*: Careful risk-benefit analysis of surgery. Otherwise follow specific management appropriate to condition

[a] Literature-identified risk factors for postoperative respiratory complications after coronary artery bypass graft surgery (CABG). Strength of association of the risk factor with adverse respiratory outcome, adequacy of that literature, and clinical response options to the presence of that risk factor are briefly outlined.

SMOKING CESSATION

Cigarette smoking exerts deleterious effects on the cardiovascular and respiratory systems in a variety of ways. It would logically follow that smoking cessation would provide significant benefit to the postoperative patient. However, a retrospective study in preoperative CABG patients from Warner et al. suggests that smoking cessation less than 8 weeks prior to surgery led to increased postoperative complications. Presumably these are consequences related to delayed improvements in mucociliary clearance. However, delaying surgery for 2 months may not be practical in a patient with active coronary disease, potentially curable lung cancer, or an active abdominal process. Even if the patient is abstinent only for hours, a potential benefit exists, as the half-life of carboxyhemoglobin is approximately 6 h. While further evaluation regarding duration of smoking cessation and postoperative pulmonary complications is necessary, current recommendations are to encourage cessation at the earliest opportunity prior to surgery.

Table 2 Preoperative Risk Factors for Respiratory Complications After Abdominal Surgery

Preoperative risk factor	Strength of association	Adequacy of literature	Perioperative options[a]
Site (proximity to diaphragm)	Strong	Adequate	*Preop*: Consider regional versus general anesthesia, laparoscopic versus laparotomy approaches, instruction on incentive spirometry, stress necessity for postop pain reporting by patient. *Postop*: Pain control, incentive spirometry, early ambulation, DVT prophylaxis.
Advanced age	Weak	Adequate	*Preop*: Risk-benefit analysis is not heavily weighed by this factor in isolation.
Morbid obesity	Weak	Inadequate	*Preop*: Massive weight loss not advised preop from respiratory standpoint.
Spirometric obstruction (COPD)	Variable	Adequate	*Preop*: Liberal use of inhaled bronchodilators, short-term steroids as needed. Avoid elective surgery in COPD patients during an exacerabation. *Postop*: Pain control, incentive spirometry, early ambulation.
Hypercarbia	Moderate	Inadequate	*Preop*: Upper abdominal surgery-laparotomy and laparoscopic—require general anesthesia, endotracheal intubation. Careful risk-benefit evaluation in this situation. Else as per COPD. *Postop*: Optimizing pain control and avoidance of sedation is optimal. Else as per COPD.
Asthma	Weak	Inadequate	*Preop*: Liberal use of inhaled bronchodilators, short-term steroids as needed. Avoid elective surgery in asthma patients during an exacerbation. Avoid endotracheal intubation if possible. *Postop*: Pain control, incentive spirometry, early ambulation.
Cystic fibrosis	Weak	Inadequate	*Preop*: Risk is generally not prohibitive. Intravenous antipseudomonal antibiotics, aggressive chest physiotherapy, bronchodilation, nutritional supplements. *Postop*: Pain control, incentive spirometry, early ambulation plus preop regimen.
Interstitial lung disease	Unknown	Absent	*Preop*: The existence of progressive interstitial disease should weigh heavily into risk-benefit analyses. No respiratory outcome data available. *Postop*: Pain control, incentive spirometry essential.
Neuromuscular disease	Unknown	Absent	*Preop*: The existence of progressive neurological/neuromuscular disease should weigh heavily into risk-benefit analyses. No respiratory outcome data available. *Postop*: Pain control, incentive spirometry.
Sleep apnea	Unknown	Inadequate	*Periop*: Continue any applied CPAP/BiPAP or tracheostomy access. Minimize sedatives.

[a] Risk factors identified in published reports for postoperative respiratory complications after abdominal surgery. Strength of association of the risk factor with adverse respiratory outcome, adequacy of that literature, and some clinical response options to the presence of that risk factor are briefly outlined.

LUNG EXPANSION TECHNIQUES

The most common etiology of hypoxemia is microatelectasis, manifest in lung volumes as a decrease in FRC. Areas that are underventilated but perfused represent ventilation/perfusion inequality leading to hypoxemia. Patient groups where this mechanism leads to significant desaturation are the obese, patients with COPD, the elderly, and patients undergoing upper abdominal or thoracic procedures. Atelectasis is the most common postoperative pulmonary complication and is more severe in thoracic and upper abdominal surgery secondary to chest wall and diaphragmatic dysfunction.

Therapeutic interventions have focused on adequate lung expansion postoperatively. Celli et al. randomized 172 patients undergoing upper abdominal surgery to three groups: incentive spirometry, deep breathing exercises, or intermittent positive-pressure breathing (IPPB). All three treatments were equally effective in preventing postoperative pulmonary complications as compared with untreated controls. This was confirmed in a recent metanalysis in patients undergoing upper abdominal surgery. Noninvasive positive-pressure masks have also been used in the postoperative period with variable success. Routine bronchoscopy for atelectasis has not been shown to improve outcome as compared with conservative therapy. Early ambulation is a more physiological method of improving lung expansion and is an essential part of any postoperative regimen. Adequate postoperative analgesia improves lung expansion by allowing more normal tidal respirations. Data on the efficacy of postoperative epidural analgesia in lowering the frequency of respiratory complications are mixed.

There are no definitive data linking postoperative atelectasis with pneumonia, although some studies and clinical experience correlate the two. The mortality of postoperative pneumonia has been reported in some series as exceeding 50%, but this varies by site of surgery, host medical status, and other factors. Aspiration precautions such as head of bed elevation, early discontinuation of nasogastric tubes, and avoidance of oversedation—in association with lung expansion techniques—are generally quite effective.

MANAGEMENT OF AIRFLOW OBSTRUCTION

Patients with obstructive lung disease often require bronchodilators to maximize pulmonary function. Early reports that bronchodilator therapy dramatically reduced postoperative pulmonary complications in those with airflow obstruction have generally been confirmed. Both ipratropium and beta$_2$ mimetics can be nebulized throughout the postoperative period until the patient has stabilized. Metered-dose inhalers (MDIs) can be substituted as the patient improves.

While theophylline use has decreased over the last decade, it has been shown to have an inotropic effect on respiratory muscles and some effectiveness in airways disease. While routine preoperative initiation is not recommended, patients currently taking theophylline with therapeutic levels (5–15 μg/mL) preoperatively should be continued postoperatively unless there are complications. In the symptomatic patient with obstructive lung disease, a short course of corticosteroids and antibiotic therapy perioperatively can be initiated with minimal toxicity. The prolonged use of high-dose corticosteroids for more than 2 weeks should be avoided as it can delay wound healing and lead to an increased incidence of infection.

PROPHYLAXIS AGAINST DEEP VEIN THROMBOSIS

Venous thromboembolism is a significant cause of morbidity and mortality in hospitalized patients. All postoperative patients represent a population at significant risk, and incidence rates vary depending upon preexisting risk factors and the type of surgery. In general, orthopedic (hip and knee), spinal cord, and multiple trauma patients have very high rates owing to prolonged immobility with subsequent venous stasis. Patients with underlying medical problems such as congestive heart failure, cor pulmonale, and malignancy are at a particularly high risk. Preventive therapy must be the cornerstone because venous thromboembolic disease can manifest with few symptoms, clinical diagnosis is insensitive, and the initial presentation may be fatal. Despite widespread knowledge of the problem, prophylaxis for deep vein thrombosis (DVT) is underutilized in many institutions. The recommendations of the American College of Chest Physicians regarding prevention of venous thromboembolism are as follows:

Low-risk general surgery patients (minor surgery, under 40 years of age, absence of clinical risk factors): No specific prophylaxis other than early ambulation is recommended.

Moderate-risk general surgery patients (major surgery, age greater than 40 years, absence of clinical risk factors): Graded compression elastic stockings (ES), intermittent pneumatic compression (IPC), or low-dose unfractionated heparin (LDUH) given subcutaneously every 12 h. It is recommended that ES and IPC be used intraoperatively, if possible, and throughout the postoperative period.

High-risk general surgical patients (major surgery, age greater than 40 years, and additional risk factors): LDUH subcutaneously every 8 h or low-molecular-weight heparin (LMWH) can be used. IPC is an acceptable alternative.

Very high-risk general surgery patients (high-risk procedure + multiple additional risk factors): Combination therapy LMWH or LDUH with IPC can be used. Perioperative warfarin may also be used in this subgroup (INR 2–3).

Total hip replacement surgery: LMWH, warfarin started pre- or immediately postoperatively (INR 2–3) *or* adjusted-dose unfractionated heparin can be used *with* IPC.

Hip fracture surgery: LMWH or warfarin (INR 2–3) with IPC.

Total knee replacement: Either LMWH or IPC can be used.

Spinal surgery: LMWH, warfarin (INR 2–3), or adjusted dose of unfractionated heparin. Additional benefit may be obtained from IPC.

Neurosurgical procedures: IPC can be used. LDUH may be an acceptable alternative. IPC and LDUH in combination may be considered in high-risk patients.

SUGGESTED READING

Anesthesia

1. Atanassoff P. Effects of regional anesthesia on perioperative outcome. J Clin Anesth 1996; 8: 446–455.
2. Jayr C, Thomas H, Rey A, Farhat F, Lasser P, Bourgain JL. Postoperative pulmonary complications: epidural analgesia using bupivacaine and opioids versus parenteral opioids. Anesthesiology 1993; 78:666–676.

Cardiac Surgery

1. Spivack SD, Shinozaki T, Albertini JJ, Deane R. Preoperative prediction of postoperative respiratory outcome: coronary artery bypass grafting. Chest 1996; 109:1222–1230.
2. Cohen A, Katz M, Katz R, Hauptman E, Schachner A. Chronic obstructive pulmonary disease in patients undergoing coronary artery bypass grafting. J Thorac Cardiovasc Surg 1995; 109: 574–581.

3. Ferraris VA, Ferraris SP. Risk factors for postoperative morbidity. J Thorac Cardiovasc Surg 1996; 111:731–738.
4. Kurki TS, Kataja M. Preoperative prediction of postoperative morbidity in coronary artery bypass grafting. Ann Thorac Surg 1996; 61:1740–1745.

Thoracic Resection

1. Kearney DJ, Lee TH, Reilly JJ, DeCamp MM, Sugarbaker DJ. Assessment of operative risk in patients undergoing lung resection. Chest 1994; 105:753–759.
2. Olsen GN. The evolving role of exercise testing prior to lung resection. Chest 1989; 95:218–225.
3. Walsh GL, Morice RC, Putnam JB, Jr, Nesbitt JC, McMurtrey MJ, Ryan MB, Reising JM, Willis KM, Morton JD, Roth JA. Resection of lung cancer is justified in high-risk patients selected by exercise oxygen consumption. Ann Thorac Surg 1994; 58:704–711.
4. Cerfolio RJ, Allen MS, Trastek VF, Deschamps C, Scanlon PD, Pairolero PL. Lung resection in patients with compromised pulmonary function. Ann Thorac Surg 1996; 62:348–351.
5. Olsen GN, Bolton JW, Weiman DS, Hornung CA. Stair climbing as an exercise test to predict the postoperative complications of lung resection. Chest 1991; 99:587–590.
6. Epstein SK, Faling J, Daly BDT, Celli BR. Inability to perform increased bicycle ergometry predicts increased morbidity and mortality after lung resection. Chest 1995; 107:311–316.
7. Mckenna RJ Jr, Fischel RJ, Brenner M, Gelb AF. Combined operations for lung volume reduction surgery and lung cancer. Chest 1996; 110:885–888.

Abdominal Surgery and Other Sites

1. Zibrak JD, O'Donnell CR. Indications for preoperative pulmonary function testing. Clin Chest Med 1993; 14:227–236.
2. Celli BR. What is the value of preoperative pulmonary function testing? Med Clin North Am 1993; 77:309–325.

Perioperative Interventions That Minimize Risk

1. Warner MA, Divertie MB, Tinker JH. Preoperative cessation of smoking and pulmonary complications in coronary artery bypass patients. Anesthesiology 1984; 60:380–383.
2. Thomas JA, McIntosh JM. Are incentive spirometry, intermittent positive pressure breathing, and deep breathing exercises effective in preventing postoperative pulmonary complications after abdominal surgery? A systematic review and meta-analysis. Phys Ther 1994; 74(1):3–7.
3. Clagett GP, Anderson FA Jr, Heit J, Levine MN, Wheeler HB. Prevention of venous thromboembolism. Chest 1995; 108 (suppl):312s–334s.

Index

About the Editors

GERALD S. DAVIS is Professor of Medicine and Director of the Pulmonary Disease and Critical Care Medicine Unit at the University of Vermont College of Medicine, Burlington, and in clinical practice through Fletcher Allen Health Care, Burlington, Vermont. The author or coauthor of over 125 professional papers and abstracts, Dr. Davis is a Fellow of the American College of Physicians and the American College of Chest Physicians, and a member of the American Thoracic Society. He received the B.S. degree (1966) from Yale University, New Haven, Connecticut, and the M.D. degree (1970) from the University of Virginia School of Medicine, Charlottesville.

THEODORE W. MARCY is Associate Professor of Medicine at the University of Vermont, Burlington, and Medical Director of Respiratory Care Services at Fletcher Allen Health Care, Burlington, Vermont. The author or coauthor of numerous professional papers, presentations, book chapters, and reviews, Dr. Marcy is a Fellow of the American College of Chest Physicians and a member of the American Thoracic Society. Dr. Marcy received the B.A. degree (1976) from Stanford University, Palo Alto, California, and the M.D. degree (1980) from the Yale University School of Medicine, New Haven, Connecticut.

ELIZABETH A. SEWARD is Clinical Assistant Professor of Medicine at the University of Vermont College of Medicine, Burlington; Attending Physician in the Department of Medicine, Fletcher Allen Health Care, Burlington, Vermont; and the Physician of Internal Medicine at the Aesculapius Medical Center in South Burlington, Vermont. A member of the American College of Physicians and the Vermont State Medical Society, Dr. Seward received the B.A. (1977), the M.S. (1985), and the M.D. (1985) degrees from the University of Vermont, Burlington.